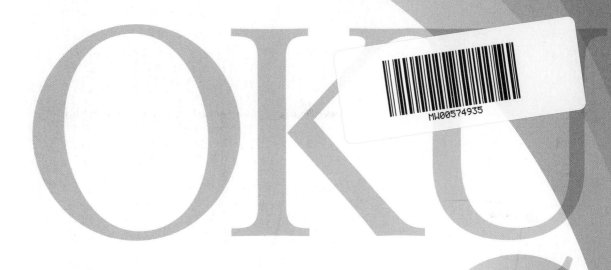

Orthopaedic Knowledge Update:
Foot and Ankle

AAOS
AMERICAN ACADEMY OF
ORTHOPAEDIC SURGEONS

OKU 5

Orthopaedic Knowledge Update:

Foot and Ankle

EDITOR:

Loretta B. Chou, MD
Professor and Chief of Foot and Ankle Surgery
Department of Orthopaedic Surgery
Stanford University
Stanford, California

Developed by the
American Orthopaedic Foot & Ankle Society

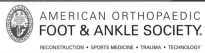

AMERICAN ORTHOPAEDIC
FOOT & ANKLE SOCIETY
RECONSTRUCTION • SPORTS MEDICINE • TRAUMA • TECHNOLOGY

AAOS

AMERICAN ACADEMY OF
ORTHOPAEDIC SURGEONS

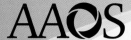

AAOS
AMERICAN ACADEMY OF ORTHOPAEDIC SURGEONS

The material presented in *Orthopaedic Knowledge Update: Foot and Ankle 5* has been made available by the American Academy of Orthopaedic Surgeons for educational purposes only. This material is not intended to present the only, or necessarily best, methods or procedures for the medical situations discussed, but rather is intended to represent an approach, view, statement, or opinion of the author(s) or producer(s), which may be helpful to others who face similar situations.

Some drugs or medical devices demonstrated in Academy courses or described in Academy print or electronic publications have not been cleared by the Food and Drug Administration (FDA) or have been cleared for specific uses only. The FDA has stated that it is the responsibility of the physician to determine the FDA clearance status of each drug or device he or she wishes to use in clinical practice.

Furthermore, any statements about commercial products are solely the opinion(s) of the author(s) and do not represent an Academy endorsement or evaluation of these products. These statements may not be used in advertising or for any commercial purpose.

Published 2014 by the
American Academy of Orthopaedic Surgeons
6300 North River Road
Rosemont, IL 60018

Copyright 2014
by the American Academy of Orthopaedic Surgeons

Library of Congress Control Number:
2014947292

ISBN 978-1-62552-279-5

Printed in the USA

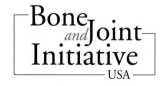

Acknowledgments

Editorial Board, Orthopaedic Knowledge Update: Foot and Ankle 5

Loretta B. Chou, MD
Professor and Chief of Foot and Ankle Surgery
Department of Orthopaedic Surgery
Stanford University
Stanford, California

Christopher P. Chiodo, MD
Foot and Ankle Division Chief
Department of Orthopaedic Surgery
Brigham and Women's Hospital/Harvard
  Medical School
Boston, Massachusetts

Bruce E. Cohen, MD
Fellowship Director-Foot and Ankle Fellowship
OrthoCarolina Foot and Ankle Institute
Charlotte, North Carolina

Andrew Haskell, MD
Co-Chair
Department of Orthopedics
Palo Alto Medical Foundation
Palo Alto, California

Susan N. Ishikawa, MD
Assistant Professor/Foot and Ankle Fellowship
  Director
Department of Orthopaedic Surgery
University of Tennessee/Campbell Clinic
Memphis, Tennessee

Clifford L. Jeng, MD
Fellowship Director
Institute for Foot and Ankle Reconstruction
Mercy Medical Center
Baltimore, Maryland

Sheldon S. Lin, MD
Associate Professor
Department of Orthopedics
Rutgers New Jersey Medical School
Newark, New Jersey

Ruth L. Thomas, MD
Professor
Department of Orthopaedic Surgery
University of Arkansas College of Medicine
Little Rock, Arkansas

AOFAS Board of Directors 2013-2014

Steven L. Haddad, MD
President

Bruce J. Sangeorzan, MD
President-Elect

Mark E. Easley, MD
Vice President

Thomas H. Lee, MD
Secretary

Jeffrey E. Johnson, MD
Treasurer

Bruce E. Cohen, MD
Member-at-Large

Timothy R. Daniels, MD
Member-at-Large

Sheldon S. Lin, MD
Member-at-Large

Selene G. Parekh, MD, MBA
Member-at-Large

Lew C. Schon, MD
Immediate Past President

Judith F. Baumhauer, MD, MPH
Past President

Contributors

Joseph Benevenia, MD
Professor and Chair
Department of Orthopaedics
Rutgers New Jersey Medical School
Newark, New Jersey

Mark J. Berkowitz, MD
Associate Staff Orthopaedic Surgeon
Orthopaedic and Rheumatologic Institute
Cleveland Clinic
Cleveland, Ohio

Gregory C. Berlet, MD
Attending
Orthopedic Foot and Ankle Center
Westerville, Ohio

Eric M. Bluman, MD, PhD
Assistant Professor
Department of Orthopaedic Surgery
Harvard Medical School
Boston, Massachusetts

Jae-Wook Byun, MD
Professor
Department of Orthopaedic Surgery
Chonnam National University Hospital
Donggu, Gwangju, Republic of Korea

Wen Chao, MD
Orthopaedic Attending
Penn Orthopaedics
University of Pennsylvania
Philadelphia, Pennsylvania

Michael J. Coughlin, MD
Director, Saint Alphonsus Foot and Ankle
  Clinic
Saint Alphonsus Regional Medical Center
Boise, Idaho

Richard J. de Asla, MD
Private Practice
Excel Orthopaedics
Harvard Medical School
Woburn, Massachusetts

Russell Dedini, MD
Surgical Fellow
Foot and Ankle Surgery
Department of Orthopaedic Surgery
University of Pennsylvania
Philadelphia, Pennsylvania

Jesse F. Doty, MD
Clinical Instructor
Department of Orthopaedic Surgery
University of Tennessee College of Medicine
Chattanooga, Tennessee

Tobin T. Eckel, MD
Staff Orthopaedic Foot and Ankle Surgeon
Walter Reed National Military Medical Center
Bethesda, Maryland

J. Kent Ellington, MS, MD
Orthopaedic Surgeon
OrthoCarolina Foot and Ankle Institute
Charlotte, North Carolina

Adolph Samuel Flemister Jr, MD
Professor
Department of Orthopaedic Surgery
University of Rochester
Rochester, New York

Erik Freeland, DO
Fellow
Department of Orthopaedic Surgery
University of Pennsylvania
Philadelphia, Pennsylvania

Michael J. Gardner, MD
Associate Professor
Department of Orthopaedic Surgery
Washington University School of Medicine
St. Louis, Missouri

David N. Garras, MD
Assistant Professor
Midwest Orthopaedics at Rush
Department of Orthopaedic Surgery
Rush University Medical Center
Chicago, Illinois

John S. Gould, MD
Professor of Surgery/Orthopaedic
Department of Orthopaedic Surgery
University of Alabama at Birmingham
Birmingham, Alabama

David J. Hak, MD, MBA, FACS
Associate Director of Orthopaedic Surgery
Denver Health Medical Center
Denver Health/University of Colorado
Denver, Colorado

Kenneth J. Hunt, MD
Assistant Professor
Department of Orthopaedics
Stanford University
Redwood City, California

Mark J. Jo, MD
Orthopaedic Surgeon
Huntington Memorial Hospital
Pasadena, California

A. Holly Johnson, MD
Orthopaedic Surgeon, Foot and Ankle
  Specialist
Massachusetts General Hospital
Department of Orthopaedics
Harvard Medical School
Boston, Massachusetts

Anish Raj Kadakia, MD
Associate Professor
Department of Orthopaedic Surgery
Northwestern University
Chicago, Illinois

Derek M. Kelly, MD
Assistant Professor
Department of Orthopaedic Surgery and
  Biomedical Engineering
University of Tennessee-Campbell Clinic
Memphis, Tennessee

David Hakbum Kim, MD
Chief, Orthopaedic Surgery
Colorado Permanente Medical Group
Lone Tree, Colorado

Todd S. Kim, MD
Assistant Clinical Professor
Department of Orthopaedic Surgery
University of California, San Francisco
San Francisco, California

John Y. Kwon, MD
Department of Orthopaedic Surgery
Massachusetts General Hospital
Boston, Massachusetts

Edward Lansang, MD, FRCSC
Clinical Assistant
Division of Orthopaedic Surgery
Toronto Western Hospital
Toronto, Ontario, Canada

Perla Lansang, MD, FRCPC
Assistant Professor
Department of Medicine
Division of Dermatology
University of Toronto
Toronto, Ontario, Canada

Johnny Lau, MD, MSc, FRCSC
Assistant Professor
Department of Surgery
University Health Network – Toronto Western
  Division
Toronto, Ontario, Canada

Keun-Bae Lee, MD, PhD
Professor
Department of Orthopaedic Surgery
Chonnam National University Medical School
  and Hospital
Donggu, Gwangju, Republic of Korea

Simon Lee, MD
Assistant Professor
Midwest Orthopaedics at Rush
Rush University Medical Center
Chicago, Illinois

Thomas H. Lee, MD
Attending
Orthopedic Foot and Ankle Center
Westerville, Ohio

J. C. Neilson, MD
Assistant Professor
Department of Orthopaedic Surgery
Medical College of Wisconsin
Milwaukee, Wisconsin

Thomas Padanilam, MD
Orthopaedic Surgeon
Toledo Orthopaedic Surgeons
Toledo, Ohio

David I. Pedowitz, MS, MD
Assistant Professor
Department of Orthopaedic Surgery
Rothman Institute
Thomas Jefferson University
Philadelphia, Pennsylvania

Terrence M. Philbin, DO
Attending
Orthopedic Foot and Ankle Center
Westerville, Ohio

Steven M. Raikin, MD
Director, Foot and Ankle Service
Professor, Orthopaedic Surgery
Rothman Institute
Thomas Jefferson University Hospital
Philadelphia, Pennsylvania

Jeffrey R. Sawyer, MD
Associate Professor
Department of Orthopaedic Surgery and
  Biomedical Engineering
University of Tennessee-Campbell Clinic
Memphis, Tennessee

Vinayak M. Sathe, MD
Assistant Professor
Department of Orthopaedic Surgery
University of Connecticut Health Center
Farmington, Connecticut

Scott B. Shawen, MD
Program Director
Department of Orthopaedic Surgery
Walter Reed National Military Medical Center
Bethesda, Maryland

G. Alexander Simpson, DO
Fellow
Orthopedic Foot and Ankle Center
Westerville, Ohio

Jeremy T. Smith, MD
Brigham Foot and Ankle Center
Brigham and Women's Hospital
Boston, Massachusetts

W. Bret Smith, DO
Attending
Moore Center for Orthopedics
Columbia, South Carolina

André Spiguel, MD
Clinical Assistant Professor
Department of Orthopaedics and
  Rehabilitation
University of Florida
Gainesville, Florida

Ruth L. Thomas, MD
Professor
Department of Orthopaedic Surgery
University of Arkansas College of Medicine
Little Rock, Arkansas

Andrea Veljkovic, MD, BComm, FRCSC
Clinical Lecturer, Staff Surgeon
Department of Orthopaedics
University of Toronto
Toronto, Ontario, Canada

Kathryn L. Williams, MD
Assistant Professor
Department of Orthopaedics and
  Rehabilitation
University of Wisconsin
Madison, Wisconsin

Brian S. Winters, MD
Orthopaedic Foot and Ankle Surgeon
Assistant Professor
Rothman Institute
Thomas Jefferson University
Egg Harbor Township, New Jersey

Preface

As a resident, I became interested in what then was the immature discipline of foot and ankle surgery. At that time, decisions were made based on the opinions of a few experts. This publication is representative of how far we have come. Much of the material in this review is based on the sound scientific studies of an international group of interested clinical scientists. The scientific literature has substantially increased in volume and breadth since the publication of the fourth edition of *OKU Foot and Ankle*. The number of submissions to the major journal focused on orthopaedic foot and ankle surgery has increased from 400 in the year 2007 to more than 800 in 2014. Also, the number of level I and II articles is increasing, and the impact factor has greatly improved.

I thank the contributors to this edition of *OKU Foot and Ankle*. The chapter authors and section editors have reviewed the current literature on orthopaedic foot and ankle surgery and disorders and provided a comprehensive evaluation and summary. The general orthopaedic surgeon will find this text helpful in keeping current with the literature and providing clinical care for his or her patients. I would like to especially thank Lisa Claxton Moore, Senior Manager, Book Program, and Rachel Winokur, Editorial Coordinator, of the AAOS Publications Department for their guidance and expertise. Finally, I thank Michael S. Pinzur, MD, Editor of *OKU Foot and Ankle 4*, who helped mentor me during the process of creating this educational resource.

I sincerely hope that the readers of *OKU Foot and Ankle 5* gain as much insight from this review as I gained in its production.

Loretta B. Chou, MD
Editor

Table of Contents

General Foot and Ankle Topics

Section Editor:

Christopher P. Chiodo, MD

Chapter 1

Biomechanics of the Foot and Ankle

Richard J. de Asla, MD

Introduction

The foot is a marvelous mechanical structure. Its unique anatomy and biomechanics allow it to play several seemingly conflicting roles. During push-off, it is a rigid lever arm for efficient propulsion. In stance, it is a stable platform for balance. It is also a part-time shock absorber that adeptly navigates uneven surfaces and terrain. The average person's foot is remarkably durable, logging more than 100 million steps during an average lifetime.

Since the development of advanced imaging, knowledge of foot and ankle biomechanics has increased tremendously.[1-5] This improved understanding of how the foot works provides better insight into disorders of the foot and ankle, which are often biomechanically based.

A thorough understanding of the biomechanics and functional anatomy of the foot and ankle is mandatory to ensure successful treatment of patients and the development and advancement of new procedures.

Structural Anatomy

The foot is divided into three regions: the forefoot, midfoot, and hindfoot. The tarsometatarsal joints (or Lisfranc joint complex) separate the forefoot from the midfoot, and the talonavicular and calcaneocuboid joints (transverse tarsal or Chopart joint) separate the midfoot from the hindfoot.

In the forefoot, the metatarsals are unique in that they are the only long bones in the body to support weight perpendicular to their long axis. In most feet, the first metatarsal is somewhat shorter than the second, with a progressive cascade of shortening from the second to the fifth metatarsal. This metatarsal break angle encourages the foot to supinate during push-off. In the sagittal plane, all metatarsals incline to some extent; the first metatarsal has the highest inclination angle (range 15° to 25°) and the remaining metatarsals demonstrate decreasing inclination angles from medial to lateral. Alterations and

subtleties in the length and position of the metatarsals affect loading patterns that may influence alignment and contribute to the development of painful callosities, metatarsalgia, and metatarsophalangeal joint pathology.

The first, fourth, and fifth metatarsals have mobility in the sagittal plane, whereas the second and third metatarsals have relatively fixed positions. The lesser metatarsal bases are connected by a series of plantar metatarsal ligaments. No such connection exists between the base of the first and second metatarsals. The absence of an intermetatarsal ligament provides the first metatarsal a degree of mobility in the transverse plane not afforded to the lesser metatarsals. This anatomic feature is exploited with hallux valgus deformities.

The forefoot is connected to the midfoot through the Lisfranc joint complex. Here, the cross-sectional wedge-shaped cuneiforms and metatarsal bases form a transverse arch across the midfoot, enhancing stability in the coronal plane (**Figure 1**). Additionally, the base of the second metatarsal is recessed proximally between the medial and lateral cuneiforms, providing stability in the horizontal plane. Stability is further enhanced by a series of very strong plantar tarsometatarsal ligaments. One of the strongest of these plantar ligaments runs obliquely from the plantar surface of the second metatarsal base to the plantar aspect of the medial cuneiform. This ligament is often referred to as the Lisfranc ligament. Disruption of the midfoot complex may result in an avulsion fracture off the base of the second metatarsal. The bony fragment, still attached to Lisfranc ligament, can be seen between the bases of the first and second metatarsals on plain radiographs—the so-called fleck sign.

The midfoot contains the navicular, the cuboid, and three cuneiform bones. These five bones are relatively immobile with respect to one another and provide a mechanical link between the hindfoot and the more mobile forefoot. The midfoot allows for the safe passage of neurovascular structures and tendons as they course from the leg to the foot. The disk-shaped navicular bone has a convex anterior surface and a concave posterior surface—both of which are covered with cartilage. Small vessels enter the navicular dorsally from the dorsalis pedis artery and medially from the posterior tibial

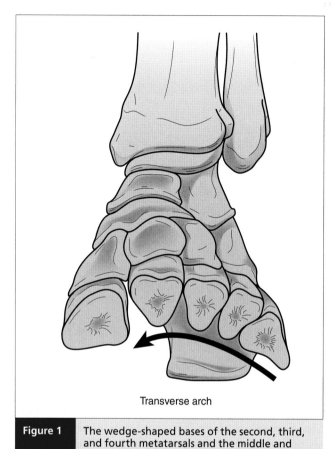

Transverse arch

| Figure 1 | The wedge-shaped bases of the second, third, and fourth metatarsals and the middle and lateral cuneiforms create a "keystone" effect that stabilizes the arch in the coronal plane. |

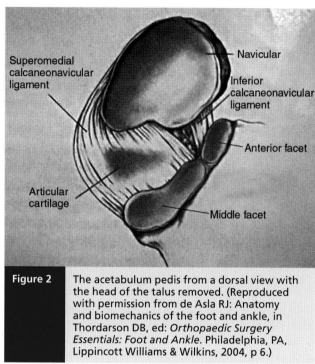

| Figure 2 | The acetabulum pedis from a dorsal view with the head of the talus removed. (Reproduced with permission from de Asla RJ: Anatomy and biomechanics of the foot and ankle, in Thordarson DB, ed: *Orthopaedic Surgery Essentials: Foot and Ankle*. Philadelphia, PA, Lippincott Williams & Wilkins, 2004, p 6.) |

artery. Blood supply to its central portion is relatively sparse. Certain foot types may accentuate shear across the central portion of the bone.[6] The navicular is also the primary attachment site of the tibialis posterior tendon. These features may combine to make the navicular bone relatively susceptible to stress fracture and poor healing.

The midfoot is separated from the hindfoot by the talonavicular and calcaneal cuboid joints, known collectively as the transverse tarsal joint or Chopart joint. The talonavicular joint is a ball-and-socket–type joint. The socket that receives the talar head is deepened by the anterior and middle facets of the calcaneus, the calcaneonavicular slip of the bifurcate ligament, and the superomedial and inferior calcaneal navicular ligaments (spring ligament). The superomedial component of the spring ligament serves to suspend the head of the talus, functioning like an anatomic hammock. This acetabulum pedis allows for transverse, sagittal, and longitudinal planes of motion and plays a vital role in foot biomechanics (Figure 2). Any motion of the talonavicular joint or subtalar joint also involves motion at the calcaneocuboid joint. Maximum congruency of the calcaneocuboid joint is achieved when the hindfoot is in varus and the forefoot

is supinated. This is the position the foot assumes with push-off.

The hindfoot consists of the calcaneus and the talus. Their articulation forms the subtalar joint as the talus sits "side saddle" over the superomedial aspect of the calcaneus. The subtalar joint consists of three separate articulations, or facets. More than 90% of all tarsal coalitions occur at either the anterior facet (calcaneonavicular coalition) or the middle facet (talocalcaneal coalition). For simplicity's sake, subtalar motion is often depicted as inversion and eversion around a mitered hinge. In reality, subtalar motion is quite complex, difficult to measure, and includes rotational motions and translations in multiple planes. The subtalar joint is stabilized by the deltoid ligament, the interosseous and cervical ligaments, and a series of lateral ligaments and structures. These lateral stabilizers include the calcaneofibular ligament (CFL), the lateral talocalcaneal ligament, and the inferior extensor retinaculum. Because of its role as a subtalar joint stabilizer, the inferior extensor retinaculum is often used in Broström-type lateral ankle ligament reconstruction procedures[7-9] (Figure 3).

The body of the talus resides in a bony housing created by the articulation between the distal fibula and tibia. The mortise is formed by the tibial plafond and medial and lateral malleoli. Composed of the talus, distal tibia, and fibula, the ankle joint includes three articulations: tibiofibular, tibiotalar, and talofibular. The tibiofibular joint represents the inferior extent of the lower

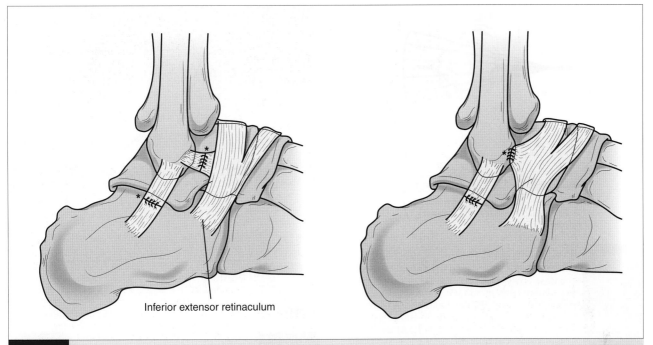

Inferior extensor retinaculum

Figure 3 | The illustrations depict a modified Broström procedure. Note that a portion of the inferior extensor retinaculum is mobilized for incorporation into the repair.

extremity syndesmosis. The syndesmosis is stabilized by four ligaments: the anterior inferior tibiofibular ligament (AITFL), the posterior inferior tibiofibular ligament, the transverse tibiofibular ligament (TTFL), and the interosseous tibiofibular ligament (IOTFL). Occasionally, a thickened accessory slip of the AITFL (Bassett ligament) may insert too distally on the fibula, causing symptoms as it impinges against the anterolateral aspect of the talar dome. The TTFL originates on the posterior aspect of the fibula and extends to the posterior margin of the medial malleolus. In between, it forms the posterior labrum, which effectively deepens the tibiotalar joint. The syndesmosis allows fibula rotation and proximal migration when the wider anterior aspect of the talar body rotates into the ankle mortise during dorsiflexion. This relationship also allows the fibula to share approximately 16% of the axial load transmitted across the ankle.[10-12]

The ankle is stabilized by the inherent bony configuration of the mortise,[13] as well as the medial and lateral ligament complexes. One author compared the articular surface of the talus to a truncated cone in which the medial aspect is oriented toward the apex and the lateral aspect is oriented toward the base. Therefore, this cone has a smaller medial radius and a larger lateral radius[14] (**Figure 4**). The articular surface of the talus is also narrower posteriorly than anteriorly. When the ankle is dorsiflexed, the widened anterior portion of the talus fills the mortise more effectively, improving bony stability. In plantar flexion, the bony contribution to

stability decreases and the surrounding ligaments must assume an increased role. The deltoid ligament complex is well configured to stabilize the medial aspect of the ankle where the apex of the deltoid meets the apex of the cone. The deltoid ligament complex is divided into two anatomically distinct layers: superficial and deep. The superficial layer is fan-shaped and has no discrete bands. It has been divided into as many as five components. The anatomically separate deep layer is short and thick and divided into two distinct ligaments: the anterior and posterior tibiotalar ligaments. Both layers act to resist valgus talar tilting and act as secondary restraints to anterior translation of the talus. The deep layer is the primary restraint to talar external rotation.

The lateral ankle ligament complex is configured more broadly to accommodate a wider radius and larger arc of rotation. The lateral ankle ligament complex comprises the anterior talofibular ligament (ATFL), the CFL, and the posterior talofibular ligament (PTFL). Lateral ankle stability depends on the orientation of the fibers of each of these ligaments, which changes with ankle position. The ATFL is an intra-articular thickening of the anterolateral ankle joint capsule. Among all lateral ligaments, the ATFL has the lowest load to failure but the highest strain; it lengthens the most before failure. When the foot is plantar flexed, the fibers of the ATFL orient parallel to the leg, providing collateral restraint to inversion. The CFL is a distinct extracapsular, cordlike ligament that spans the ankle and the subtalar joints. This ligament is

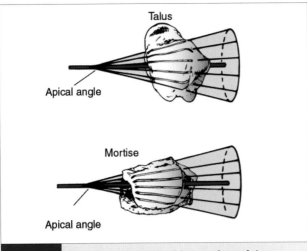

Figure 4 The cone-shaped trochlear surface of the talus. The apex is oriented medially whereas the base is oriented laterally. (Adapted with permission from Inman VT: *The Joints of the Ankle.* Baltimore, MD, Williams and Wilkins, 1976 and reproduced with permission from Haskell A, Mann RA: Biomechanics of the foot and ankle, in Coughlin MJ, Mann RA, Saltzman CL, eds: *Surgery of the Foot and Ankle,* ed 8. Philadelphia, PA, Mosby, 2007, p 3-36.)

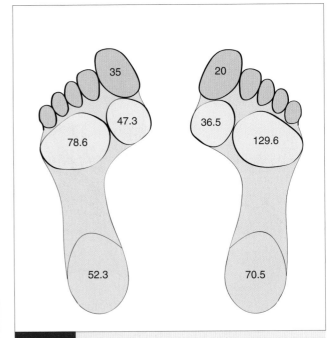

Figure 5 Peak forces, in newtons, measured on the plantar foot before and after silicone arthroplasty of the first metatarsalphalangeal joint. (Adapted from Beverly MC, Horan FT, Hutton WC: Load cell analysis following silastic arthroplasty of the hallux. *Int Orthop* 1985;9[2]:101-104.)

always perpendicular to and stabilizes the subtalar joint. However, when the ankle is plantarflexed, this ligament assumes a relatively horizontal orientation with respect to the tibiotalar joint, rendering it ineffective as a stabilizer. When the foot dorsiflexes, the roles of the ATFL and CFL are reversed.[15,16]

Clinical Biomechanics

At its most basic level, the foot can be conceptualized as a tripod. In stance, weight is distributed collectively between the head of the first metatarsal, the heel, and the four lesser metatarsal heads. Malalignment and alterations in biomechanics may disrupt this balance, resulting in painful conditions (**Figure 5**). For example, a cavus foot type is more prone to increased loading under the first metatarsal head and lateral aspect of the foot. A patient with a dorsiflexion malunion of a metatarsal fracture is at increased risk for a painful callus under another metatarsal head. Furthermore, foot deformity and position may ultimately affect more proximal joints, as seen in patients with planovalgus foot deformities. The rotational forces created by the planovalgus foot may eventually result in attenuation of the deltoid ligament and valgus tilting of the talus. When a foot and ankle surgeon attempts to correct deformity, the tripod concept must be kept in mind.

The true axis of rotation of the tibiotalar joint consists of a series of instant centers of rotation as the talus translates in the horizontal plane with dorsiflexion and plantar flexion. However, for most purposes, this axis can be estimated using a line that passes through the distal aspects of both malleoli. This empirical axis lies in approximately 20° to 30° of external rotation with respect to the coronal plane and is obliquely oriented at approximately 82° from the axis of the tibia (**Figure 6**). With the foot free and the leg in a fixed position, the oblique ankle joint axis causes the foot to externally rotate with dorsiflexion and internally rotate with plantar flexion (**Figure 7**). Conversely, when the foot is fixed to the floor, the oblique axis imposes an internal rotation force to the leg as the body passes over the foot, and the foot dorsiflexes. As the foot pushes off, ankle plantar flexion results in external rotation of the leg. Rotation of the tibia is coupled with the inversion and eversion motion of the subtalar joint. One study suggests that when tibiotalar motion is markedly reduced by arthritis, the normal motion coupling seen in healthy ankle joints breaks down.[17]

Motion of the subtalar joint has been compared to a mitered hinge. Its axis passes obliquely from the plantar surface laterally to dorsomedially, deviating from the horizontal plane by approximately 41° and from the sagittal plane by approximately 23°.[14,18] The subtalar axis

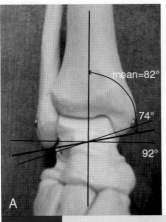
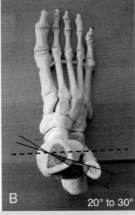

Figure 6 **A,** Ankle joint axis of rotation as viewed in the coronal plane. **B,** Ankle joint axis of rotation as viewed from the horizontal plane. (Reproduced with permission from de Asla RJ: Anatomy and biomechanics of the foot and ankle, in Thordarson DB, ed: *Orthopaedic Surgery Essentials: Foot and Ankle.* Philadelphia, PA, Lippincott Williams and Wilkins, 2004, p 18.)

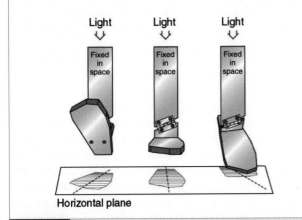

Figure 7 With the leg fixed in position and the foot free, the oblique ankle joint axis causes outward rotation with dorsiflexion and inward rotation with plantar flexion. (Reproduced with permission from Haskell A, Mann RA: Biomechanics of the foot and ankle, in Coughlin MJ, Mann RA, Saltzman CL, eds: *Surgery of the Foot and Ankle,* ed 8. Philadelphia, PA, Mosby, 2007, pp 3-36.)

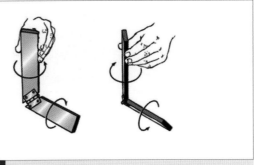

Figure 8 A mitered joint hinge is shown. (Reproduced with permission from Haskell A, Mann RA: Biomechanics of the foot and ankle, in Coughlin MJ, Mann RA, Saltzman CL, eds: *Surgery of the Foot and Ankle,* ed 8. Philadelphia, PA, Mosby 2007, pp 3-36.)

of rotation is highly variable between patients. Using the model in **Figure 8** as a visual aid, a more horizontally oriented axis appears to translate to more rotation of the horizontal component with every degree of vertical component rotation. The reverse is true with a more vertically oriented axis. Clinically, it is recognized that patients with flatter feet (a more horizontal axis) have more subtalar motion, while patients with a cavus foot type (a more vertical axis) tend to experience stiffer motion.

The transverse tarsal joint allows for hindfoot motion while the forefoot remains plantigrade to the ground. This relationship is facilitated by the acetabulum pedis. The heel strikes the ground in varus and then quickly everts. Anatomically, the everted hindfoot places the axis of rotation of the calcaneal cuboid joint parallel to the axis of rotation of the talonavicular joint. This parallel configuration permits motion across the transverse tarsal joint, which accommodates uneven terrain and absorb impact forces. As the body's center of mass moves forward over the foot the tibia externally rotates, causing the hindfoot to rotate into varus through coupled motion. The changing position of the hindfoot causes the once-parallel axes of the transverse tarsal joints to converge. This convergence effectively "locks" the transverse tarsal joint, effectively changing the foot from an accommodating platform for stance into a rigid lever arm for efficient push-off.

Motion of the subtalar joint and transverse tarsal joint (also called the triple joint complex) are inextricably linked, with the talonavicular joint playing the key role. In conditions requiring arthrodesis of the talonavicular joint, motion through the remaining joints of the triple joint complex is virtually nonexistent.[19] Acting in conjunction with the bony architecture of the foot and ankle is a series of dynamic and static soft-tissue stabilizers. At heel strike, the tibialis anterior tendon eccentrically contracts to control foot descent, serving to dissipate forces and prevent slapping of the foot against the ground. The tibialis posterior tendon plays a vital role in producing hindfoot inversion during push-off through its action across the transverse tarsal joint. The pull of the tibialis posterior tendon adducts the navicular over the head of the talus, helping to invert the calcaneus, which follows the cuboid. The ability to perform an efficient heel rise depends on the tibialis posterior tendon's ability to secure the transverse tarsal joint in adduction. At heel rise, the

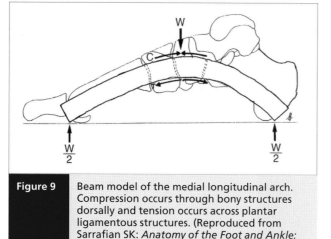

Figure 9	Beam model of the medial longitudinal arch. Compression occurs through bony structures dorsally and tension occurs across plantar ligamentous structures. (Reproduced from Sarrafian SK: *Anatomy of the Foot and Ankle: Descriptive, Topographic, Functional*, ed 2. Philadelphia, PA, Lippincott, Williams & Wilkins, 1993, p 560.)

Figure 10	Truss model of the medial longitudinal arch. The bony architecture of the foot is conceptualized as two beams connected by the plantar fascia, which functions as a tie rod. (Reproduced from Sarrafian SK: *Anatomy of the Foot and Ankle: Descriptive, Topographic, Functional*, ed 2. Philadelphia, PA, Lippincott, Williams and Wilkins, 1993, p 559.)

triceps surae pulls the Achilles tendon to become the strongest hindfoot inverter. This ensures the midfoot will remain locked for toe-off.

When disease renders the posterior tibial tendon ineffective, the transverse tarsal midfoot locking mechanism is compromised. When the midfoot fails to lock, the stability of the medial longitudinal arch becomes solely dependent on plantar soft-tissue static stabilizers for support. Without dynamic stabilization and bony protection of the transverse tarsal joint, these stabilizers will attenuate and eventually fail under tension, resulting in progressive collapse of the medial longitudinal arch, and the hindfoot will fail to invert. As a consequence, the Achilles tendon will pull on an everted hindfoot to ensure that midfoot locking does not occur. In this scenario, the Achilles tendon becomes a deforming force that leads to further and accelerated deformity.

The medial longitudinal arch is a dynamic structure that aids in shock absorption and terrain accommodation on heel strike and in midstance, and then allows for efficient propulsion at toe-off. Two models have been proposed to help describe the biomechanics of the medial longitudinal arch.[20] In one model, the arch is conceptualized as a curved, segmented beam. The beam comprises the calcaneus, talus, navicular, cuneiforms, and the medial three metatarsals. The segments are stabilized by static plantar ligamentous connections. With weight bearing, compression forces develop on the dorsal aspect of the beam while tensile forces are created on the plantar aspect. The dorsal compression forces are resisted by the bony architecture of the arch, whereas plantar tensile forces are resisted by the ligaments (**Figure 9**).

The beam model of the medial longitudinal arch does not consider the role of the plantar fascia. This structure is incorporated in the truss model of the arch (**Figure 10**). In the truss model, the arch is conceptualized as a triangular structure composed of two oblique beams with a dorsal pivot connected plantarly by a tie rod. Anatomically, the plantar fascia functions as a tie rod, originating from the posterior calcaneal tuberosity and inserting onto the sesamoids and the bases of the proximal phalanges of the lesser toes. With loading, the plantar fascia resists the plantarly generated tensile forces.[21] Total or partial release of the plantar fascia may decrease arch height.[22]

During late midstance and toe-off, the hallux and lesser toes dorsiflex, which effectively tightens the plantar fascia and adds to the stability of the midfoot. The mechanism by which this occurs has been likened to a windlass device (**Figure 11**). A windlass is used to transport or lift objects vertically. It makes use of a lever arm (the hallux and lesser toes) that is attached to a cable or rope (the plantar fascia) wound around a cylinder (the metatarsophalangeal joints), which acts as a fulcrum.

Gait

Human gait is defined as the process by which the lower extremities are used for forward locomotion. Many biomechanical events unfold during human gait that simply occur too rapidly to evaluate clinically. Numerous techniques developed in the field of biomechanics can potentially quantitatively assess body segment motions and forces. Such techniques, however, usually necessitate the use of a formal gait laboratory and a dedicated team. Techniques include video gait analysis, force plates, fluoroscopic imaging, three-dimensional reconstruction software, electromyography, and a host of other technologies.

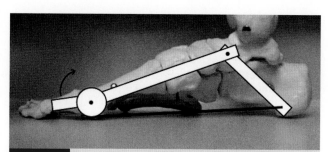

Figure 11 Windlass mechanism. A truss is shown superimposed over a skeletal model of the foot. As the toes dorsiflex, the drum (metatarsophalangeal joints) rotates, applying tension to the tie rod (plantar fascia) and effectively supporting the arch. (Reproduced with permission from de Asla RJ: Anatomy and biomechanics of the foot and ankle, in Thordarson DB, ed: *Orthopaedic Surgery Essentials: Foot and Ankle*. Philadelphia, PA, Lippincott Williams & Wilkins, 2004, p 21.)

Despite the accuracy of certain gait analysis techniques, widespread clinical use has yet to occur and debate remains as to their clinical relevance. Criteria have been proposed regarding the inclusion of gait analysis as a routine part of an orthopaedic examination.[23,24]

Normal human gait is extremely efficient with regard to energy and oxygen consumption. The gait cycle is a pattern of recurring predefined events that can be analyzed in terms of "stride." A single stride starts from the moment of heel strike to the moment the same heel strikes the ground again. Stride length is defined as the distance covered between these two consecutive heel strikes. A step is the distance between the heel strike of one foot and the heel strike of the opposite foot. Cadence is defined by the number of steps taken during a given unit of time. In walking, a single stride is divided into two phases: the stance phase and the swing phase. The stance phase begins when the foot strikes the ground and continues until the toes of the same foot leave the ground (or toe-off). This represents approximately 60% of the gait cycle. Swing phase is the remaining 40% of the cycle and extends from toe-off until the heel strikes the ground.

The stance phase is further divided into three intervals. The first interval starts at heel strike and ends at foot flat. This segment is characterized by weight acceptance and rapid ankle plantar flexion under eccentric control of the anterior leg musculature. The second interval extends from foot flat opposite foot strike. During this interval, the body's center of gravity passes forward of the plantar foot. This "controlled fall" is halted when the contralateral heel strikes the ground. The final interval extends from the end of the second interval through toe-off. This interval is characterized by rapid ankle plantar flexion

and the cascade of biomechanical events that creates a rigid foot for efficient push-off.

Electromyographic measurements provide insight into muscle function during gait analysis. At heel strike, the anterior muscles of the leg actively control the descent of the foot to avoid slapping. This eccentric action also absorbs ground reaction forces. Activity of the extensor muscle group is largely replaced by activity of the flexor groups. Flexor activity starts with the tibialis posterior tendon preparing the foot for heel rise. The peroneal tendons provide varus stability as the ankle rotates in dorsiflexion during single-limb stance. The triceps surae activates, followed by recruitment of the toe flexors, causing heel rise, rapid plantar flexion, and eventual toe-off. In the early swing phase, the plantar muscles relax and the extensors act to dorsiflex the foot again, allowing for clearance and preparation for the next heel strike. As the foot progresses from foot strike to toe-off, the center of load progresses from the center of the heel through the hallux.

Running alters the gait cycle in several important ways. Running gait adds two float phases. During walking, one foot is always in contact with the ground. During float phase, both feet are off the ground. Additionally, there is no longer a period of double-limb support. During running gait, ground reaction force increases, the phasic activity of muscles is altered, and the range of motion of the lower extremity joints increases.

Alterations of normal gait can result in gait dysfunction. In general, a dysfunctional gait pattern leads to insufficiencies that cause increased energy and oxygen consumption. Pain is probably the most common cause of gait disturbance. One study demonstrated that patients with ankle arthritis who underwent either ankle arthroplasty or arthrodesis returned to a more normal gait pattern.[25] In another study, patients who underwent ankle arthrodesis had decreased stride length.[26] Among patients who have undergone amputation, the more proximal the amputation, the higher the required energy expenditure for gait.[27]

Many disorders of the foot and ankle result in discernible and characteristic patterns in human gait. An antalgic gait results from pain and is defined by the shortened stance phase of the affected limb. A steppage gait results from foot drop or weakness of the anterior musculature of the leg. It is characterized by lifting the affected limb higher during the swing phase so the foot adequately clears the ground. A calcaneal gait is characterized by exaggerated heel weight bearing and results from weakness or paralysis of the posterior compartment musculature. A waddling gait is the result of proximal myopathy and is characterized by a broad-based stance with the pelvis drooping toward the leg being raised during the swing phase. This gait abnormality is in contrast to a Trendelenburg gait, which is caused by weakness of the hip abductors and results in compensatory lurching of the trunk toward the weakened side during stance.

Summary

With the advent of new technologies and techniques over the decades, the ability to measure foot and ankle biomechanics has substantially expanded. If surgeons are to create and optimize new treatment options for patients, the knowledge base must continue to expand.

Annotated References

1. Arndt A, Westblad P, Winson I, Hashimoto T, Lundberg A: Ankle and subtalar kinematics measured with intracortical pins during the stance phase of walking. *Foot Ankle Int* 2004;25(5):357-364.

2. de Asla RJ, Wan L, Rubash HE, Li G: Six DOF in vivo kinematics of the ankle joint complex: Application of a combined dual-orthogonal fluoroscopic and magnetic resonance imaging technique. *J Orthop Res* 2006;24(5):1019-1027.

3. Fassbind MJ, Rohr ES, Hu Y, et al: Evaluating foot kinematics using magnetic resonance imaging: From maximum plantar flexion, inversion, and internal rotation to maximum dorsiflexion, eversion, and external rotation. *J Biomech Eng* 2011;133(10):104502.

   In this study the authors describe a method for quantifying foot bone motion from maximum plantar flexion, inversion, and internal rotation to maximum dorsiflexion, eversion, and external rotation using a foot plate with an electromagnetic sensor, a custom-built MRI-compatible device to hold patient's foot during scanning, and three-dimensional rendering software.

4. Kitaoka HB, Crevoisier XM, Hansen D, Katajarvi B, Harbst K, Kaufman KR: Foot and ankle kinematics and ground reaction forces during ambulation. *Foot Ankle Int* 2006;27(10):808-813.

5. Lundberg A: Kinematics of the ankle and foot. In vivo roentgen stereophotogrammetry. *Acta Orthop Scand Suppl* 1989;233:1-24.

6. Torg JS, Pavlov H, Cooley LH, et al: Stress fractures of the tarsal navicular. A retrospective review of twenty-one cases. *J Bone Joint Surg Am* 1982;64(5):700-712.

7. Harper MC: The lateral ligamentous support of the subtalar joint. *Foot Ankle* 1991;11(6):354-358.

8. Ringleb SI, Dhakal A, Anderson CD, Bawab S, Paranjape R: Effects of lateral ligament sectioning on the stability of the ankle and subtalar joint. *J Orthop Res* 2011;29(10):1459-1464.

   The authors used a six-degree-of-freedom loading device to collect kinematic data from sensors attached to the calcaneus, talus, and tibia by keeping all the ligaments intact and by serially sectioning the ATFL, CFL, cervical ligament, and talocalcaneal interosseus ligament. They found the ATFL and CFL contributed to tibiotalar stability. The interosseous ligament was found to contribute most to subtalar joint stability. The authors concluded that diagnosing subtalar joint instability by physical examination is difficult.

9. Heilman AE, Braly WG, Bishop JO, Noble PC, Tullos HS: An anatomic study of subtalar instability. *Foot Ankle* 1990;10(4):224-228.

10. Beumer A, van Hemert WL, Swierstra BA, Jasper LE, Belkoff SM: A biomechanical evaluation of the tibiofibular and tibiotalar ligaments of the ankle. *Foot Ankle Int* 2003;24(5):426-429.

11. Hoefnagels EM, Waites MD, Wing ID, Belkoff SM, Swierstra BA: Biomechanical comparison of the interosseous tibiofibular ligament and the anterior tibiofibular ligament. *Foot Ankle Int* 2007;28(5):602-604.

12. Nester CJ, Findlow AF, Bowker P, Bowden PD: Transverse plane motion at the ankle joint. *Foot Ankle Int* 2003;24(2):164-168.

13. Tochigi Y, Rudert MJ, Saltzman CL, Amendola A, Brown TD: Contribution of articular surface geometry to ankle stabilization. *J Bone Joint Surg Am* 2006;88(12):2704-2713.

14. Inman VT: *The Joints of the Ankle.* Baltimore, MD, Williams & Wilkins, 1976.

15. Fujii T, Kitaoka HB, Luo ZP, Kura H, An KN: Analysis of ankle-hindfoot stability in multiple planes: An in vitro study. *Foot Ankle Int* 2005;26(8):633-637.

16. Ozeki S, Kitaoka H, Uchiyama E, Luo ZP, Kaufman K, An KN: Ankle ligament tensile forces at the end points of passive circumferential rotating motion of the ankle and subtalar joint complex. *Foot Ankle Int* 2006;27(11):965-969.

17. Kozanek M, Rubash HE, Li G, de Asla RJ: Effect of post-traumatic tibiotalar osteoarthritis on kinematics of the ankle joint complex. *Foot Ankle Int* 2009;30(8):734-740.

   In this in vivo study, the authors use a combined dual orthogonal fluoroscopic and MRI technique to measure six-degree-of-freedom kinematics of the arthritic tibiotalar joint and its effect on the kinematics of the subtalar joint. The study suggests that subtalar joint motion in the sagittal, coronal, and transverse rotational planes tends to occur in opposite directions in patients with tibiotalar arthritis when compared with ankle control. These findings demonstrate a breakdown in the normal motion coupling seen in healthy ankle joints.

18. Inman VT: *Human Walking.* Baltimore, MD, Williams & Wilkins, 1981.

19. Astion DJ, Deland JT, Otis JC, Kenneally S: Motion of the hindfoot after simulated arthrodesis. *J Bone Joint Surg Am* 1997;79(2):241-246.

20. Sarrafian SK: Functional anatomy of the foot and ankle, in Sarafian SK, ed: *Anatomy of the Foot and Ankle: Descriptive, Topographic, Functional,* ed 2. Philadelphia, PA, Lippincott-Williams & Wilkins, 1993.

21. Hicks JH: The mechanics of the foot. II. The plantar aponeurosis and the arch. *J Anat* 1954;88(1):25-30.

22. Cheung JT, An KN, Zhang M: Consequences of partial and total plantar fascia release: A finite element study. *Foot Ankle Int* 2006;27(2):125-132.

23. Brand RA: Can biomechanics contribute to clinical orthopaedic assessments? *Iowa Orthop J* 1989;9:61-64.

24. Brand RA, Crowninshield RD: Comment on criteria for patient evaluation tools. *J Biomech* 1981;14(9):655.

25. Flavin R, Coleman SC, Tenenbaum S, Brodsky JW: Comparison of gait after total ankle arthroplasty and ankle arthrodesis. *Foot Ankle Int* 2013;34(10):1340-1348.

The authors prospectively studied gait kinematics in three dimensions using a 12-camera digital motion capture system in patients who had undergone either ankle arthrodesis or ankle arthroplasty. Analysis was performed both preoperatively and postoperatively with findings compared with those of a volunteer control group. The authors concluded that patients in both the arthrodesis and arthroplasty groups had substantial improvements in various parameters of gait when compared with their own preoperative function. Neither group functioned as well as the control group. Total ankle arthroplasty produced a more symmetric vertical ground reaction force curve, which was closer to that of the control group than was the curve of the ankle arthrodesis group. Level of evidence: II.

26. Thomas R, Daniels TR, Parker K: Gait analysis and functional outcomes following ankle arthrodesis for isolated ankle arthritis. *J Bone Joint Surg Am* 2006;88(3):526-535.

27. Waters RL, Perry J, Antonelli D, Hislop H: Energy cost of walking of amputees: The influence of level of amputation. *J Bone Joint Surg Am* 1976;58(1):42-46.

Chapter 2

Shoes and Orthoses

Jesse F. Doty, MD   Michael J. Coughlin, MD

Introduction

Patients and various healthcare professionals expect orthopaedic providers to be familiar with shoe wear and bracing biomechanics and lower extremity pathologic conditions. A successful foot and ankle bracing experience often is the result of an evolution that produced the final product. Ideally, an experienced orthotist sees a patient regularly during the brace manufacturing process, and he or she modifies the brace based on observation. This chapter discusses shoe and orthosis design and bracing, and provides updates and fundamentals that can be applied to numerous foot and ankle conditions. Knowledge of these basic topics helps physicians communicate effectively with orthotists regarding their clinical goals for a brace. The orthotist will often make recommendations and incorporate modifications based on their personal experience and patient feedback.

Shoes

The past several decades have been characterized by substantial changes in shoe design, with the development of more specialized shoe wear driven by market demand. Appropriate shoes protect feet from the environment as a first priority, but current options and modifications

offer advantages for specific environments. A steel-toe, stiff-soled shoe that is worn in the workplace may protect a laborer, whereas a soft-soled, cushioned shoe can prevent skin ulcers in patients with diabetes. As technology improves, athletic shoes have become more customized and are designed to be sport-specific. A recent survey of adolescent cross-country runners revealed that 73% identified arch-type compatibility with shoe design as the most important factor in choosing a shoe. Another 74% reported not knowing how many miles they had logged in a single pair of running shoes before replacement.[1]

Running sports have vastly expanded, and research and development efforts have resulted in specialized trail and "barefoot-style" running shoes (**Figure 1**). Some of these concepts have been driven by market demand with little evidence for their safety and efficacy. In the case of barefoot-style running, well-designed studies are necessary to prove whether this minimalist running style is beneficial or harmful to overall foot and ankle health. Some studies support the notion that peak ground forces are reduced as a runner changes his gait pattern from a hindfoot strike typical of shod runners to a forefoot strike typical of barefoot runners.[2] A 2011 study[3] evaluated people who ran barefoot, in minimalist shoes, and in cushioned running shoes. The study reported that, both statically on a slantboard and dynamically on a treadmill, runners could estimate direction and amplitude of support slope more accurately with a minimalist shoe model. No substantial differences were found between runners using the minimalist shoe model and those who ran barefoot. The authors claimed that their data supports the assumption that cushioned shoes substantially impair foot position awareness compared to less-structured shoes or barefoot conditions. Secondary claims of minimalist running advantages including increased coordination and improved intrinsic muscle foot strength are associated with less clinical evidence and are based on opinions and anecdotal evidence.[4]

Now that injury prevention and playing field surface type are major topics in professional sports, organizations such as the National Football League have provided substantial financial support for shoe research and development, with an emphasis on performance and protection

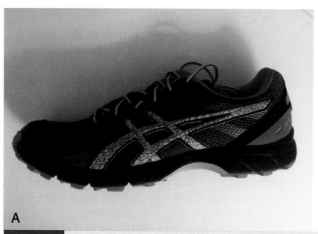
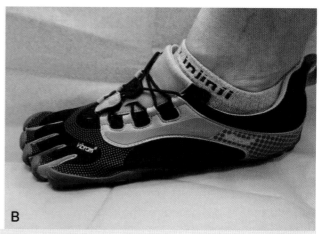

Figure 1   **A,** A trail-running shoe with a protective cover shields toes from protruding branches and rocks. The mesh upper is designed of lightweight, breathable material that can dry quickly without sacrificing protection or a snug fit. The aggressive outsole is designed to provide traction and stability on naturally uneven terrain. This particular shoe has a water drainage system incorporated through the sole to eliminate shoe saturation when crossing water hazards. **B,** A barefoot-style running shoe with an outsole only thick enough to protect the skin and with little or no cushion. Advocates claim this minimalist style of running results in a more natural gait that strengthens the foot and lower leg muscles.

for athletes.[5,6] A 2011 study[7] reported that thicker soles evoke a stronger protective eversion response from the peroneal muscles to counter the increasing moment arm at the ankle-subtalar joint complex following sudden foot inversion. The study's authors suggested that thicker soles are likely to increase risk for lateral ligament injury at the ankle when the protective response of the peroneal tendons is overwhelmed.

The influence of high-fashion footwear on foot and ankle biomechanics and pathoanatomy has long been a subject of concern. A 2013 study[8] found that habitual high-fashion shoe wearers showed decreased range of motion in dorsiflexion and eversion compared to flat-shoe wearers. The study's authors recommended intensive ankle stretching exercises for habitual high-heeled shoe wearers. Another team of 2013 investigators[9] performed electromyography of different muscle groups in high-heeled shoe wearers and found that high heels adversely affect muscle control and reduce loads in the quadriceps and spine musculature. These authors suggested that the addition of a total-contact insert to a shoe might improve comfort rating and foot stability.

Even with advances in technology introduced by the shoe industry, many of the basic components that make up a shoe remain the same (Table 1).

Shoe Modifications

Until recently, off-the-shelf shoes were generally designed with no pathologic considerations in mind. Research and development driven by the shoe industry has resulted in a plethora of shoe options. Now patients with less severe

Table 1

Basic Shoe Components

Upper	Portion of the shoe enclosing the dorsum of the foot above the insole; includes the toe box, vamp, and quarter
Lower	Portion of the shoe plantar to the foot; includes the insole, midsole, and outsole
Toe Box	Distal portion of the upper that provides space for the toes
Vamp	Midsection of the upper that covers the dorsum of the midfoot
Quarter	Posterior portion of the upper that covers the hindfoot posteriorly and laterally; may have a reinforced area around the heel known as the heel counter
Insole	Part of the lower that directly contacts the plantar surface of the foot and is frequently removable
Midsole	Cushioned area between the insole and outsole that is designed for shock absorption
Outsole	Portion of the lower that contacts the ground and provides traction

pathology may be able to achieve pain relief through strategic footwear selection. Those with mild forefoot malalignment have a large selection of wide toe box athletic shoes to choose from that may relieve pressure over

Table 2

Shoe Types and Modifications

In-depth shoe	Additional 0.25- to 0.375-inch depth to accommodate deformity; often manufactured with factory insoles that can easily be exchanged
Custom shoe	May provide the best accommodation and protection because they are fabricated from a positive model of a mold or a CT scan
Relasting	This refers to customization of an off-the-shelf shoe to accommodate deformity without sacrificing the normal appearance to the casual observer. The outsole is removed and a cut is made through the remaining sole. Material is added into the cut to fill the gap and to widen the shoe and a new outsole is applied.
Flare	A firm strip of material added as an outrigger to provide a wider base of support on the shoe surface for increased stability
Shank	Steel or carbon composite embedded in the layers of the sole to stiffen it from heel to toe; used to decrease bending in the shoe
Rocker sole	Additional material generally is added in the midsole to create a rocker intended to allow the foot to roll over from heel strike to toe-off with decreased bending. Multiple types exist, but generally the apex of the rocker is placed proximal to the area where pressure relief is desired.

forefoot deformities. Many athletic shoe manufacturers market styles with varied degrees of arch support to accommodate runners with either pes planus or pes cavus. These shoes may increase comfort, especially for active patients with mild cavus or planus in what would otherwise be considered a normal plantigrade foot. Patients with diabetes now have easier access to therapeutic in-depth shoes with soft uppers and cushioned insoles, which can relieve pressure over bony prominences. In-depth shoes feature an additional 0.25 to 0.375 inches of depth and can be easily modified by removing the factory inlay and inserting a foot orthosis without affecting overall fit.[10]

Although such a wide array of off-the-shelf footwear is available, orthopaedic specialists consult with patients who may benefit from footwear customizations (Table 2). Shoes can be modified to increase ambulation efficiency; compensate for decreased motion secondary to pain, fusion, arthritis, or deformity; increase stability; or offload areas of high pressure.[10] Shoe modifications may be less tolerated by younger, active patients, but these alterations may delay the need for surgical intervention in patients who are sedentary or provide temporal relief for poor surgical candidates. The upper portion of a standard shoe can be stretched to accommodate a deformity; for example, a "ball-and-ring stretcher" can be placed on a shoe to soften the upper material and make room for a bony prominence such as a hallux valgus deformity or a hammer toe. Modifications to offload bony prominences also may be made to shoe insoles. A factory insole can be supplemented or removed and replaced with an over-the-counter insole or a custom insole. When a metatarsal bar pad is added to an insole transversely and proximally to the metatarsal heads, this offloads this area during gait.

Metatarsal pads are manufactured in multiple sizes, and patients can shape pads before adding them to an insole depending on the location of their pain.

Pads can also be positioned on insoles for use as "wedges" or "posts" with which to address varus or valgus deformities or forces at the forefoot and hindfoot. A medial heel wedge provides a varus moment to the hindfoot, which may decrease lateral impingement or help correct hindfoot valgus in patients with pes planus. Runners with pes planus have reported a decreased incidence of foot and knee pain when a medial heel wedge was added to their soft insole.[11] A lateral heel wedge provides a valgus moment to the hindfoot, which may relieve tension on the peroneal tendons or decrease lateral instability. Posting the forefoot may also alter hindfoot position. Medial posting of a varus forefoot can decrease the valgus moment transferred to the hindfoot from the malaligned forefoot. Lateral posting of a valgus forefoot can decrease the varus moment transferred to the hindfoot from the malaligned forefoot[12] (Figure 2).

Exchanging a thin, standard factory insole with a thick gel, foam, or air-cushioned insole may help relieve metatarsalgia, heel pain, or generalized foot discomfort. Some conditions may be relieved by retaining a cushioned insole and reducing shoe flexibility by adding a carbon fiber plate plantar to the insole. This strategy is used to eliminate bending forces transferred to the foot from the shoe during gait. The addition of a carbon fiber plate may stiffen a shoe enough to relieve pain from hallux rigidus, metatarsalgia, and midfoot arthritis by decreasing the excursion of the painful joints (Figure 3).

A cobbler or pedorthotist may add a rocker bottom to the shoe sole, and some shoes are manufactured with

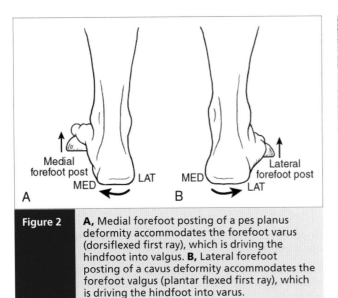

Figure 2 **A,** Medial forefoot posting of a pes planus deformity accommodates the forefoot varus (dorsiflexed first ray), which is driving the hindfoot into valgus. **B,** Lateral forefoot posting of a cavus deformity accommodates the forefoot valgus (plantar flexed first ray), which is driving the hindfoot into varus.

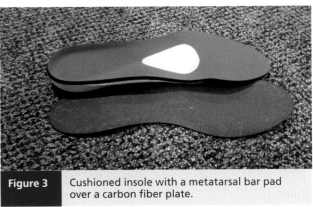

Figure 3 Cushioned insole with a metatarsal bar pad over a carbon fiber plate.

an incorporated rocker bottom. A rocker bottom is created by adding material that usually is placed in the midsole region between the heel and toe. This material allows patients to roll over the foot, thereby decreasing floor-reaction forces and bending forces on the foot. The rocker-bottom modification is useful for patients with limited or painful joint excursion because of arthritis, metatarsalgia, or other disorders. Similarly, a rocker bottom may improve gait in patients with limited excursion of their joints after arthrodesis procedures.[13] In a recent study evaluating foot kinematics during gait with a rocker-bottom sole, the authors reported that a rocker bottom is effective in reducing the "windlass effect" and may be useful in treating plantar fasciitis.[14]

Modifications aside, the primary clinical goal of shoe selection and shoe fitting is to choose a shoe that fits a patient appropriately. The shoe must be the correct shape and depth and be at least 0.375 inches longer than the longest toe to accommodate additional devices such as an orthosis.[10]

Orthoses

An orthosis is an orthopaedic device used to support, align, prevent, or correct deformities or to improve functions of body motion. Many different types of orthoses exist. The clinical portion of orthosis development must be biomechanically accurate for the orthosis to work appropriately. A basic understanding of the terminology and the clinical applications of orthoses allows a clinician to provide direction to the orthotist to ensure effective fabrication and treatment. An experienced orthotist often incorporates his or her personal algorithms, modifications, and materials into the orthosis based on

the clinician diagnosis. The clinician must first determine the goal to be accomplished with the orthosis. An orthosis is generally prescribed to either alter the biomechanics of the foot and ankle or to achieve comfort and protection by offloading certain areas and distributing weight to a broader surface area. The clinician should designate whether the orthosis is to be accommodative, supportive, or corrective. An accommodative orthosis is generally made of softer material shaped much like the patient's native anatomy to distribute weight along the plantar surface of the foot for cushioning and pressure relief. A supportive orthosis may be used to help stabilize a flexible deformity such as supple pes planus treated with an arch support. A corrective orthosis is manufactured to intentionally alter alignment and biomechanics, possibly with purposeful deviation from a patient's anatomy. Molded thermoplastic is typically used by the orthotist to provide and preserve the shape of the orthosis. When writing a prescription for the orthotist, it also helps if the clinician designates orthosis length. A full-length orthosis extends to the tip of the toes, a sulcus-length orthosis extends to the base of the toes, and a three-quarter-length orthosis ends proximal to the metatarsal heads. Ankle and hindfoot pathology often can be treated with a three-quarter-length orthosis. However, when forefoot posting is desired, a full-length or sulcus-length orthosis may better accomplish treatment goals.

A foot orthosis extends from the heel to the forefoot area, whereas an ankle-foot orthosis (AFO) extends above the ankle joint. Even when pathology is primarily localized to the midfoot or hindfoot, it may be more effectively treated by extending the orthosis or brace above the ankle. This can be done without sacrificing ankle motion by using an articulated AFO, which allows patients to plantarflex and dorsiflex the ankle while decreasing varus and valgus forces at the hindfoot and ankle. An articulated AFO can be considered for treatment of tendon pathology such as tibialis posterior tendon dysfunction or peroneal tendon dysfunction.[15]

A nonarticulated or solid-ankle AFO is manufactured to more completely immobilize the ankle joint and can be used for ankle arthritis treatment. A wrap across the dorsum of the midfoot can be incorporated on the foot portion of an AFO to add rotational control in the event that more varus or valgus stability of the midfoot and hindfoot would be beneficial. An articulated AFO with a dorsal midfoot wrap can substantially decrease rotational stresses for patients with painful subtalar or midfoot arthritis while allowing them to maintain their ankle motion (Figure 4). Other potential AFO modifications are listed in Table 3. Although an AFO may allow for the most patient-specific customization, noncustomized devices are commercially available and may be effective and reduce costs.

Multiple published studies evaluate the effectiveness of orthoses. In a review of 11 randomized controlled trials, it was reported that custom foot orthoses may produce clinically important improvements in select patients.[16] Custom foot orthoses appeared to be at least slightly beneficial in juvenile idiopathic arthritis (JIA), rheumatoid arthritis, pes cavus, and hallux valgus deformities. However, surgical treatment can be more beneficial for hallux valgus deformities, and prefabricated orthoses were just as effective as custom orthoses for JIA.[16,17] Both a meta-analysis and randomized controlled trial on the use of foot orthoses for the treatment of plantar fasciitis reported that custom and prefabricated orthoses are equally effective in diminishing pain but did not completely resolve symptoms.[18,19] In another study, the authors found that when a foot orthosis was combined with a rocker-bottom sole, it was more effective in reducing plantar fasciitis pain.[20] A study on the use of night AFOs in treating plantar fasciitis pain reported that an anterior orthosis positioned at neutral was more comfortable for sleeping and more effectively decreased pain than a posterior orthosis with dorsiflexion force.[21]

A comprehensive literature review on foot orthoses and ankle instability concluded that a foot orthosis has a positive impact on chronically unstable ankles because it likely influences multiple levels of somatosensory feedback and neuromuscular control.[22] Another study on ankle instability found that a cavus foot orthosis that included a recess at the first metatarsal head and a ramp at the lateral forefoot was effective in reducing ankle instability by decreasing forefoot-driven hindfoot varus.[12] In a report on the use of a foot orthoses to slow the progression of hallux valgus deformities, authors found no difference in progression of the deformity while using an orthosis (versus not using an orthosis) at 12-month follow-up.[23] In 2007, authors presented a well-designed study[24] on foot orthoses and their use in children with bilateral flexible severe pes planus. The authors randomized

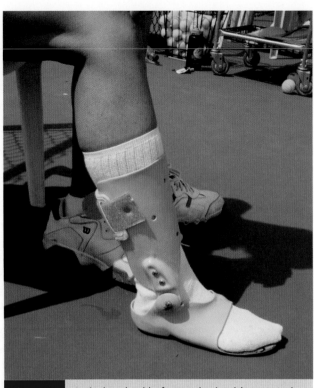

Figure 4 Articulated ankle-foot orthosis with an anterior in-step piece. (Courtesy of Richard Alvarez, MD, Chattanooga, TN.)

160 children ages 7 to 11 years of age to control, custom orthosis, and prefabricated orthosis treatment groups. At 3- and 12-month follow-ups, the authors evaluated motor proficiency, self-perception, exercise efficiency, and pain and found no evidence to justify the use of in-shoe orthoses for this condition. In a 2007 comprehensive meta-analysis of foot orthoses for lower limb overuse conditions[25] investigators revealed no difference in custom versus prefabricated orthoses, and investigators demonstrated that either type is acceptable for injury prevention. Although an orthosis appears to help prevent a first incidence of lower limb overuse conditions, little evidence supports or refutes this intervention's effectiveness after the overuse condition has developed.

In a 2008 study,[26] investigators looked at 25 feet and ankles with Charcot arthropathy in an attempt to identify an alternative to the Charcot Restraint Orthotic Walker and total contact casting. They reported that a prefabricated pneumatic removable walker brace (Aircast) fitted with a custom insole can successfully be used to manage the foot and ankle with Charcot arthropathy. The brace was effective in immobilizing the foot and ankle during healing and was associated with a high satisfaction rate and safety profile.

One prospective study evaluated the efficacy of a newly introduced brace to treat stage II flexible tibialis

Table 3

Ankle-Foot Orthosis Types and Modifications

Solid-ankle AFO	Trimlines fully enclose the malleoli to substantially decrease mobilization of the foot and ankle complex
Semisolid-ankle AFO	Trimlines enclose the posterior soft tissues but do not project anteriorly along the malleoli; allows limited ankle motion with weight-bearing but dampens ground reaction forces
Posterior leaf spring AFO	Trimlines are generally narrow posteriorly and are flexible enough to allow normal weight-bearing motion; retains enough shape memory to assist in foot dorsiflexion during the swing-through phase
Articulated AFO	Separate foot and leg segments are connected by an articulating mechanism aligned with the axis of the ankle to allow controlled dorsiflexion and plantar flexion. The hinge mechanism can be adjusted or modified to restrict or assist in certain motions.
Wrap-around AFO	Completely encloses the foot, ankle, and lower leg; maximizes skin contact area and may more effectively maintain desired alignment
Double upright AFO	Often attaches to the exterior of the patient's shoes; skin contact is avoided, which may be more desirable for patients with varied amounts of swelling or skin breakdown
Carbon fiber AFO	Incorporates many of the same designs and functions of plastic AFOs; the carbon allows the orthosis to be less bulky and provides energy storage in recoil, which returns force to the patient during gait
Post	Wedge under the medial or lateral forefoot used to bring the floor up to a fixed varus or valgus deformity or used in the hindfoot medially or laterally to tilt the heel
Cutout	Cutout, well, recess, or depression that can be used in the forefoot, midfoot, or hindfoot to unload a specific area
Lift	Generally used as a neutral heel wedge to generate equinis and relax the Achilles tendon
Cushion	Foam or other soft material used plantarly in the forefoot, midfoot, or hindfoot to relieve plantar pressure at painful areas
Extension	Rigid extension to the tips of the toes to decrease bending forces of the midfoot and forefoot
Flange	Semirigid rim or lip extension on the orthosis to help support or build up a certain area such as a collapsed arch
Metatarsal bar	Pad placed proximal to the metatarsal heads to unload plantar pressure at the area distal to the pad

AFO = ankle-foot orthosis.

posterior tendon dysfunction.[27] Patients were fitted with a custom-molded foot orthosis termed a "shell brace" that extended up to the malleolar area proximally for added support.[27] The authors reported that hindfoot flexibility was maintained in most patients and that functional outcomes and patient satisfaction scores were higher than average[27] (Figure 5).

High-energy extremity trauma is common in combat, and the Operation Enduring Freedom and Operation Iraqi Freedom conflicts have been characterized by high-energy explosive wound patterns primarily affecting the extremities. The high incidence of these injuries has encouraged researchers to develop surgical advances and rehabilitation programs to pursue limb salvage to address injuries once considered unsalvageable. The Intrepid Dynamic Exoskeletal Orthosis (IDEO, TechLink) was created to improve functional capabilities of the limb-salvage wounded warrior population and to be used in a high-intensity rehabilitation program known as the Return to Run clinical pathway.[28] The IDEO is a custom energy-storing AFO in which a proximal orthosis cuff helps offload the extremity and the foot-plate limits extremes of ankle motion. The IDEO's plantar flexion shape and carbon fiber material store and deliver energy

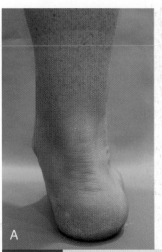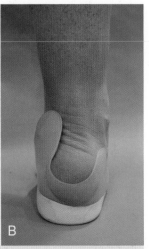

Figure 5   **A,** Adult-acquired flatfoot deformity with severe hindfoot valgus. **B,** Correction of tibialis posterior tendon dysfunction using the shell brace.

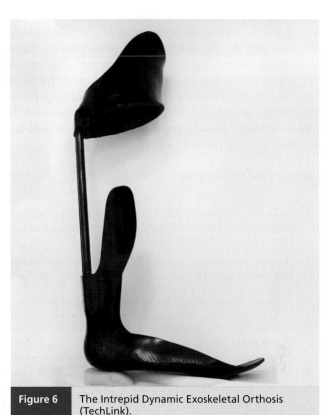

Figure 6   The Intrepid Dynamic Exoskeletal Orthosis (TechLink).

that simulates plantar flexion power[29] (Figure 6). Researchers compared functional performance of the IDEO to a standard carbon fiber AFO, a posterior leaf spring AFO, and no brace in 18 subjects with lower extremity fusion or weakness.[30] Among these patients, 13 had originally considered amputation. Substantial improvements were seen in functional tests such as ambulation on rocky terrain, the 40-yard dash, and stair ascent rates.[30] After completion of the Return to Run clinical pathway, of the 13 patients who had considered amputation, 8 opted for limb salvage, 2 were undecided, and 3 chose amputation.[30]

A recently developed brace, the Toad Medical Anti-Gravity (TAG) Foot Brace (Toad Medical Corporation, Bedford Heights, OH), uses a prosthetic suspension fit that includes a 3-mm silicone liner to protect the skin and allow weight-bearing to be distributed through the tibia so the foot is bypassed. Advocates of the TAG brace contend that it is designed to allow normal ambulation while unweighting the foot and ankle. Through its modular design, pressure on the lower extremity can be slowly increased throughout the healing cycle. Clinical studies are underway but have not yet been published on this antigravity brace (Figure 7).

Summary

Many patients may find long-term bracing cumbersome, embarrassing, or intolerable and may opt for surgical treatment. Wearing an AFO changes walking speed, step length, and cadence and creates asymmetry between the limbs when only one limb is braced.[31] However, among those with mild symptoms and patients who are poor

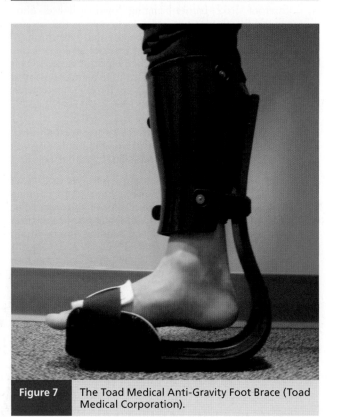

Figure 7   The Toad Medical Anti-Gravity Foot Brace (Toad Medical Corporation).

surgical candidates, an orthosis, brace, or shoe modification may be an effective form of treatment. Basic knowledge of bracing allows orthopaedic surgeons to accurately communicate guidelines to an orthotist who can then manufacture an appropriate device to achieve the desired clinical goals. Recent exciting developments in lower extremity bracing provide promising new options for both civilian and military rehabilitation.

Annotated References

1. Enke RC, Laskowski ER, Thomsen KM: Running shoe selection criteria among adolescent cross-country runners. *PM R* 2009;1(9):816-819.

   Among survey participants, 73% identified arch-type compatibility with shoe design as the most important factor in choosing a running shoe. However, only 57% reported knowing their arch type. Among respondents, 74% did not know how many miles they had accrued in a single pair of running shoes before replacement. Level of evidence: V.

2. Lieberman DE, Venkadesan M, Werbel WA, et al: Foot strike patterns and collision forces in habitually barefoot versus shod runners. *Nature* 2010;463(7280):531-535.

   Barefoot endurance runners often land on their forefoot (forefoot strike) before bringing down their heel. Shod runners mostly rearfoot strike, facilitated by the elevated and cushioned heel. Analyses show that even on hard surfaces, barefoot runners who forefoot strike generate smaller collision forces than shod rearfoot strikers. This difference primarily is caused by more plantar flexion at landing and more ankle compliance during impact. Level of evidence: V.

3. Squadrone R, Gallozzi C: Effect of a five-toed minimal protection shoe on static and dynamic ankle position sense. *J Sports Med Phys Fitness* 2011;51(3):401-408.

   Static ankle joint position sense was assessed in the sagittal and frontal planes by asking runners to estimate the perceived direction and amplitude of a support slope surface board placed under their foot. Dynamic measures were performed with the subjects running on a treadmill and then evaluating the treadmill slope. A minimalist shoe, a cushioned protective running shoe, and a barefoot condition were compared. The static trials had significantly more angle error underestimation ($P < 0.05$) with the running shoe, while no significant differences were found between minimalist-shoe and barefoot conditions. The treadmill surface slope was more accurately estimated with use of a minimalist shoe than in the other two conditions ($P < 0.05$).

4. Hsu AR: Topical review: Barefoot running. *Foot Ankle Int* 2012;33(9):787-794.

   The literature appears to support changes in gait pattern from hindfoot to forefoot strike with a reduction in peak forces when altering form to barefoot running style. Level of evidence: V.

5. Hennig EM: The influence of soccer shoe design on player performance and injuries. *Res Sports Med* 2011;19(3):186-201.

   Soccer shoe design can influence shooting speed and accuracy. Future research on soccer shoe optimization must address injury prevention and improved performance. Level of evidence: V.

6. Smeets K, Jacobs P, Hertogs R, et al: Torsional injuries of the lower limb: An analysis of the frictional torque between different types of football turf and the shoe outsole. *Br J Sports Med* 2012;46(15):1078-1083.

   Peak torque generated during a controlled rotation of the foot was measured in this study. Six parameters that could influence frictional forces were considered: the sports surface, shoe outsole cleat design, weather conditions, weight, presence of an impact, and direction of rotation. Football turf without infill demonstrated substantially lower frictional torques than natural grass, whereas football turf with sand/rubber infill produced higher torques.

7. Ramanathan AK, Parish EJ, Arnold GP, Drew TS, Wang W, Abboud RJ: The influence of shoe sole's varying thickness on lower limb muscle activity. *Foot Ankle Surg* 2011;17(4):218-223.

   Electromyographic recordings of peroneus longus muscle activity following unanticipated inversion of the foot in a tilting platform were collected. Test conditions included barefoot activity and activity in standard shoes and shoes with 2.5-cm and 5.0-cm sole adaptation. Compared to the barefoot condition, there was an increase in the magnitude of muscle contraction when wearing shoes (which further increases with thickening shoe soles). The peroneus longus was responding earlier in the shod conditions when compared to barefoot, although the results were variable within the three shod conditions.

8. Kim Y, Lim JM, Yoon B: Changes in ankle range of motion and muscle strength in habitual wearers of high-heeled shoes. *Foot Ankle Int* 2013;34(3):414-419.

   Habitual wearers of high-heeled shoes and flat shoes were recruited. Range of motion, maximal voluntary isometric force, and concentric ankle contraction power were measured. Wearers of high-heeled shoes showed more ankle range of motion on plantar flexion and inversion than flat-shoe wearers ($P < 0.05$) but displayed decreased dorsiflexion and eversion. Concentric contraction power in ankle eversion was also two times higher in wearers of high-heeled shoes ($P < 0.05$).

9. Hong WH, Lee YH, Lin YH, Tang SF, Chen HC: Effect of shoe heel height and total-contact insert on muscle loading and foot stability while walking. *Foot Ankle Int* 2013;34(2):273-281.

   High-heel wearers walked under six conditions formed by the cross-matching of shoe insert and heel height.

Measures of interest were rearfoot kinematics, muscle activities as assessed by electromyography, and subjective comfort rating as assessed by the visual analogue scale. Elevated heel height substantially increased plantar flexion and inversion at heel strike, prolonged tibialis anterior co-contraction, and the quadriceps activation period.

10. Janisse DJ, Janisse E: Shoe modification and the use of orthoses in the treatment of foot and ankle pathology. *J Am Acad Orthop Surg* 2008;16(3):152-158.

   Shoe modification and foot orthoses can play an important role in the management of foot and ankle pathology. Therapeutic footwear may be used to treat patients with diabetes, arthritis, neurologic conditions, traumatic injuries, congenital deformities, and sports-related injuries. These modalities may improve patient gait and increase level of ambulation. Level of evidence: V.

11. Shih YF, Wen YK, Chen WY: Application of wedged foot orthosis effectively reduces pain in runners with pronated foot: A randomized clinical study. *Clin Rehabil* 2011;25(10):913-923.

   In this study, a rearfoot medially wedged insole was a useful intervention to prevent or reduce painful knee or foot symptoms during running in athletes with pronated foot. Immediately after wearing the foot orthosis, pain incidence reduced in the treatment group but not in the control group (P = 0.04). The pain intensity score decreased significantly after orthosis application. Level of evidence: II.

12. LoPiccolo M, Chilvers M, Graham B, Manoli A II: Effectiveness of the cavus foot orthosis. *J Surg Orthop Adv* 2010;19(3):166-169.

   This study reveals an average precavus foot orthosis pain score of 7.22 and average postcavus foot orthosis pain score of 2.41 (P < 0.0005). Among patients reporting ankle instability, 92% experienced a decrease in the frequency of instability events postcavus foot orthosis. Level of evidence: IV.

13. Arazpour M, Hutchins SW, Ghomshe FT, Shaky F, Karami MV, Aksenov AY: Effects of the heel-to-toe rocker sole on walking in able-bodied persons. *Prosthet Orthot Int* 2013;37(6):429-435.

   Gait analysis was performed under two conditions: walking with either a baseline shoe with a flat sole or a modified shoe adapted with a heel-to-toe rocker sole. Substantial differences were observed between rocker sole conditions during initial double-limb support and second double-limb support in the stance phase. In frontal plane movement, substantial differences were observed between the rocker sole conditions, but only during the second double-limb support phase. The heel-to-toe rocker sole may be useful for conditions including ankle arthrodesis and for use with solid ankle-foot orthoses but may not be suitable for patients with reduced balance or unstable posture.

14. Lin SC, Chen CP, Tang SF, Wong AM, Hsieh JH, Chen WP: Changes in windlass effect in response to different shoe and insole designs during walking. *Gait Posture* 2013;37(2):235-241.

   The authors performed a biomechanical study of 10 healthy volunteers evaluating shoe and insole combinations. Rocker-sole shoes are effective in reducing the windlass effect regardless of the type of insole inserted.

15. Kulig K, Reischl SF, Pomrantz AB, et al: Nonsurgical management of posterior tibial tendon dysfunction with orthoses and resistive exercise: A randomized controlled trial. *Phys Ther* 2009;89(1):26-37.

   Participants were randomly assigned to one of three groups to complete a 12-week program of orthotic wear and stretching (the O group); orthotic wear, stretching, and concentric progressive resistive exercise; or orthotic wear, stretching, and eccentric progressive resistive exercise (the OE group). Foot Functional Index scores (total, pain, and disability) decreased in all groups after the intervention. The OE group demonstrated the most improvement in each subcategory, and the O group demonstrated the least improvement. Pain immediately after the 5-minute walk test was substantially reduced across all groups after the intervention. Level of evidence: II.

16. Hawke F, Burns J, Radford JA, du Toit V: Custom-made foot orthoses for the treatment of foot pain. *Cochrane Database Syst Rev* 2008;3:CD006801.

   Eleven trials involving 1,332 participants were included in this review: five trials evaluated custom-made foot orthoses for plantar fasciitis; three trials evaluated foot pain in rheumatoid arthritis; and one trial each was conducted for foot pain in pes cavus, hallux valgus, and JIA. Comparisons to custom-made foot orthoses involved sham orthoses; no intervention; standardized interventions given to all participants; noncustom (prefabricated) foot orthoses; combined manipulation, mobilization or stretching; night splints; and surgery. Follow-up durations ranged between 1 week and 3 years. Custom-made foot orthoses were effective for painful pes cavus, rearfoot pain in rheumatoid arthritis, foot pain in JIA, and painful hallux valgus. However, surgery was even more effective for hallux valgus and noncustom foot orthoses appeared as effective as custom for JIA. Level of evidence: I.

17. Hawke F, Burns J: Brief report: Custom foot orthoses for foot pain: What does the evidence say? *Foot Ankle Int* 2012;33(12):1161-1163.

   The evidence base for prescription custom foot orthoses is limited, with many types of foot pain yet to be tested in randomized controlled trials.

18. Anderson J, Stanek J: Effect of foot orthoses as treatment for plantar fasciitis or heel pain. *J Sport Rehabil* 2013;22(2):130-136.

   This meta-analysis reviewed four studies on the effectiveness of a foot orthosis to treat plantar fasciitis: a randomized controlled trial, retrospective cohort study, prospective repeated measures study, and prospective cohort study are included in the analysis. Level of evidence: III.

19. Baldassin V, Gomes CR, Beraldo PS: Effectiveness of prefabricated and customized foot orthoses made from low-cost foam for noncomplicated plantar fasciitis: A randomized controlled trial. *Arch Phys Med Rehabil* 2009;90(4):701-706.

When participants returned to at least one follow-up evaluation, there was a significant improvement in both study groups (*P* < 0.05) but no difference in modified Foot Function Index pain at 4 and 8 weeks. Level of evidence: II.

20. Fong DT, Pang KY, Chung MM, Hung AS, Chan KM: Evaluation of combined prescription of rocker sole shoes and custom-made foot orthoses for the treatment of plantar fasciitis. *Clin Biomech (Bristol, Avon)* 2012;27(10):1072-1077.

Subjects performed walking trials that consisted of one unshod condition and four shod conditions while wearing baseline shoes, rocker-sole shoes, baseline shoes with foot orthotics, and rocker-sole shoes with foot orthotics. A combination of rocker-sole shoes and foot orthoses produced a substantially lower visual analog scale pain score than rocker-sole shoes (30.9 mm) and foot orthoses. With regard to baseline shoes, this combination also substantially reduced the most medial heel peak pressure (–34%) without overloading other plantar regions when compared to rocker-sole shoes (–8%) and foot orthoses (–29%). The findings suggest that a combined prescription of a rocker-sole shoe and a custom-made foot orthoses had more immediate therapeutic effects compared to when each treatment was individually prescribed.

21. Attard J, Singh D: A comparison of two night ankle-foot orthoses used in the treatment of inferior heel pain: A preliminary investigation. *Foot Ankle Surg* 2012;18(2):108-110.

Each participant was given a questionnaire with which to evaluate their satisfaction with their orthosis regarding comfort, ease of use, and appearance and describe if their foot pain was reduced and at what stage the pain had decreased. Two-thirds of all participants confirmed that morning pain and stiffness was less severe after wearing an AFO; both orthosis types were relatively easy to don and doff, but the posterior orthosis was more uncomfortable and disrupted sleep. On average, the anterior AFO reduced heel pain more substantially than the posterior orthosis. Level of evidence: V.

22. Richie DH Jr: Effects of foot orthoses on patients with chronic ankle instability. *J Am Podiatr Med Assoc* 2007;97(1):19-30.

23. Reina M, Lafuente G, Munuera PV: Effect of custom-made foot orthoses in female hallux valgus after one-year follow-up. *Prosthet Orthot Int* 2013;37(2):113-119.

Women with mild to moderate hallux valgus were divided into two groups: the experimental group used custom-made foot orthoses and the control group had no treatment. First intermetatarsal and hallux abductus angles were measured at the beginning of the study and after 12 months of follow-up. There were no significant intra-group differences in the initial and follow-up angles. Level of evidence: III.

24. Whitford D, Esterman A: A randomized controlled trial of two types of in-shoe orthoses in children with flexible excess pronation of the feet. *Foot Ankle Int* 2007;28(6):715-723.

25. Collins N, Bisset L, McPoil T, Vicenzino B: Foot orthoses in lower limb overuse conditions: A systematic review and meta-analysis. *Foot Ankle Int* 2007;28(3):396-412.

26. Verity S, Sochocki M, Embil JM, Trepman E: Treatment of Charcot foot and ankle with a prefabricated removable walker brace and custom insole. *Foot Ankle Surg* 2008;14(1):26-31.

Twenty-five ankles with Charcot arthropathy were treated with a prefabricated pneumatic removable walker brace fitted with a custom orthotic insole. Follow-up data were collected from patient interview, examination, and radiography. At follow-up, 17 (68%) feet and ankles had consolidation (Stage III) of Charcot arthropathy (average duration of brace use was 29 weeks) and patients were subsequently treated with rocker-sole shoes, insoles, and ankle-foot orthoses; 8 (32%) feet and ankles received ongoing brace treatment. Three feet developed a new deformity during brace treatment, but average radiographic parameters of hindfoot to forefoot alignment had minimal change between initial and final radiographs an average of 36 weeks after initial radiographic evaluation. Level of evidence: IV.

27. Krause F, Bosshard A, Lehmann O, Weber M: Shell brace for stage II posterior tibial tendon insufficiency. *Foot Ankle Int* 2008;29(11):1095-1100.

This is a prospective case series of 18 patients with flexible Stage II tibialis posterior tendon dysfunction who were fitted with a new custom-molded foot orthosis. At a mean follow-up of 61.4 months, functional results were assessed with the American Orthopaedic Foot and Ankle Society ankle hindfoot score and clinical or radiographic progression. Scores improved substantially from a mean of 56 points to a mean of 82 points. Three patients (16%) had clinical progression to a fixed deformity (Stage III) and a radiographic increase of their deformity. All the other patients were satisfied with the brace's comfort and noted improvement in their mobility. Level of evidence: IV.

28. Patzkowski JC, Blanck RV, Owens JG, Wilken JM, Blair JA, Hsu JR: Can an ankle-foot orthosis change hearts and minds? *J Surg Orthop Adv* 2011;20(1):8-18.

The Intrepid Dynamic Exoskeletal Orthosis device has substantially improved the functional capabilities of the limb-salvage wounded warrior population when combined with a high-intensity rehabilitation program. Clinical and biomechanical research is currently underway to fully identify potential benefits all of the devices.

29. Hsu JR, Bosse MJ: Challenges in severe lower limb injury rehabilitation. *J Am Acad Orthop Surg* 2012;20(suppl 1):S39-S41.

The Return to Run clinical pathway, an integrated orthotic and rehabilitation initiative, is an example of goal-oriented rehabilitation with periodic assessment to restore wounded warriors to high-level performance following severe lower extremity trauma. Level of evidence: V.

30. Patzkowski JC, Blanck RV, Owens JG, et al; Skeletal Trauma Research Consortium: Comparative effect of orthosis design on functional performance. *J Bone Joint Surg Am* 2012;94(6):507-515.

Eighteen subjects with unilateral dorsiflexion and/or plantar flexion weakness were evaluated with six functional tests while they were wearing the IDEO, rocker brace, posterior leaf spring, or no brace. Tests included a four-square step test, a sit-to-stand five times test, tests of self-selected walking velocity over level and rocky terrain, and a timed stair ascent. Subjects also completed one trial of a 40-yard (37-meter) dash, completed a satisfaction questionnaire, and indicated whether they had ever considered amputation (and, if so, if they still intended to proceed with it). Level of evidence: IV.

31. Guillebastre B, Calmels P, Rougier P: Effects of rigid and dynamic ankle-foot orthoses on normal gait. *Foot Ankle Int* 2009;30(1):51-56.

Two AFO models with different mechanical concepts (a rigid-AFO [R-AFO] and dynamic-AFO [D-AFO]) were worn by subjects. Velocity, step time, and step length were assessed for each of the five conditions during which subjects walked barefoot and wore an R-AFO or a D-AFO.

1: General Foot and Ankle Topics

Chapter 3

Imaging Studies of the Foot and Ankle

Steven M. Raikin, MD   Brian S. Winters, MD

Introduction

Imaging studies are a component of the clinical evaluation of a patient with a condition affecting the foot or ankle. After completion of a careful history and physical examination, imaging studies usually are obtained as the next step in determining a diagnosis and treatment plan. Each of the available imaging modalities has appropriate indications and applications.

Plain Radiography

Plain radiography is the foundation of most diagnostic foot and ankle imaging. Bone anatomy, integrity, and alignment as well as joint congruency can be assessed through a routine set of radiographs, which usually can be obtained during the patient's initial office visit. Weight-bearing radiographs must be obtained whenever possible. Although a patient with an acute traumatic injury may only tolerate non–weight-bearing radiography to assess structural anatomy and rule out the presence of fracture, these radiographs do not show the foot or ankle in a physiologic position and therefore may not facilitate detection of malalignment or some pathologic conditions.

The popularity of digital radiology has eclipsed that of printed radiographic studies during the past few years. Radiographs are captured digitally in two ways.[1] Computed radiography is affordable, offers excellent image quality, and uses existing radiography systems.

This chapter is adapted from Raikin SM: Imaging, in Pinzur MS, ed: Orthopaedic Knowledge Update Foot and Ankle, ed 4. Rosemont, IL, American Academy of Orthopaedic Surgeons, 2008, pp 25–36. Dr. Raikin or an immediate family member serves as a paid consultant to Biomet, and has received research or institutional support from Biomimetic. Neither Dr. Winters nor any immediate family member has received anything of value from or has stock or stock options held in a commercial company or institution related directly or indirectly to the subject of this chapter.

True digital radiography requires more expensive technology than traditional radiography or computerized modification, but offers greater efficiency and the capacity for higher image quality and a lower radiation dosage. Images are stored in a picture archiving and communication system rather than on hard-copy film. The most commonly used format for medical images is Digital Imaging and Communication in Medicine (DICOM), which allows safe, high-quality off-site viewing and analysis of radiographs. Digital radiography also allows computer-assisted measurements of distances or angles to be generated for use in diagnosing pathologic foot and ankle conditions.

The Foot

Routine radiography of the foot includes the AP, lateral, and oblique views. The internal (medial) oblique view usually is part of the routine three-view set and is useful for showing the lateral tarsometatarsal joints and detecting a possible calcaneonavicular coalition. The external (lateral) oblique view should be ordered to more clearly show perinavicular joints or identify an accessory navicular bone.

In specific circumstances, other views can be used to obtain additional information about the bony anatomy. The sesamoid axial projection can reveal sesamoid-metatarsal arthritis, fracture or osteonecrosis of the hallux sesamoids, or sesamoid alignment relative to the crista on the plantar aspect of the metatarsal head. The calcaneal axial (Harris-Beath) view is obtained at a 45° angle from posterior to proximal. This view allows analysis of the posterior and middle facet of the subtalar joint to detect arthritis or a tarsal coalition. The Broden views are a sequence of angled radiographs centered over the sinus tarsi and taken at a 10° to 40° cephalic tilt. These views reliably show the posterior facet of the subtalar joint in calcaneal fracture management or subtalar fusion. The talar neck view provides a true AP view and is useful in assessing talar neck fractures. This view is obtained with the foot internally rotated 15° and the beam angled 15° cephalad while centered over the talar neck.

The Ankle

A three-view weight-bearing set of radiographs is routinely recommended for analysis of the ankle, including the AP, lateral, and mortise views. For the AP view, the ankle, mortise is aligned in approximately 20° of external rotation relative to the sagittal plane. A true mortise view, in which the x-ray beam is oriented perpendicular to the intermalleolar axis, is therefore obtained with the leg internally rotated. This view allows the best assessment of mortise congruity and the talar dome.

Several ankle-specific views also are used to evaluate the ankle joint. The 50° external rotation view is optimal for the detection of posterior malleolar fracture fragments. The hindfoot alignment view is obtained with the patient standing on a raised platform and the x-ray beam directed from behind and angled 20° caudally, with the cassette placed perpendicular to the beam.

Stress views are used to assess ankle instability. While a lateral radiograph is being obtained, an anterior drawer test is performed (the evaluator's hands are protected by lead gloves, or a mechanical jig is used). Anterior displacement of the talus of more than 10 mm (or more than 5 mm than that of the stressed uninvolved ankle) is consistent with lateral ankle ligament dysfunction. Similarly, varus or valgus stress radiographs are used to assess the integrity of the lateral ligament complex or deltoid ligament, respectively. A 10° difference in the talar tilt of the injured and normal extremities is considered pathologic. However, the reliability and reproducibility of stress testing is questionable because of the wide variation in test findings in normal ankles and healthy patients, tester-dependent variation in forces applied against the ankle, and variation in patients' resistance to the force. Therefore, the results of stress testing alone should not determine the treatment of ankle instability.

Fluoroscopy has become a vital tool for assessing joint or bone alignment and positioning internal hardware during surgery. Technical advances have resulted in great improvement in fluoroscopic image quality as well as the size and ease of handling of the machine. The small C-arm units used by many foot and ankle surgeons expose the surgical team and patient to minimal radiation (outside of the direct path of the beam).[2]

Radiographic Measurements

Many radiographic measurements have been described for evaluating the alignment of the foot and ankle, several of which are particularly important. Computer-assisted measurement of digital radiographs has resulted in improved accuracy. A smartphone goniometer application is extremely accurate for measuring certain angles.[3] All measurements are most accurate if based on weight-bearing radiographs.

The hallux valgus angle and the first-second intermetatarsal angle are the mainstay measurements for assessing the severity of hallux valgus deformity. These measurements have good intraobserver and interobserver reliability when standard methods are used. The first and second metatarsal axes are each drawn by connecting the midpoint of the shaft of the metatarsal 2 cm from the proximal and distal articular surfaces. The axis of the phalanx is drawn through the shaft midpoints 0.5 cm from each of its articulations. The hallux valgus interphalangeal angle is drawn between the phalangeal axis of the proximal and distal phalanges of the hallux. The distal metatarsal articular angle is the angle subtended by a line drawn perpendicular to the long axis of the first metatarsal and a line corresponding to the distal articular surface of the first metatarsal. Compared with the hallus valgus and first-second intermetatarsal angle, the distal metatarsal articular angle is less reliable and reproducible for determining joint congruency.[4] These measurements can be computer enhanced, but this step usually is not necessary.

The talus–first metatarsal angle, also called the Meary angle, is drawn through the long axes of the talus and the first metatarsal on the lateral radiograph. This angle is useful for assessing arch height and recently was found to be reliable for measuring adult flatfoot deformity.[5] The talonavicular coverage angle measures the lateral subluxation of the navicular at the talar head or the extent to which the talar head is uncovered, and it is useful for evaluating forefoot abduction in pes planovalgus deformities. On a weight-bearing AP radiograph of the foot, a line is created joining the two ends of the articular surface of the talar head, and another line joins the matching two ends of the joint surface of the navicular. The angle created by perpendicular lines drawn from the midpoints of each of these two lines is the talonavicular coverage angle; a normal value is less than 7°.

Tenography

Plain radiographs can be used to observe secondary changes caused by tendon dysfunction but cannot be used to evaluate the tendons themselves. Tenography involves the injection of contrast material into the tendon sheath under fluoroscopy, often followed by a steroid injection. Tenosynovitis, stenosing tenosynovitis, and a tendon tear or rupture can be seen. Tenography can be particularly useful in a posttraumatic setting in which the value of other diagnostic modalities is limited by the presence of anatomic deformity or associated hardware (for example, in peroneal impingement after calcaneal fracture).[6] In the absence of a tendon tear, intrasheath steroid injection with tenography relieves symptoms in some patients with tenosynovitis around the foot and ankle.[7] This cost-effective but invasive technique is associated with a small risk of tendon rupture. Tenography has been less frequently used for diagnostic purposes since the widespread adoption of MRI.

Ultrasonography

Ultrasonographic evaluation of tendons around the foot and ankle offers several advantages over other modalities. Ultrasonography is cost-effective, safe, noninvasive, and not based on radiation. Structures are evaluated in real time. Dynamic evaluation of tendon function allows conditions such as peroneal subluxation or dislocation to be directly visualized. The transducer can be manipulated to avoid interference from any metallic implant in the ankle. This ability is useful in evaluating tendon injury after hardware placement in the foot or ankle, which would create interference during MRI. Ultrasonography also avoids the possibility of the so-called magic angle phenomenon on MRI (artifact seen in tendons oriented 54.7° to the magnetic field), which can inaccurately suggest the presence of intratendinous pathology. Ultrasonography is slightly less sensitive than MRI for use in diagnosing tibialis posterior tendon pathology, but a recent study found that discrepancies did not result in altered clinical management.[8] Ultrasonography has high sensitivity and specificity for detecting peroneal tendon tears and 100% positive predictive value for detecting peroneal subluxation, as correlated with intraoperative findings.[9]

For evaluating tears in the lateral ankle ligament, ultrasonography has sensitivity and specificity comparable to that of MRI. Morton neuroma, recurrent interdigital neuroma, and other soft-tissue masses or cysts can be detected on ultrasonography after an equivocal clinical evaluation.

Most modern ultrasound machines are able to evaluate regional blood flow. The movement of blood cells within the vessels causes a change in the pitch of reflected sound waves called the Doppler effect. A computer converts the Doppler sounds into colors that are overlaid on the musculoskeletal ultrasonographic image. The presence of local hyperemia secondary to inflammation can confirm that the ultrasonographic findings are consistent with the pathology or symptoms.

The primary disadvantage of ultrasonography is that it is a technician-dependent modality. Many medical centers lack a radiologist trained and experienced in interpreting the results of musculoskeletal ultrasonographic studies. Ultrasonography offers only poor visualization of bone. Because direct skin contact and the application of gel are required, ultrasonography cannot be used through a cast or splint.

Recent advances in technology have led to improvements in the quality, portability, and cost of ultrasound machines, and office-based ultrasonography is now feasible. To complement the clinical examination and standard radiographic evaluation, a diagnostic ultrasonographic examination can be done during the patient's initial visit to the foot and ankle surgeon. Ultrasonography can be particularly useful in making a subtle diagnosis and planning treatment; for example, a determination that the patient has a Morton neuroma in the second web space rather than early plantar plate dysfunction precludes the use of a cortisone injection, which can cause metatarsophalangeal instability.[10] In-office ultrasonography also can be used to identify tendinosis, a tendon injury around the foot and ankle, a mass or tumor, or a nonradiopaque foreign body such as a wood splinter. Ultrasonography can be used to improve the accuracy of diagnostic injections in the foot or ankle, guide injections for a condition such as Morton neuroma or plantar fasciitis, and guide the aspiration of cysts. The use of ultrasonography was found to improve the accuracy and outcome of therapeutic injections and thereby reduce the need for additional procedures.[11]

Computed Tomography

CT provides high-resolution thin-slice studies of the foot and ankle. The development and implementation of multidetector-row slip-ring technology has resulted in improved imaging of osseous structures. Source images acquired in the axial, coronal, or sagittal plane allow three-dimensional views of the bony anatomy for diagnosis and therapeutic planning. Relatively new computer software creates multiplane reconstructions without increasing the patient's exposure to ionizing radiation; for example, coronal images can be constructed from axial images, and three-dimensional reconstruction models can be created from the initial source images (**Figure 1**). Around the foot and ankle, studies with 3-mm or thinner slices are routinely recommended. The foot position in the scanner is important because the source image planes are obtained parallel to the osseous structures of the foot in each plane using a tomographic scout localizer image. The presence of cast or splinting material around the region does not interfere with CT but may create difficulty in positioning the foot. The advent of multidetector-row systems has permitted rapid image acquisition and high-quality three-dimensional reconstruction to be achieved with decreased radiation dosages.

In the foot and ankle, CT is most commonly used to assess bony abnormalities and is particularly useful in providing fine osseous detail not obtainable with plain radiography. Fracture, infection, osteochondral injury

1: General Foot and Ankle Topics

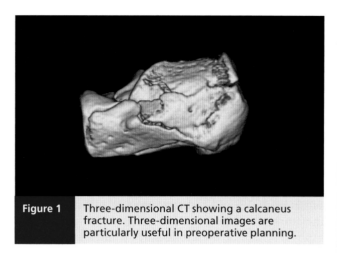

Figure 1 Three-dimensional CT showing a calcaneus fracture. Three-dimensional images are particularly useful in preoperative planning.

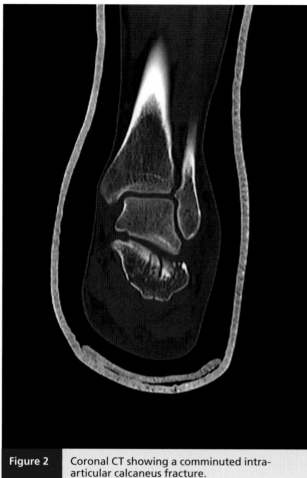

Figure 2 Coronal CT showing a comminuted intra-articular calcaneus fracture.

(requiring accurate assessment of the bony anatomy and lesion size), arthritis, osteonecrosis, and osseous tumor or congenital abnormality can be diagnosed using CT. This is particularly useful in suspected subtle fracture, joint diastasis, or articular incongruity not detectable on plain radiography, as in suspected Lisfranc injuries, syndesmotic injuries, and tibial plafond fractures. In addition, CT can be used to assess the extent of joint comminution in calcaneal or plafond fractures and to assist in preoperative planning (**Figure 2**).

CT has high accuracy and sensitivity for the detection of fracture nonunion and is more reliable than serial radiographic studies for assessing the extent of union after surgical arthrodesis[12] (**Figure 3**). The use of micro-CT and nano-CT technology is likely to further enhance the accuracy of this modality. The interpretation of postoperative CT can be negatively influenced by metallic artifact or scatter from internal hardware. Relatively new software uses metal deletion techniques to limit this effect and improve the accuracy of study interpretation.

Current CT scanners use multidetector configurations in which a narrow, fan-shaped x-ray beam and detector rotates around the patient to quickly acquire multiple image sections. This technology cannot be used with the patient in a weight-bearing stance, as is needed to evaluate extremity alignment and deformity during physiologic loading. Axial loads can be applied to joints to simulate weight bearing when the patient is supine, but the resulting studies have questionable accuracy. The recently developed cone-beam CT technology uses a pyramid-shaped x-ray beam and a large-area detector to obtain volumetric data from multiple projections through a single rotation around the patient, who is in a standing, weight-bearing position.[13] The technique for image reconstruction is similar to that used for multidetector CT. The three-dimensional data obtained from cone-beam CT allows a much-improved quantitative analysis

of many pathologies. Other advantages of cone-beam CT over multidetector CT include more rapid acquisition of images, superior image quality, and lower radiation dosages (approximately 9 mGy compared with 27 to 40 mGy). The compact, portable design of the cone-beam CT machine has positive implications for workflow and storage. Cone-beam CT technology has the potential to be extremely valuable in musculoskeletal extremity imaging from both clinical and economic viewpoints.

Nuclear Medicine

Nuclear medicine studies involve the intravenous administration of a radioactive tracer and subsequent scanning with a gamma camera that detects a concentration of the tracer in the anatomic area of study. Conventional nuclear medicine studies of the musculoskeletal system (bone scans) involve the administration of technetium Tc-99m methylene diphosphonate, which binds to hydroxyapatite crystals during bone formation. Bone turnover caused by occult fracture, stress fracture, tumor, infection, or a metabolic disorder can be detected. Scanning is done

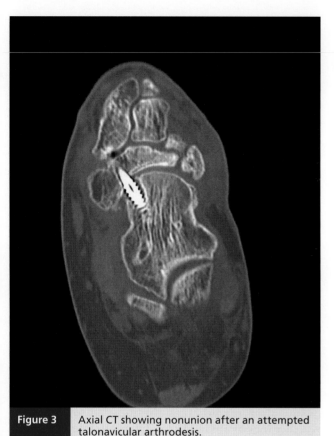

Figure 3 Axial CT showing nonunion after an attempted talonavicular arthrodesis.

or technetium Tc-99m exametazine include a smaller radiation dosage and a shorter interval before scanning than required using Indium[111] (4 hours compared with 24 hours). Delayed scanning identifies areas of increased leukocyte uptake, which signify inflammation or infection. Synchronous uptake in the same area on both a leukocyte-labeled and a standard three-phase bone scan specifically indicates bone activity caused by infection. To identify bone marrow infection, technetium Tc-99m sulfur colloid scanning is used. The addition of a leukocyte-labeled study increases the specificity of the study.

Positron emission tomography (PET) is a relatively new technique that usually involves intravenous injection of [18]fluorodeoxyglucose (FDG) followed by a scan for positron emission decay 1 hour later. In a study of patients with Charcot foot, FDG PET was found to exclude bone or soft-tissue infection in the presence of a foot ulcer with overall sensitivity of 100% and accuracy of 93.8%.[15] FDG PET also was found to be more accurate for diagnosing active chronic osteomyelitis than indium-111–labeled scanning.

Nuclear medicine imaging allows arterial limb perfusion to be assessed, particularly in the presence of calcified vessels that may have a spuriously elevated ankle brachial index. Thallium-210 scanning detects deficiencies in muscle perfusion reserves and perfusion abnormalities in patients with asymptomatic diabetes who have clinically normal perfusion.[16] FDG PET accurately assesses the extent of atherosclerosis in the extremities of patients with diabetes.[17]

The combination of single photon-emission CT and CT (SPECT-CT) is a relatively new imaging modality in which highly detailed CT is analyzed with the functional information from a triple-phase radionuclide bone scan using a gamma camera.[18] SPECT-CT is not yet widely used but can enable detection of arthritis around the foot and particularly the differentiation of involved joints around the midfoot. In addition, SPECT-CT has potential in diagnosing clinically indeterminable soft-tissue impingement syndromes, excluding nonunion or arthritis seen on other radiographic modalities, and locating clinically relevant pathology in multifocal disease. Although some studies have supported the widespread use of SPECT-CT, most data do not justify its routine use.[18-20]

Magnetic Resonance Imaging

Other than conventional radiography, MRI is the most frequently used modality for imaging the foot and ankle. MRI has the ability to evaluate bone, ligament, tendon, and muscle injuries about the foot and ankle, using a standard noncontrast protocol. Injury can be characterized based on known patterns of abnormal signal that indicate

in three phases. The first scan, the blood flow phase, is done within 1 minute of tracer administration to identify increased blood flow caused by inflammation. The second phase is obtained 5 minutes after tracer administration and detects blood pooling. The third, delayed phase is obtained 4 hours after injection of the tracer and detects bone turnover. The entire body can be scanned, or the scan can be restricted to pinhole views of the area of interest. Bone scans are highly sensitive but have poor specificity because many conditions affect blood flow and bone turnover. In some conditions, such as sympathetically mediated complex regional pain syndrome, increased tracer may appear in the affected area in all three phases of the study. It is important to note that bone scan results return to normal no earlier than 6 months after a fracture and that 10% of uncomplicated fractures still have increased local tracer uptake 2 years after the injury.[14]

Leukocyte labeling can be used to increase the specificity of bone scans for infection. Peripheral blood is aspirated from the patient, and the white blood cells are labeled with radioactive tracer several hours before scanning. The commonly used labels include technetium Tc-99m hexamethyl propylene amine oxide and indium-111 oxime. The advantages of labeling with technetium Tc-99m hexamethyl propylene amine oxide stress along a specific biomechanical axis. The advantages inherent to MRI in comparison with other imaging modalities include its multiplanar capabilities, sensitivity for both osseous and soft-tissue edema, and use of a magnetic field to generate images, without exposure of tissue to ionizing radiation. The disadvantages include its cost and the relatively long time period required for imaging. Some patients who have an implanted ferromagnetic device, such as a cardiac pacemaker, an automatic defibrillator, a biostimulator, an implanted infusion device, cerebral aneurysm clips, internal hearing aids, or metallic foreign bodies about the orbits, are not candidates for MRI. Many types of recently implanted medical devices and fixation hardware are nonferromagnetic, however, and thus are MRI compatible. Although the use of MRI in the foot and ankle has increased dramatically over the past decade, it is still not typically used as a first-line diagnostic modality. Most commonly, MRI of the foot and ankle is indicated if radiographic or CT findings are inconclusive or inconsistent with clinical symptoms, a primary soft-tissue process such as tendon or ligament dysfunction is suspected, or pain atypically persists during a treatment course.

MRI of the foot or ankle should include both fluid-sensitive (T2-weighted) and anatomy-specific (T1-weighted) sequences. Optimally, MRI of the foot or ankle should include at least two fat-suppressed sequences to maximize fluid sensitivity. MRI studies dedicated to the ankle should be distinct from those dedicated to the foot. Ankle MRI studies should begin proximal to the tibiotalar joint and proceed to the midfoot level, including the tibialis posterior and peroneus brevis insertions. In contrast, a foot MRI should begin at the talar head and proceed through the toes. All MRI protocols for imaging the ankle or foot should include three anatomic planes. At the ankle, the recommended protocols use two sagittal sequences, including one fluid-sensitive fat suppression sequence and one anatomy-specific sequence (T1-weighted spin-echo), as well as two axial sequences with similar parameters. A coronal fluid-sensitive sequence should be tailored to evaluate for potential osteochondral lesions at the tibiotalar joint. Acquisition of these five sequences can be accomplished on most systems in approximately 20 minutes. For MRI dedicated to the foot, optimal plane selection can be difficult because of varying definitions of terms such as coronal and axial; for this reason, descriptive terms are recommended for plane selection, including short axis, long axis, and sagittal. Both fluid-sensitive and anatomy-specific short axis sequences (so-called bread slice sequences) should be acquired for showing metatarsal and intermetatarsal pathology. Inversion recovery sequences often provide the most homogeneous fat suppression in the sagittal plane, and a long axis

fluid-sensitive sequence should be acquired along the metatarsals to simulate an AP radiographic view.

Intravenous gadolinium contrast occasionally is indicated in foot and ankle MRI. Precontrast and postcontrast imaging sequences are used in evaluating for a soft-tissue mass or osteomyelitis. Other relative indications for the use of intravenous contrast in foot or ankle MRI include inflammatory arthropathy, stenosing tenosynovitis, postoperative scarring, and intermetatarsal neuroma. Severe renal insufficiency is a relative contraindication for the use of a gadolinium-based contrast agent because of a suspected association with development of nephrogenic systemic fibrosis. An intra-articular contrast injection may prove useful as part of a dedicated arthrographic MRI protocol for a specific purpose, such as assessing the integrity of the lateral ankle ligaments or the stability of an osteochondral lesion.[21] The use of a circumferential receiver coil design, such as a head or an extremity coil, can be effective for generating adequate signal throughout the ankle or foot.

The use of one protocol with acquisition of images in a large field of view for both the foot and ankle is discouraged except for specific indications including reflex sympathetic dystrophy. The patient history and clinical examination should allow the clinician to determine whether foot or ankle MRI is indicated. If injury affecting both the ankle and the forefoot is suspected, the use of two separate MRI protocols is recommended.

Numerous MRI system designs and field strengths are available, but some have limitations arising from patient characteristics such as claustrophobia and large body habitus. These factors usually do not need to be considered in imaging the foot or ankle. MRI should be acquired at standard- or high-field strength (1.5 or higher) to obtain adequate resolution of ligaments, tendons, and articular surfaces in the distal lower extremity. For the rare patient who cannot tolerate a standard closed 1.5-Tesla MRI unit, a high-field strength dedicated extremity system should be used in preference to a low-field strength (0.2- or 0.3-Tesla) open system.

The development of ultra–high-field MRI has resulted in continuing improvement in diagnostic accuracy; both 3-Tesla units and high-field strength, extremity-specific coils produce superior image quality.[22] Musculoskeletal structures exhibit a low signal-to-noise ratio at 1.5 Tesla, but the ratio is almost doubled at 3 Tesla. The application of relatively new techniques such as parallel acquisition improves both resolution and acquisition time; the decrease in imaging time is almost fourfold. Three-dimensional sequences obtained using a low-field scanner are characterized by a suboptimal signal-to-noise ratio and poor-contrast images that frequently are further degraded by artifacts. In comparison with 1.5-Tesla imaging, 3-Tesla imaging produces higher spatial resolution, smaller cut (almost halved) image thickness, and an increased contrast-to-noise ratio, which further improve the anatomic detail of the image.

Higher Tesla MRI has the disadvantage of greater energy deposition, which can result in substantial artifacts, the most problematic of which are chemical shift and metal artifacts. Chemical shift artifact is noticeable at fat-water interfaces and particularly at bone-cartilage interfaces, where it may appear to represent abnormal cartilage thickness. Metal artifact is much more evident at 3 Tesla than at 1. 5 Tesla, and it markedly degrades the image quality. Although techniques such as shortened echo time, parallel imaging with transmit-receive joint-specific multichannel coils, and widening of the receiver bandwidth can counteract the artifact effect, patients with implanted hardware in the field of view should undergo MRI with a 1.5-Tesla magnet.

Some centers now offer 7-Tesla MRI, which has been shown to further increase the signal-to-noise and contrast-to-noise ratios and thereby increase the accuracy of an ankle MRI evaluation.[23] These units are not yet widely available for clinical use, however. It is important to remember that regardless of field strength, MRI is limited by the quality and efficiency of the receiver coil. The use of a dedicated extremity coil or ankle coil is preferable for adequate MRI of the foot and ankle.

Osseous Injury

Displaced fractures most commonly are diagnosed using plain radiography or CT. In contrast, nondisplaced fractures and contusions about the foot and ankle can best be identified on MRI. Both types of fracture appear on fluid-sensitive, fat-suppressed MRI sequences as T2 hyperintense signal. The T2 hyperintense signal should be more focal and more intense in a fracture than in an osseous contusion, and it may have a linear morphology. Abnormal signal on T1-weighted sequences is characteristic of fractures and helps distinguish a fracture from a contusion. In a patient with known trauma, linear hypointense T1-weighted signal in the location of T2 hyperintensity can be interpreted as fracture with some certainty. Osteochondral impaction injury is characterized by abnormal T2 hyperintense and T1 hypointense signal extending in a sunburst pattern from an articular surface. The term osteochondral impaction injury is relatively nonspecific because in acute trauma a discrete osteochondral lesion can be difficult to distinguish from an osteochondral contusion.

MRI routinely is used for the diagnosis of osteochondral lesions or defects. Typical signal characteristics include a subchondral osseous T1 hypointense crescent (or a T2 hyperintense signal), which indicates fluid

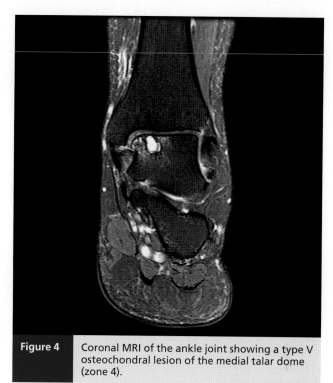

Figure 4 Coronal MRI of the ankle joint showing a type V osteochondral lesion of the medial talar dome (zone 4).

undercutting the bone fragment and implies instability (**Figure 4**). Osteochondral lesions on the talar dome are almost twice as likely to be medial (at the anterior-to-posterior equator) than lateral.[24] Medial talar dome lesions involve a larger surface area and tend to have deeper craniocaudal dimensions than their lateral counterparts. Less commonly, osteochondral lesions about the foot and ankle are located in the talar head, the tibial plafond, the calcaneocuboid joint, or the metatarsal heads. These lesions also can be effectively diagnosed with MRI.

Specific mechanisms of traumatic ankle and foot injuries often have a characteristic pattern of bony contusion on MRI. Analysis can result in a better understanding of the injury mechanism and diagnosis of associated soft-tissue injury. In an inversion ankle injury, the common locations of T2 hyperintense osseous contusions are the tip of the fibula, the entire medial malleolus, the anterior process and anterolateral body of the calcaneus, the talar neck or anteromedial talus extending to the middle subtalar joint, and the proximal cuboid at the calcaneocuboid articulation. An eversion injury causes bony contusion of the proximal aspect of the cuboid at the calcaneocuboid joint as well the malleoli. Bone marrow edema in the distal fibula tends to be diffuse and ill-defined, and bone marrow edema in the medial malleolus tends to be isolated to its tip, suggesting an avulsion injury.

MRI of the foot also is useful in assessing subtle bone injuries that can be difficult to detect with plain radiography alone. Bone contusion and osteochondral injury involving the distal articular surfaces of the cuneiforms and proximal articular surfaces of the metatarsals should increase suspicion for Lisfranc ligament injury. MRI is extremely sensitive for acute nondisplaced or stress fractures of the metatarsals, which are easily identified on short axis sequences through the forefoot, where they appear as diffuse abnormal medullary T2 hyperintensity. Plantar plate injury can be diagnosed on MRI by identifying T2 hyperintensity within the metatarsal head and a breach in the soft-tissue structures intimately plantar to the plantar aspect of each metatarsal head. Osseous injury of the first metatarsophalangeal sesamoids can be identified on MRI and characterized as fracture, contusion, or osteonecrosis.

Ligamentous Injury

Normal ligaments should appear hypointense or dark on all MRI sequences. In an acute sprain, ligaments have poor definition as well as periligamentous fluid signal. Diffuse enlargement, attenuation, or complete disruption can indicate a subacute or chronic high-grade injury. It is difficult to establish the clinical competence of a sprained ligament solely on the basis of MRI.

Acute injury of the distal tibiofibular syndesmosis generally appears as focal enlargement and edema of ligamentous structures on axial MRI sequences. Although the anteroinferior tibiofibular ligament often is disrupted, the posterior syndesmosis rarely is abnormal on nonweight-bearing images. After injury, syndesmotic structures ossify over time and appear diffusely dark, thickened, and heterogenous on axial MRI.

MRI can help diagnose injuries of the lateral ligaments of the ankle. Because inversion injury and subsequent trauma are common, the anterior talofibular ligament rarely appears normal on MRI. Establishing a diagnosis of acute or subacute sprain of this ligament requires the ill-defined or enlarged ligament to be accompanied by bone contusions or edema within the lateral soft tissues. Chronic anterior talofibular ligament injury appears as diffuse ligament hypertrophy with scar tissue, as in anterolateral impingement, or as complete absence of the ligament, which suggests lateral instability. The calcaneofibular ligament is less frequently abnormal on MRI than the anterior talofibular ligament. The calcaneofibular ligament should appear as a thin, hypointense, linear structure that runs deep to the peroneal tendons in the subfibular region. This ligament is best assessed on sequential coronal sequences, and a normal insertion on the lateral calcaneus should be documented on every ankle MRI. Acute injury often appears as disruption of the ligament from the calcaneal periosteum with surrounding soft-tissue edema; chronic injury can appear as diffuse

ligamentous enlargement. Although MRI has suboptimal sensitivity for diagnosing medial deltoid ligament injury, an osseous contusion pattern indicating eversion injury may be correlated with a sprain of the deltoid ligament. With a high-grade deltoid injury, the ligament can be seen on coronal MRI as entirely disrupted from its medial malleolus origin.

MRI is useful for diagnosing a ligament sprain in the foot, particularly a subtle or clinically confusing sprain. If a Lisfranc ligament injury is suspected, long axis sequences should be acquired in the plane of the Lisfranc (medial cuneiform–second and third metatarsal [C1-M2M3]) ligament to allow assessment of the morphology and signal pattern.[25] The Lisfranc ligament can be assessed from these sequences by directly identifying intraligamentous edema, partial tearing, or complete disruption. MRI detection of disruption of the plantar C1-M2M3 ligament portion of the Lisfranc ligamentous complex was found to be highly correlated with Lisfranc instability, as confirmed by gold-standard stress radiographs obtained under anesthesia.[26] In the forefoot, a sprain or tear of the plantar plate of the first metatarsophalangeal joint (turf toe) is recognizable on T2-weighted MRI sequences. MRI can differentiate ligamentous from osseous injury or complete tears from partial sprains.

Tendinous Injury

MRI is ideal for assessing the tendons of the foot and ankle. Structures are shown in the cross-sectional axial or sagittal plane, and normal tendons should appear hypointense with homogenous signal and smooth contours. Tenosynovitis appears as peritendinous high signal intensity consistent with fluid. An abnormal tendon appears heterogenous with intratendinous medium signal intensity as well as abnormal morphology such as hypertrophy, thickening, marked attenuation, or complete absence in a rupture. MRI can confirm a clinical diagnosis of tendon pathology and quantify the severity of disease.

MRI examination of the ankle can be used in assessing a degenerative tibialis posterior tendon.[27] Conventional nonweight-bearing MRI may show abnormal valgus alignment of the hindfoot on coronal images at the level of the middle subtalar joint. Sagittal MRI sequences may show midfoot sag, which is the analogue of an abnormal Meary angle. Axial sequences may show uncovering of the talar head by the navicular. Tibialis posterior tendon dysfunction is confirmed by the presence of this triad of malalignments. MRI is less sensitive for tendon degeneration relatively early in the course of tibialis posterior tendinopathy. On axial MRI sequences, the normal appearance of the distal insertion is characterized as resembling an inverted Hershey's Kiss candy. The navicular insertion of the tibialis posterior tendon blends with the medial bundle of the spring ligament to create a broad footprint. More proximally, the spring ligament is directed medially. The tibialis posterior tendon tapers quickly on axial sequences to an ovoid configuration that appears slightly larger than the adjacent flexor hallucis longus tendon. The absence of this rapid tapering and a broader configuration proximal to the navicular (a so-called Tootsie Roll configuration) can be the earliest clues to insertional tibialis posterior tendinopathy. Tibialis posterior tendinopathy also can develop more proximally behind the medial malleolus. Enlargement and intratendinous heterogeneity as well as subcortical malleolar marrow edema are hallmarks of advanced degeneration of the tendon. Tibialis posterior tendon pathology commonly is seen as a hypertrophic appearance or marked attenuation of the tendon; less commonly, a complete rupture appears as absence of the tendon within its sheath.

At the lateral ankle, numerous peroneal tendon pathologies can be reliably diagnosed using MRI (**Figure 5**). In the retrofibular or subfibular region, a peroneus brevis split tear can appear as a wishbone-shaped tendon on axial sequences or even as a splitting into two tendon bellies. At the level of the lateral malleolus, peroneal instability can be seen as redundancy or tearing of the superior peroneal retinaculum, stripping of the retinaculum off the periosteum of the malleolus, or frank dislocation of the peroneus longus tendon out of the groove and adjacent to the lateral malleolus itself. With degenerative peroneal tendon conditions, either tendon may show diffuse enlargement (in tendinosis) or longitudinal, intratendinous high signal on T2-weighted sequences (in interstitial tearing). A distal peroneus longus tendon tear can mimic other plantar soft-tissue injuries; to diagnose a dorsiflexion injury, it is important to follow the peroneus longus tendon under the calcaneocuboid joint and the midfoot to its insertion on the plantar surface of the first metatarsal.

Accessory ossicles around the foot and ankle are prone to injury that may not be discernible on plain radiographs. In injury to the os trigonum posterior to the talus, MRI may show fluid collection on T2-weighted sequences or increased signal intensity within the synchondrosis. Similarly painful os peroneum syndrome can be diagnosed on MRI by signal intensity change within the os peroneum, which lies within the peroneus longus tendon at the level of the calcaneal cuboid joint. Signal intensity changes indicate inflammatory changes, a stress fracture, or osteonecrosis of the ossicle.

Ankle MRI is an accurate diagnostic modality for traumatic and degenerative pathologies involving the Achilles and anterior tibial ankle tendons (**Figure 6**). Achilles tendon injury can be located in the critical zone

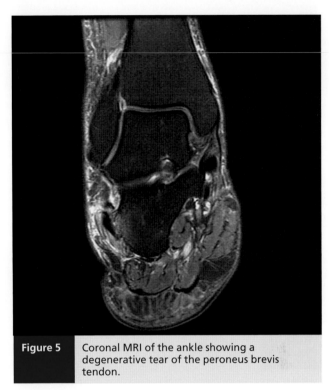

Figure 5 Coronal MRI of the ankle showing a degenerative tear of the peroneus brevis tendon.

or tendon insertion, or result in enthesial pathologies including retrocalcaneal bursitis, bone marrow edema in the dorsal calcaneus associated with Haglund exostosis, and insertional spurring, all of which can be detected and differentiated on MRI. Tendinosis can be seen on MRI as morphologic thickening of the tendon, signal change within the substance of the tendon itself, or linear splits within the tendon, which suggest degenerative tearing. In addition to diagnostic assistance, MRI can provide guidance in the management of insertional Achilles tendinopathy. A rupture in the tendon usually can be diagnosed by clinical evaluation alone, but MRI can be beneficial in confirming the rupture and quantifying any retraction gapping between the tendon ends.

Cartilage Injury

MRI has become the imaging study of choice for assessing the integrity of articular cartilage. Standard MRI studies do not evaluate the cartilage itself but instead detect decreased joint space (thinning of the articular cartilage) or periarticular bone marrow edema. The edema suggests abnormal biology of the adjacent cartilage, as occurs with osteochondral lesions and arthritis.

Routine MRI does not permit quantification of early degenerative changes, but in recent years the T2 mapping technique has been used to assess the cartilage of the ankle joint in several foot and ankle pathologies. In the knee, T2 mapping was found to specifically quantify cartilage water content and collagen fiber orientation.[28]

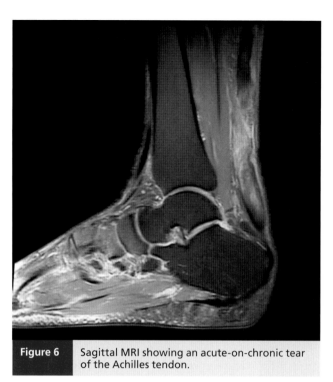

Figure 6 Sagittal MRI showing an acute-on-chronic tear of the Achilles tendon.

T2 mapping is a color-coded method of quantifying the T2-weighted relaxation curve. T2 relaxation is an exponential decay function reflecting the loss of signal that occurs rapidly during the dephasing of the excited nuclei after a disturbing radiofrequency pulse is applied. The signal is influenced by the structural anisotropy of the collagen, where a well-defined relationship exists between the excited hydrogen atoms and the long axis of the magnetic field. When the angle between the external field and the spinning hydrogen atoms within the collagen reaches approximately 55°, there is an expected prolongation of T2 relaxation time, which is clinically manifested as increased signal intensity. Increased T2 relaxation time has been associated with the breakdown of the cartilage architecture, including loss of collagen fiber integrity, altered water content, and subsequent osteoarthritis.

Tissues that decay slowly can display a signal that is apparent on standard MRI. In contrast, some substances decay rapidly and thus have a very short T2 relaxation time that precludes their measurement on standard MRI sequences. To obtain a very short signal, as in the collagen found within tendons, ligaments, menisci, and cartilage, the use of a specialized pulse sequence is necessary. This ultrashort echo time can be obtained using the relatively new 3-Tesla or higher magnet technology.[29]

Other Indications

MRI can be used to identify sources of ankle pain related to impingement of soft-tissue structures, including infiltration of the sinus tarsi, mass effect within the tarsal tunnel causing nerve compression, and intra-articular anterolateral or anteromedial ankle impingement. MRI can identify atraumatic osseous pathologies including os trigonum syndrome as well as patchy bone marrow edema related to altered biomechanics or stress response. MRI has an essential role in the workup of symptomatic midfoot or hindfoot coalition because of its ability to show osseous morphology as well as the sequelae of the resulting abnormal weight distribution.

MRI of the foot is a useful tool for patients with soft-tissue or osseous pathology and for those with acute injury or a degenerative condition. MRI is useful in the evaluation of refractory plantar fasciitis because of its ability to identify fascial tears and reactive bone marrow edema at the plantar calcaneus. MRI is the imaging modality of choice for many other common soft-tissue conditions of the foot, including plantar fibromatosis, intermetatarsal neuromas, ganglion cysts of tendon sheaths or joint capsules, and synovial chondromatosis of the ankle. With inflammatory arthropathies, MRI delineates the extent of both osseous erosion and periarticular synovitis. Finally, MRI has evolved into a modality of choice for imaging foot infections such as osteomyelitis because of its ability to accurately identify the presence and extent of osseous involvement as well as any soft-tissue abscess or phlegmon.

Summary

Appropriate imaging of the foot and ankle is essential to the orthopaedic surgeon's ability to diagnose and guide the treatment of many lower extremity pathologies. An understanding of the available imaging modalities and their advantages and disadvantages contributes to an optimal outcome for patients with a foot or ankle disorder.

Annotated References

1. Gallet J, Titus H: CR/DR systems: What each technology offers today; what is expected for the future. *Radiol Manage* 2005;27(6):30-36.

2. Giordano BD, Baumhauer JF, Morgan TL, Rechtine GR II: Patient and surgeon radiation exposure: Comparison of standard and mini-C-arm fluoroscopy. *J Bone Joint Surg Am* 2009;91(2):297-304.

   The safety of mini-C-arm radiographic imaging in the operating room was compared with that of standard imaging. The conclusion was that whenever possible, mini-C-arm imaging should be used to lower the radiation exposure of the surgical team and patient.

3. Ege T, Kose O, Koca K, Demiralp B, Basbozkurt M: Use of the iPhone for radiographic evaluation of hallux valgus. *Skeletal Radiol* 2013;42(2):269-273.

Radiographs of 32 patients with hallux valgus deformity were assessed. Angular deformity was measured by computer-assisted techniques and through a smartphone application. The maximum mean difference between the two techniques was 1.25° (SD, ±1.02°) for the hallux varus angle, 0.92° (±0.92°) for the first-second intermetatarsal angle, and 1.10° (±0.82°) for the distal metatarsal articular angle, with excellent intraobserver and interobserver reliability.

4. Chi TD, Davitt J, Younger A, Holt S, Sangeorzan BJ: Intra- and inter-observer reliability of the distal metatarsal articular angle in adult hallux valgus. *Foot Ankle Int* 2002;23(8):722-726.

5. Sensiba PR, Coffey MJ, Williams NE, Mariscalco M, Laughlin RT: Inter- and intraobserver reliability in the radiographic evaluation of adult flatfoot deformity. *Foot Ankle Int* 2010;31(2):141-145.

The talus–first metatarsal angle is an accurate radiographic identifier of adult symptomatic flatfoot deformity, although the medial cuneiform–fifth metatarsal distance and the calcaneal pitch angle were found to have the highest interobserver reliability.

6. Chen W, Li X, Su Y, et al: Peroneal tenography to evaluate lateral hindfoot pain after calcaneal fracture. *Foot Ankle Int* 2011;32(8):789-795.

Seventy-four patients with hindfoot pain after healing of a calcaneus fracture underwent peroneal tenography, and 51 (69%) were found to have peroneal impingement. The severity of lateral hindfoot pain was directly correlated with tendon sheath impingement and indirectly related to calcaneal widening.

7. Schreibman KL: Ankle tenography: What, how, and why. *Semin Roentgenol* 2004;39(1):95-113.

8. Jain NB, Omar I, Kelikian AS, van Holsbeeck L, Grant TH: Prevalence of and factors associated with posterior tibial tendon pathology on sonographic assessment. *PM R* 2011;3(11):998-1004.

In ultrasonographic evaluation of 217 patients with tibialis posterior tendon pathology, 80% of grade 2 tears were seen in the supramalleolar or retromalleolar area.

9. Neustadter J, Raikin SM, Nazarian LN: Dynamic sonographic evaluation of peroneal tendon subluxation. *AJR Am J Roentgenol* 2004;183(4):985-988.

10. Carlson RM, Dux K, Stuck RM: Ultrasound imaging for diagnosis of plantar plate ruptures of the lesser metatarsophalangeal joints: A retrospective case series. *J Foot Ankle Surg* 2013;52(6):786-788.

The sensitivity and specificity of ultrasonographic examination for plantar plate tears of the lesser metatarsophalangeal joint were 100% and 60%, respectively, with a positive predictive value of 60%. These results were comparable to those of MRI, but the cost of the examination was considerably lower.

11. Reach JS, Easley ME, Chuckpaiwong B, Nunley JA II: Accuracy of ultrasound guided injections in the foot and ankle. *Foot Ankle Int* 2009;30(3):239-242.

In a cadaver study, ultrasonographic guidance was used during injection of methylene blue to the metatarsophalangeal, subtalar, and ankle joints; peritendinous injections around the Achilles, tibialis posterior, and flexor hallucis longus tendons also were administered. All injections were 100% accurate except that the subtalar injection was 90% accurate.

12. Coughlin MJ, Grimes JS, Traughber PD, Jones CP: Comparison of radiographs and CT scans in the prospective evaluation of the fusion of hindfoot arthrodesis. *Foot Ankle Int* 2006;27(10):780-787.

13. Tuominen EK, Kankare J, Koskinen SK, Mattila KT: Weight-bearing CT imaging of the lower extremity. *AJR Am J Roentgenol* 2013;200(1):146-148.

Cone-beam CT technology allows both supine and weight-bearing imaging of the lower extremities, with a reasonable radiation dosage and excellent image quality. Weight-bearing CT can provide important new clinical information.

14. Frater C, Emmett L, van Gaal W, Sungaran J, Devakumar D, Van der Wall H: A critical appraisal of pinhole scintigraphy of the ankle and foot. *Clin Nucl Med* 2002;27(10):707-710.

15. Basu S, Chryssikos T, Houseni M, et al: Potential role of FDG PET in the setting of diabetic neuro-osteoarthropathy: Can it differentiate uncomplicated Charcot's neuroarthropathy from osteomyelitis and soft-tissue infection? *Nucl Med Commun* 2007;28(6):465-472.

16. Lin CC, Ding HJ, Chen YW, Huang WT, Kao A: Usefulness of thallium-201 muscle perfusion scan to investigate perfusion reserve in the lower limbs of Type 2 diabetic patients. *J Diabetes Complications* 2004;18(4):233-236.

17. Basu S, Zhuang H, Alavi A: Imaging of lower extremity artery atherosclerosis in diabetic foot: FDG-PET imaging and histopathological correlates. *Clin Nucl Med* 2007;32(7):567-568.

18. Singh VK, Javed S, Parthipun A, Sott AH: The diagnostic value of single photon-emission computed tomography bone scans combined with CT (SPECT-CT) in diseases of the foot and ankle. *Foot Ankle Surg* 2013;19(2):80-83.

Fifty patients with an unclear clinical diagnosis were evaluated using SPECT-CT. In 39 patients (78%) the findings were not exactly correlated with the initial clinical diagnosis, and a change in the treatment plan was required. Accuracy, sensitivity, specificity, and positive predictive value were 94%, 95.5%, 83.3%, and 97.6%, respectively.

19. Claassen L, Uden T, Ettinger M, Daniilidis K, Stukenborg-Colsman C, Plaass C: Influence on therapeutic decision making of SPECT-CT for different regions of the foot and ankle. *Biomed Res Int* 2014;2014:927576.

   Eighty-six patients underwent SPECT-CT scans of the foot and ankle. In at least 65% of cases, the result of the SPECT-CT had a direct effect on the clinical treatment decision. There was a greater influence on scans of the Chopart and Lisfranc joints than on the subtalar and ankle joints.

20. Chicklore S, Gnanasegaran G, Vijayanathan S, Fogelman I: Potential role of multislice SPECT/CT in impingement syndrome and soft-tissue pathology of the ankle and foot. *Nucl Med Commun* 2013;34(2):130-139.

   Of 209 patients undergoing SPECT-CT scans, 43 (21%) were found to have soft-tissue impingement. Only 24 of these 43 cases (56%) had a prior suspected clinical diagnosis of impingement prior to their SPECT-CT study. The diagnosis was made in 12 cases (28%) using standard technetium bone scans, which were performed to evaluate for bony impingement. The study concluded that SPECT-CT was useful in localizing and characterizing soft-tissue impingement syndrome around the ankle region in patients with pain of unknown etiology.

21. Cerezal L, Abascal F, García-Valtuille R, Canga A: Ankle MR arthrography: How, why, when. *Radiol Clin North Am* 2005;43(4):693-707, viii.

22. Collins MS, Felmlee JP: 3T magnetic resonance imaging of ankle and hindfoot tendon pathology. *Top Magn Reson Imaging* 2009;20(3):175-188.

   Relatively new 3-Tesla MRI units allow optimal fast spin-echo imaging with lower echo spacing for longer echo train lengths and minimal image blurring.

23. Juras V, Welsch G, Bär P, Kronnerwetter C, Fujita H, Trattnig S: Comparison of 3T and 7T MRI clinical sequences for ankle imaging. *Eur J Radiol* 2012;81(8):1846-1850.

   Ten volunteers underwent MRI evaluation using 3- and 7-Tesla magnets. A substantial benefit was found to using ultrahigh-field 7-Tesla MRI with routine clinical sequences. Scanners with high signal-to-noise and contrast-to-noise ratios may be useful for ankle imaging in clinical

practice. However, careful protocols and dedicated extremity coils are necessary for obtaining optimal results.

24. Elias I, Zoga AC, Morrison WB, Besser MP, Schweitzer ME, Raikin SM: Osteochondral lesions of the talus: Localization and morphologic data from 424 patients using a novel anatomical grid scheme. *Foot Ankle Int* 2007;28(2):154-161.

25. Potter HG, Deland JT, Gusmer PB, Carson E, Warren RF: Magnetic resonance imaging of the Lisfranc ligament of the foot. *Foot Ankle Int* 1998;19(7):438-446.

26. Raikin SM, Elias I, Dheer S, Besser MP, Morrison WB, Zoga AC: Prediction of midfoot instability in the subtle Lisfranc injury: Comparison of magnetic resonance imaging with intraoperative findings. *J Bone Joint Surg Am* 2009;91(4):892-899.

   MRI examination of 21 feet was followed by stress radiography under anesthesia to assess for Lisfranc instability after a suspected ligamentous injury. Disruption of the plantar C1-M2M3 ligament was the greatest predictor of instability. Sensitivity, specificity, and positive predictive value were 94%, 75%, and 94%, respectively. MRI allowed correct classification of the Lisfranc joint complex in 19 (90%) of the 21 patients.

27. Lim PS, Schweitzer ME, Deely DM, et al: Posterior tibial tendon dysfunction: Secondary MR signs. *Foot Ankle Int* 1997;18(10):658-663.

28. Potter HG, Black BR, Chong R: New techniques in articular cartilage imaging. *Clin Sports Med* 2009;28(1):77-94.

   Three-dimensional modeling techniques allow the semi-automated creation of models of the joint surface and thickness for use in templating before joint resurfacing or focal cartilage repair. Quantitative MRI techniques provide noninvasively obtained information about cartilage and repair tissue biochemistry.

29. Marik W, Apprich S, Welsch GH, Mamisch TC, Trattnig S: Biochemical evaluation of articular cartilage in patients with osteochondrosis dissecans by means of quantitative T2- and T2-mapping at 3T MRI: A feasibility study. *Eur J Radiol* 2012;81(5):923-927.

   Ten patients with grade 1 or 2 osteochondral lesions of the talus were evaluated using T2 mapping, which can be useful in assessing the microstructural composition of cartilage overlying osteochondral lesions.

Chapter 4

Foot and Ankle Conditions in Children and Adolescents

Jeffrey R. Sawyer, MD   Derek M. Kelly, MD

Introduction

Most foot and ankle conditions in children and adolescents are self-limiting and can be successfully treated using modalities such as an orthosis, activity modification, and physical therapy. Surgery usually is not necessary to treat an accessory navicular, tarsal coalition, or flatfoot deformity, but it can be effective for relieving pain and improving function in the few of patients who have persistent symptoms. To determine the appropriate treatment, it is mandatory to identify the exact cause of the symptoms.

Accessory Navicular

An accessory navicular (os naviculare) is found in 10% to 14% of asymptomatic normal feet.[1] Three types have been identified (Figure 1). A type I accessory navicular is a small, round ossicle of bone that lies completely separate from the navicular within the substance of the tibialis posterior tendon at its insertion into the navicular. Type II typically is a larger bone that connects to the navicular tuberosity by a synchondrosis. A type II accessory navicular constitutes a large portion of the tibialis posterior tendon. Type III is similar to type II in appearance except for the absence of the synchondrosis; instead, the navicular is completely fused to the accessory ossicle.[2]

Description

An accessory navicular typically is found in early adolescence when the patient experiences progressively

worsening medial midfoot pain. Occasionally, the symptoms begin with a sprain of the foot or ankle, and the pain often is exacerbated by sports activities or shoe wear. A flexible pes planovalgus deformity is present in 50% of patients with a symptomatic accessory navicular.[3] The patient typically reports tenderness to palpation over the medial prominence. The pain often can be exacerbated by resisted tibialis posterior tendon contraction. The patient and parents may be concerned about the size and appearance of the bump on the medial arch (Figure 2).

Radiographic Evaluation

The standard standing AP, internal oblique, and lateral radiographic views usually are sufficient for detecting the accessory bone (Figure 3). It is important to identify any associated abnormalities, such as pes planus or a calcaneonavicular coalition. A reverse (external) oblique radiograph of the foot also is used to identify the accessory ossicle. Advanced imaging such as CT, MRI, or nuclear scintigraphy usually is unnecessary. In a patient with symptoms, a bone scan is likely to show signal intensity at the site of the ossicle in a type II deformity. MRI is excellent for defining the soft-tissue anatomy of the tibialis posterior tendon insertion and identifying a synchondrosis. A symptomatic accessory navicular sometimes is found on MRI obtained to determine the cause of ankle pain of unclear etiology.[4] In a symptomatic accessory navicular, MRI often reveals edema in the synchondrosis and nearby bony structures.[5]

Nonsurgical Treatment

Patients with an insidious onset of symptoms often can achieve pain relief by avoiding the offending activity, wearing an over-the-counter soft orthosis, and/or using NSAIDs. A rigid arch-support orthosis can be painful because of pressure over the accessory navicular. Patients with associated flatfoot deformity and a contracture of the gastrocnemius or Achilles tendon can benefit from a stretching program. A period of immobilization in a walking cast or boot may help relieve symptoms that began acutely or are not resolved after other treatments.

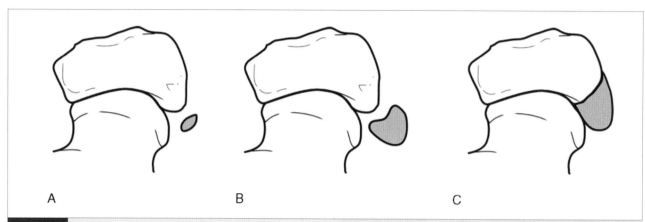

Figure 1 Illustrations showing the classification of the accessory navicular. **A,** Type I, in which a small, round ossicle is completely separate from the navicular. **B,** Type II, in which a larger ossicle is connected to the navicular by a synchondrosis. **C,** Type III, which is similar to type II except for the absence of a synchondrosis.

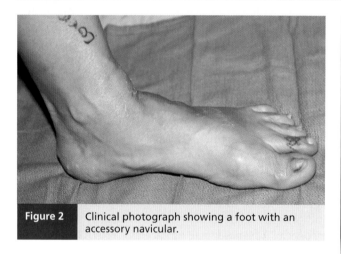

Figure 2 Clinical photograph showing a foot with an accessory navicular.

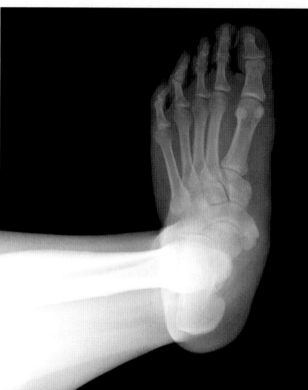

Figure 3 AP radiograph showing an accessory navicular. An external oblique view sometimes helps detect or fully delineate the accessory bone.

Most patients can be successfully treated using these nonsurgical measures.[1,6]

Surgical Treatment

Surgical treatment is an option if an extended course of nonsurgical treatment does not result in relief of symptoms. The original Kidner procedure involved excision of the accessory ossicle and advancement of the tibialis posterior tendon to the medial cuneiform.[7] Most experts now prefer a modified Kidner procedure that entails simple excision of the ossicle and side-to-side repair, rather than advancement, of the tibialis posterior tendon.[8-10]

A type I accessory navicular ossicle can be simply excised through a longitudinal split in the tibialis posterior tendon. A type II or III deformity requires subperiosteal dissection from the tibialis posterior tendon insertion. Care should be taken to avoid violating the talonavicular capsule. The tibialis posterior tendon can be repaired in a side-to-side fashion. Resection of a large type II or III deformity may require nearly complete detachment of the tibialis posterior tendon insertion to achieve adequate bony decompression. The detached tendon can be reattached to the residual navicular using suture anchors (Figure 4). Two recent studies found no significant difference in outcomes or complications after simple excision with or without advancement of the tibialis posterior tendon.[11,12]

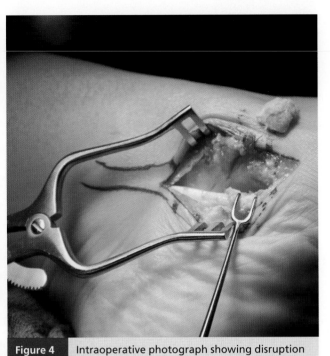

| Figure 4 | Intraoperative photograph showing disruption of the tibialis posterior tendon insertion after excision of an accessory navicular. Reattachment with suture anchors is required. |

Arthrodesis of a large ossicle to the native navicular with screw fixation has the apparent advantage of avoiding disruption of the insertion of the tibialis posterior tendon.[13-15] Although a 20% rate of nonunion was reported in one study, overall patient satisfaction was high.[15] Studies with large numbers of patients and lengthy follow-up are necessary to determine the role of fusion in the treatment of an accessory navicular.

Surgical treatment of associated flatfoot deformity and Achilles contracture at the time of accessory navicular excision remains controversial.[11,16] A gastrocnemius recession often is adequate to release an associated contracture. Flatfoot deformity can be treated with medial displacement calcaneal osteotomy, lateral column lengthening, or subtalar arthroereisis. It is unclear whether these additional procedures result in better outcomes than simple excision.

Tarsal Coalition

Tarsal coalition is an abnormal connection between the bones of the hindfoot or midfoot and is caused by failure of mesenchymal segmentation. A coalition can be fibrous, cartilaginous, or bony, and it can occur in isolation or as a component of a genetic syndrome.[17,18] Progression from fibrous to cartilaginous and ultimately to bony tissue occurs during skeletal maturation, coinciding with a gradual onset of symptoms. This process explains why a symptomatic coalition is rare in young children. An association between rigid pes planus and tarsal coalition has been described, and classic studies have linked peroneal spastic flatfoot with talocalcaneal coalitions.[19] Calcaneonavicular and talocalcaneal coalitions, especially of the middle facet, are most common. Coalitions between other tarsal bones occur less often.[20-23] Fifty percent of coalitions are bilateral. Multiple coalitions are rare, but it is essential to consider this possibility before undertaking surgical treatment.[24] Tarsal coalition is reported to be transmitted in an autosomal dominant fashion with variable penetrance.[19] The true prevalence of tarsal coalition is unknown because many coalitions are asymptomatic, but it may be as high as 11%.[20]

Description

A calcaneonavicular coalition usually is discovered in a child age 8 to 12 years, often after an acute ankle sprain caused by impaired subtalar mobility. Patients report lateral hindfoot pain and tenderness in the sinus tarsi and often have peroneal muscle spasms secondary to pain. Hindfoot motion usually is limited, especially in patients with a complete bony coalition. Pes planovalgus deformity is typical and often is associated with an Achilles tendon or gastrocnemius muscle contracture. On single-limb heel rise test, the foot has poor restoration of the medial longitudinal arch and persistence of hindfoot eversion.

A talocalcaneal coalition usually is found in a child age 12 to 16 years. Patients often seek treatment after an ankle sprain or another minor trauma. Hindfoot range of motion often is more limited than in children with a calcaneonavicular coalition, and hindfoot valgus often is more severe. Patients rarely have a cavovarus deformity. The classic finding of peroneal muscle spasm is most common in talocalcaneal coalitions. Other causes of peroneal spastic flatfoot should be considered, however, including an osteochondral lesion of the talus, inflammatory arthritis, infection, fracture, and tumor.

Radiographic Evaluation

The initial radiographic evaluation includes the weight-bearing AP, lateral, and 45° internal oblique views of the foot as well as an axial (Harris) view of the hindfoot. Talar beaking (a dorsal osteophyte) at the talonavicular joint often is seen in a talocalcaneal or calcaneonavicular coalition and is not typically associated with true talonavicular arthritis. A calcaneonavicular coalition is best seen on a 45° internal oblique radiograph. A lateral radiograph may reveal prominence of the anterior process of the calcaneus toward the navicular (the so-called anteater's nose sign; Figure 5). A talocalcaneal coalition is best seen on the axial view as an irregularity and an oblique orientation of the middle subtalar facet.

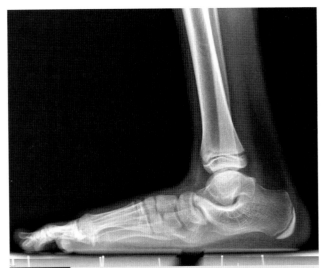

Figure 5 Lateral radiograph showing a calcaneonavicular coalition and an anteater's nose sign.

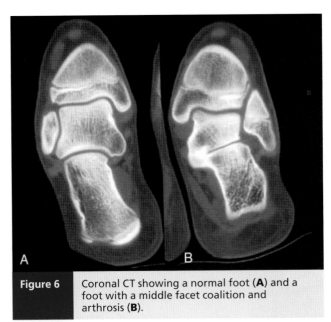

Figure 6 Coronal CT showing a normal foot (**A**) and a foot with a middle facet coalition and arthrosis (**B**).

A talocalcaneal coalition is less consistently seen on the lateral view, usually because the valgus obliquity of the subtalar joint causes it to be poorly defined.

The difficulty of diagnosing a tarsal coalition using plain radiographs, especially a talocalcaneal coalition, has resulted in the increased use of CT and MRI. CT can be used to identify the coalition, determine its extent, differentiate a bony from a fibrous coalition, and identify arthritis or additional coalitions in other parts of the foot (**Figure 6**). CT also is useful for evaluating the foot for other structural abnormalities that are difficult to see on plain radiographs such as an accessory anterior facet or a calcaneofibular impingement, which often accompanies a talocalcaneal coalition.[25,26] MRI is the preferred modality for evaluating young patients, who are likely to have a fibrous coalition because ossification is incomplete. In addition, reducing exposure to ionizing radiation is particularly desirable in young patients.[27]

Nonsurgical Treatment
Initial nonsurgical treatment is recommended for all patients with a tarsal coalition. The modalities include rest, activity modification, and a period of immobilization in a cast, boot, or brace. After the symptoms subside, the patient can progress to using a custom orthosis and slowly resume activities. A stretching program for the Achilles tendon and gastrocnemius should be considered for patients with a gastrocnemius-soleus complex contracture. Subsequent treatment may include the use of a University of California Biomechanics Laboratory orthosis. Although this device is more effective for controlling hindfoot eversion than an over-the-counter

orthosis, achieving compliance in an active adolescent can be difficult.

Surgical Treatment
Calcaneonavicular coalitions are excised through a longitudinal incision over the sinus tarsi. The adequacy of the excision is assessed both clinically and radiographically; full hindfoot motion should be obtained intraoperatively. Care must be taken not to injure the talonavicular joint and the talar head. The extensor digitorum brevis muscle belly and fascia can be advanced and interposed into the excision site. The use of fat graft also has been shown to be effective and may avoid skin cosmesis issues or inadequate coverage of the resection site associated with extensor digitorum brevis interposition.[28] The long-term results are somewhat less than encouraging, however. As many as 25% of patients were found to require further surgical intervention, American Orthopaedic Foot and Ankle Society (AOFAS) outcome scores were only fair (mean, 78.1), and pain, walking distance, and range of motion outcomes also were only fair.[29] An associated gastrocnemius-soleus complex contracture should be treated at the time of surgical resection. Isolated gastrocnemius contracture can be treated with a gastrocnemius recession, and combined gastrocnemius and soleus contracture can be treated with percutaneous Achilles lengthening.

Surgical procedures for treating talocalcaneal coalitions include arthrodesis, coalition resection, and osteotomy without resection. The long-held criteria for determining whether a coalition should be resected include size of less than 30% to 50% of the posterior facet, hindfoot valgus of 16° to 21°, and little or no narrowing

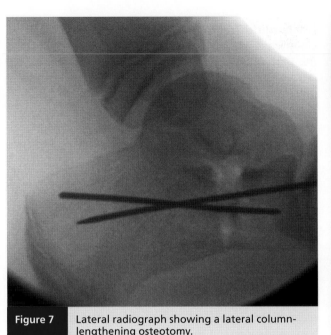

Figure 7   Lateral radiograph showing a lateral column-lengthening osteotomy.

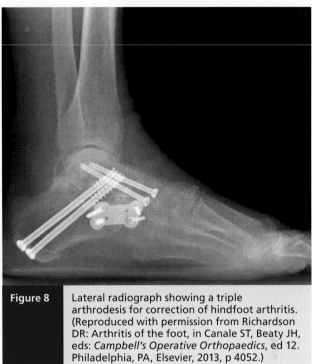

Figure 8   Lateral radiograph showing a triple arthrodesis for correction of hindfoot arthritis. (Reproduced with permission from Richardson DR: Arthritis of the foot, in Canale ST, Beaty JH, eds: *Campbell's Operative Orthopaedics*, ed 12. Philadelphia, PA, Elsevier, 2013, p 4052.)

or degeneration of the posterior facet of the subtalar joint.[30-32] The site of the pain and the severity of the valgus deformity may be at least as important as the size of the coalition, however.[33] Calcaneal lengthening osteotomy was preferred over arthrodesis for a painful talocalcaneal coalition and advanced hindfoot valgus[33] (Figure 7).

Talocalcaneal coalitions are excised through a medial approach between the flexor digitorum longus and flexor hallucis longus tendons. Care must be taken to avoid the medial neurovascular bundle. It is crucial that the coalition be adequately resected, particularly from anterior to posterior. Careful inspection of the anterior and posterior subtalar facets is necessary after removal of the coalition. Most surgeons prefer to interpose bone wax and local fat in the resected coalition site, although other interpositional materials, including tendon and de-epithelialized skin, also have been used. Local fat graft can be obtained anterior to the Achilles tendon.[34] A recent study of a large number of patients treated with resection and fat interposition reported good deformity correction and high AOFAS ankle and hindfoot scale scores; subsequent realignment was needed in 34% of patients, however.[35] Similar short-term results were reported after flexor hallucis tendon interposition. Most experts recommend single-stage coalition resection and flatfoot reconstruction rather than arthrodesis as an initial treatment of moderate to severe coalitions.[33,36] Correction of calcaneofibular impingement is another potential advantage of deformity correction and calcaneal lengthening. Calcaneofibular impingement often is present in patients with a talocalcaneal coalition, and

further investigation is needed to determine the relationship between impingement and symptoms. Arthroscopic resection of talocalcaneal coalitions has been described, but further evaluation of its safety and efficacy is needed, compared with well-established open techniques.[37,38]

Although surgical treatment of a tarsal coalition usually results in improvement in pain and function, numerous studies have found that normal kinematics and pedobarographic parameters are not fully restored.[29,39,40] Extensive involvement of the middle facet leads to relatively poor outcomes after talocalcaneal coalition excision.[31,32,41] One study found no association between the size of a talocalcaneal coalition or a hindfoot valgus angle and the long-term functional outcome.[42] These findings do not appear to apply to anterior and middle facet coalitions. A decision on surgical reconstruction with subtalar fusion or triple arthrodesis should be based on the presence of arthritic changes, hindfoot rigidity, and the severity of planovalgus deformity. Although triple arthrodesis is a reliable salvage procedure, isolated hindfoot fusion generally is preferable in adults to avoid stress transfer to the ankle joint and the development of degenerative arthritis.[33] Triple arthrodesis was recommended only for feet with Chopart arthritis[33] (Figure 8).

Flexible Pediatric Flatfoot

Flexible pes planovalgus (flatfoot) deformity is found in as many as 80% of young children, but its prevalence decreases with age to approximately 10% to 20% of adults.[43] Children who are obese are at increased risk for pain as well as worsening of the deformity.[44-46] Children with flexible flatfoot deformity, especially when it is painful, often have an associated Achilles tendon or gastrocnemius contracture.[47] Muscle activity appears to have minimal influence on the development or persistence of flexible flatfoot deformity.[48]

Description

Most children with flexible flatfoot deformity do not have symptoms. The parents often seek an orthopaedic evaluation because of concern about the appearance of the child's feet. The supple deformity consists of loss of the normal medial longitudinal arch and hindfoot valgus. The talar head often is palpable medially, secondary to navicular uncovering. On examination, the deformity is easily reducible. With heel rise, the arch is restored and the hindfoot inverts. The arch also is restored with the Jack toe raise test and passive dorsiflexion of the first metatarsophalangeal joint. Patients with symptoms have tenderness along the talonavicular joint or medial longitudinal arch in the region of the midsubstance of the plantar fascia. Skin changes such as calluses may be present over the uncovered talar head. The patient may have night pain in the medial leg, gastrocnemius-soleus complex, and plantar foot.[46] In a patient with severe deformity, sinus tarsi pain can develop secondary to calcaneofibular abutment. It is important to clinically assess the patient's entire lower extremity for rotational malalignment.

Radiographic Evaluation

Although radiographic differences appear in children with flexible flatfoot, little evidence supports the routine use of radiography in the absence of symptoms. When radiographic evaluation is necessary, it includes the weight-bearing AP, 45° internal oblique, and lateral views. Weight-bearing AP ankle and axial hindfoot views occasionally are used to evaluate for other potential sources of the valgus appearance of the foot. Patients with pes planovalgus have an increased talar declination and an increased convex-downward Meary (talar–first metatarsal) angle on the lateral radiograph. The weight-bearing AP view shows uncovering of the talar head with lateral subluxation of the navicular. Patients with an Achilles tendon or gastrocnemius contracture have a decreased calcaneal pitch. The considerable interobserver and intraobserver error in radiographic measurements of pes planus is proportional to the number of steps required to obtain the measurement.[49] The amount of talar head coverage is the only clinically relevant measurement that differs based on the presence or absence of symptoms.[50]

Nonsurgical Treatment

Counseling and education as to the benign nature of flexible flatfoot are the mainstay responses to the condition. No high-level evidence supports any form of nonsurgical intervention in the absence of symptoms.[51,52] In a patient with an Achilles tendon or gastrocnemius contracture, a stretching program may be useful for relief of symptoms, but no long-term studies have proved the benefit of such a program. A prescription orthosis or scaphoid pad can be used, but there are no long-term studies documenting the benefit of a custom orthosis for treating the condition. Orthoses, braces, or corrective shoes have not been shown to correct the deformity or prevent its progression in patients without symptoms.

Surgical Treatment

Surgery should be considered for the few patients who have persistent pain after nonsurgical treatment. Arthroereisis (insertion of an implant into the sinus tarsi) has had some success. A foreign body reaction to the original polymeric silicone implants in the sinus tarsi necessitated the development of metallic implants. Radiographic parameters have improved with the use of relatively new implants, and patient satisfaction rates now range from 79% to 100%.[53] However, rates of complications and unplanned reoperation have been high.[53,54] Improved outcomes were reported when arthroereisis was performed in conjunction with gastrocnemius recession.[55] After unsuccessful subtalar arthroereisis, revision with a lateral column calcaneal lengthening osteotomy can be considered at the time of implant removal or can be performed in a staged fashion. Talonavicular fusion at one time was considered an option for treating flexible pediatric planus but now is reserved for patients with painful neuromuscular pes planus.[56]

After unsuccessful nonsurgical treatment, many patients can be treated with a lateral column-lengthening osteotomy.[57] Care must be taken to protect the sural nerve and peroneal tendons during lateral dissection of the calcaneal wall. A saw or osteotome is used under fluoroscopic guidance for a lateral-to-medial calcaneal osteotomy starting in the Gissane angle and angling medially between the anterior and middle facets of the subtalar joint. The medial wall can be left intact. A lamina spreader is used to distract the osteotomy, with care taken to avoid subluxation of the calcaneocuboid joint, which can be prophylactically pinned before distraction. An 8- to 10-mm wedge-shaped autograft or allograft is inserted. Graft placement and foot positioning are crucial for correction of midfoot abduction as well as any residual supination. Compression screws, lateral plating, or threaded Kirschner wires are chosen for fixation depending on the size and bone quality of the patient. Excessive dorsal graft within the sinus tarsi must be trimmed to prevent impingement. Autograft has not been shown to be clearly superior to allograft.

A comparison of outcomes at midterm follow-up after a calcaneal lengthening osteotomy or combined calcaneal-cuboid-cuneiform osteotomies found good clinical and radiographic results after both procedures.[57] Patients who underwent lateral column lengthening had greater postoperative talar head coverage but also had a slightly higher complication rate. A talonavicular capsulotomy, spring ligament repair, and flexor digitorum longus transfer can be added to improve deformity correction and inversion strength in patients who are skeletally mature and have severe deformity and weak inversion.

Apophysitis

Sever Disease

Sever disease (calcaneal apophysitis) was first described in 1912 as "apophysitis of the os calcis" in five children.[58] This condition is most common in children age 9 to 12 years. Patients typically report pain at the Achilles tendon insertion into the os calcis, in the calcaneal apophysis itself, or near the origin of the plantar fascia. Symptoms often are exacerbated by aggressive sports activities but can occur with simple walking. Associated Achilles tendon or gastrocnemius contracture is common, and constant tension from a tight gastrocnemius-soleus complex may be a contributing factor. Pedobarographic analysis found an association between high plantar pressures, hindfoot equinus, and symptoms of calcaneal apophysis, but a cause-and-effect relationship has not been established.[59] Unlike Osgood-Schlatter disease, Sever disease has no classic radiographic findings. The diagnosis is primarily clinical.[60] Imaging sometimes is considered useful for ruling out other causes of heel pain in children, such as a stress fracture or benign bone lesion. One study found a 1.4% rate of abnormal radiographic findings in children with heel pain and concluded that routine imaging is unnecessary to establish a clinical diagnosis of calcaneal apophysitis.[61] Another study found a 5% rate, however, and this report concluded that a single lateral radiograph of the calcaneus is justified in the initial evaluation of pediatric heel pain.[61,62]

Symptoms typically resolve with closure of the calcaneal apophysis. Surgery rarely is indicated. The treatment options include activity modification, silicone heel wedges, postactivity icing, NSAIDs, and a stretching program for the gastrocnemius-soleus complex. A brief period of cast or boot immobilization occasionally is required if other treatments have been unsuccessful. The waxing and waning course of Sever disease can be frustrating for patients and their families, who must be instructed about the natural history of the disease and the treatment options. Frequent reassurance may be necessary until the child reaches skeletal maturity.

Iselin Disease

Iselin disease, another type of traction apophysitis in the immature foot, first was described in 1912 as pain and radiographic changes at the "tuberositas metatarsi quinti" in a 13-year-old girl.[63] The apophysis at the fifth metatarsal base first appears radiographically as a small sliver of bone in 12-year-old boys and 10-year-old girls; these ages are typical for the onset of symptoms[64] (Figure 9). Chronic symptoms can result from overuse, and acute symptoms can be the result of an inversion injury. Although the pain is located at the base of the fifth metatarsal, it can radiate down the lateral border of the foot. Examination reveals tenderness to palpation over the fifth metatarsal base apophysis at the insertion of the peroneus brevis tendon. This pain can be reproduced by eversion of the foot against resistance. Radiographic evaluation is necessary to rule out a fracture of the proximal metaphysis of the fifth metatarsal. The fifth metatarsal base apophysis often is confused with an avulsion fracture, particularly after an acute injury. Contralateral radiographs can be useful if there is concern that the bony apophysis might represent an avulsion fracture.

The treatment of Iselin disease includes rest (often with a short period of boot immobilization), icing, and NSAIDs. Surgery rarely is indicated for Iselin disease but may be necessary for an established nonunion.[64]

Osteochondrosis

Symptomatic necrosis can occur in almost any bone of the foot during childhood or adolescence.[65,66] The etiology of these avascular events or osteochondroses remains a mystery. The two most common types of osteochondrosis in pediatric patients involve the navicular and the metatarsal head.

Köhler Disease

Navicular osteochondrosis in a pediatric patient was first described in 1908.[67] Patients often have pain in the medial midfoot, occasionally have swelling over the navicular, and often walk with a limp. Boys are more commonly affected than girls. The symptoms and abnormal radiographic appearance typically resolve within 6 months to 1 year[68] (Figure 10). The treatment is based on the severity of symptoms. Patients with mild symptoms can be treated with activity modification and NSAIDs. Patients with more severe pain may require a period of cast or boot immobilization for adequate relief of pain.

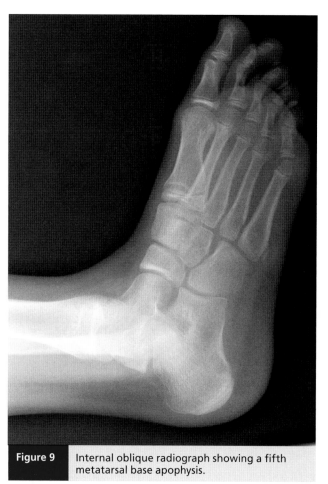

Figure 9 Internal oblique radiograph showing a fifth metatarsal base apophysis.

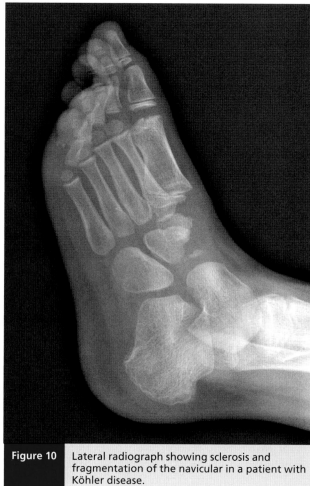

Figure 10 Lateral radiograph showing sclerosis and fragmentation of the navicular in a patient with Köhler disease.

Freiberg Infraction

Radiographic osteonecrosis in the second metatarsal head was first described in 1914.[69] The second metatarsal head is most commonly affected, but changes also may be seen in any of the other metatarsals. Unlike Köhler disease, which tends to occur in young boys and appears to be unrelated to the level of physical activity, Freiberg infraction is most common in adolescent girls who are athletes. Patients often report pain and swelling over the affected metatarsophalangeal joint or point tenderness over the plantar aspect of the metatarsal head during weight bearing. The radiographic evaluation may reveal sclerosis, metatarsal head flattening, and enlargement of the metatarsal epiphysis. The exact cause of Freiberg infraction is unknown, but it seems to be related to repetitive trauma that results in vascular insult of the metatarsal epiphysis. Most patients can expect symptoms to resolve after treatment with activity modification, NSAIDs, and soft shoe inserts. Patients who have severe symptoms or who do not receive relief with more simple measures may require a brief period of immobilization. Symptoms of Freiberg infraction and associated radiographic changes typically are spontaneously resolved over the course of 2 years. Surgery may be necessary if the patient has residual symptoms after the healing phase or mechanical symptoms from a malformed metatarsal head or loose bodies. The possible surgical procedures include removal of loose bodies, local synovectomy, and débridement of osteophytes or necrotic bone.[70] A dorsal wedge osteotomy of the metatarsal neck can be used to move normal plantar cartilage into a position of articulation with the proximal phalanx.[71] Osteochondral autograft plug transplantation has been described for replacing the damaged metatarsal head articular cartilage.[72,73] Metatarsal head resection is not recommended because it can result in continued pain, transfer metatarsalgia, and joint instability.

Summary

Disorders of the foot and ankle affecting children and adolescents usually improve and may be treated with observation, activity modification, physical therapy, and shoe inserts. If surgical treatment is required, a favorable outcome usually can be expected. Understanding the anatomy of the skeletally immature foot and establishing the correct diagnosis are key to choosing the appropriate treatment.

Annotated References

1. Grogan DP, Gasser SI, Ogden JA: The painful accessory navicular: A clinical and histopathological study. *Foot Ankle* 1989;10(3):164-169.

2. Sella EJ, Lawson JP, Ogden JA: The accessory navicular synchondrosis. *Clin Orthop Relat Res* 1986;209:280-285.

3. Sullivan JA, Miller WA: The relationship of the accessory navicular to the development of the flat foot. *Clin Orthop Relat Res* 1979;144:233-237.

4. Issever AS, Minden K, Eshed I, Hermann KG: Accessory navicular bone: When ankle pain does not originate from the ankle. *Clin Rheumatol* 2007;26(12):2143-2144.

5. Sizensky JA, Marks RM: Imaging of the navicular. *Foot Ankle Clin* 2004;9(1):181-209.

6. Smith TR: Management of dancers with symptomatic accessory navicular: 2 case reports. *J Orthop Sports Phys Ther* 2012;42(5):465-473.

   Two adolescent female dancers with a symptomatic accessory navicular were successfully treated. One patient underwent surgical excision, and the other was treated with a graduated physical therapy program and orthoses. Level of evidence: V.

7. Kidner FC: The pre-hallux (accessory scaphoid) and its relation to flat-foot. *J Bone Joint Surg* 1929;11:831-837.

8. Lee KT, Kim KC, Park YU, Park SM, Lee YK, Deland JT: Midterm outcome of modified Kidner procedure. *Foot Ankle Int* 2012;33(2):122-127.

   Fifty patients had pain relief and a high satisfaction rate 7 years after undergoing a modified Kidner procedure. Level of evidence: IV.

9. Micheli LJ, Nielson JH, Ascani C, Matanky BK, Gerbino PG: Treatment of painful accessory navicular: A modification to simple excision. *Foot Ankle Spec* 2008;1(4):214-217.

   Eleven of 13 patients had an excellent result at long-term follow-up after a modified Kidner procedure. Level of evidence: IV.

10. Jasiewicz B, Potaczek T, Kacki W, Tesiorowski M, Lipik E: Results of simple excision technique in the surgical treatment of symptomatic accessory navicular bones. *Foot Ankle Surg* 2008;14(2):57-61.

    Twenty of 21 patients treated with simple excision of a symptomatic accessory navicular had total or complete pain relief at 5-year follow-up. Level of evidence: IV.

11. Cha SM, Shin HD, Kim KC, Lee JK: Simple excision vs the Kidner procedure for type 2 accessory navicular associated with flatfoot in pediatric population. *Foot Ankle Int* 2013;34(2):167-172.

    Fifty patients with flatfoot and an accessory navicular did well with simple excision or modified Kidner procedure without concomitant flatfoot surgery. Level of evidence: IV.

12. Pretell-Mazzini J, Murphy RF, Sawyer JR, et al: Surgical treatment of symptomatic accessory navicular in children and adolescents. *Am J Orthop (Belle Mead NJ)* 2014;43(3):110-113.

    A comparison of 14 feet treated with isolated excision and 18 feet with excision plus tendon advancement found no substantial difference in outcomes. However, there was a trend toward more complications and more reoperations after tendon advancement. Level of evidence: III.

13. Chung JW, Chu IT: Outcome of fusion of a painful accessory navicular to the primary navicular. *Foot Ankle Int* 2009;30(2):106-109.

    Union was obtained in 28 (82%) of 34 feet, but 6 feet required excision of the accessory navicular after screw loosening resulted in nonunion. Functional outcomes were excellent in 22 feet, good in 5, fair in 1, and poor in 6. Level of evidence: IV.

14. Malicky ES, Levine DS, Sangeorzan BJ: Modification of the Kidner procedure with fusion of the primary and accessory navicular bones. *Foot Ankle Int* 1999;20(1):53-54.

15. Scott AT, Sabesan VJ, Saluta JR, Wilson MA, Easley ME: Fusion versus excision of the symptomatic Type II accessory navicular: A prospective study. *Foot Ankle Int* 2009;30(1):10-15.

    A comparison of 10 patients who underwent arthrodesis with 10 patients who underwent the modified Kidner procedure found similar improvement in AOFAS scores. After arthrodesis, there were two nonunions and one painful implant. After the Kidner procedure, three patients had persistent midfoot pain and progressive loss of the longitudinal arch. Level of evidence: II.

16. Garras DN, Hansen PL, Miller AG, Raikin SM: Outcome of modified Kidner procedure with subtalar arthroereisis for painful accessory navicular associated with planovalgus deformity. *Foot Ankle Int* 2012;33(11):934-939.

    Substantial improvements in pain and function were obtained with the modified Kidner procedure and subtalar arthroereisis in 10 patients with an accessory navicular and flatfoot deformity. Level of evidence: IV.

17. Agochukwu NB, Solomon BD, Benson LJ, Muenke M: Talocalcaneal coalition in Muenke syndrome: Report of

a patient, review of the literature in FGFR-related cranio-synostoses, and consideration of mechanism. *Am J Med Genet* 2013;161(3):453-460.

A 7-year-old girl with Muenke syndrome and bilateral symptomatic talocalcaneal coalitions was successfully treated with resection of the coalitions. Although tarsal coalitions are a distinct feature of Muenke syndrome, most are asymptomatic. Level of evidence: V.

18. Ellington JK, Myerson MS: Surgical correction of the ball and socket ankle joint in the adult associated with a talonavicular tarsal coalition. *Foot Ankle Int* 2013;34(10):1381-1388.

    In a study of 13 patients with a talonavicular tarsal coalition, 4 patients were treated with arthrodesis and 9 with supramalleolar osteotomy. Nine patients had a good result (four after arthrodesis, five after osteotomy). Four patients had a fair result after osteotomy. The mean AOFAS score improved from 30 to 78 after osteotomy and from 24 to 60 after arthrodesis. Level of evidence: III.

19. Leonard MA: The inheritance of tarsal coalition and its relationship to spastic flat foot. *J Bone Joint Surg Br* 1974;56(3):520-526.

20. Nalaboff KM, Schweitzer ME: MRI of tarsal coalition: Frequency, distribution, and innovative signs. *Bull NYU Hosp Jt Dis* 2008;66(1):14-21.

    A review of MRI of 574 ankles found tarsal coalitions in 66 patients. Most of the coalitions (71%) were calcaneonavicular; 56% of these were cartilaginous, and 44% were fibrous. Level of evidence: III.

21. Ross JR, Dobbs MB: Isolated navicular-medial cuneiform tarsal coalition revisited: A case report. *J Pediatr Orthop* 2011;31(8):e85-e88.

    Isolated navicular–medial cuneiform tarsal coalition in a patient was described. The 9-year-old girl was treated with resection and free-fat interposition rather than arthrodesis. At 2-year follow-up, she was pain free with a full range of motion. Level of evidence: V.

22. Staser J, Karmazyn B, Lubicky J: Radiographic diagnosis of posterior facet talocalcaneal coalition. *Pediatr Radiol* 2007;37(1):79-81.

23. Sarage AL, Gambardella GV, Fullem B, Saxena A, Caminear DS: Cuboid-navicular tarsal coalition: Report of a small case series with description of a surgical approach for resection. *J Foot Ankle Surg* 2012;51(6):783-786.

    Three of four patients with a cuboid-navicular coalition had a history of ankle sprains. After coalition resection and fat-graft interposition, all were pain free and able to return to earlier levels of activity. Level of evidence: IV.

24. Masquijo JJ, Jarvis J: Associated talocalcaneal and calcaneonavicular coalitions in the same foot. *J Pediatr Orthop B* 2010;19(6):507-510.

Three patients with concurrent talocalcaneal and calcaneonavicular coalitions were treated with coalition resection and extensor digitorum brevis interposition. The incidence of multiple tarsal bars and the importance of CT in preoperative planning were described. Level of evidence: IV.

25. Martus JE, Femino JE, Caird MS, Hughes RE, Browne RH, Farley FA: Accessory anterolateral facet of the pediatric talus: An anatomic study. *J Bone Joint Surg Am* 2008;90(11):2452-2459.

    A survey of 79 osteologic specimens found an accessory anterolateral talar facet in 34%. The presence of the facet was associated with increased age (17 versus 11 years), male sex, and a smaller Gissane angle.

26. Kernbach KJ, Blitz NM: The presence of calcaneal fibular remodeling associated with middle facet talocalcaneal coalition: A retrospective CT review of 35 feet. Investigations involving middle facet coalitions: Part II. *J Foot Ankle Surg* 2008;47(4):288-294.

    Calcaneal fibular remodeling, a pathologic component of middle facet talocalcaneal coalition, was found in 19 of 35 feet (54%). Calcaneal fibular remodeling is believed to contribute to the symptoms of painful middle facet talocalcaneal coalition and may require surgical procedures in addition to resection. Level of evidence: IV.

27. Guignand D, Journeau P, Mainard-Simard L, Popkov D, Haumont T, Lascombes P: Child calcaneonavicular coalitions: MRI diagnostic value in a 19-case series. *Orthop Traumatol Surg Res* 2011;97(1):67-72.

    Radiographs were normal in 10 of 19 feet with pediatric calcaneonavicular coalition. Four of seven bone scans were considered normal. CT resulted in a correct diagnosis in seven patients, but the coalition was missed in four patients. All MRIs resulted in a positive diagnosis of tarsal coalition. Level of evidence: III.

28. Mubarak SJ, Patel PN, Upasani VV, Moor MA, Wenger DR: Calcaneonavicular coalition: Treatment by excision and fat graft. *J Pediatr Orthop* 2009;29(5):418-426.

    At 1-year follow-up after resection of 96 feet, 87% of patients had returned to sports or other earlier activities; 5% had symptomatic regrowth that required repeat resection. A cadaver study found that the extensor digitorum brevis was able to fill only 65% of the resection gap. Level of evidence: IV.

29. Skwara A, Zounta V, Tibesku CO, Fuchs-Winkelmann S, Rosenbaum D: Plantar contact stress and gait analysis after resection of tarsal coalition. *Acta Orthop Belg* 2009;75(5):654-660.

    Surgical treatment of tarsal coalition achieved a fair clinical and radiographic result in 15 feet but did not restore physiologic gait and foot loading. Level of evidence: IV.

30. Comfort TK, Johnson LO: Resection for symptomatic talocalcaneal coalition. *J Pediatr Orthop* 1998;18(3):283-288.

31. Luhmann SJ, Schoenecker PL: Symptomatic talocalcaneal coalition resection: Indications and results. *J Pediatr Orthop* 1998;18(6):748-754.

32. Wilde PH, Torode IP, Dickens DR, Cole WG: Resection for symptomatic talocalcaneal coalition. *J Bone Joint Surg Br* 1994;76(5):797-801.

33. Mosca VS, Bevan WP: Talocalcaneal tarsal coalitions and the calcaneal lengthening osteotomy: The role of deformity correction. *J Bone Joint Surg Am* 2012;94(17):1584-1594.

   Calcaneal lengthening osteotomy combined with gastrocnemius or Achilles tendon lengthening fully corrected valgus deformity and provided short- to intermediate-term pain relief in nine feet with an unresectable coalition. Level of evidence: IV.

34. Sperl M, Saraph V, Zwick EB, Kraus T, Spendel S, Linhart WE: Preliminary report: Resection and interposition of a deepithelialized skin flap graft in tarsal coalition in children. *J Pediatr Orthop B* 2010;19(2):171-176.

   De-epithelialized skin flap interposition was effective in treating six tarsal coalitions. AOFAS scores were excellent in two patients and good in four. Preservation of surrounding muscles and tendons is an advantage of the technique, but the need for a large skin incision is a disadvantage. Level of evidence: IV.

35. Gantsoudes GD, Roocroft JH, Mubarak SJ: Treatment of talocalcaneal coalitions. *J Pediatr Orthop* 2012;32(3):301-307.

   Excision and fat graft interposition resulted in a good to excellent result in 42 of 49 feet (85%) with a talocalcaneal coalition. At average 43-month follow-up, 1 patient had a recurrence requiring repeat excision, and 11 had required surgery to correct alignment. Level of evidence: IV.

36. Lisella JM, Bellapianta JM, Manoli A II: Tarsal coalition resection with pes planovalgus hindfoot reconstruction. *J Surg Orthop Adv* 2011;20(2):102-105.

   In eight feet with a talocalcaneal coalition, hindfoot reconstruction in addition to coalition resection increased motion, corrected malalignment, and decreased pain. Hindfoot reconstruction with resection was recommended for patients with a coalition and painful planovalgus hindfoot deformity. Level of evidence: IV.

37. Knörr J, Accadbled F, Abid A, et al: Arthroscopic treatment of calcaneonavicular coalition in children. *Orthop Traumatol Surg Res* 2011;97(5):565-568.

   At 12-month follow-up of children with a calcaneonavicular coalition, the mean AOFAS score had improved from 58 to 91, and there were no recurrences. The suggested advantages of arthroscopic resection included more rapid recovery and a better cosmetic result. Level of evidence: IV.

38. Singh AK, Parsons SW: Arthroscopic resection of calcaneonavicular coalition/malunion via a modified sinus tarsi approach: An early case series. *Foot Ankle Surg* 2012;18(4):266-269.

   At approximately 6-month follow-up of four patients treated with arthroscopic resection for a calcaneonavicular coalition or malunion, complete excision was confirmed, there were no recurrences, and symptoms had improved. Level of evidence: IV.

39. Hetsroni I, Ayalon M, Mann G, Meyer G, Nyska M: Walking and running plantar pressure analysis before and after resection of tarsal coalition. *Foot Ankle Int* 2007;28(5):575-580.

40. Hetsroni I, Nyska M, Mann G, Rozenfeld G, Ayalon M: Subtalar kinematics following resection of tarsal coalition. *Foot Ankle Int* 2008;29(11):1088-1094.

   Patients who were awaiting tarsal coalition resection or who had undergone bar resection 2 to 4 years earlier were compared with control subjects. Passive subtalar motion and AOFAS scores improved after surgery, but normal foot kinematics were not restored. Level of evidence: III.

41. Scranton PE Jr: Treatment of symptomatic talocalcaneal coalition. *J Bone Joint Surg Am* 1987;69(4):533-539.

42. Khoshbin A, Law PW, Caspi L, Wright JG: Long-term functional outcomes of resected tarsal coalitions. *Foot Ankle Int* 2013;34(10):1370-1375.

   Follow-up 13 to 15 years after resection of a talocalcaneal or calcaneonavicular coalition in 32 feet found no association between the size of the talocalcaneal coalition or hindfoot valgus angle and the long-term functional outcome. Level of evidence: IV.

43. Staheli LT, Chew DE, Corbett M: The longitudinal arch: A survey of eight hundred and eighty-two feet in normal children and adults. *J Bone Joint Surg Am* 1987;69(3):426-428.

44. Chen KC, Tung LC, Yeh CJ, Yang JF, Kuo JF, Wang CH: Change in flatfoot of preschool-aged children: A 1-year follow-up study. *Eur J Pediatr* 2013;172(2):255-260.

   At 1-year follow-up, flatfoot had improved to normal in 38% of 580 children, but 10% of children with originally normal feet had developed flatfoot. The risk factors for flatfoot development were relatively young age, male sex, obesity, and excessive joint laxity. Level of evidence: III.

45. Chen KC, Yeh CJ, Tung LC, Yang JF, Yang SF, Wang CH: Relevant factors influencing flatfoot in preschool-aged children. *Eur J Pediatr* 2011;170(7):931-936.

   In 1,598 children, the prevalence of bilateral flatfoot decreased substantially with age from 54% of 3-year-olds to 21% of 6-year-olds. A substantial association was found between bilateral flatfoot and age, sex, obesity, joint laxity, and a W-sitting position. Level of evidence: III.

46. Benedetti MG, Ceccarelli F, Berti L, et al: Diagnosis of flexible flatfoot in children: A systematic clinical approach. *Orthopedics* 2011;34(2):94.

    Evaluation of 53 children with flexible flatfoot found foot symptoms in 65% and functional limitations in 68%. Body mass index was positively correlated with the presence of symptoms and their severity. Functional assessment by specific tests was recommended. Level of evidence: III.

47. Mosca VS: Flexible flatfoot in children and adolescents. *J Child Orthop* 2010;4(2):107-121.

    Comprehensive review of flexible flatfoot, including epidemiology, clinical and radiographic features, and treatment. Level of evidence: V.

48. Basmajian JV, Stecko G: The role of muscles in arch supports of the foot. *J Bone Joint Surg Am* 1963;45:1184-1190.

49. Metcalfe SA, Bowling FL, Baltzopoulos V, Maganaris C, Reeves ND: The reliability of measurements taken from radiographs in the assessment of paediatric flat foot deformity. *Foot (Edinb)* 2012;22(3):156-162.

    An assessment of the interrater and intrarater reliability of 10 key radiographic measures found wide variation, with a strong negative correlation between reliability and the number of steps required for the measurement. Level of evidence: III.

50. Moraleda L, Mubarak SJ: Flexible flatfoot: Differences in the relative alignment of each segment of the foot between symptomatic and asymptomatic patients. *J Pediatr Orthop* 2011;31(4):421-428.

    A review of 135 patients with flexible flatfoot found no differences between symptomatic and asymptomatic feet in alignment of the hindfoot, longitudinal arch, lateral column length, or pronation-supination of the forefoot. Lateral displacement of the navicular appeared to be related to onset of symptoms. Level of evidence: III.

51. Jane MacKenzie A, Rome K, Evans AM: The efficacy of nonsurgical interventions for pediatric flexible flat foot: A critical review. *J Pediatr Orthop* 2012;32(8):830-834.

    A systematic literature review found only limited evidence for the efficacy of nonsurgical interventions. This lack of good-quality evidence should be considered in decision making for the management of pediatric flatfoot. Level of evidence: IV.

52. Rome K, Ashford RL, Evans A: Non-surgical interventions for paediatric pes planus. *Cochrane Database Syst Rev* 2010;7:CD006311.

    A review determined that evidence from randomized controlled studies is too limited for drawing conclusions about the use of nonsurgical interventions for pediatric flatfoot. Level of evidence: I.

53. Metcalfe SA, Bowling FL, Reeves ND: Subtalar joint arthroereisis in the management of pediatric flexible flatfoot: A critical review of the literature. *Foot Ankle Int* 2011;32(12):1127-1139.

    In a literature review, eight of nine radiographic parameters showed substantial improvement after subtalar arthroereisis in pediatric patients with flexible flatfoot. Static arch height and joint congruency were increased. Rates of patient satisfaction ranged from 79% to 100%. The complications included sinus tarsi pain, device extrusion, and undercorrection. Complication rates ranged from 5% to 19%, and unplanned removal rates from 7% to 19%. Level of evidence: IV.

54. Scharer BM, Black BE, Sockrider N: Treatment of painful pediatric flatfoot with Maxwell-Brancheau subtalar arthroereisis implant: A retrospective radiographic review. *Foot Ankle Spec* 2010;3(2):67-72.

    Of 68 feet with a Maxwell-Brancheau subtalar arthroereisis implant, 10 feet (15%) had a complication requiring reoperation. The implant was exchanged in 9 feet because of implant migration, undercorrection, or overcorrection. Radiographic evaluation revealed improvement in talonavicular joint coverage and lateral and anterior-posterior talocalcaneal angles. Level of evidence: IV.

55. Jay RM, Din N: Correcting pediatric flatfoot with subtalar arthroereisis and gastrocnemius recession: A retrospective study. *Foot Ankle Spec* 2013;6(2):101-107.

    Treatment of equinus deformity with gastrocnemius recession and arthroereisis in 20 children (34 feet) reduced pain and improved function in all 34 feet. The AOFAS score increased an average of 21 points after surgery. Level of evidence: IV.

56. de Coulon G, Turcot K, Canavese F, Dayer R, Kaelin A, Ceroni D: Talonavicular arthrodesis for the treatment of neurological flat foot deformity in pediatric patients: Clinical and radiographic evaluation of 29 feet. *J Pediatr Orthop* 2011;31(5):557-563.

    Talonavicular arthrodesis led to satisfactory results in 28 of 29 feet with neurologic flatfoot deformity. At an average 3-year follow-up, improvements in radiographic measurement angles were maintained. Level of evidence: IV.

57. Moraleda L, Salcedo M, Bastrom TP, Wenger DR, Albiñana J, Mubarak SJ: Comparison of the calcaneo-cuboid-cuneiform osteotomies and the calcaneal lengthening osteotomy in the surgical treatment of symptomatic flexible flatfoot. *J Pediatr Orthop* 2012;32(8):821-829.

    Comparison of calcaneal-cuboid-cuneiform osteotomies and the calcaneal lengthening osteotomy found that calcaneal lengthening osteotomy attained greater improvement in the relationship of the navicular to the head of the talus but was associated with more frequent and more severe complications. Level of evidence: III.

58. Sever JW: Apophysitis of the os calcis. *NY Med J* 1912;95:1025.

59. Becerro de Bengoa Vallejo R, Losa Iglesias ME, Rodríguez Sanz D, Prados Frutos JC, Salvadores Fuentes P, Chicharro JL: Plantar pressures in children with and without Sever's disease. *J Am Podiatr Med Assoc* 2011;101(1):17-24.

A comparison of 22 boys with symptoms of calcaneal apophysitis and 24 control subjects used clinical examination and pedobarographic analysis. A relationship was found among hindfoot equinus, high plantar foot pressures, and heel pain. Level of evidence: III.

60. Kose O, Celiktas M, Yigit S, Kisin B: Can we make a diagnosis with radiographic examination alone in calcaneal apophysitis (Sever's disease)? *J Pediatr Orthop B* 2010;19(5):396-398.

Eighty feet (50 with and 30 without Sever disease) were radiographically assessed. Without clinical information, the ability to make a true diagnosis, as well as interobserver and intraobserver reliability, was fair at best. Level of evidence: III.

61. Kose O: Do we really need radiographic assessment for the diagnosis of non-specific heel pain (calcaneal apophysitis) in children? *Skeletal Radiol* 2010;39(4):359-361.

A benign calcaneal cyst was identified in one of 71 radiographs obtained in patients with a diagnosis of calcaneal apophysitis. Level of evidence: IV.

62. Rachel JN, Williams JB, Sawyer JR, Warner WC, Kelly DM: Is radiographic evaluation necessary in children with a clinical diagnosis of calcaneal apophysitis (Sever disease)? *J Pediatr Orthop* 2011;31(5):548-550.

Radiographic abnormalities were found in 5 of 96 patients (5%) with heel pain. Abnormal findings resulted in more aggressive treatment of these patients, including immobilization and radiographic follow-up. Level of evidence: IV.

63. Iselin H: Wachstumbeschwerden zur Zeit der Knocheren Entwicklung der Tuberositas metatarsi quinti. [In German] *Deut Z Chi* 1912;117:529.

64. Canale ST, Williams KD: Iselin's disease. *J Pediatr Orthop* 1992;12(1):90-93.

65. Atbasi Z, Ege T, Kose O, Egerci OF, Demiralp B: Osteochondrosis of the medial cuneiform bone in a child: A case report and review of 18 published cases. *Foot Ankle Spec* 2013;6(2):154-158.

A 6-year-old boy with medial foot pain and radiographic evidence of bilateral medial cuneiform osteochondrosis

was successfully treated with activity modification and analgesia. Level of evidence: V.

66. Klein R, Burgkart R, Woertler K, Gradinger R, Vogt S: Osteochondrosis juvenilis of the medial malleolar epiphysis. *J Bone Joint Surg Br* 2008;90(6):810-812.

A 12-year-old boy with bilateral pes planus and osteochondrosis of the medial malleoli was successfully treated nonsurgically. Level of evidence: V.

67. Köhler A: Ueber eine haufige bisher anscheinend unbekannte Erkrankung einzelner Kinklicherkernochen. [In German] *Muchen Med Wochnschr* 1908;55:1923.

68. Ippolito E, Ricciardi Pollini PT, Falez' F: Köhler's disease of the tarsal navicular: Long-term follow-up of 12 cases. *J Pediatr Orthop* 1984;4(4):416-417.

69. Freiberg AH: Infraction of the second metatarsal bone: A typical injury. *Surg Gynecol Obstet* 1914;19:191-193.

70. Cerrato RA: Freiberg's disease. *Foot Ankle Clin* 2011;16(4):647-658.

A review of Freiberg disease included the proposed etiologies, diagnosis, and surgical and nonsurgical treatment options. Level of evidence: V.

71. Chao KH, Lee CH, Lin LC: Surgery for symptomatic Freiberg's disease: Extraarticular dorsal closing-wedge osteotomy in 13 patients followed for 2-4 years. *Acta Orthop Scand* 1999;70(5):483-486.

72. Miyamoto W, Takao M, Uchio Y, Kono T, Ochi M: Late-stage Freiberg disease treated by osteochondral plug transplantation: A case series. *Foot Ankle Int* 2008;29(9):950-955.

Four girls (average age, 12 years) were treated with osteochondral plug transplantation from the ipsilateral knee to the damaged metatarsal head. At 1-year follow-up, radiographic and arthroscopic examination results were satisfactory. Level of evidence: IV.

73. Tsuda E, Ishibashi Y, Yamamoto Y, Maeda S, Kimura Y, Sato H: Osteochondral autograft transplantation for advanced stage Freiberg disease in adolescent athletes: A report of 3 cases and surgical procedures. *Am J Sports Med* 2011;39(11):2470-2475.

The surgical techniques for osteochondral autograft plug transplantation in three patients with advanced collapse were described in detail. At 2-year follow-up, all three patients had a good clinical result. Level of evidence: V.

Neuromuscular Disease

SECTION EDITOR:

RUTH L. THOMAS, MD

Chapter 5

Cavovarus Deformity

A. Holly Johnson, MD

Introduction

The cavovarus foot involves a complex array of deformities of the hindfoot, midfoot, and forefoot. The elevated medial longitudinal arch is caused by hyperplantar flexion of the first ray (forefoot equinus) and relative dorsiflexion of the calcaneus (calcaneocavus). The hindfoot is in varus, and the forefoot is pronated. Claw toes develop, and the plantar metatarsal fat pad migrates distally. These characteristic deformities result from muscle imbalance secondary to a neurologic, traumatic, or other cause. Altered foot and ankle mechanics and the resulting abnormal gait cause a multitude of issues, including lateral instability, bony overload and stress fracture, loss of motion, and possibly a fixed arthritic limb. Treatment is guided by the relative flexibility of the foot and the extent of deformity

Etiology

Cavovarus foot deformities have several etiologies. In the past, approximately one third of incidences were classified as idiopathic, but improved diagnostic methods have determined that many of these incidences are attributable to a neurologic disease.[1] Charcot-Marie-Tooth (CMT) disease is the most common cause of pes cavovarus, but other etiologies also have been identified[2,3] (Table 1).

The most common neurologic causes of pes cavus are hereditary motor sensory neuropathies, which are responsible for CMT disease as well as other, less common syndromes and diseases. CMT disease encompasses several genetically varied syndromes with similar clinical manifestations. Jean-Martin Charcot, a French neurologist and anatomist, described the disease with Pierre Marie in 1886. Also in 1886, Howard Tooth, an English physician, described the same disorder as peroneal muscular atrophy.[4]

Neither Dr. Johnson nor any immediate family member has received anything of value from or has stock or stock options held in a commercial company or institution related directly or indirectly to the subject of this chapter.

The CMT neuropathies result from a mutation in one of more than 40 genes that affect Schwann cells and neurons. The disease has demyelinating (CMT1 and CMT4), axonal (CMT2 and CMT4), and intermediate (CMTX, CMT2E, and CMT) forms.[5-7] The classic phenotype of the most common form, CMT1, emanates from an abnormality in the peripheral myelin protein-22 (*PMP22*) gene and is characterized by axonal demyelination that causes distal sensory loss, weakness, and skeletal deformity.[5] Patients with CMT disease typically have abnormalities before they reach age 20 years and often before age 10 years. The peripheral neuropathy leads to distal muscle weakness, with intrinsic muscle degeneration that over time selectively spreads proximally to larger muscle groups, leading to imbalances in forces around the foot and ankle and eventually to cavovarus deformity.[8]

Neurologic conditions including other hereditary motor sensory neuropathies unrelated to CMT disease, amyotrophic lateral sclerosis, Huntington disease, cerebral palsy, spinal cord lesions, and other cerebral injuries also can lead to pes cavovarus.[3] In a child with pes cavus, the clinician must consider a spinal cord anomaly, especially if the deformities are unilateral.[9] Congenital causes of pes cavovarus, such as congenital talipes equinovarus (clubfoot) and arthrogryposis, can be identified from birth. Arthrogryposis typically causes early rigid deformity, but other causes of rigid cavovarus in adolescence or young adulthood can be avoided if they are treated effectively during childhood.[10] In the past, poliomyelitis, which affects the anterior horn cells of the spinal cord, was a common cause of foot and ankle deformity.

Trauma to the lower extremity can cause cavovarus deformity. Malunion of a talar neck fracture leads to shortening of the medial column and a fixed varus position of the talonavicular joint and the hindfoot. An untreated calcaneus fracture can heal in a varus malunion. Superficial peroneal nerve injury can cause foot drop and posterior tibial tendon overdrive. Any isolated tendon injury can leave the strength of the opposing tendon unchecked, causing deformity over time. A burn injury or a compartment syndrome causing muscle contraction and neurologic injury can lead to cavovarus deformity. Some incidences of cavovarus deformity have no obvious etiology and may be the result of an as-yet undetected peripheral neuropathy. Treatment of the deformity and imbalance is not determined, however.

Anatomy and Pathomechanics

Pes cavovarus can be seen as the product of any of several different etiologies arising in an imbalance of both the intrinsic and extrinsic musculature of the foot.[11] Depending on the muscles involved and the etiology of the disorder, the appearance of the deformity varies. Many deformities continue to progress over time.

In the normal foot, proper function is maintained by pairs of muscles working in opposition to each other. These agonist-antagonist pairs keep the foot balanced. If one muscle is disturbed, relative overdrive of the opposing muscle results, and a deformity develops. Understanding the normal anatomy and function of the muscle groups is essential to comprehending the pathologic cavovarus foot (Table 2).

The tibialis anterior, which inserts on the navicular and medial cuneiform, acts as a primary dorsiflexor and secondary inverter of the ankle. The antagonist of the tibialis anterior is the peroneus longus, which acts as a plantar flexor and weak evertor; it inserts on the plantar aspect of the medial cuneiform and the first metatarsal base. The tibialis posterior, with its wide insertion along the medial and plantar medial aspect of the medial column, inverts the foot primarily and plantar flexes secondarily. The tibialis posterior is opposed by the peroneus brevis, a strong evertor that inserts at the base of the fifth metatarsal.

The intrinsic muscles, including the lumbricals and the interossei, insert into the extensor mechanism at the proximal phalanx; they flex the metatarsophalangeal (MTP) joints and extend the proximal and distal interphalangeal joints. The extrinsic extensor muscles, including the extensor digitorum longus, extensor hallucis longus, extensor digitorum brevis, and extensor hallucis brevis, extend the toes through the MTP, proximal interphalangeal, and distal interphalangeal joints. The extrinsic long flexors (including the flexor digitorum longus and flexor hallucis longus) and the short flexors (including the flexor digitorum brevis and flexor hallucis brevis) flex the toes at the proximal and distal interphalangeal joints.

CMT disease is the most commonly used template for cavovarus deformity. In the most widely accepted etiology, weakness in the peroneus brevis and tibialis anterior is primarily responsible for the deformity. As these two muscle groups deteriorate, the peroneus longus and tibialis posterior initially are spared and increase in strength. Dorsiflexion through the tibialis anterior and long toe extensors and eversion through the peroneus brevis are compromised. The opposing muscles are left unrestrained. The overpull of the tibialis posterior leads to medial displacement of the talonavicular and calcaneal cuboid joints and locks the subtalar joint in supination.[4] The peroneus longus pulls the first ray into plantar flexion. As the tibialis anterior becomes unable to dorsiflex the ankle, the long toe extensors attempt to act as a substitute, and they hyperextend the toes at the MTP joints. Weakness of the intrinsic muscles contributes to the clawing of the toes and distal migration of the plantar fat pad. Forefoot equinus and plantar flexion of the first ray cause forefoot pronation. As the forefoot deformity becomes fixed, the hindfoot becomes fixed in varus to keep the foot plantigrade[10,12] (Figure 1).

The mechanism of development may be different in cavovarus stemming from another etiology. In poliomyelitis, triceps surae involvement causes weak push-off

Table 2

Muscles of the Foot and Ankle

Muscle	Insertion	Function	Antagonist
Tibialis anterior	Navicular, medial cuneiform	Strong dorsiflexion, weak inversion	Peroneus longus
Tibialis posterior	Medial column (wide insertion at medial and plantar midfoot and forefoot)	Strong inversion, weak plantar flexion	Peroneus brevis
Peroneus longus	First metatarsal base, medial cuneiform	Strong plantar flexion of the first metatarsal, weak eversion	Tibialis anterior
Peroneus brevis	Fifth metatarsal base	Eversion	Tibialis posterior
Intrinsics (lumbricals, interossei)	Proximal phalanges (extensor expansions)	Flexion of metatarsophalangeal joints, extension of proximal and distal interphalangeal joints	Extrinsic long extensors and flexors
Extrinsic long extensors (extensor digitorum longus, extensor hallucis longus, extensor digitorum brevis, extensor hallucis brevis)	Extensor hood at metatarsophalangeal joint, distal phalanges	Extension of metatarsophalangeal joints, proximal and distal interphalangeal joints	Intrinsics, extrinsic long flexors
Extrinsic long flexors (flexor digitorum longus, flexor hallucis longus, flexor digitorum brevis, flexor hallucis brevis)	Flexor sheath, plantar aspect of distal phalanges	Toe flexion at proximal and distal interphalangeal joints	Extrinsic long extensors

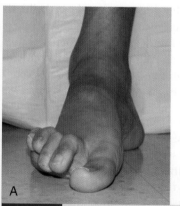 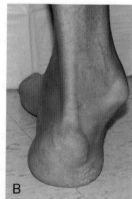

Figure 1 Photographs show a cavovarus foot in a patient with Charcot-Marie-Tooth disease. **A,** Anterolateral view shows the high medial longitudinal arch and clawing of the toes. **B,** Posterior view shows the varus position of the hindfoot. (Reproduced from Johnson AH, May CJ: Adult cavovarus foot. *Orthopaedic Knowledge Online Journal* 2012;10[4]. http://orthoportal.aaos.org/oko/article.aspx?article=OKO_FOO042. Accessed September 4, 2014.)

strength. The long toe flexors are recruited, leading to forefoot plantar flexion and the development of cavus. A deep posterior compartment syndrome with subsequent muscle contracture can lead to tibialis posterior overpull with equinus and cavovarus. Understanding the etiology of the disorder and identifying the affected nerves and muscles usually allows the pathomechanics to be understood.

Diagnosis

Patients typically have pain and/or instability in the foot and ankle. Foot pain may be caused by lateral bony overload at the base of the fifth metatarsal or cuboid or at the sesamoids with hyperplantar flexion of the first ray. There may be a stress fracture at the fifth metatarsal base; recurrent stress fracture can occur in a subtle cavovarus foot or with a fixed deformity.[13] Pain beneath the metatarsal heads may be caused by distal migration of the plantar fat pad associated with subluxated or dislocated MTP joints and claw toes. Late in the disease, when the deformities are fixed, the cause of pain may be secondary to degenerative changes in the joints (particularly the subtalar, midfoot, and ankle joints). Instability typically results from eversion weakness. Hindfoot varus leads to lateral instability at the ankle and subtalar joint. The patient may have frequent ankle sprains and damage to the collateral ligaments.

Children with minimal symptoms of pes cavus are often referred for evaluation. The presence of clinical features such as weakness, unsteady gait, family history, or other neurologic deficits can obviate the need for further testing.[14]

History and Physical Examination

A careful history is an important first step in diagnosing the cause of a cavovarus deformity. The family history can be useful because the patient often describes a sibling or parent with similar physical characteristics. Identification of a family member with pes cavovarus suggests a hereditary neuropathy. A unilateral deformity, especially if it is severe or accompanied by other neurologic abnormalities, may indicate a spinal cord abnormality.[9]

The patient should be examined standing and walking, with the limbs unclothed. During the swing phase of gait, foot drop or recruitment of the toe extensors indicates tibialis anterior weakness. The lower extremities should be compared while the patient is standing. From behind, the position of the heel is noted relative to the midfoot and forefoot; hindfoot varus is more apparent from this viewpoint. The Coleman block test is critical to understanding whether the hindfoot deformity is rigid and whether the deformity is driven by the forefoot or hindfoot. If the heel is corrected to neutral or a few degrees of valgus, the hindfoot is flexible, and correction of the forefoot deformity also will correct the hindfoot deformity. If the hindfoot remains in varus, the deformity is rigid, and a hindfoot and forefoot procedure probably will be necessary for deformity correction[15] (Figure 2).

Joint motion is examined to identify an equinus contracture. If the contracture is not corrected with the knee flexed, the cause may be a tight soleus and/or gastrocnemius, or it may be a mechanical block to dorsiflexion, such as a tibial or talar bone spur or a medialized talus. If dorsiflexion increases when the knee is bent, the gastrocnemius is contracted. A thorough neurologic examination is critical. Vibration, position, sensation, and reflexes as well as muscle strength should be checked, and any muscle atrophy or weakness should be noted. A child should be examined to detect spinal skin dimples, a hair patch, or another sign of occult spinal disease.

Any patient with lateral instability, weakness, frequent sprains, peroneal tendon tear or pain, or fifth metatarsal fracture must be evaluated for a cavovarus deformity. Even a subtle deformity can lead to lateral overload and

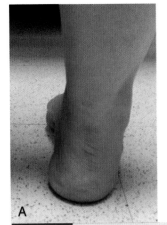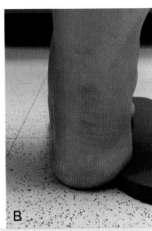

Figure 2 Posterior photographs show a cavovarus deformity before (**A**) and during (**B**) the Coleman block test. With the Coleman block in place, the hindfoot is corrected to neutral, and the hindfoot deformity is found to be flexible.

subsequent deformity. In some patients, alignment must be considered in addition to the acute diagnosis.[16]

The diagnosis of CMT disease typically is based on physical examination findings, neurologic testing, family history, and genetic testing. A physician may be alerted to the presence of pes cavus by physical examination findings consistent with the disorder, such as a high arch, weak extensors, claw toes, and even foot drop. Electromyography and nerve conduction studies can be used to identify patterns of deficiency often seen with CMT disease. If a familial link appears to be present, genetic testing is indicated for purposes of determining the prognosis, a need for family planning, and eligibility for a clinical study.[14,17] Algorithms for neurologic and genetic testing have been developed and published.[18] Nerve biopsies typically are unnecessary for diagnosis.

Imaging Studies

AP, oblique, and lateral weight-bearing radiographs of the foot and ankle are the essential initial imaging studies. An axial heel view, a Canale view of the talar neck, and a Cobey-Saltzman view to evaluate hindfoot alignment may be useful.[19] CT is useful for assessing the extent of joint degeneration and understanding bony alignment. MRI can be used in determining the ligamentous and tendinous integrity of the foot and ankle.

The weight-bearing lateral radiograph is perhaps the most useful study for evaluating and understanding a cavovarus deformity. An understanding of the appearance of a normal lateral radiograph and the commonly measured angles (Meary, Hibb, and calcaneal pitch) is helpful for identifying radiographic abnormalities and variations[20] (Figure 3). A subtle abnormality, such as a

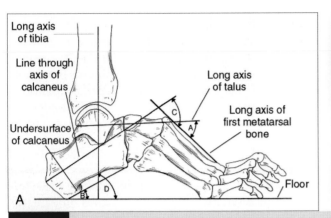
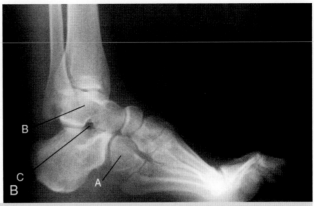

Figure 3 **A,** Schematic drawing shows the angles used to evaluate the cavovarus foot. A = Meary angle, B = calcaneal pitch angle, C = Hibb angle, D = tibioplantar angle. Lateral weight-bearing radiograph (**B**) demonstrates characteristic findings. A = bell-shaped cuboid, B = double talar dome, C = open sinus tarsi. (Panel A adapted with permission from Sabir M, Lyttle D: Pathogenesis of pes cavus in Charcot-Marie-Tooth disease. *Clin Orthop Relat Res* 1983;175:173-178. Panel B adapted from Johnson AH, May CJ: Adult cavovarus foot. *Orthopaedic Knowledge Online Journal* 2012;10[4]. http://orthoportal.aaos.org/oko/article.aspx?article=OKO_FOO042. Accessed September 4, 2014.)

bell-shaped cuboid, a double talar dome, or an open sinus tarsi, also can be identified on a weight-bearing lateral radiograph. If a spinal cord abnormality is suspected, imaging of the hips and spine may be indicated.

Nonsurgical Treatment

The goal of treating a cavovarus foot is to restore normal function and allow the patient to ambulate with a painless plantigrade foot. The treatment varies with the extent of the deformity and its relative flexibility. Nonsurgical treatment may be attempted, but surgery often is necessary. The patient must understand the realistic expectation for success.

Nonsurgical treatment of a cavovarus foot includes the use of orthotic devices and bracing. An off-the-shelf insert, with or without a lateral post, may be beneficial for a foot with mild hindfoot varus, but a custom-molded semirigid orthotic device typically is necessary. Metatarsal pads can be added to offload painful metatarsal heads. Lace-up ankle supports or an Arizona brace can be used to treat ankle instability or pain from degenerative joint changes. A custom-molded ankle-foot orthosis is useful for treating severe ankle and/or subtalar instability, rigid deformity, arthritic pes cavus, or foot drop. Care must be taken to avoid skin breakdown and ulceration, especially in a patient with neuropathy. The patient must be instructed about the potential for skin breakdown.

Shoe modifications and the use of extra-depth shoes may be necessary to accommodate the high arch and claw toes of a cavovarus foot. Special shoes also may be required to allow sufficient room for seating an ankle brace or other orthotic device.

Surgical Treatment Planning

A surgical intervention is chosen based on the extent, etiology, and rigidity of the deformity as well as other variables. The surgical plan should be tailored to the individual patient's needs. The surgeon must clearly communicate the surgical goals, probable recovery time, and reasonable short-term and long-term expectations with the patient.

Careful preoperative planning is crucial. Flexible joints should be preserved, but rigid arthritic joints may require fusion. In a patient with muscle imbalance, tendon transfers and realigning osteotomies lead to better outcomes than fusion.[21,22] Patients who underwent triple arthrodesis during childhood often return in young adulthood with arthritic ankles and few viable options for reconstruction. Contracted tendons should be released or lengthened, and contracted joints should be released.[2] Some surgeons prefer early surgical intervention to prevent progressive deformity in patients with identified muscle imbalance.

Preoperative planning must include thorough imaging and diagnostic studies. Standard radiographs including three weight-bearing views of the foot and ankle are mandatory. CT may be necessary for understanding the three-dimensional anatomy of the foot and gauging the extent of joint degeneration. MRI is useful for evaluating ligament and tendon integrity and assessing the cartilaginous surface of the joints to determine whether fusion or joint salvage is preferable. If tendon transfers are being considered and physical examination findings are equivocal, electromyography may be needed to assess tendon strength and viability.

Soft-Tissue Procedures

Plantar Fascia Release

The plantar fascia in a cavovarus foot often is contracted as a result of the calcaneovarus and the first ray plantar flexion. A plantar fascia release (Steindler procedure) often is the first step in cavovarus reconstruction.[23] The patient is positioned supine, and a thigh or calf tourniquet is used. An oblique incision of approximately 3 cm is made at the glabrous fold medially at the level of the medial insertion point of the plantar fascia. Meticulous dissection is done through the fat to the fascia of the abductor hallucis, and the fascia is released. The tight plantar fascia is identified and isolated with thyroid retractors or Freer elevators above and below. The fascia is released sharply using a No. 15 blade transversely. The wound is irrigated and closed. The postoperative protocol is based on the requirements of other foot procedures done at the same time.

Gastrocnemius Recession

Depending on the extent of the equinus component, a heel cord lengthening is likely to be part of any cavovarus foot reconstruction. Gastrocnemius tightness may limit the ability of other procedures, such as calcaneal osteotomy, to correct the deformity.[24,25] If the hindfoot is in varus, the Achilles tendon is effectively shortened, and the type of lengthening depends on the extent of Achilles tendon involvement. A preoperative Silfverskiöld test helps determine whether the contracture is coming from the gastrocnemius or the Achilles tendon.[26] Ankle dorsiflexion is assessed with the knee first held straight and then flexed 90°. If the gastrocnemius is tight, dorsiflexion is limited with the knee extended (the gastrocnemius is stretched) and is improved with the knee flexed (the gastrocnemius is relaxed). If ankle dorsiflexion is limited with the knee either flexed or extended, the Achilles tendon is tight.

Gastrocnemius recession is done with the patient supine and the use of a thigh tourniquet. A 4- to 5-cm longitudinal incision is made in the midcalf. The dissection is carried down to the fascia, with care to avoid and protect the saphenous nerve and vein. The fascia is incised the length of the incision. Blunt dissection is used to identify the gastrocnemius muscle at the point before it joins the soleus at the Achilles tendon. The gastrocnemius is isolated with retractors or a speculum, and the gastrocnemius fascia is released medially to laterally as the ankle is held in dorsiflexion. Care should be taken to identify and protect the sural nerve, which often is just posterior to the fascia. After the release, the ankle is gently stretched in dorsiflexion. The fascia should be reapproximated to avoid muscle herniation.

Heel Cord Lengthening

If Achilles tendon contracture is responsible for the equinus component of the cavovarus deformity, the tendon can be lengthened in an open or percutaneous procedure. Percutaneous lengthening usually is adequate, but occasionally an open lengthening is necessary to gain adequate length. In percutaneous lengthening, the patient is prone or supine, depending on the concomitant procedures. Three small stab incisions are made longitudinally 1.5 to 2 cm apart along the center of the tendon, starting 1.5 to 2 cm proximal to the tendinous insertion. Through the stab incision, a No. 15 blade is turned 90°, and the lateral half of the tendon is released transversely. Through another stab incision, the medial half of the tendon is released 1.5 cm proximally. Finally, in the same manner, the lateral half is released 1.5 cm proximally. The ankle is tensioned in dorsiflexion, and the tendon slowly is Z-lengthened. Open lengthening usually is done through a medial incision.

Modified Jones Procedure

With loss of tibialis anterior strength, the extensor hallucis longus overcompensates to aid in ankle dorsiflexion. The result is hyperdorsiflexion of the first MTP joint and clawing of the big toe. The pulling of the peroneus longus to plantar flex the first ray contributes to the deformity. Traditionally, this deformity has been treated using the modified Jones procedure.[27] Fusing the interphalangeal joint and transferring the extensor hallucis longus to the metatarsal head largely corrects the deformity.[28] The interphalangeal joint is fused first. Through a small dorsal incision, the interphalangeal joint is prepared, compressed, and fixed with crossing screws or a single 4.0 screw across the joint. The extensor hallucis longus is released from its insertion. The distal metatarsal is exposed, and a transverse drill hole is made across the level of the distal third of the joint. The extensor hallucis longus is threaded through the hole and sewn back onto itself while the ankle is held in 10° of dorsiflexion.

An alternative to the Jones procedure involves harvesting the flexor hallucis longus, which is released through a medial incision at the MTP joint as far distally as possible. The tendon is passed plantar to dorsal through a 2.5-mm drill hole in the plantar base of the proximal phalanx, and then sewn back to itself or to the periosteum. The extensor hallucis longus may need to be lengthened, and the MTP capsule may need to be released.[29,30]

Peroneus Brevis to Peroneus Longus Tenodesis and Lateral Ligament Reconstruction

Lateral instability typically is present with peroneus brevis weakness and relative peroneus longus overdrive, as seen in CMT disease. In other disorders causing pes cavovarus, such as peroneal nerve injury, traumatic tendon rupture, and chronic ankle instability, hindfoot varus and peroneal deficiency can lead to mechanical lateral instability. If the peroneus longus remains intact and functional, it can act as an evertor after tenodesis to the remaining peroneus brevis tendon.

The peroneal tendons are exposed laterally at the ankle and hindfoot. The peroneus longus is sewn side to side to the peroneus brevis at the level of the ankle joint posterior to the fibula, using a strong nonabsorbable suture. If the peroneus brevis is damaged, it should be resected just distal to the tenodesis site. An intact peroneus brevis can remain, and tenodesis of the peroneus longus can be done distally, close to its insertion on the fifth metatarsal. Torn but viable lateral ligaments should be imbricated and reattached to their footprints on the distal fibula using suture anchors. The extensor retinaculum can be mobilized and oversewn to reinforce the repair (the Broström-Gould technique).[31]

Posterior Tibial Tendon Transfer

The tendon is harvested through a medial incision from its broad insertion along the navicular and medial column. Another small incision is made 8 to 10 cm above the ankle joint adjacent to the medial tibia, through which the tendon is pulled proximally. A lateral incision is made 3 to 4 cm distal to this, and the tendon is tunneled through the interosseus membrane, exiting in the anterior compartment. Finally, the tendon is tunneled under the soft tissue, under the retinaculum to the middle or lateral cuneiform, and is fixed with a biotenodesis screw. Care is taken to fix the tendon while the ankle is held in a neutral position to provide adequate tension. Final fixation of the tendon should be delayed until the end of the surgery, after any concomitant procedures are completed.

Other Tendon Transfers

Other tendon transfers may be considered, depending on the etiology of the deformity and the extent of weakness, even though these transfers may not be traditional for cavovarus deformity. For example, there may be a need to transfer an anterior tibial tendon laterally to the middle or lateral cuneiform so that it will not continue to contribute to inversion. The extensor digitorum longus can be used for dorsiflexion of the foot if the posterior tibial tendon is weak. The tendon slips can be released distally and sutured together, and then routed to the dorsal midfoot at the middle or lateral cuneiform and secured with a biotenodesis screw or through a bone tunnel. Releasing the long extensors distally helps to correct toe clawing.[29]

Bony Procedures

First Metatarsal Dorsiflexion Osteotomy

If the primary cause of a cavovarus deformity is in the forefoot, as is typical in CMT disease, a first metatarsal dorsiflexion osteotomy is needed for correction. With a hyperplantar-flexed first ray in CMT disease or another disorder, the patient may report plantar forefoot pain and have clawing of the of the first MTP joint. A longitudinal incision is made over the dorsum of the base of the first metatarsal, the osteotomy is made 1 cm distal to the first tarsometatarsal joint, and a 4- to 5-mm dorsal wedge is removed. The gap is closed and fixed with a 2.7-mm plate or with 2.7- or 3.5-mm screws. Alternatively, the first tarsometatarsal joint can be fused in dorsiflexion, with similar results.

Calcaneal Osteotomy

A hindfoot varus deformity that is not passively correctable manually or with the Coleman block test should be treated using a calcaneal osteotomy. The osteotomy moves the heel into a physiologically neutral or slightly valgus position. The Achilles tendon often must be lengthened through gastrocnemius recession or direct tendon lengthening to allow the tuber to shift laterally and thereby shift the Achilles tendon moment arm laterally. Calcaneal osteotomy not only corrects hindfoot varus but also shifts the center of force laterally at the ankle joint.[32]

The Dwyer closing-wedge osteotomy shortens the calcaneus, can weaken the Achilles tendon, and often undercorrects the hindfoot varus.[33-36] A lateral slide osteotomy can achieve a powerful correction without shortening the calcaneus (Figure 4). In this procedure, the incision is made laterally on the heel extending from the anterior aspect of the Achilles tendon insertion to the anterior edge of the calcaneal tuber. The cut should be perpendicular to the long axis of the calcaneus. Two 1.25-mm guidewires can be used superiorly and inferiorly to mark the intended location of the osteotomy, which can be confirmed on lateral fluoroscopy. A sagittal saw is used to make the cut, and a wide osteotome or laminar spreader is used to spread the periosteum medially to allow the heel to slide 1 cm laterally. The posterior fragment can also be moved superiorly to decrease the calcaneal pitch. The osteotomy is fixed with two screws placed anteriorly through the posterior tuber. Overhanging lateral bone is tamped down or resected for bone graft (Figure 5).

The Z-shaped osteotomy is another powerful procedure to correct hindfoot varus.[33] This version of the calcaneal lateral slide allows multiplanar correction[34] (Figure 6). A Z-shaped cut is made laterally into the calcaneus. The superior vertical limb is cut about 1.5 cm anterior to the Achilles insertion at the slope of the

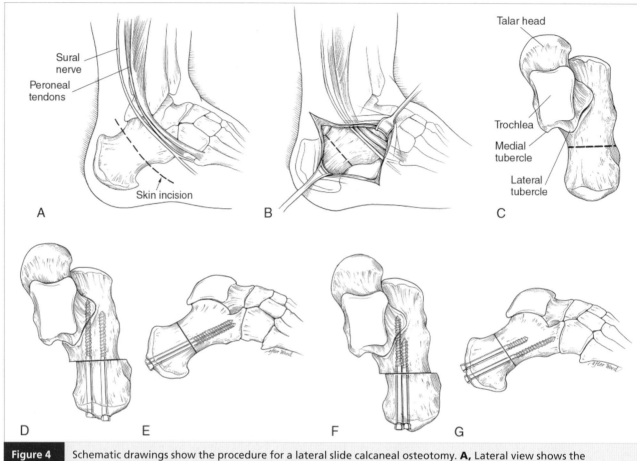

Figure 4 Schematic drawings show the procedure for a lateral slide calcaneal osteotomy. **A,** Lateral view shows the posterior lateral incision. **B,** Lateral view shows placement of the calcaneus cut with a saw after the soft tissues have been retracted, **C,** Oblique coronal view of the osteotomy, which avoids penetrating close to the sustentaculum tali. **D** and **E** show the osteotomy held with two side-by-side transcalcaneal screws. **F** and **G** show alternative screw positioning with superior and inferior screws. Dashed line = incision, solid line = osteotomy. (Adapted with permission from Hansen ST Jr, ed: *Functional Reconstruction of the Foot and Ankle*. Philadelphia, PA, Lippincott Williams & Wilkins, 2000, p. 369.)

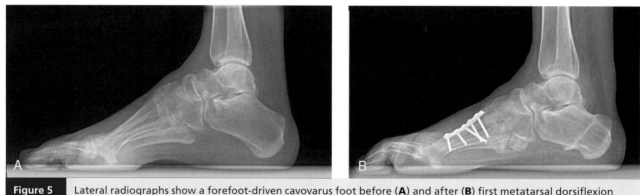

Figure 5 Lateral radiographs show a forefoot-driven cavovarus foot before (**A**) and after (**B**) first metatarsal dorsiflexion osteotomy, lateral ligament reconstruction with peroneus longus–to–peroneus brevis tenodesis, calcaneal osteotomy, and gastrocnemius recession.

superior calcaneal cortex. The inferior vertical limb is cut at the posterior extent of the posterior facet. A horizontal saw cut joins the cut limbs, and a lateral-based wedge is removed to increase the valgus correction. The heel is moved laterally and may also be externally rotated. One or two screws are used for fixation (**Figure 7**).

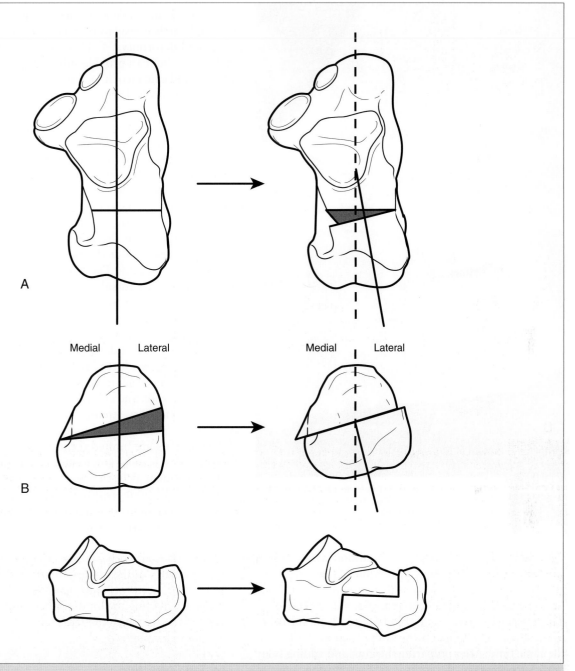

A

Medial   Lateral   Medial   Lateral

B

Figure 6 Schematic drawings show steps in a Z-shaped osteotomy. This triplanar osteotomy allows both translation and rotation for a more powerful correction of the hindfoot varus. The solid vertical lines on the left drawings and the dashed lines on the right drawings represent the central axis of the calcaneus in each plane. **A,** Axial view of the calcaneal osteotomy (left), then shows the lateral rotation of the osteotomy with medial gapping (right). **B,** Posterior view of the calcaneus shows the lateral wedge cut (left) then removed and closed down creating valgus through the cut (right). **C,** Lateral view of the calcaneus shows the lateral wedge cut (left), then the wedge removed and closed down creating valgus through the cut (right).

Fusion

Fusion is indicated if the deformities are rigid or arthritic and symptomatic, and a plantigrade, stable foot cannot be achieved through osteotomy, tissue releases, and tendon transfers alone. Arthrodesis cannot be used in isolation in the presence of deforming muscular forces, however, or further deformity may occur. Muscle balancing must be concomitant with fusion to maintain the neutral position achieved at the time of surgery.[2]

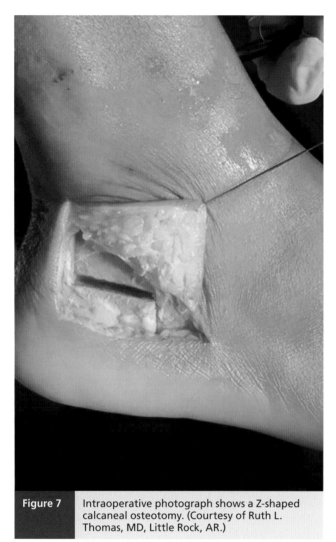

Figure 7 Intraoperative photograph shows a Z-shaped calcaneal osteotomy. (Courtesy of Ruth L. Thomas, MD, Little Rock, AR.)

Subtalar fusion is used if rigid hindfoot varus coexists with degenerative changes in the joint. The varus can be corrected through the joint by removing lateral bone or adding a bone block to the medial side of the joint. The approach to the subtalar joint depends on the other procedures to be done on the lateral side of the foot at the same time. After preparing the joint and adding bone graft, if necessary, the joint is stabilized with internal fixation and is assessed clinically and radiographically. If residual varus remains, a calcaneal slide osteotomy can be added before final fixation with two screws from the heel into the talar dome and neck.

A triple arthrodesis is indicated if degenerative changes are seen at the talonavicular, calcaneocuboid, and/or subtalar joint. Often the medial capsule and a portion of the posterior tibial tendon must be released to rotate the talus medially in relation to the navicular joint. The joints are prepared and fixed in the standard fashion, and concomitant forefoot procedures are done as needed.

The Siffert beak triple arthrodesis combines osteotomy and triple arthrodesis to correct varus and cavus in severe, rigid deformity.[37,38] This correction is technically challenging but can provide substantial correction. The subtalar and calcaneocuboid joints are prepared through a lateral approach. Through a medial approach, the capsule over the talonavicular joint is elevated without stripping the blood supply to the talus. Step cuts are made in the plantar aspect of the talar head and in the adjacent dorsal navicular, with more bone taken dorsally, and the two bones are linked into each other. The lateral side is shortened through the calcaneocuboid joint. The joints are fixed with screws and/or plates.[37]

Midfoot osteotomies with fusion can be useful for correcting cavus. In the Jahss osteotomy, dorsal bone wedges are resected at the tarsometatarsal joints, and the joints are fused.[39] The Cole and Japas osteotomies correct cavus with dorsal closing-wedge osteotomies and navicular cuneiform fusion.[4] The Siffert beak triple arthrodesis incorporates closing wedge osteotomies at the talonavicular, calcaneocuboid, and subtalar joints as part of a triple arthrodesis to correct severe rigid deformity.[38] These procedures can be challenging, and fusion may be difficult to achieve. Newer procedures including navicular excision and cuboid closing-wedge osteotomies for severe deformity attempt to salvage any motion and avoid fusion in relatively young patients.[40]

The options are limited if the foot deformity is rigid and the ankle is in a symptomatic arthritic varus state. Pantalar fusion may be the only viable option to straighten the foot and ankle (Figure 8). Some surgeons use total ankle replacement in combination with triple arthrodesis or foot reconstruction in some patients with cavovarus and ankle arthritis[41] (Figure 8). Total ankle replacement should be selected with caution because any remaining varus deformity in the ankle can lead to abnormal patterns of wear on the prosthesis and early failure of components. Correcting the hindfoot deformity and plantar flexion of the first ray was reported to help realign the ankle out of varus.[42]

Claw Toe Correction

Claw toes result from extensor overload at the MTP joints and flexor overload at the proximal interphalangeal joints. Dynamic deformities can be resolved with correction of the deforming forces after a cavovarus reconstruction of the foot.[6] Flexor-to-extensor transfer can be useful for flexible deformities that persist. The Taylor procedure and its iterations essentially involve transferring the flexor digitorum longus to the extensor digitorum longus dorsally at the MTP joint.[43,44] Through a dorsal incision at the MTP joint, the long flexor is carefully dissected and then released as far distally as possible. The tendon

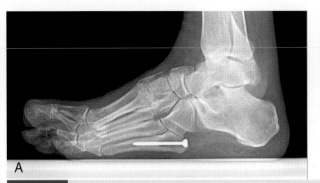
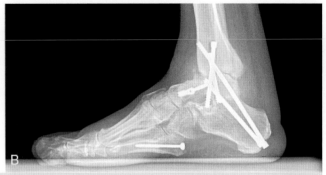

Figure 8 Lateral radiographs show severe, rigid cavovarus in a patient with multiple sclerosis. **A,** The patient had a prior fifth metatarsal stress fracture from lateral overload fixated with a screw. **B,** Image taken after a pantalar fusion to reestablish a plantigrade, stable weight-bearing foot.

is brought up on the lateral side of the joint or split and sutured, each end to the medial and the lateral side of the extensor expansion. Rigid claw toes require formal correction with MTP releases, proximal interphalangeal resections, and pinning to fuse and straighten the toes.

Summary

The cavovarus foot is characterized by hindfoot varus, a high medial longitudinal arch, and claw toes caused by muscle imbalances. The clinical findings vary depending on the etiology and severity of the deformity. Cavovarus foot can be caused by a neurologic disorder, trauma, a congenital deformity, or an unknown cause. A neurologic workup should be considered if the cause is unknown or the deformity is bilateral. The treatment is based on the extent of deformity and the flexibility of the foot. The goals are to preserve motion, if possible, and to establish a plantigrade, pain-free foot. Surgery may be indicated if nonsurgical treatment is unsuccessful or the deformity progresses. Soft-tissue and bony procedures including tendon transfers and osteotomies should be tailored to the characteristics of the foot. Arthrodesis can be used to treat arthritic or rigid deformity. The surgical plan must be well thought out and individualized to reestablish function and preserve motion, if possible, with careful consideration of the patient's needs and the possibility of future intervention.

Annotated References

1. Piazza S, Ricci G, Caldarazzo Ienco E, et al: Pes cavus and hereditary neuropathies: When a relationship should be suspected. *J Orthop Traumatol* 2010;11(4):195-201.

   Pes cavus was described as a spy sign in hereditary peripheral neuropathies, especially in patients with a positive family history, abnormal gait, bilateral deformities, or neurologic symptoms.

2. Younger AS, Hansen ST Jr: Adult cavovarus foot. *J Am Acad Orthop Surg* 2005;13(5):302-315.

3. Lovell WW, Morrissy RT, Winter RB, eds: *Lovell and Winter's Pediatric Orthopaedics*, ed 3. Philadelphia, PA, Lippincott Williams & Wilkins, 1990.

4. Wenz W, Dreher T: Charcot-Marie-Tooth disease and the cavovarus foot, in Pinzur MS, ed: *Orthopaedic Knowledge Update: Foot and Ankle 4*. Rosemont, IL, American Academy of Orthopaedic Surgeons, 2008, pp 291-306.

   A review chapter of Charcot-Marie-Tooth disease and the cavovarus foot designed for orthopaedic education and learning. Level of evidence: IV.

5. Patzkó A, Shy ME: Update on Charcot-Marie-Tooth disease. *Curr Neurol Neurosci Rep* 2011;11(1):78-88.

   Underlying pathomechanisms, diagnostic methods, and emerging therapeutic strategies in Charcot-Marie-Tooth disease were reviewed.

6. Thomas PK, Griffin JW, Low P, Poduslo J, Dyck PJ, eds: *Peripheral Neuropathy*, ed 3. Philadelphia, PA, WB Saunders, 1993.

7. Bird TD, Ott J, Giblett ER, Chance PF, Sumi SM, Kraft GH: Genetic linkage evidence for heterogeneity in Charcot-Marie-Tooth neuropathy (HMSN type I). *Ann Neurol* 1983;14(6):679-684.

8. Holmes JR, Hansen ST Jr: Foot and ankle manifestations of Charcot-Marie-Tooth disease. *Foot Ankle* 1993;14(8):476-486.

9. Miller A, Guille JT, Bowen JR: Evaluation and treatment of diastematomyelia. *J Bone Joint Surg Am* 1993;75(9):1308-1317.

10. Alexander IJ, Johnson KA: Assessment and management of pes cavus in Charcot-Marie-Tooth disease. *Clin Orthop Relat Res* 1989;246:273-281.

2: Neuromuscular Disease

11. Samilson RL, Dillin W: Cavus, cavovarus, and calcaneocavus: An update. *Clin Orthop Relat Res* 1983;177:125-132.

12. McCluskey WP, Lovell WW, Cummings RJ: The cavovarus foot deformity: Etiology and management. *Clin Orthop Relat Res* 1989;247:27-37.

13. Bluth B, Eagan M, Otsuka NY: Stress fractures of the lateral rays in the cavovarus foot: Indication for surgical intervention. *Orthopedics* 2011;34(10):e696-e699.

    The incidence of fifth metatarsal stress fracture is increasing in patients with cavovarus deformity. Surgical intervention was recommended for patients with an active lifestyle who have severe deformity or subtle pes cavus, so as to decrease the risk of fracture recurrence and further morbidity. Level of evidence: IV.

14. Karakis I, Gregas M, Darras BT, Kang PB, Jones HR: Clinical correlates of Charcot-Marie-Tooth disease in patients with pes cavus deformities. *Muscle Nerve* 2013;47(4):488-492.

    Clinical features can help predict whether a patient has Charcot-Marie-Tooth (CMT) disease, thereby allowing expensive and often painful nerve and muscle testing to be avoided. Family history as well as weakness, gait unsteadiness, and other neurologic signs associated with pes cavus were strongly linked to a diagnosis of CMT disease in more than half of 70 pediatric patients. Level of evidence: II.

15. Coleman SS, Chesnut WJ: A simple test for hindfoot flexibility in the cavovarus foot. *Clin Orthop Relat Res* 1977;123:60-62.

16. Maskill MP, Maskill JD, Pomeroy GC: Surgical management and treatment algorithm for the subtle cavovarus foot. *Foot Ankle Int* 2010;31(12):1057-1063.

    This case control study of 23 patients who underwent various procedures including calcaneal osteotomy, peroneus longus to brevis transfer, Achilles lengthening, and first metatarsal osteotomy showed average postoperative American Orthopaedic Foot and Ankle Society hindfoot score improvement from 45 to 90, and improved radiographic parameters. Level of evidence: III

17. Miller LJ, Saporta AS, Sottile SL, Siskind CE, Feely SM, Shy ME: Strategy for genetic testing in Charcot-Marie-disease. *Acta Myol* 2011;30(2):109-116.

    A retrospective study of more than 1,000 patients with Charcot-Marie-Tooth disease analyzed family history, phenotypes, and prevalence to create algorithms designed to guide genetic testing. Level of evidence: II.

18. Murphy SM, Laura M, Fawcett K, et al: Charcot-Marie-Tooth disease: Frequency of genetic subtypes and guidelines for genetic testing. *J Neurol Neurosurg Psychiatry* 2012;83(7):706-710.

    Genetic sequencing for 1,607 patients with Charcot-Marie-Tooth (CMT) disease found that four genes account for 90% of the CMT subtypes. Guidelines for genetic testing of patients suspected to have CMT disease were based on these data. Level of evidence: II.

19. Saltzman CL, el-Khoury GY: The hindfoot alignment view. *Foot Ankle Int* 1995;16(9):572-576.

20. Schwend RM, Drennan JC: Cavus foot deformity in children. *J Am Acad Orthop Surg* 2003;11(3):201-211.

21. Ward CM, Dolan LA, Bennett DL, Morcuende JA, Cooper RR: Long-term results of reconstruction for treatment of a flexible cavovarus foot in Charcot-Marie-Tooth disease. *J Bone Joint Surg Am* 2008;90(12):2631-2642.

    Twenty-five patients post reconstructive procedures without fusions for cavovarus deformity associated with Charcot-Marie-Tooth disease were followed for an average of 26.1 years. Compared with triple arthrodesis, reconstructed patients demonstrated less radiographic progression of degenerative arthritis and a lower reoperation rate. Level of evidence: IV.

22. Leeuwesteijn AE, de Visser E, Louwerens JW: Flexible cavovarus feet in Charcot-Marie-Tooth disease treated with first ray proximal dorsiflexion osteotomy combined with soft tissue surgery: A short-term to mid-term outcome study. *Foot Ankle Surg* 2010;16(3):142-147.

    A retrospective evaluation of short-term to midterm surgical results of 33 patients with Charcot-Marie-Tooth disease and a cavovarus foot found that 90% were satisfied with the result. The surgeries included dorsiflexion osteotomy of the first ray and calcaneal osteotomy with tendon transfers in flexible deformities. Level of evidence: IV.

23. Steindler A: The treatment of pes cavus (hollow claw foot). *Arch Surg* 1921;2(2):325-337.

24. Strayer LM Jr: Recession of the gastrocnemius: An operation to relieve spastic contracture of the calf muscles. *J Bone Joint Surg Am* 1950;32(3):671-676.

25. Strayer LM Jr: Gastrocnemius recession: Five-year report of cases. *J Bone Joint Surg Am* 1958;40(5):1019-1030.

26. Silfverskiold N: Reduction of the uncrossed two-joints muscles of the leg to one-joint muscles in spastic conditions. *Acta Chir Scand* 1924;56:315-328.

27. Breusch SJ, Wenz W, Döderlein L: Function after correction of a clawed great toe by a modified Robert Jones transfer. *J Bone Joint Surg Br* 2000;82(2):250-254.

28. Tynan MC, Klenerman L: The modified Robert Jones tendon transfer in cases of pes cavus and clawed hallux. *Foot Ankle Int* 1994;15(2):68-71.

29. Ryssman DB, Myerson MS: Tendon transfers for the adult flexible cavovarus foot. *Foot Ankle Clin* 2011;16(3):435-450.

This article reviews tendon transfer options and describes the surgical techniques to address flexible cavovarus deformity in the adult.

30. Myerson MS: Cavus foot correction and tendon transfers for management of paralytic deformity, in Myerson MS, ed: *Reconstructive Foot and Ankle Surgery: Management of Complications,* ed 2. Philadelphia, PA, Elsevier-Saunders, 2010, pp 155-189.

The author describes different techniques to manage deformity in patients with cavus associated with paralytic disease. Level of evidence: IV.

31. Gould N, Seligson D, Gassman J: Early and late repair of lateral ligament of the ankle. *Foot Ankle* 1980;1(2):84-89.

32. Krause FG, Sutter D, Waehnert D, Windolf M, Schwieger K, Weber M: Ankle joint pressure changes in a pes cavovarus model after lateralizing calcaneal osteotomies. *Foot Ankle Int* 2010;31(9):741-746.

Three types of calcaneal osteotomies were done in eight cadaver specimens with a simulated cavovarus deformity. Evaluation of the change in pressure force through the calcaneus and peak pressure through the tibiotalar joint at half body weight found that lateralized osteotomies helped reestablish normal ankle joint pressures. Level of evidence: V.

33. Knupp M, Horisberger M, Hintermann B: A new Z-shaped calcaneal osteotomy for 3-plane correction of severe varus deformity of the hindfoot. *Tech Foot Ankle Surg* 2008;7(2):90-95.

The authors describe their technique to lateralize the calcaneus with a variation on the traditional oblique calcaneal osteotomy. The Z-shaped cut allows for translation as well as rotation to gain a more powerful correction of hindfoot varus. Level of evidence: V.

34. Malerba F, De Marchi F: Calcaneal osteotomies. *Foot Ankle Clin* 2005;10(3):523-540, vii.

35. Dwyer FC: Osteotomy of the calcaneum for pes cavus. *J Bone Joint Surg Br* 1959;41(1):80-86.

36. Dwyer FC: The present status of the problem of pes cavus. *Clin Orthop Relat Res* 1975;106:254-275.

37. Siffert RS, Forster RI, Nachamie B: "Beak" triple arthrodesis for correction of severe cavus deformity. *Clin Orthop Relat Res* 1966;45:101-106.

38. Siffert RS, del Torto U: "Beak" triple arthrodesis for severe cavus deformity. *Clin Orthop Relat Res* 1983;181:64-67.

39. Jahss MH: Tarsometatarsal truncated-wedge arthrodesis for pes cavus and equinovarus deformity of the fore part of the foot. *J Bone Joint Surg Am* 1980;62(5):713-722.

40. Mubarak SJ, Dimeglio A: Navicular excision and cuboid closing wedge for severe cavovarus foot deformities: A salvage procedure. *J Pediatr Orthop* 2011;31(5):551-556.

A new technique was used to treat severe stiff cavovarus in children. The navicular was excised and a closing-wedge osteotomy of the cuboid was done as a salvage procedure in 16 feet. Level of evidence: IV.

41. Jung HG, Jeon SH, Kim TH, Park JT: Total ankle arthroplasty with combined calcaneal and metatarsal osteotomies for treatment of ankle osteoarthritis with accompanying cavovarus deformities: Early results. *Foot Ankle Int* 2013;34(1):140-147.

At 1- to 4-year follow-up of 10 ankles after total ankle arthroplasty with concomitant procedures to correct cavovarus deformity of the hindfoot and forefoot, the results were promising in terms of preserving function and implant life. The ankles had an average underlying preoperative varus of 19°. Level of evidence: IV.

42. Krause FG, Henning J, Pfander G, Weber M: Cavovarus foot realignment to treat anteromedial ankle arthrosis. *Foot Ankle Int* 2013;34(1):54-64.

Sixteen patients who underwent symptomatic medial ankle arthrosis and cavovarus malalignment were studied at an average 84-month follow-up. Osteotomies and tendon transfers, as needed to correct the cavovarus deformity, and excision of anteromedial tibiotalar spurring, causing impingement, led to improvement in symptoms related to the ankle. Level of evidence: IV.

43. Taylor RG: The treatment of claw toes by multiple transfers of flexor into extensor tendons. *J Bone Joint Surg Br* 1951;33(4):539-542.

44. Barbari SG, Brevig K: Correction of clawtoes by the Girdlestone-Taylor flexor-extensor transfer procedure. *Foot Ankle* 1984;5(2):67-73.

Chapter 6

Diabetic Foot Disease

Ruth L. Thomas, MD

Introduction

Diabetes mellitus first was recognized and described approximately 1,500 years ago, but the course of the disease dramatically changed with the discovery of insulin in 1922. Diabetes causes comorbidities affecting multiple systems. Foot morbidity is the most common reason for hospitalization of patients with diabetes in the United States and is responsible for substantial consumption of health care resources.

Diabetic foot disease is associated with the risk of ulceration, infection, foot deformity, neuroarthropathy, and amputation. The success of orthopaedic care depends on the vascularity of the limb as well as patient cooperation in glycemic control and foot care. It is recommended that care be provided by a team that includes an orthopaedic surgeon, an endocrinologist, an infectious disease specialist, a vascular surgeon, a plastic surgeon, a physical therapist, an orthotist, and a pedorthist.

Epidemiology

Diabetes once was considered to be a disease of the West, but its prevalence is now increasing at alarming rates worldwide. Approximately 7% of the world's population is estimated to have diabetes, and the percentage is expected to reach 8.3% by 2030.[1] The increasing incidence in the United States is a direct reflection of the increasing rate of obesity.[2] The number of individuals in the United States in whom diabetes was diagnosed is 18.8 million (8.3% of the population). In addition, an estimated 7 million individuals have diabetes but the disease has not been diagnosed. More than 79 million people in the United States are considered to be prediabetic. Diabetes is most common among individuals older than 65 years,

and the aging of the population is correlated with the increasing prevalence of the disease. The direct medical cost of caring for patients with diabetes in the United States was $176 billion in 2012. This figure represents a 41% increase over the preceding 5 years and amounts to 10% of all expenditures for direct medical care in the United States.[3]

Complications associated with diabetic foot disease are the most common reason patients with diabetes are admitted to the hospital. In the United States, the annual incidence of foot ulcers in patients with diabetes is 4% to 6%, and the lifetime incidence is 15%. Patients with diabetes undergo almost 80,000 lower extremity amputations per year.[1]

Etiology

Diabetic neuropathy is the most important factor in the development of diabetic foot disease. As the severity of neuropathy increases, so does the risk of ulceration, amputation, and death. With increasing neuropathy, the patient's functional ability, balance, and coordination decline. Neuropathy probably is the result of both metabolic and vascular factors. Sensation, motor control, and autonomic function are disturbed with diabetic neuropathy, and these changes occur simultaneously. The risk of neuropathy in a patient with diabetes increases over time; the incidence is approximately 8% at the time of diagnosis but is 50% 25 years after diagnosis.[4] Sensory neuropathy affects 75% of patients with diabetes.[5]

The neuropathy begins distally and progresses proximally in a stocking glove pattern. Somatic sensory neuropathy is length dependent; it affects the longest nerves and is related to the patient's height (a tall patient is at greatest risk). Disturbance of large sensory fibers is reflected in a decreased awareness of light touch and diminished proprioception. Disturbance of small sensory fibers is reflected in a loss of pain and temperature perception. Almost one-third of patients with neuropathy report pain that is worse in the evening. The pain commonly is bilateral and symmetric, and it may be characterized in terms of burning, tingling, allodynia, electric shock, deep shooting pain, cramping, or aching.

Over time, vibratory sensation is lost, and deep tendon reflexes disappear. Surgical decompression can be helpful if identifiable nerve compression is present, but only limited research supports this recommendation.[6-8] A task force of the American Diabetes Association found the procedure to have negligible evidentiary support.[6]

Motor neuropathy can result in clawing and hammering of the toes secondary to loss of intrinsic muscle balance. Fixed toe deformities often result in pressure over the proximal interphalangeal joints and beneath the metatarsal heads. Progressive Achilles tendon contracture further increases forefoot pressures. These deformities increase the risk of pressure ulceration.

Autonomic neuropathy occurs in 20% to 40% of patients with diabetes.[5] The major clinical manifestations of autonomic neuropathy include resting tachycardia, exercise intolerance, orthostatic hypotension, constipation, gastroparesis, erectile dysfunction, sudomotor dysfunction, impaired neurovascular function, so-called brittle diabetes, and hypoglycemic autonomic failure.[9] Autonomic dysfunction affects control of sweat glands, blood vessel tone, and thermoregulation. The normal hyperemic response, which is necessary to fight infection, is lost. The skin becomes dry and scaly, cracks and fissures develop, and bacteria are able to invade, causing infection.

When a person is standing, foot pressures can become very high. In the absence of sufficient blood flow to the underlying skin and tissue, cell oxygenation is inadequate and tissue dies. The result is ulceration beneath the points of greatest pressure. Ulceration can occur during less than 1 hour of constant standing. Repetitive mild trauma, as in walking, can cause preulcerative conditions that over time progress to complete ulceration. The triad of neuropathy, foot deformity, and repetitive trauma creates a high risk of ulcer formation.

Vascular disease is extremely common in patients with diabetes. Heart disease continues to be the leading cause of death in patients with diabetes; approximately 73% of patients with diabetes have concurrent hypertension.[1]

The risk of cerebrovascular accident is as much as four times greater in patients with diabetes than in the general population.[1] The typical atherosclerotic findings in patients with diabetes include diffuse, circumferential, often bilateral involvement, with plaque formation in the medial layer of blood vessels. Atherosclerosis in the nondiabetic population usually is patchy, with plaque formation occurring in the intimal layer of blood vessels. Patients with diabetes are affected by atherosclerosis at a younger age, and the disease progression is more rapid. The iliac and femoral vessels often are affected. Typically, involvement occurs at or just distal to the popliteal trifurcation involving the anterior tibialis, posterior tibialis,

and peroneal arteries. Compromised blood flow to either lower extremity, combined with neuropathy, dramatically increases the risk for subsequent foot ulceration.

Evaluation of the Foot and Ankle in Patients With Diabetes

Obtaining a thorough history is crucial in a patient with diabetes. The identification of peripheral neuropathy and/or vascular disease, followed by appropriate intervention, can decrease the risk of subsequent infection and ulceration.

Examination of the foot and ankle should begin with an evaluation of the patient's gait, posture, range of motion, muscle strength, and skin coverage. Limited joint mobility can increase plantar pressures, resulting in foot ulceration. Thin, shiny, atrophic, and hairless skin is indicative of diminished vascularity. Any corns, calluses, or ulcerations should be documented by size, location, margins, and depth. It is also important to observe any exposure of a tendon and to determine whether an ulceration can be probed to bone. Areas with intradermal hemorrhage or blistering represent preulceration. Thick toenails indicate vascular or fungal disease. Any deformities of the foot and ankle should be noted, and the presence or absence of protective sensation should be documented. The accepted threshold for normal sensation is the ability to perceive a Semmes-Weinstein size 5.07 nylon monofilament wire applied perpendicular to the skin. However, two recent studies found that vibration perception threshold testing has greater sensitivity for detecting impaired sensation.[10,11] Pulses and capillary refill should be documented because adequate vascularity is critical for healing. The fit and material of the patient's shoes also should be evaluated. The interior of the shoes should be checked for foreign objects, and the insole removed to look for blood or other fluid discharge. Examination of the sole of the shoe may reveal an abnormal wear pattern related to deformity.

Imaging

The imaging of the diabetic foot begins with plain radiography, which primarily is used to evaluate major structural changes. Radiographs can provide information on joint alignment, soft-tissue gas, vascular calcifications, foreign bodies, and osteomyelitis. Focal demineralization, a reflection of underlying marrow changes, is the earliest radiographic change related to neuroarthropathy or osteomyelitis. The classic triad of osteomyelitis, which includes periosteal reaction, osteolysis, and bone destruction, may not be evident during the early stages of the disease (the first 20 days).[12] Ultrasonography rarely is used in the diagnosis of osteomyelitis, but it can help identify a foreign body or with identifying and aspirating an abscess. If there is a need to differentiate between infected and uninfected fluid surrounding a tendon sheath, ultrasonography can reveal the abnormal internal echogenicity characteristic of infected fluid collection.[13] CT is preferable to plain radiography for identifying cortical erosions, but it has limited value in diagnosing early osteomyelitis. CT also is unable to distinguish between the changes of chronic infection and neuroarthropathy. Because of its multiplanar capability and high spatial and contrast resolution, MRI is considered the best modality for evaluating the soft-tissue and bone marrow changes often seen with diabetic foot infection.[14-16] MRI has high sensitivity for the detection of early bone marrow edema associated with neuroarthropathy and osteomyelitis. The MRI-revealed basis of a diagnosis of osteomyelitis includes abnormal bone marrow signals typified by confluent hypointensity on T1-weighted images, which reflect infiltration of the infectious process. Gadolinium contrast injection can improve the ability to detect the abscess or necrosis associated with osteomyelitis. MRI also can be used to differentiate osteomyelitis from neuroarthropathy or reactive bone marrow edema or to differentiate a sterile joint effusion from septic arthritis.[14,17] It can be challenging to differentiate between midfoot neuroarthropathy and osteomyelitis. Secondary findings such as direct spread from an ulcer associated with rocker-bottom deformity or the presence of a sinus tract can contribute to the diagnosis. With midfoot septic arthritis, a diagnosis of osteomyelitis is supported by proximal extension of edema beyond subchondral bone and hypointense signal in the adjacent marrow on T1-weighted images.

If the use of MRI is contraindicated, radionuclide studies can contribute to the differentiation of neuropathic joint disease from osteomyelitis. Triple-phase bone scanning using technetium Tc-99m (^{99}Tc) phosphonates has 94% sensitivity and 95% specificity for the diagnosis of osteomyelitis of the bone in the absence of another abnormality.[13,18] However, specificity is reduced to 33% in the presence of neuroarthropathy, trauma, recent surgery, or tumor. ^{99}Tc bone scanning is advantageous because its high sensitivity results in a high negative predictive value; a negative bone scan essentially rules out infection. Indium 111 white blood cell (WBC) scintigraphy in general is more accurate than ^{99}Tc bone scanning for diagnosing osteomyelitis; a negative result strongly supports the absence of infection. Complementary ^{99}Tc sulfur colloid bone marrow imaging allows labeled leukocyte uptake associated with bone marrow to be distinguished from that caused by infection.

Other white blood cell labeling options include radiolabeled granulocytes, antigranulocyte monoclonal antibody fragment, radiolabeled polyclonal immunoglobulin, and Tc-99m hexamethylpropylene amine oxime–labeled WBCs.[19] Positron emission tomography (PET)–CT with-^{18}fluorodeoxyglucose, which indicates an increase in glucose metabolism, also can be used to detect diabetic infection of soft tissue or bone. This modality has high accuracy and specificity for the differentiation of osteomyelitis from neuroarthropathy and is superior to leukocyte-labeled studies for the diagnosis of chronic osteomyelitis.[20,21]

Laboratory Studies and Vital Signs

If cellulitis or a deeper infection is suspected, appropriate laboratory testing should be done. An elevated WBC count indicates infection, but the WBC count can be normal even if an infection is present, possibly secondary to an impaired immune response.[22] Leukocytosis higher than 11 x 10^9/L was associated with a 2.6-fold increase in the risk of amputation, and fever higher than 100.5°F (38°C) was associated with a 1.3-fold increase of 1.3 times in the risk of amputation.[23] Another study found that more than 50% of patients with acute osteomyelitis of the foot had a normal WBC count, and 82% had a normal oral body temperature.[24] An evaluation of 400 patients with moderate or severe diabetic foot infection found a mean WBC count of 8.24 x 10^9/L; those who were unsuccessfully treated had a mean WBC count of 9.977 x 10^9/L, and those who favorably responded to treatment had a mean WBC count of 7.933 x 10^9/L.[25] A total lymphocyte count higher then 1.5 x 10^9/L is correlated with immunocompetence in wound healing. Albumin levels above 30 g/dL support a nutritional status satisfactory for healing; healing can occur but is less predictable with lower levels.[26] Patients requiring transtibial amputation had substantially lower serum albumin levels than patients who underwent successful limb salvage.[27] An elevated erythrocyte sedimentation rate often is correlated with inflammation or infection; usually, a level less than 40 is more common with cellulitis or a local soft-tissue infection. A level higher than 60 suggests underlying osteomyelitis. The C-reactive protein level is highly sensitive but not specific for inflammation, and it can be normal even in a patient with a deep infection.[22] C-reactive protein level is a better parameter than WBC count or neutrophil count for diagnosis and monitoring of treatment in deep diabetic foot infections.[28] Worsening glycemic control is one of the earliest signs of diabetic foot infection. Hyperglycemia (measured at 11.1 mmol/L) was used as a variable to distinguish moderate from severe infection.[27] In combination with other study results, this information can be helpful in judging whether a patient's infection is improving or worsening.

Complications and Treatment

Diabetic Ulcer

Pressure ulceration is a serious complication in patients with diabetes. Foot ulceration occurs during the lifetime of 15% of patients with diabetes and is the leading cause of lower extremity amputation in these patients.[28] Prompt identification and early treatment are crucial. Infected and/or ischemic diabetic foot ulcers account for approximately 25% of all hospital stays by patients with diabetes.[1]

The causes of ulceration are multifactorial and include loss of skin integrity, neuropathy, decreased vascularity, foot deformity, increased body weight, poor vision, malnutrition, poor glucose regulation, need for insulin, impaired leukocyte function, use of immunosuppressive drugs, and tobacco use. In a comparison of 32 patients with diabetes and 32 healthy control subjects, the patients with diabetes had a thicker Achilles tendon and stiffer plantar soft tissue than the control subjects.[29] As much as a fivefold increase in the mechanical stiffness of the plantar soft tissues has been reported in patients with diabetic foot disease.[30] The findings confirmed the previous study showing increased stiffness in the plantar soft tissues in patients with diabetic pheripheral neuropathy, resulting in increased tissue hydrostatic pressure in the loaded foot and effectively reducing the blood supply to the areas of highest pressure. [29]

The most common reasons a diabetic ulcer does not heal include decreased vascular supply, deep infection, and failure to unload the affected area. Wound size, wound duration, and wound grade are directly associated with the likelihood of wound healing by the 20th week of care.[31] The Brodsky classification system, which is based on ulcer depth and ischemia, helps determine the need for hospitalization and possible surgery[32] (Figure 1). The Scottish Foot Ulcer Risk Score, which classifies an ulcer as mild, moderate, or high risk based on palpable pulses, sensory neuropathy, foot deformity, and a history of ulcer or amputation, can be used to predict ulcer development and ulcer healing.[33] A prospective analysis of 1,000 patients was used to develop a diabetic ulcer severity score in which the examiner assigns one point for each of four parameters: inability to palpate a pedal pulse, ability to probe to bone, presence of an ulcer anywhere other than a toe, and multiple ulcerations.[34] A relatively high score was associated with an increased risk of amputation, and an increase of one point in a patient's score predicted a 35% decrease in the likelihood of healing. A higher score was correlated with a larger initial wound area, a longer wound history, and a greater likelihood that surgery or hospitalization will be required.

The first step in ulcer management is to remove all necrotic tissue and surrounding callus formation. This step converts a chronic wound into an acute wound and encourages healing. Elliptical wounds usually heal better than circular wounds. The wound should be débrided weekly or more frequently. The second step is to offload pressure by distributing it over a larger surface area, thus decreasing the pressure concentration and the risk of tissue failure. Although offloading can be accomplished by avoiding weight bearing on the involved extremity, patient compliance is problematic. Total contact casting remains the gold standard and is the most commonly used method of pressure offloading. A shorter healing time and a better rate of healing were found when a diabetic healing cast was used rather than a half shoe or a removable cast walker.[35] Although total contact casting is highly successful, the reported complication rates are as high as 17%.[36] The time required for ulcer healing progressively increases with its location from toe to midfoot to heel.[37]

Hyperbaric oxygen therapy has been available as an adjunct treatment of diabetic foot ulcers for more than 20 years, but it is costly, available only in a limited number of centers, and of unproved effectiveness. Guidelines of both the American Diabetes Association and the Infectious Diseases Society of America (IDSA) suggest that the use of hyperbaric oxygen therapy should be limited to patients who respond to an oxygen challenge. Transcutaneous oxygen tension at the affected extremity level is increased when the patient is placed into a total body chamber.[31,38] Irrespective of the method used to heal an ulcer, the risk of recurrence is as high as 57%.[36]

After the ulcer has healed, it is important that the patient wear shoes with insoles that continue to offload the pressure site. With terminally augmented biofeedback, 21 patients were able to learn a new walking strategy that decreased the peak plantar pressure under a previously defined at-risk zone.[39] The clinical value of this technique in a large population of patients with diabetes has not been proved.

Infection

In comparison with individuals without diabetes, those with diabetes are at an 80% greater risk for cellulitis, a fourfold greater risk for osteomyelitis, a twofold greater risk for sepsis and death resulting from infection, and a tenfold greater risk of amputation.[1] The use of antibiotics should be considered if infection is present. An infection that does not threaten the limb can be treated with oral antibiotics. Oral antibiotics have been used to keep osteomyelitis in remission under certain circumstances but have not been uniformly successful.[40] An infection that does not respond to wound management and the use of

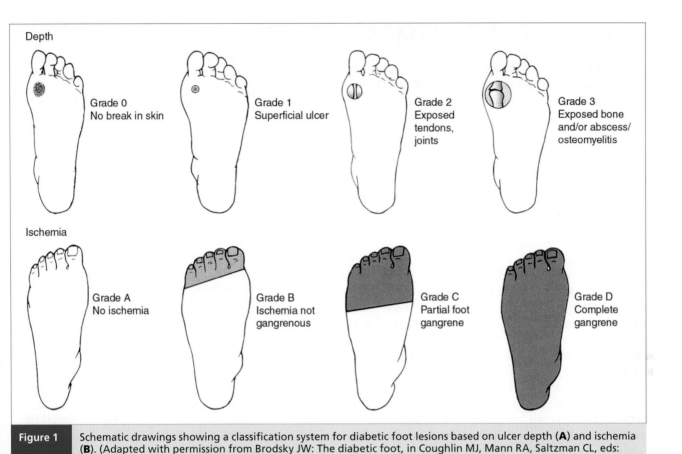

Figure 1 Schematic drawings showing a classification system for diabetic foot lesions based on ulcer depth (**A**) and ischemia (**B**). (Adapted with permission from Brodsky JW: The diabetic foot, in Coughlin MJ, Mann RA, Saltzman CL, eds: *Surgery of the Foot and Ankle*, ed 8. Philadelphia, PA, Mosby, 2007, vol 2, pp 1281-1368.)

oral antibiotics is limb threatening and can be life threatening. Surgical management should be the primary focus for these patients, with adjunctive intravenous antibiotic therapy. Parenteral first-generation cephalosporin can be administered empirically until the results of surgically obtained tissue cultures are available to dictate subsequent antibiotic therapy.

The use of topical antibiotics alone is not recommended for treating an infected ulcer, but topical metronidazole has been used to control odor in the presence of extensive tissue devitalization.[22] In a double-blind randomized controlled study, pexiganan acetate cream, a synthetic analogue of the antimicrobial cationic peptide magainin 2 (a host-defense peptide isolated from frog skin), appeared to be as effective as oral ofloxacin for treating mildly infected ulcers.[41] The use of topical silver-containing dressings has been recommended because of the antibacterial properties of silver ion, but their clinical efficacy has not been proved.[42,43] Bacterial biofilm production can interfere with ulcer healing, and removal of this biofilm is an extremely important aspect of wound management. Surgical irrigation using detergents improves the efficacy of débridement, and topical agents to facilitate biofilm removal are available for clinical use.[44,45]

Swab culturing is notoriously inaccurate because of the risk of contamination. Culture specimens can be most accurately obtained in the operating room after surgical preparation. Deep tissue, including bone or granulation tissue, should be obtained, rather than the tissue that can be obtained by swabbing. Most diabetic foot ulcers have polymicrobial contamination; 75% were found to have a mean 2.4 organisms per wound.[46] Aerobic gram-positive cocci, especially staphylococci, are the most common causative organisms.[46] Aerobic gram-negative bacilli often are copathogens in infections that are chronic or occur after antibiotic treatment. Obligate anaerobes can be copathogens in ischemic or necrotic wounds. With increasing ulcer depth, anaerobic bacteria become more abundant than staphylococci. Bacterial diversity, species richness, and relative abundance of proteobacteria increase as the age of the ulcer increases.[47] The risk of ulcer-associated infection is increased with hyperglycemia, which has a deleterious effect on neutrophils and granulocytes.[48] Poor glycemic control is associated with ulcer cluster, and very poor glycemic control is associated with an increase in the concentration of *Staphylococcus*-rich and *Streptococcus*-rich ulcer clusters.[47] The risk of multidrug-resistant bacteria in diabetic foot ulcers increases with deep and recurrent ulcers, history of previous hospitalization, elevated HbA1c level, nephropathy, and retinopathy.[49]

It is important to initially determine the type and severity of infection.[27,50,51] A 2004 consensus report of the IDSA described four grades of severity in diabetic foot infection.[52] An almost-identical severity classification was established by the International Working Group on the Diabetic Foot (IWGDF) in 2012.[51] Recently IDSA and IWGDF agreed that a severe diabetic foot infection is accompanied by two or more of the signs of a systemic inflammatory response: a body temperature higher than 39° or lower than 36°C, a heart rate higher than 90 bpm, a respiratory rate higher than 20 breaths per minute or a $PaCO_2$ less than 32 mm Hg, and a WBC count higher than 12×10^9/L or lower than 4×10^9/L [53] (Table 1). The earlier guidelines included hyperglycemia, azotemia, and acidosis, but these were dropped from the IDSA-IWGDF consensus. Other groups have established different guidelines for severe diabetic foot infection.[22]

Wet gangrene or soft-tissue emphysema represents severe infection. The most commonly isolated pathogens in osteomyelitis are gram-positive organisms, especially *Staphylococcus aureus*. However, a review of 341 patients found that 44% of bone cultures contained gram-negative pathogens alone or in combination with a gram-positive organism.[54] Infections with gram-negative pathogens more often were associated with a fetid odor, necrotic tissue, and clinical signs of severe infection than those with gram-positive pathogens.[54]

Weight bearing on an infected foot should be discouraged because the infection will spread from an area of high pressure (the infection site) to areas of lower pressure (uninfected sites), most commonly from the plantar foot to the dorsal foot. Infections spread through the foot along tendons within their sheaths. Infection spread is observed when purulent drainage is expressed through the ulcer during palpation at a distant location. As each compartment within the foot becomes involved, pressures within the compartment increase and can cause extensive tissue damage. As part of the surgical débridement, the involved compartment must be opened and all necrotic tissue removed.

Simple surgical intervention may include abscess drainage, aggressive débridement of ulcers, and application of negative pressure wound therapy. Negative pressure wound therapy is more effective than topical moist wound dressings and can be safely applied after an infected diabetic ulcer is débrided.[28] More aggressive surgical intervention can include exostectomy, deformity correction, muscle or microvascular free flaps, or

Table 1

International Consensus on the Classification of Diabetic Foot Wound Infections

Grade	Characteristics
I	No symptoms, no signs of infection
	Lesion involving only the skin (no subcutaneous tissue lesion or systemic disorder) with local warmth and erythema of 0.5 to 2.0 cm
II	Local tenderness or pain
	Local swelling or induration
	Purulent discharge (thick, opaque to white, or sanguineous)
	Erythema more than 2 cm plus one of the following: local tenderness or pain, local swelling or induration, or purulent discharge
	Elimination of other causes of inflammation of the skin (for example, trauma, gout, acute Charcot arthropathy, fracture, thrombosis, venous stasis)
III	Local infection involving structures beneath the skin and subcutaneous tissue, as in deep abscess, lymphangitis, osteomyelitis, septic arthritis, or fasciitis
	No systemic inflammatory response
	Regardless of local infection, the presence of systemic signs corresponding to body temperature greater than 39°C or less than 36°C and pulse >90 bpm
IV	Respiratory rate greater than 20/min
	$PaCO_2$ less than 32 mm Hg
	Leukocytes greater than 12 or less than x 10^9/L
	Proportion of immature leukocytes greater than 10%

Adapted with permission from Richard JL, Sotto A, Lavigne JP: New insights in diabetic foot infection. *World J Diabetes* 2011;2(2):24-32.

amputation. Staged reconstructive surgical procedures sometimes are necessary. Lengthening of the Achilles tendon can decrease plantar pressure and allow forefoot ulcers to heal.[55,56] However, overcorrection can lead to an increase in peak pressure under the heel, a calcaneal gait, and a subsequent heel ulcer that eventually may require partial calcanectomy or transitibial amputation.[55] Plantar fascia release recently was found to result in healing of forefoot ulcers.[57]

Amputation

Nonhealing foot wounds are a factor in 85% of lower extremity amputations. Even minor trauma can result in amputation.[58] A strong correlation exists between morbid obesity and diabetes-associated morbidity.[59] The risk of amputation is highest in patients who live in poverty, belong to a racial or ethnic minority group, are older than 50 years, are men rather than women, or smoke tobacco.[60-62] A retrospective control cohort study of 100 patients with diabetes at one academic institution found that patients admitted with severe foot infection had a hospital stay that was 60% longer than that of patients with a moderate infection.[27] The risk of amputation was 55% in patients with severe infection and 42% in those with moderate infection. The rate of major amputation was three times higher in patients with severe diabetic foot infection. Moderate foot infection was differentiated from severe infection based on the IDSA consensus (Table 1); fever, heart rate, respiratory rate, and WBC count were considered as indicative of the systemic inflammatory response syndrome.

After amputation, an inverse relationship exists between the amount of energy consumption and the length of the residual limb; more energy is consumed if the patient has a shorter residual limb. Thirty percent of patients with a unilateral amputation undergo amputation of the contralateral limb within 3 years.[36] Two-thirds of patients die within 5 years of the amputation. In choosing the level of amputation, the surgeon must consider both the optimal level for healing (the vascular supply) and optimal residual limb function. The factors contributing to the decision include the quality of the tissue, the extent of the infection, the vascularity of the limb, and the patient's nutritional, immune, and ambulatory status. The levels of amputation are identified as partial digital, digital, ray resection transmetatarsal, Chopart, Syme, transtibial, and transfemoral. Osteomyelitis of the heel is more likely to require transtibial amputation than osteomyelitis of the forefoot or midfoot.[63] Midfoot amputation may require tendon lengthening or releases and possibly tendon transfers to balance the foot. After metatarsal head resection, the greatest risk of reulceration is at the first metatarsal head, and the lowest risk is at the fifth metatarsal head.[64] An 84.5% healing rate was reported after a first Syme amputation.[26] The risk of major reamputation after minor foot amputation in patients with diabetes is strongly associated with the presence of peripheral vascular disease.[65] Transtibial amputation is associated with high rates of morbidity and mortality. Nonetheless, a comparison with partial foot amputation found that after 1 and 3 years only transmetatarsal amputation resulted in a statistically lower mortality rate than transtibial amputation.[66]

Transmetatarsal and Chopart amputations resulted in better ambulatory ability and longer durability than other partial foot amputations. During the past decade the rate of lower extremity amputations has declined among patients with diabetes in the Medicare population.[67] The rates of decrease have been most significant in proximal level amputations rather than distal level limb-conserving amputations. Simultaneously, the use of orthopaedic interventions such as total-contact casting and Achilles tendon lengthening has increased.

Vascular Disease

Vascular disease is 30 times more common in patients with diabetes than in other individuals.[36] It is important for the examiner to determine the patient's palpable tibialis posterior pulse, dorsalis pedis pulse, and capillary filling time. Any evidence of ischemia or a nonhealing wound warrants a vascular evaluation. Arterial Doppler ultrasonography is effective in assessing the adequacy of circulation. This test is reproducible and is not operator dependent. The results are reported in terms of toe pressures and the ratio of ankle pressure to arm Doppler arterial pressure. An acceptable level for healing is toe pressures higher than 40 mm Hg or an ankle-brachial index higher than 45 mm Hg. Absolute toe pressures are a better predictor of healing than the ankle-brachial index.[68] A triphasic waveform is present within normal vessels. When the vessel is calcified, the waveform is monophasic, and the reading can be falsely elevated. Transcutaneous oxygen tension values higher than 30 mm Hg indicate an acceptable potential for healing; this technique does not produce false readings with calcified vessels. If screening reveals limb ischemia, arteriography can identify the site of occlusion. This test is expensive, however, and has possible complications including allergic dye reaction, pseudoaneurysm, and acute renal failure in patients with compromised renal function or dehydration.

No screening tool is 100% accurate. When vascular compromise is documented, a vascular consultation should be obtained to determine whether revascularization is a viable option. The options for revascularization include percutaneous transluminal angioplasty and vascular bypass.

Charcot Neuroarthropathy

Charcot neuroarthropathy involves progressive destruction of the joints, most commonly in the feet and ankles. The reported incidence of this complication is less than 1% in the general population of patients with diabetes and is as high as 13% in high-risk patients with diabetes. Men and women are at equal risk. Thirty percent of patients with this complication have bilateral involvement.[32]

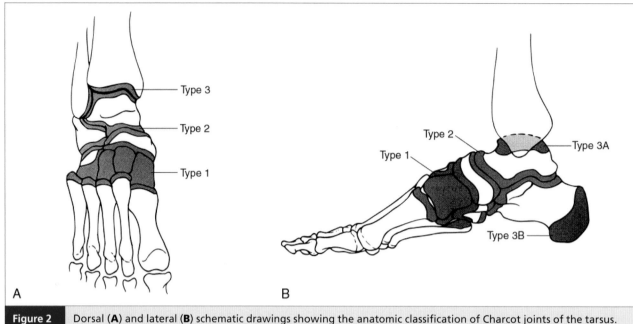

| Figure 2 | Dorsal (**A**) and lateral (**B**) schematic drawings showing the anatomic classification of Charcot joints of the tarsus. Type 1 (midfoot) involves the tarsometatarsal and naviculocuneiform joints. Type 2 (hindfoot) involves the subtalar, talonavicular, and calcaneocuboid joints. Type 3A (ankle) involves the tibiotalar joint. Type 3B (calcaneus involves a pathologic fracture of the tubercle of the calcaneus. (Adapted with permission from Brodsky JW: The diabetic foot, in Coughlin MJ, Mann RA, Saltzman CL, eds: *Surgery of the Foot and Ankle*, ed 8. Philadelphia, PA, Mosby, 2007, vol 2, pp 1281-1368.) |

Two theories are proposed to explain the development of Charcot neuroarthropathy. The theory of neurotraumatic destruction states that joint destruction is the result of cumulative trauma unrecognized by an insensate foot. In contrast, the theory of neurovascular destruction states that bone resorption and ligament laxity are secondary to a neurally controlled vascular reflex. Most experts believe that a combination of these pathways is responsible for the destruction seen in the affected diabetic foot or ankle.

Several studies supported the role of osteopenia in diabetic neuroarthropathy. Localized osteopenia increases the risk of fracture with continued weight bearing. Excessive osteoclastic activity was found in Charcot-reactive bone, with cytokine mediators inciting bone resorption.[69] Increased expression of nuclear transcription factor NF-κB resulted in increased osteoclastogenesis, thus confirming the role of inflammatory cytokines.[70] These findings suggest the possibility of using pharmacologic agents to limit cytokine activation and osteoclastic resorption. Patients with Charcot dislocation often have normal bone density, and those with Charcot fracture often have decreased bone density. The severity of diabetes is not correlated with the risk of Charcot neuroarthropathy. Charcot neuroarthropathy can develop in patients with mild diabetes who are being treated with oral hypoglycemic medications or diet control.

Charcot neuroarthropathy has three classic stages.[71] Stage I, the fragmentation phase, is clinically characterized by hyperemia, edema, increased warmth, and erythema around the affected joint. Stage I is radiographically characterized by fragmentation of bone associated with fracture and joint subluxation. In stage II, the subacute or coalescence phase, the acute inflammatory findings decrease. Radiographs show evidence of bone debris and new bone formation. Stage III is the chronic or consolidation phase. Swelling and warmth surrounding the joint resolves, but there may be considerable residual deformity. On radiographs the fragmentation is seen to have consolidated, but residual joint deformity and bone loss are evident.

Charcot involvement of the foot and ankle is described in terms of the four commonly affected anatomic areas[32] (**Figure 2**). Type I which occurs in 60% of patients, affects the midfoot, tarsometatarsal, and naviculocuneiform joints. The subsequent collapse most commonly results in a residual deformity involving a plantar medial bony exostosis that places the foot at risk of pressure ulceration. Type II, which affects 30% to 35% of patients, involves the hindfoot, with subsequent instability resulting in foot subluxation and ulcer formation. Type IIIA, which affects 5% of patients, involves the ankle joint and is the most unstable pattern. Type IIIB involves fracture of the calcaneal tuberosity and results in weak

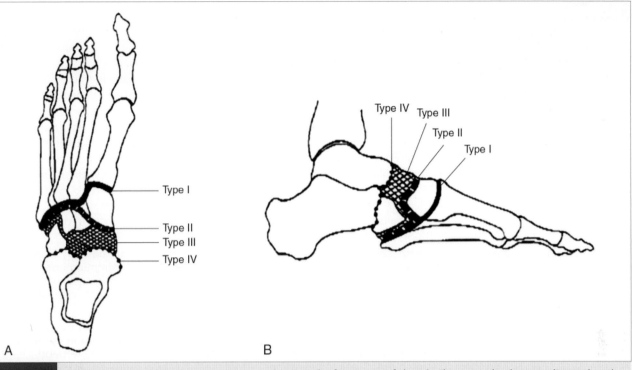

Figure 3   AP (**A**) and lateral (**B**) schematic drawings showing the four types of chronic Charcot rocker bottom. (Reproduced with permission from Schon LC, Weinfeld SB, Horton GA, Resch S: Radiographic and clinical classification of acquired midfoot tarsus. *Foot Ankle Int* 1998:19;394-404.)

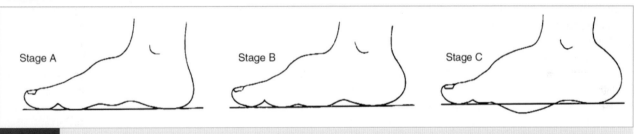

Figure 4   Schematics showing the three stages of chronic Charcot rocker bottom deformity. (Reproduced with permission from Schon LC, Weinfeld SB, Horton GA, Resch S: Radiographic and clinical classification of acquired midfoot tarsus. *Foot Ankle Int* 1998:19; 394-404.)

pushoff, pes planus, and risk of ulceration associated with the avulsed bony prominence. In general, the more proximal the Charcot joint involvement, the higher the risk of subsequent joint instability.

In a second classification, type I is described as destruction of the metatarsophalangeal joint, with medial plantar prominence and abduction deformity[72] (**Figure 3**). Type II involves the naviculocuneiform joint, with residual plantar lateral prominence under the fourth and fifth metatarsocuboid joints. Type III affects the navicular and the medial column, with collapse resulting in an adducted-supinated deformity and a plantar lateral prominence under the cuboid. Type IV involves the transverse tarsal joints with associated prominence under the calcaneocuboid and talonavicular joints. Substage A, B,

or C is assigned based on the severity of the rocker-bottom sole (**Figure 4**).

Regardless of the classification system, the goal of treatment after stage III (the consolidation phase) is for the foot to be stable, plantigrade, and amenable to bracing or accommodative orthotic devices and shoes. Any residual deformity should be treated to enable these goals to be reached and to keep the foot free of ulceration and infection. The nonsurgical treatment of a foot at stage I includes rest, elevation, and protection. A total contact cast with weekly cast changes and minimal protected weight bearing can be useful until the acute process begins to resolve. As the foot improves, the cast can be changed every 2 weeks. During the transition to stage II, the swelling and temperature begin to stabilize. A

2: Neuromuscular Disease

Table 2

Foot Care Instructions for Patients With Diabetes

Washing your feet	Wash your feet daily. Dry them carefully, especially between the toes. Do not soak your feet (unless instructed to do so by your health care provider). If your feet are dry, apply a very thin coat of lubricant (oil or cream) after bathing and drying them. Don't put oil or cream between your toes.
Inspecting your feet	Inspect your feet daily. Use an unbreakable mirror to help see the bottom of your feet. Check for scratches, cuts, or blisters. Always check between your toes. If your vision is impaired, ask someone to check your feet for you.
Cutting your toenails	Cut your toenails by following the contour of the nail. Smooth the corners with an emery board. Don't trim into the corners of your toenails or cut ingrown toenails. If redness appears around your toenails, see your healthcare provider immediately.
Treating corns and calluses	Do not cut corns or calluses. Do not use corn plasters or chemicals for removing corns or calluses. Do not use strong antiseptic solutions or adhesive tape on your feet.
Avoiding heat and cold	Avoid extreme temperatures. Test water with your hand or elbow before bathing. Don't walk on hot surfaces, such as sand at the beach or cement around a swimming pool. In winter, wear wool socks and protective foot gear such as fleece-lined boots. Do not apply a hot water bottle or heating pad to your feet. If your feet are cold at night, wear socks.
Choosing shoes	Don't walk barefoot, even indoors. Don't wear sandals with thongs between your toes. Don't wear shoes without stockings or socks. Inspect the inside of your shoes every day for foreign objects, nail points, torn linings, and rough areas. Shoes should be comfortable at the time of purchase. Don't buy shoes that are too tight and depend on them to stretch out. Break in new shoes before wearing them regularly. Ask your podiatrist or other health care provider about the types of shoes most appropriate for you.
Avoiding harm to your legs	Don't wear restrictive clothing on your legs (such as leg garters). Avoid crossing your legs. Doing so can cause pressure on the nerves and blood vessels in the legs.
Avoiding tobacco and alcohol	Do not smoke. Do not drink alcohol excessively.
Talking to your health care providers	See your health care provider regularly, and be sure your feet are examined at least four times a year. Tell your podiatrist or other health care provider at once if you develop a blister or sore on your foot. Be sure to tell your podiatrist that you have diabetes.

removable boot walker or ankle-foot orthosis can be substituted for the total-contact cast, with continued limitation of forefoot and midfoot pressures. During stage III, the use of accommodative shoes with a custom-molded protective orthotic device can be initiated.

Residual deformity can result in chronic pressure and subsequent ulceration. If shoe wear modification and bracing do not prevent recurrent episodes of ulceration, surgical intervention is required. Orthopaedic foot and ankle surgeons have a growing interest in the correction of acquired deformities to improve the patient's walking independence and quality of life. Internal fixation, external fixation, or a combination can be used to achieve this goal.

Surgical Complications

After an ankle fracture, patients with diabetes are at risk of complications including failure of wound healing, infection, malunion, delayed union, nonunion, and Charcot neuroarthropathy.[73,74] Charcot ankle neuroarthropathy most commonly occurs in patients with diabetes who have a delayed diagnosis and/or delayed immobilization or who have a nonsurgically treated displaced ankle fracture.[75] In a review of 160,000 patients with ankle fracture, the incidence of diabetes was 5.7%.[76] The patients with diabetes were found to have a significantly longer-than-average hospital length of stay as well as higher rates of in-hospital mortality, in-hospital postoperative complications, and nonroutine discharge ($P < 0.001$ for all factors). Similar complication rates were reported in multiple reviews of elective arthrodesis procedures in patients with diabetes.[77-79] To assess the risk factors associated with nonunion, delayed union, and malunion, the outcomes of 165 patients with diabetes who had undergone arthrodesis, osteotomy, or fracture reduction were reviewed.[80] Peripheral neuropathy, duration of surgery, and glycohemoglobin levels higher than 7% were found to be significant for bone-healing complications, with

Table 3

Categories of Risk for Foot Complications

Category	Risk Factors	Treatment Recommendations
0	No history of ulceration No deformity No previous amputation Pedal pulses present No sensory loss	Instruction in basic foot care Annual foot examination Regular footwear
1	No history of ulceration No deformity No previous amputation Pedal pulses present Sensory loss	Daily foot self-examination Instruction in diabetic foot care Foot examination by physician every 6 months Depth shoes or running shoes Nonmolded, soft inlays Possible total-contact orthotic devices
2	No history of ulceration Moderate (prelesion) deformity (for example, hallux rigidus, metatarsal head prominence, claw toes or hammer toes, callus, plantar bony prominence, hallux valgus, dorsal exostosis) Pedal pulses present Single lesser ray amputation Sensory loss	Daily foot self-examination Instruction in diabetic foot care Foot examination by physician every 4 months Depth shoes or running shoes Custom-molded orthotic devices Possible adjuncts including silicon toe sleeves, lamb's wool, foam toe separators, hammer toe crests, metatarsal pads External shoe modifications including metatarsal bars, rocker-bottom soles, extended steel shanks, medial or lateral heel wedges
3	History of ulceration Presence of deformity (for example, Charcot arthropathy, hallux rigidus, metatarsal head prominence, claw toes, hammer toes, callus, plantar bony prominence, hallux valgus, dorsal exostosis) Previous amputation (multiple ray, first ray, transmetatarsal, Chopart) Pedal pulses present or absent Sensory loss	Daily foot self-examination Instruction in diabetic foot care for at-risk patients Foot examination by physician every 2 months Custom-fabricated, pressure-dissipating accommodative foot orthotic devices Inlay-depth, soft-leather, adjustable-lacing shoes External shoe modifications including rocker-bottom soles, extended steel shanks, solid ankle-cushion heels well filled with low-density material Offloading orthotic devices including patellar tendon–bearing brace, ankle-foot orthoses Immediate clinical evaluation of any new skin or nail issue Possible evaluation by orthopaedic foot and ankle surgeon

(Adapted from Philbin TM: The diabetic foot, in Pinzur MS, ed: *Orthopaedic Knowledge Update: Foot and Ankle,* ed 4. Rosemont, IL, American Academy of Orthopaedic Surgeons, 2008, pp 273-290.)

peripheral neuropathy having the strongest association. Surgical treatment of these patients at high risk should emphasize optimal glycemic control, maximization of limb vascularity, meticulous soft-tissue care, and prolonged avoidance of weight bearing after the surgery.[73,76]

Establishing Risk and Preventive Care

Amputation rates can be reduced by 45% to 85% if patients participate in a comprehensive foot care program that includes risk assessment, foot care education, and preventive therapy, with treatment of foot problems and referral to a specialist when indicated.[81] All patients with diabetes should undergo an annual foot examination.[82] These patients should be taught the importance of blood glucose monitoring and self-examination of the feet (Table 2). The physician is able to predict the risk of future foot complications based on the patient's history and physical examination. The risk factors for development of a diabetic ulcer include loss of sensation, diminished pulses, foot deformity, abnormal reflexes, advanced age, history of a foot ulcer or other treatment, and an abnormal neuropathy disability score.

The risk of foot complications is scored from 0 to 3 (Table 3). A normal-appearing foot with normal sensation and no more than minor deformity is assigned to risk category 0. The patient should have basic knowledge of foot care, receive an annual examination, and wear ordinary footwear. In contrast, an insensate foot with deformity and a history of ulceration is assigned to risk category 3. The patient requires foot risk education and should perform a foot self-examination three to four times daily. Protective shoes should be worn during walking and while standing. Cross-sectional studies support the use of rocker sole footwear and custom orthotic devices to reduce plantar pressure, but longitudinal studies are needed to confirm this benefit.[83] Most centers that care for patients with diabetic foot disease recommend extra-depth shoes constructed of soft leather or another accommodative material, with minimal seams, adjustable lacing, and custom-fabricated, pressure-dissipating insoles. Rigid orthotic devices should be avoided. For some patients, a brace is necessary to provide stability, limit motion, unload pressure, distribute forces evenly throughout the foot, and accommodate deformities.

Patients at high risk should undergo a foot examination by a physician every 2 months and a visual inspection of the feet during every encounter with a healthcare provider. In addition, any new skin or nail issue should immediately be clinically evaluated. Foot infection in patients with diabetes almost always follows trauma, and it is associated with a high risk of hospitalization and possible amputation. Accordingly, patients with diabetes who have foot trauma, especially those with peripheral vascular disease, should be targeted for rapid intervention to prevent infection.

Racial, ethnic, and sex disparities in preventive diabetes care have been well documented.[84-87] Prevention programs should concentrate on patient compliance with medications and clinical follow-up, especially in patients who are members of a racial or ethnic minority. A multidisciplinary team approach to the management of diabetic foot disease has repeatedly been shown to improve clinical outcomes.[27,53,88,89]

Summary

The global health burden of diabetic foot disease is steadily increasing. Continuing research into effective management strategies remains critical. Patient education and early intervention are most likely to result in a successful outcome when a multidisciplinary team approach is used.

Annotated References

1. American Diabetes Association: Statistics about diabetes: Diabetes from the National Diabetes Statistics Report, 2014 (released June 10, 2014). http://www.diabetes.org/diabetes-basics/statistics/. Accessed September 3, 2014.

2. Hebert JR, Allison DB, Archer E, Lavie CJ, Blair SN: Scientific decision making, policy decisions, and the obesity pandemic. *Mayo Clin Proc* 2013;88(6):593-604.

   Epidemic rates of obesity are contributing to the rising rate of type 2 diabetes. Obesity has become a major public health problem.

3. American Diabetes Association: Economic costs of diabetes in the U.S. in 2012. *Diabetes Care* 2013;36(4):1033-1046.

4. Berlet GC, Philbin TM: The diabetic foot and ankle, in Lieberman JR, ed: *AAOS Comprehensive Orthopaedic Review.* Rosemont, IL, American Academy of Orthopaedic Surgeons, 2009, pp 1217-1224.

5. Ross MA: Neuropathies associated with diabetes. *Med Clin North Am* 1993;77(1):111-124.

6. Cornblath DR, Vinik A, Feldman E, Freeman R, Boulton AJ: Surgical decompression for diabetic sensorimotor polyneuropathy. *Diabetes Care* 2007;30(2):421-422.

7. Dellon AL, Muse VL, Scott ND, et al: A positive Tinel sign as predictor of pain relief or sensory recovery after decompression of chronic tibial nerve compression in patients with diabetic neuropathy. *J Reconstr Microsurg* 2012;28(4):235-240.

   Patients with diabetic neuropathy who had a positive Tinel sign over the tibial nerve at the tarsal tunnel were evaluated before and after surgical decompression of the tarsal tunnel. A positive Tinel sign predicted substantial relief of pain and improvement in plantar sensibility.

8. Valdivia Valdivia JM, Weinand M, Maloney CT Jr, Blount AL, Dellon AL: Surgical treatment of superimposed, lower extremity, peripheral nerve entrapments with diabetic and idiopathic neuropathy. *Ann Plast Surg* 2013;70(6):675-679.

   A retrospective review of 158 consecutive patients (96 with diabetes and 62 with idiopathic neuropathy) found that neurolysis of multiple sites of chronic nerve compression in the lower extremity resulted in improvement in sensation in 88% of patients with preoperative numbness and 81% of patients with impaired balance.

9. Vinik AI, Maser RE, Mitchell BD, Freeman R: Diabetic autonomic neuropathy. *Diabetes Care* 2003;26(5):1553-1579.

10. Wienemann T, Chantelau EA: The diagnostic value of measuring pressure pain perception in patients with diabetes mellitus. *Swiss Med Wkly* 2012;142:w13682.

The authors determined that pressure algometry was not superior to measuring vibration perception threshold in patients with diabetes with or without painless plantar ulcers.

11. Richard JL, Reilhes L, Buvry S, Goletto M, Faillie JL: Screening patients at risk for diabetic foot ulceration: A comparison between measurement of vibration perception threshold and 10-g monofilament test. *Int Wound J* 2014;11(2):147-151.

Vibration perception threshold testing and a 10-g Semmes-Weinstein monofilament wire testing were performed in 400 consecutive patients with diabetes. Vibration perception threshold testing identified a much higher number of patients at risk for foot ulceration than Semmes-Weinstein monofilament testing.

12. Donovan A, Schweitzer ME: Current concepts in imaging diabetic pedal osteomyelitis. *Radiol Clin North Am* 2008;46(6):1105-1124, vii.

13. Loredo R, Rahal A, Garcia G, Metter D: Imaging of the diabetic foot: Diagnostic dilemmas. *Foot Ankle Spec* 2010;3(5):249-264.

The authors determined that no single best test for the evaluation of the diabetic foot exists and that multiple studies should be used.

14. Kapoor A, Page S, Lavalley M, Gale DR, Felson DT: Magnetic resonance imaging for diagnosing foot osteomyelitis: A meta-analysis. *Arch Intern Med* 2007;167(2):125-132.

15. Schweitzer ME, Daffner RH, Weissman BN, et al: ACR Appropriateness Criteria on suspected osteomyelitis in patients with diabetes mellitus. *J Am Coll Radiol* 2008;5(8):881-886.

16. Rozzanigo U, Tagliani A, Vittorini E, Pacchioni R, Brivio LR, Caudana R: Role of magnetic resonance imaging in the evaluation of diabetic foot with suspected osteomyelitis. *Radiol Med* 2009;114(1):121-132.

MRI has high sensitivity for the detection of osteomyelitis in a diabetic foot but has lower specificity compared with Charcot neuropathic joint destruction.

17. Toledano TR, Fatone EA, Weis A, Cotten A, Beltran J: MRI evaluation of bone marrow changes in the diabetic foot: A practical approach. *Semin Musculoskelet Radiol* 2011;15(3):257-268.

Both osteomyelitis and reactive marrow edema show an increased T2-weighted MRI signal, but osteomyelitis can be confirmed by T1 hypointensity in the bone marrow. A diagnosis of osteomyelitis is supported by the presence of a localized or contiguously spreading forefoot focus of abnormal bone marrow away from the subchondral surface and adjacent to a skin ulcer, cellulitis, abscess, or sinus tract.

18. Ranachowska C, Lass P, Korzon-Burakowska A, Dobosz M: Diagnostic imaging of the diabetic foot. *Nucl Med Rev Cent East Eur* 2010;13(1):18-22.

MRI is the gold standard for diagnostic imaging of the diabetic foot. The role of bone scanning is decreasing, but it can be helpful in the early stages of osteitis or Charcot neuro-osteoarthropathy. Inflammation-targeted scintigraphy is useful, and PET will become increasingly common.

19. Poirier JY, Garin E, Derrien C, et al: Diagnosis of osteomyelitis in the diabetic foot with a 99mTc-HMPAO leucocyte scintigraphy combined with a 99mTc-MDP bone scintigraphy. *Diabetes Metab* 2002;28(6, Pt 1):485-490.

20. Kumar R, Basu S, Torigian D, Anand V, Zhuang H, Alavi A: Role of modern imaging techniques for diagnosis of infection in the era of 18F-fluorodeoxyglucose positron emission tomography. *Clin Microbiol Rev* 2008;21(1):209-224.

PET with [18]fluorodeoxyglucose was reviewed for detecting and monitoring infection. This modality is effective for evaluation of osteomyelitis, infected prostheses, fever of unknown origin, and AIDS.

21. Nawaz A, Torigian DA, Siegelman ES, Basu S, Chryssikos T, Alavi A: Diagnostic performance of FDG-PET, MRI, and plain film radiography (PFR) for the diagnosis of osteomyelitis in the diabetic foot. *Mol Imaging Biol* 2010;12(3):335-342.

An ongoing study of 110 patients with diabetes with suspected infection compared surgical and microbial findings with the preoperative interpretation of [18]fluorodeoxyglucose PET studies. Although not as sensitive as MRI, PET was more specific.

22. Richard JL, Sotto A, Lavigne JP: New insights in diabetic foot infection. *World J Diabetes* 2011;2(2):24-32.

A review of the diagnosis and management of diabetic foot infections reported recent data on identification, assessment, and antibiotic therapy of diabetic foot infections.

23. Bone RC, Sibbald WJ, Sprung CL: The ACCP-SCCM consensus conference on sepsis and organ failure. *Chest* 1992;101(6):1481-1483.

24. Armstrong DG, Lavery LA, Sariaya M, Ashry H: Leukocytosis is a poor indicator of acute osteomyelitis of the foot in diabetes mellitus. *J Foot Ankle Surg* 1996;35(4):280-283.

25. Lipsky BA, Sheehan P, Armstrong DG, Tice AD, Polis AB, Abramson MA: Clinical predictors of treatment failure for diabetic foot infections: Data from a prospective trial. *Int Wound J* 2007;4(1):30-38.

26. Pinzur MS, Stuck RM, Sage R, Hunt N, Rabinovich Z: Syme ankle disarticulation in patients with diabetes. *J Bone Joint Surg Am* 2003;85(9):1667-1672.

27. Wukich DK, Hobizal KB, Brooks MM: Severity of diabetic foot infection and rate of limb salvage. *Foot Ankle Int* 2013;34(3):351-358.

A retrospectively controlled cohort study identified 100 patients with diabetic foot infection who required hospital admission. Patients with severe infection had an amputation rate of 55% compared with 42% for those with moderate infection, and their hospital stay was 60% longer.

28. Dzieciuchowicz L, Kruszyna L, Krasiński Z, Espinosa G: Monitoring of systemic inflammatory response in diabetic patients with deep foot infection treated with negative pressure wound therapy. *Foot Ankle Int* 2012;33(10):832-837.

Acutely débrided deep diabetic foot infection in 10 patients was safely treated with negative pressure wound therapy. Only one-half of the patients had an elevated WBC count and neutrophil concentration. C-reactive protein level was elevated in 9 patients and was the preferable parameter for both diagnosis and monitoring of treatment.

29. Cheing GL, Chau RM, Kwan RL, Choi CH, Zheng YP: Do the biomechanical properties of the ankle-foot complex influence postural control for people with Type 2 diabetes? *Clin Biomech (Bristol, Avon)* 2013;28(1):88-92.

A handheld ultrasonographic indentation system was used to measure the soft-tissue biomechanical properties of the Achilles tendon and plantar soft tissue of the foot in 32 patients with diabetes and 32 individuals without diabetes. Patients with or without neuropathy had a thicker Achilles tendon and stiffer plantar soft tissue than the healthy control subjects. These findings were correlated with the use of vestibular, somatosensory, or visual inputs to maintain balance in patients with diabetes.

30. Sun JH, Cheng BK, Zheng YP, Huang YP, Leung JY, Cheing GL: Changes in the thickness and stiffness of plantar soft tissues in people with diabetic peripheral neuropathy. *Arch Phys Med Rehabil* 2011;92(9):1484-1489.

This is a continuation of work by Zheng using ultrasonography to measure the thickness and stiffness of the plantar soft tissues comparing normal healthy controls to patients with diabetic peripheral neuropathy.

31. Margolis DJ, Gupta J, Hoffstad O, et al: Lack of effectiveness of hyperbaric oxygen therapy for the treatment of diabetic foot ulcer and the prevention of amputation: A cohort study. *Diabetes Care* 2013;36(7):1961-1966.

A longitudinal observational cohort study compared the effectiveness of hyperbaric oxygen therapy with that of other therapies for treating diabetic foot ulcer and preventing lower extremity amputation. All 6,259 enrollees had adequate lower limb arterial perfusion and a foot ulcer that extended through the dermis. Hyperbaric oxygen therapy was not found to improve outcomes.

32. Brodsky JW: The diabetic foot, in Coughlin MJ, Mann RA, Saltzman CL, eds: *Surgery of the Foot and Ankle*, ed 8. Philadelphia, PA, Mosby, 2007, pp 1281-1368.

33. Leese G, Schofield C, McMurray B, et al: Scottish foot ulcer risk score predicts foot ulcer healing in a regional specialist foot clinic. *Diabetes Care* 2007;30(8):2064-2069.

34. Beckert S, Witte M, Wicke C, Königsrainer A, Coerper S: A new wound-based severity score for diabetic foot ulcers: A prospective analysis of 1,000 patients. *Diabetes Care* 2006;29(5):988-992.

35. Armstrong DG, Nguyen HC, Lavery LA, van Schie CH, Boulton AJ, Harkless LB: Off-loading the diabetic foot wound: A randomized clinical trial. *Diabetes Care* 2001;24(6):1019-1022.

36. Philbin TM: The diabetic foot, in Pinzur MS, ed: *Orthopaedic Knowledge Update Foot and Ankle*, ed 4. Rosemont, IL, American Academy of Orthopaedic Surgeons, 2008, pp 273-290.

37. Pickwell KM, Siersma VD, Kars M, Holstein PE, Schaper NC; Eurodiale consortium: Diabetic foot disease: Impact of ulcer location on ulcer healing. *Diabetes Metab Res Rev* 2013;29(5):377-383.

The influence of ulcer location on time to healing of diabetic foot ulcers was studied in 1,000 patients using a multivariate Cox regression analysis. Time to ulcer healing increased progressively from toe to midfoot to heel but was not different for plantar and nonplantar ulcers.

38. Health Quality Ontario: Hyperbaric oxygen therapy for non-healing ulcers in diabetes mellitus: An evidence-based analysis. *Ont Health Technol Assess Ser* 2005;5(11):1-28.

39. De León Rodriguez D, Allet L, Golay A, et al: Biofeedback can reduce foot pressure to a safe level and without causing new at-risk zones in patients with diabetes and peripheral neuropathy. *Diabetes Metab Res Rev* 2013;29(2):139-144.

The usefulness of biofeedback was evaluated in 21 patients with diabetes and peripheral neuropathy who learned a walking strategy designed to reduce points of high plantar pressure during gait.

40. Embil JM, Rose G, Trepman E, et al: Oral antimicrobial therapy for diabetic foot osteomyelitis. *Foot Ankle Int* 2006;27(10):771-779.

41. Lamb HM, Wiseman LR: Pexiganan acetate. *Drugs* 1998;56(6):1047-1052, discussion 1053-1054.

42. Bergin SM, Wraight P: Silver based wound dressings and topical agents for treating diabetic foot ulcers. *Cochrane Database Syst Rev* 2006;1:CD005082.

43. Vermeulen H, van Hattem JM, Storm-Versloot MN, Ubbink DT: Topical silver for treating infected wounds. *Cochrane Database Syst Rev* 2007;1:CD005486.

44. Anglen JO: Comparison of soap and antibiotic solutions for irrigation of lower-limb open fracture wounds: A prospective, randomized study. *J Bone Joint Surg Am* 2005;87(7):1415-1422.

45. Lipsky BA, Hoey C: Topical antimicrobial therapy for treating chronic wounds. *Clin Infect Dis* 2009;49(10):1541-1549.

 Clinically relevant information was provided on topical antimicrobial agents used for the treatment of nonhealing wounds. Using a newer, relatively nontoxic antiseptic was preferred to using topical antibiotics, especially those available for systemic use.

46. Pinzur MS, Gil J, Belmares J: Treatment of osteomyelitis in Charcot foot with single-stage resection of infection, correction of deformity, and maintenance with ring fixation. *Foot Ankle Int* 2012;33(12):1069-1074.

 In 178 patients who underwent surgical correction of Charcot deformity, 73 had evidence of osteomyelitis at the time of surgery. The most common organisms were staphylococci. The cultures positive for *S aureus* were divided between methicillin-susceptible and methicillin-resistant organisms.

47. Gardner SE, Hillis SL, Heilmann K, Segre JA, Grice EA: The neuropathic diabetic foot ulcer microbiome is associated with clinical factors. *Diabetes* 2013;62(3):923-930.

 Microbiomes were profiled from 52 neuropathic non-ischemic diabetic foot ulcers without clinical evidence of infection using high-throughput sequencing of the bacterial 16S ribosomal RNA gene. Wound cultures vastly underrepresent microbial load, microbial diversity, and the presence of potential pathogens. Deeper ulcers were associated with ulcer cluster and abundance of anaerobic bacteria. Longer duration was correlated with bacterial diversity, species richness, and relative abundance of proteobacteria. Poor glycemic control was associated with ulcer cluster and with poorest control increasing concentrations of *Staphylococcus*-and *Streptococcus*-rich ulcer clusters.

48. Wilson RM: Neutrophil function in diabetes. *Diabet Med* 1986;3(6):509-512.

49. Richard JL, Sotto A, Jourdan N, et al; Nîmes University Hospital Working Group on the Diabetic Foot (GP30): Risk factors and healing impact of multidrug-resistant bacteria in diabetic foot ulcers. *Diabetes Metab* 2008;34(4, Pt 1):363-369.

50. Aragón-Sánchez J: A review of the basis of surgical treatment of diabetic foot infections. *Int J Low Extrem Wounds* 2011;10(1):33-65.

 An expert examination of the basis of nonvascular surgical treatment of diabetic foot infections emphasized the importance of anatomic concepts, the variety of possible clinical presentations, and the concepts of surgical timing

51. Lipsky BA, Peters EJ, Senneville E, et al: Expert opinion on the management of infections in the diabetic foot. *Diabetes Metab Res Rev* 2012;28(Suppl 1):163-178.

 This update from the IWGDF offers a systematic review of diabetic foot infection management. MRI offers the most accurate means of diagnosing bone infection, but bone biopsy for culture and histopathology remains the standard. Culture-based identification of the infecting organism allows the optimal antibiotic treatment to be chosen. Appropriate surgical treatment and ulcer management are important. Adjunctive therapies are available, but the data supporting them are weak.

52. Lipsky BA, Berendt AR, Deery HG, et al; Infectious Diseases Society of America: Diagnosis and treatment of diabetic foot infections. *Clin Infect Dis* 2004;39(7):885-910.

53. Lipsky BA, Berendt AR, Cornia PB, et al; Infectious Diseases Society of America: Executive summary: 2012 Infectious Diseases Society of America clinical practice guideline for the diagnosis and treatment of diabetic foot infections. *Clin Infect Dis* 2012;54(12):1679-1684.

 The authors summarize the clinical practice guideline, which includes a classification system and a vascular assessment.

54. Aragón-Sánchez J, Lipsky BA, Lázaro-Martínez JL: Gram-negative diabetic foot osteomyelitis: Risk factors and clinical presentation. *Int J Low Extrem Wounds* 2013;12(1):63-68.

 The most common pathogens in 341 incidences of diabetic foot osteomyelitis were gram-positive organisms, especially *S aureus*. Gram-negative organisms were isolated in 44% (alone or with a gram-positive organism). Patients whose bone samples contained gram-negative organisms had a higher prevalence of leukocytosis and higher WBC counts than those with gram-positive organisms.

55. Colen LB, Kim CJ, Grant WP, Yeh JT, Hind B: Achilles tendon lengthening: Friend or foe in the diabetic foot? *Plast Reconstr Surg* 2013;131(1):37e-43e.

 Two groups of diabetic patients with plantar forefoot or midfoot ulceration underwent soft-tissue reconstruction from 1983 to 1991 or from 1996 to 2004. The relative risk of ulcer recurrence was reduced by 94% with the addition of Achilles tendon lengthening to the original wound closure procedure.

56. Mueller MJ, Sinacore DR, Hastings MK, Strube MJ, Johnson JE: Effect of Achilles tendon lengthening on neuropathic plantar ulcers: A randomized clinical trial. *J Bone Joint Surg Am* 2003;85(8):1436-1445.

57. Kim JY, Hwang S, Lee Y: Selective plantar fascia release for nonhealing diabetic plantar ulcerations. *J Bone Joint Surg Am* 2012;94(14):1297-1302.

Sixty patients with diabetes were treated using a selective plantar fascia release for nonhealing diabetic neuropathic ulcers in the forefoot. Patients with preoperative metatarsophalangeal joint motion of 5° to 30° had an increase of at least 13° after the plantar fascia release healed.

58. Smith DG, Assal M, Reiber GE, Vath C, LeMaster J, Wallace C: Minor environmental trauma and lower extremity amputation in high-risk patients with diabetes: Incidence, pivotal events, etiology, and amputation level in a prospectively followed cohort. *Foot Ankle Int* 2003;24(9):690-695.

59. Pinzur M, Freeland R, Juknelis D: The association between body mass index and foot disorders in diabetic patients. *Foot Ankle Int* 2005;26(5):375-377.

60. Wachtel MS: Family poverty accounts for differences in lower-extremity amputation rates of minorities 50 years old or more with diabetes. *J Natl Med Assoc* 2005;97(3):334-338.

61. Moura Neto A, Zantut-Wittmann DE, Fernandes TD, Nery M, Parisi MC: Risk factors for ulceration and amputation in diabetic foot: Study in a cohort of 496 patients. *Endocrine* 2013;44(1):119-124.

Of 496 patients, 461 (92.9%) had diabetic neuropathy. Predictors of amputation were male sex and a neuroischemic diabetic foot. The combination of neuropathy and peripheral vascular disease added substantially to the risk of amputation. Men with combined risk factors should receive particular attention in the foot clinic.

62. Anderson JJ, Boone J, Hansen M, Spencer L, Fowler Z: A comparison of diabetic smokers and non-smokers who undergo lower extremity amputation: A retrospective review of 112 patients. *Diabet Foot Ankle* 2012 [published online ahead of print October 16].

A retrospective study of 46 nonsmokers and 66 smokers at risk for amputation because of diabetic foot ulcers found that the smokers underwent more amputations and more proximal amputations than the nonsmokers. Increased smoking in terms of pack years was correlated with an increased risk of proximal amputation.

63. Faglia E, Clerici G, Caminiti M, Curci V, Somalvico F: Influence of osteomyelitis location in the foot of diabetic patients with transtibial amputation. *Foot Ankle Int* 2013;34(2):222-227.

In an Italian study of 350 patients with diabetes treated for osteomyelitis, the rate of transtibial amputation was higher if the osteomyelitis involved the heel rather than the midfoot or forefoot.

64. Molines-Barroso RJ, Lázaro-Martínez JL, Aragón-Sánchez J, García-Morales E, Beneit-Montesinos JV, Álvaro-Afonso FJ: Analysis of transfer lesions in patients who underwent surgery for diabetic foot ulcers located on the plantar aspect of the metatarsal heads. *Diabet Med* 2013;30(8):973-976.

After Cox regression model analysis, a review of 119 patients who underwent resection of at least one metatarsal head found the highest risk of reulceration after amputation of the first metatarsal head and the least risk after amputation of the fifth metatarsal head.

65. Nerone VS, Springer KD, Woodruff DM, Atway SA: Reamputation after minor foot amputation in diabetic patients: Risk factors leading to limb loss. *J Foot Ankle Surg* 2013;52(2):184-187.

A review of 163 patients with diabetes who underwent a minor foot amputation and later underwent at least one subsequent major or minor lower extremity amputation analyzed possible risk factors including age, glycemic control, kidney function, previous kidney or kidney-pancreas transplantation, smoking history, and presence and severity of peripheral arterial disease. Only patients with peripheral arterial disease had a statistically significant relationship between conversion from minor foot amputation to major limb amputation. It is important to assess peripheral vascular status in all patients with diabetes before surgical intervention.

66. Brown ML, Tang W, Patel A, Baumhauer JF: Partial foot amputation in patients with diabetic foot ulcers. *Foot Ankle Int* 2012;33(9):707-716.

The longevity, outcome, and mortality of partial foot amputations was examined as an alternative to transtibial amputation. Patients with transmetatarsal and Chopart amputations had high ambulatory levels and durability.

67. Belatti DA, Phisitkul P: Declines in lower extremity amputation in the U.S. Medicare population, 2000–2010. *Foot Ankle Int* 2013;34(7):923-931.

The complete Medicare Part B claims database from 2000 to 2010 was searched for all codes designating lower extremity amputation as well as specific orthopaedic treatments of diabetic foot infection.

68. Apelqvist J, Castenfors J, Larsson J, Stenström A, Agardh CD: Prognostic value of systolic ankle and toe blood pressure levels in outcome of diabetic foot ulcer. *Diabetes Care* 1989;12(6):373-378.

69. Baumhauer JF, O'Keefe RJ, Schon LC, Pinzur MS: Cytokine-induced osteoclastic bone resorption in Charcot arthropathy: An immunohistochemical study. *Foot Ankle Int* 2006;27(10):797-800.

70. Jeffcoate WJ, Game F, Cavanagh PR: The role of proinflammatory cytokines in the cause of neuropathic osteoarthropathy (acute Charcot foot) in diabetes. *Lancet* 2005;366(9502):2058-2061.

71. Eichenholtz SN: *Charcot Joints.* Springfield, IL, Thomas,1966.

72. Schon LC, Marks RM: The management of neuroarthropathic fracture-dislocations in the diabetic patient. *Orthop Clin North Am* 1995;26(2):375-392.

73. Bibbo C, Lin SS, Beam HA, Behrens FF: Complications of ankle fractures in diabetic patients. *Orthop Clin North Am* 2001;32(1):113-133.

74. McCormack RG, Leith JM: Ankle fractures in diabetics: Complications of surgical management. *J Bone Joint Surg Br* 1998;80(4):689-692.

75. Chaudhary SB, Liporace FA, Gandhi A, Donley BG, Pinzur MS, Lin SS: Complications of ankle fracture in patients with diabetes. *J Am Acad Orthop Surg* 2008;16(3):159-170.

76. Ganesh SP, Pietrobon R, Cecílio WA, Pan D, Lightdale N, Nunley JA: The impact of diabetes on patient outcomes after ankle fracture. *J Bone Joint Surg Am* 2005;87(8):1712-1718.

77. Papa J, Myerson M, Girard P: Salvage, with arthrodesis, in intractable diabetic neuropathic arthropathy of the foot and ankle. *J Bone Joint Surg Am* 1993;75(7):1056-1066.

78. Perlman MH, Thordarson DB: Ankle fusion in a high risk population: An assessment of nonunion risk factors. *Foot Ankle Int* 1999;20(8):491-496.

79. Stuart MJ, Morrey BF: Arthrodesis of the diabetic neuropathic ankle joint. *Clin Orthop Relat Res* 1990;253:209-211.

80. Shibuya N, Humphers JM, Fluhman BL, Jupiter DC: Factors associated with nonunion, delayed union, and malunion in foot and ankle surgery in diabetic patients. *J Foot Ankle Surg* 2013;52(2):207-211.

A retrospective study reviewed surgical complications in 165 patients with diabetes who had undergone arthrodesis, osteotomy, or fracture reduction. After adjusting for covariates, peripheral neuropathy, surgery duration, and glycohemoglobin were found to be significantly associated with bone-healing complications. Peripheral neuropathy had the strongest association.

81. Centers for Disease Control and Prevention: 2011 National Diabetes Fact Sheet. http://www.cdc.gov/diabetes/pubs/factsheet11.htm. Accessed August 28, 2014.

82. Singh N, Armstrong DG, Lipsky BA: Preventing foot ulcers in patients with diabetes. *JAMA* 2005;293(2):217-228.

83. Healy A, Naemi R, Chockalingam N: The effectiveness of footwear as an intervention to prevent or to reduce biomechanical risk factors associated with diabetic foot ulceration: A systematic review. *J Diabetes Complications* 2013;27(4):391-400.

The effectiveness of footwear in preventing ulceration has not been examined, and findings conflict on the effectiveness of footwear interventions. The value of rocker-sole footwear and custom orthotic devices in plantar pressure reduction was supported in cross-sectional studies, but longitudinal studies are required.

84. Blumberg SN, Warren SM: Disparities in initial presentation and treatment outcomes of diabetic foot ulcers in a public, private and VA hospital. *J Diabetes* 2014;6(1):68-75.

A retrospective chart review of patients with diabetes newly diagnosed with a foot ulcer found that patients treated in a Veterans Administration hospital had significantly higher amputation rates than those treated at adjacent private and public hospitals. The veterans were older than the patients at the other hospitals (mean age, 72.5 years), most were members of a racial minority, and most had a gangrenous ulcer.

85. Pu J, Chewning B: Racial difference in diabetes preventive care. *Res Social Adm Pharm* 2013;9(6):790-796.

The 2008 Medical Expenditure Panel Survey outcome data on diabetic preventive care were assessed by reviewing participants' self-reports. Patients least likely to receive three elements of diabetes preventive care were identified as uninsured, Hispanic, relatively young, living in a rural area, or having a low family income.

86. Kim G, Ford KL, Chiriboga DA, Sorkin DH: Racial and ethnic disparities in healthcare use, delayed care, and management of diabetes mellitus in older adults in California. *J Am Geriatr Soc* 2012;60(12):2319-2325.

The 2009 California Health Interview Survey descriptive statistics and logistic regression analyses were used in weighing data from a sample of 3,003 adults age 60 years or older with a self-reported diagnosis of diabetes mellitus. The findings revealed a need for racial and ethnic-specific interventions to reduce disparities in diabetes management.

87. Yu MK, Lyles CR, Bent-Shaw LA, Young BA: Sex disparities in diabetes process of care measures and self-care in high-risk patients. *J Diabetes Res* 2013;2013:575814.

Sex differences in processes of diabetes care and self-care activities were assessed in a cross-sectional analysis. Women were less likely than men to undergo dyslipidemia screening, reach a low-density lipoprotein goal, and use statins. No sex differences were observed in glycohemoglobin testing, microalbuminuria screening, or angiotensin-converting enzyme inhibitor use. Women were less likely to report regular exercise but had better adherence to healthy diet, glucose monitoring, and foot self-examination.

88. Kuehn BM: Prompt response, multidisciplinary care key to reducing diabetic foot amputation. *JAMA* 2012;308(1):19-20.

A multidisciplinary team approach to the management of diabetic foot infections was recommended by the IDSA .

89. Maderal AD, Vivas AC, Zwick TG, Kirsner RS: Diabetic foot ulcers: Evaluation and management. *Hosp Pract (1995)* 2012;40(3):102-115.

2: Neuromuscular Disease

Chapter 7

Peripheral Nerve Disease

Vinayak M. Sathe, MD

Introduction

Peripheral nerve entrapments in the foot and ankle are rare when compared with the upper limb and as such tend to remain underdiagnosed. These injuries can cause substantial impairment in foot and ankle function and may result in chronic, disabling conditions that subsequently are harder to treat. A detailed patient history and clinical examination and judicious use of various investigations now available can result in a diagnosis of the clinical condition in most situations. This chapter discusses the most common peripheral nerve entrapments seen in the foot and ankle and their presentations, evaluation, and treatment.

Interdigital Plantar Neuralgia

Interdigital plantar neuralgia was first described as early as 1845 for pain in relation to the third interspace. This entity, commonly referred to as Morton neuroma, was described by Thomas Morton in 1876. He actually reported a peculiar, painful affection of the fourth metatarsophalangeal joint, which was treated with resection of that joint with the additional removal of soft tissue surrounding the joint including digital branches of the third and fourth web space nerves. He described removing the swollen portion of the tissue, thinking this was a neuroma. It is now known that it is not a true tumor of the nerve. The histologic findings describe interstitial sclerohyalinosis, degeneration of nerve fibers without wallerian degeneration, intraneural and perineural fibrosis, and stromal changes with increased elastic fibers.[1,2] This condition has also been referred to as compression neuropathy.

Anatomy

There is still no clear explanation of the etiology of this condition. Multiple theories have been proposed. The deep transverse metatarsal ligament has been implicated as the site and cause of the nerve compression. The pathologic findings, including intraneural fibrosis and degeneration, occur distal to the intermetatarsal ligament (IMTL), supporting the theory of direct compression by the IMTL.[2] In another study, the distance between the common digital nerve bifurcation and the deep transverse metatarsal ligament was examined. It was noted that the area of pathology was always distal to the deep transverse metatarsal ligament (DTML) during gait in the heel-off and midstance phases.[3] Nerve biopsy specimens were obtained from patients with interdigital neuralgia and compared with those from asymptomatic nerves at autopsy. This study showed no substantial difference between interdigital plantar neuralgia biopsy specimens and those of normal nerves obtained at autopsy.[4]

The plantar aspect of the foot is supplied by the medial plantar nerve (MPN), which branches into the first, second, and third digital nerves and the lateral plantar nerve (LPN), which provides the common digital nerve to the fourth interspace and a proper digital branch to the lateral side of the fifth toe. One study postulated that the nerve in the third web space composed of communicating branches from the MPN and LPN is thicker and consequently more susceptible to injury,[5] but this has not been supported clinically. Another study observed that the second and third intermetatarsal spaces are narrower than the first and fourth and theorized that this could be the reason for the more common entrapment of the nerves in these interspaces.[6] A communicating branch between the third and fourth common digital nerves is present in up to 28% of feet and an injury to one of these communicating branches could result in pain, which might be responsible for recurrent pain after neuroma resection.[7]

Another proposed contributing factor is the difference in mobility between the medial three rays compared to the lateral two rays. The first, second, and third metatarsals are more firmly fixed to the corresponding cuneiforms, whereas the fourth and fifth metatarsals have more movement with their cuboid articulation. This

Neither Dr. Sathe nor any immediate family member has received anything of value from or has stock or stock options held in a commercial company or institution related directly or indirectly to the subject of this chapter.

2: Neuromuscular Disease

difference may expose the common digital nerve to trauma. Although this theory can be argued for the third web space, it is negated by the presence of neuromas in the second interspace.[8]

Other causes of interdigital plantar neuralgia include direct injuries to the interdigitial nerve such as stepping on sharp objects, and crushing or traction injuries. It has also been proposed that repetitive activities such as prolonged standing or walking on hard surfaces with uncushioned shoes might result in interdigital neuralgia. In runners, dancers, or athletes, high forefoot forces during cutting, twisting, spinning, or jumping activities might result in overuse injury of the interdigital nerve. Similarly, modern footwear can promote excessive dorsiflexion of the metatarsophalangeal (MTP) joint, causing forced plantar flexion of the metatarsals and subsequent trauma to the nerves.[9] Fat pad atrophy may make the nerve more vulnerable. Rarely, the transverse metatarsal ligament may become thickened or have an aberrant band that will resolve the symptoms of interdigital neuroma when released.[9] Other extrinsic causes of nerve injury include ganglion, lipoma, or MTP joint instability. In approximately 10% to 15% of patients, MTP joint capsule attenuation allows medial deviation of the third toe and consequent lateral shifting of the third metatarsal, reducing the third intermetatarsal space and causing interdigital plantar neuralgia.[9] Injury to the plantar plate with subluxation or dislocation of the MTP joint may put additional strain on the nerve. Patients with proximal nerve compression may experience double crush syndrome whereby the distal nerve becomes more sensitive to any pressure. Arthritis and synovitis of the MTP joints due to various causes and fracture sequelae such as malunion may result in interdigital plantar neuralgia.

History and Physical Examination

The most common age for presentation of interdigital plantar neuralgia is reportedly 55 years (range, 29 to 81 years). Interdigital plantar neuralgia is 4 to 15 times more likely to be diagnosed in women than men.[8,10] Typically, the presenting symptoms are in the second or third interspace. The occurrence of symptoms in the first or fourth interspace is rare and atypical. Unilateral involvement is more common, but there is a 15% incidence of bilateral neuromas. A 3% incidence of two neuromas in the same foot has been reported.[11] Patients report burning, stabbing, tingling, electric-type shooting pain radiating into the affected toes. Removing tight-fitting shoes often relieves the symptoms. Walking barefoot on soft surfaces also helps to ease the pain. Some patients describe fullness under the toes. The normal gait pattern of heel strike, then rolling onto the ball of the foot, may be lost as patients try to curl the toes during stance to reduce the pain.

When starting the physical examination it is important to observe for foot alignment while standing to detect deviations in the toes, clawing, and swelling or fullness in the interspace compared to the contralateral side. The skin both dorsally and plantarly is closely examined for the presence of corns, calluses, or erythema. It is also important to inspect the patient's shoes because tight-fitting footwear is common. Careful palpation of the foot should be performed. Any areas of tenderness and/or fullness are noted. Each MTP joint is evaluated for synovitis, range of motion, laxity, and instability. An MTP joint drawer test is done to assess stability. This is important to rule out pathology in the MTP joints as responsible for the painful symptoms. The intermetatarsal spaces are then examined individually with compression to identify the origin of pain.

Various tests and examination techniques have been described for interdigital plantar neuralgia. The most commonly reported clinical findings include plantar tenderness in 95%, radiation of pain into the toes in 46%, a palpable mass in 12%, and numbness and widening of the interspace in 3%.[9] Another recent study showed that web space tenderness was positive in 95%, foot squeeze test positive in 88%, plantar percussion positive in 61%, and toe tip sensation deficit present in 67%.[12] A digital nerve stretch test has also been described with 100% sensitivity and 95% positive predictive value. To perform this test, both ankles are held in full dorsiflexion and the lesser toes on either side of the suspected web space are passively fully extended on both feet. The test is positive if the patient reports discomfort in the web space of the affected foot.[13] The Mulder test is done by compression with mediolateral pressure to the corresponding metatarsal heads while palpating the plantar webspace. A palpable "click" or "clunk" that reproduces patient symptoms is considered supportive of interdigital plantar neuralgia.[14] Palpation of the affected toes rarely shows loss of sensation.

A gross motor examination, including motor function and reflexes to rule out lumbar radiculopathy, is performed. Sensation is then tested for the sural, saphenous, and superficial peroneal nerves.

Diagnostic Studies

AP, lateral, and oblique radiographs are obtained to evaluate for dislocation, subluxation, arthritis, foreign body, or other abnormalities. Additional modalities that have been used for diagnosis of interdigital plantar neuralgia include ultrasonography (US) and MRI. Both are controversial in regard to their routine use in diagnosing interdigital plantar neuralgia. The size of the lesion is very important in detecting interdigital neuroma using these modalities. In one study, both US and MRI were found to be inaccurate. Specifically, US was shown to have inaccuracies for lesions less than 5 mm.[15] This study also concluded that relying on US or MRI would have led to inaccurate diagnosis in 18 of 19 cases. A detailed clinical examination was found to be the most sensitive and specific diagnostic modality. Another report found US to be very good at detecting intermetatarsal interdigital plantar neuralgia with 92% accuracy.[16]

No reliable electrodiagnostic studies are available to document the evidence of an interdigital plantar neuralgia. In one study using near-nerve needle sensory nerve conduction, an abnormal dip phenomenon was the most characteristic electrophysiologic diagnostic marker for interdigital plantar neuralgia.[17] Overall, electrodiagnostic studies are mainly used for detection of more proximal nerve compression or if there is suspicion for radiculopathy.

Selective injections into the painful intermetatarsal space can be used as a diagnostic tool. Although complete relief may be obtained, it is advisable not to interpret this as a confirmation of interdigital plantar neuralgia without further support through the physical examination.

Nonsurgical Treatment

Early treatment involves fitting the patient with a wide, soft, laced shoe, preferably with a low heel. This type of footwear allows the toes to spread, thereby relieving local pressure and also eliminating chronic hyperextension of the MTP joints. A soft metatarsal support pad just proximal to the metatarsal heads may provide relief from pressure in the area and offload the forefoot, reducing painful symptoms.

The use of corticosteroid injections may be helpful, but usually does not provide long-lasting relief. Substantial pain relief can be obtained after local injection in 60% to 80% of patients, with relief lasting up to 2 years in 30%.[18] In a recent patient-blinded randomized trial, 40 mg methylprednisolone with 1% lidocaine was injected under US control by a radiologist. Compared with the control group, global assessment of foot health was better in the corticosteroid group at 3 months. The study concluded that corticosteroid injections for interdigital plantar neuralgia can often provide symptomatic benefit for at least 3 months.[19] However, corticosteroid injections can be associated with serious side effects, especially if the injection is given at the wrong site. Injections should be used with some degree of caution. Atrophy of the subcutaneous fat pad and skin discoloration have been reported. Disruption of the joint capsule with resultant damage to the collateral ligaments and subsequent deviation of the toe medially or laterally can be a serious problem.

Neuroma alcohol sclerosing therapy has been reported to be safe and effective, although multiple injections have been used as treatment. In one study, 61% success was quoted after US-guided injection for interdigital plantar neuralgia.[20] In a follow-up study of 101 cases using alcohol injection for interdigital plantar neuralgia under US guidance, partial or total symptom improvement was reported in 94% of patients, with 84% becoming totally pain free. Thirty of these patients also had follow-up US 6 months later, which showed a 30% decrease in the size of the neuroma.[21] However, authors of a level II prospective case series reporting on results with 5-year follow-up stated that alcohol injection did not provide permanent resolution of symptoms for most patients and can be associated with considerable morbidity.[22] Other described nonsurgical options include NSAIDs, oral vitamin B_6 (200 mg daily for 3 months and then 100 mg daily), off-label use of tricyclic antidepressants, serotonin uptake inhibitors, and antiseizure medications. Overall, between 60% to 70% of patients in whom interdigital plantar neuralgia are diagnosed eventually undergo surgical intervention after failure of nonsurgical treatment.[12]

Surgical Treatment

If nonsurgical treatment fails, surgical intervention is indicated. Successful results after surgery have been reported to be between 51% and 93%.[1,8,23-26] Surgical excision of the nerve is the most frequent technique used to relieve pain from interdigital plantar neuralgia. Other options include neurectomy combined with burying the nerve stump into nearby nerve or muscle, nerve transposition, transverse intermetatarsal ligament release with or without neurolysis, and endoscopic decompression of the transverse metatarsal ligament. Endoscopic decompression has been reported to provide excellent pain relief with low rate of complications.[27] An alternate technique without endoscopy was performed in 14 patients (17 nerve decompressions) using instrumentation designed for carpal tunnel release. The authors of this study reported complete pain relief in 11 of 14 patients 26 months after surgery.[28]

Typically, a dorsal incision is used for primary surgery but plantar incision has been described as well. A recent level I prospective randomized controlled study trial of plantar and dorsal incisions for surgical treatment of primary Morton neuroma was done. The results demonstrated clinically good outcomes with both approaches, 87% plantar and 83% dorsal, with no difference in regard to pain, restrictions of daily activities, and scar tenderness. However, although scar complications were more commonly reported in the plantar group, resection of artery rather than nerve, wound infection

2: Neuromuscular Disease

and dehiscence, and postneurectomy pain were more commonly reported in the dorsal group[29] (**Figure 1**).

If the point of tenderness is very proximal, in revision cases a plantar approach can be useful (**Figure 2**). This approach provides excellent exposure of the nerve because the nerve is very plantar (**Figure 3**). It is important to place the incision between the metatarsal heads to prevent a tender scar on the weight-bearing surface of the foot.

Regardless of the incision approach, care must be taken to identify and resect all plantar nerve branches because these branches will tether the interdigital nerve, preventing its proximal retraction off the weight-bearing area of the forefoot. It is important to transect the nerve well proximal to the level of the metatarsal heads. An uncut retained branch that originates proximally may be a conduit for persistent neuritic symptoms. Excising interdigital plantar neuralgia from adjacent spaces should be avoided whenever possible because it may lead to dense sensory loss in the central toe.[30] A retrospective analysis of 674 consecutive primary neuroma excision surgeries showed that 38.9% pathology specimens included a digital artery.[31]

There are various outcome studies after surgical excision. In one study, in 56 patients with 76 interdigital plantar neuralgias, 71% became asymptomatic, 9% had substantial improvement, 6% had marginal improvement, and 14% failed. Still, 65% of the satisfied patients had residual plantar pain and 32% reported normal sensation in the web space.[8] Another study reported on 66 patients with 5.8 years follow-up and an 85% satisfaction rate. Approximately 70% of these patients needed some modification in their footwear to remain pain free.[23] A 2008 study including 120 patients with an average follow-up of 5.6 years used the Giannini neuroma score to

evaluate results. Fifty-one percent had good to excellent results, 10% fair results, and 40% had poor results. The average visual analog score was 2.5. A second web space interdigital plantar neuralgia was a prognostic indicator for poor outcome. The authors concluded that long-term outcomes are not as good as previously reported, possibly secondary to residual toe numbness.[26]

Recurrent neuromas are not uncommon and the presenting symptoms are often identical to those of the initial presentation. Recurrent symptoms can result from inadequate proximal nerve resection or incomplete resection of tethering plantar nerve branches.[25,32,33] The bulb neuroma, which forms at the end of the nerve, takes approximately 12 months to become large enough to cause pain. Accordingly, patients may present with recurrence of symptoms several months to years after the index surgery.

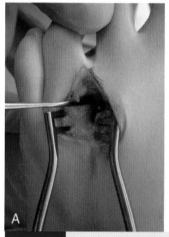
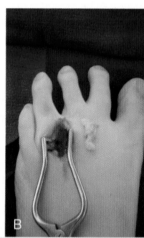

Figure 1   **A,** Dorsal approach showing intermetatarsal ligament. **B,** Excised neuroma.

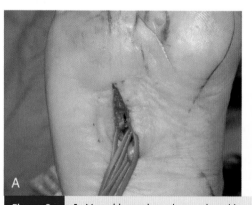
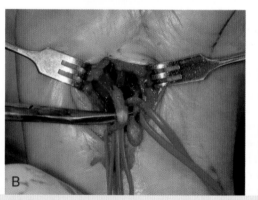
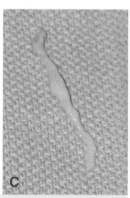

Figure 2   **A,** Vessel loops have been placed beneath three nerves that were found in the area immediately deep to the plantar fascia within the adipose tissue between the flexor digitorum longus tendons. **B,** Retraction enables excellent visualization of these structures. **C,** Resected plantar nerve from a patient with suspected recurrent and adjacent neuroma. (Panel **A** and **B** reproduced from Title CI, Schon LC: Morton's neuroma. http://orthoportal.aaos.org/oko/article.aspx?article=OKO-FO010. Accessed August 26, 2014. **C** reproduced from Title CI, Schon LC: Morton neuroma: Primary and secondary neurectomy. *J Am Acad Orthop Surg* 2008;16:550-557.)

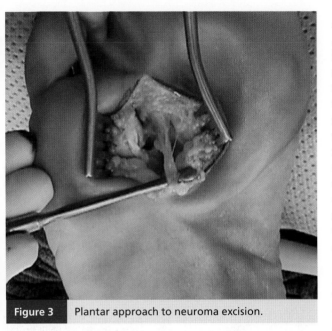

Figure 3 Plantar approach to neuroma excision.

Usually, patients with persistent or recurrent neuromas have a well-localized area of plantar tenderness. Palpation produces a Tinel sign with electric-like pain. Adjacent metatarsal head tenderness may be caused by the regenerating nerve innervations of the skin over the metatarsal heads. One option for revision surgery is the implantation of the nerve stump into the intrinsic muscles of the foot, which has been reported to provide pain relief in 80% of patients.[34]

Revision surgery should be undertaken with caution because the results are not as predictable as primary surgery. When evaluating the patient with recurrent symptoms of interdigital plantar neuralgia, the clinician should be suspicious of inadequate initial resection, formation of a true stump neuroma, misdiagnosis of correct web space, adjacent web space neuroma, and a proximal tarsal tunnel syndrome or nerve entrapment resulting from spine pathology.

Tarsal Tunnel Syndrome

Tarsal tunnel syndrome (TTS) is an entrapment neuropathy of the tibial nerve or one of its branches as it passes through the tarsal tunnel. Originally described in 1960, the condition was dubbed tarsal tunnel syndrome in 1962.[35] This syndrome can result from space-occupying lesions or constriction of the posterior tibial nerve. It has been compared with carpal tunnel syndrome in the hand because of name similarity, but in reality these two entities have little in common.

Anatomy

At the level of the ankle the flexor retinaculum or laciniate ligament is composed of the deep and superficial aponeuroses of the leg and creates a fibro-osseous tunnel posterior to the medial malleolus. Contents passing through this tunnel include the posterior tibial tendon, flexor digitorum longus tendon, flexor hallucis longus tendon, the posterior tibial artery, nerve, and vein. The floor of the tunnel is formed by the superior aspect of the calcaneus, the medial wall of the talus, and the distal-medial aspect of the tibia. The proximal and inferior borders of the tunnel are delineated by the inferior and superior margins of the flexor retinaculum. Within the tunnel, the posterior tibial nerve lies between the tendons of the flexor digitorum longus and flexor hallucis longus.

The tibial nerve ends by bifurcating into the medial and lateral plantar nerves. This usually occurs within the tarsal tunnel (93% to 96%), with the remaining 4% to 7% occurring more proximally. Proximal division is considered a risk factor for TTS because of the increased volume of two nerves entering the canal-narrowing.[36] The medial calcaneal nerve usually branches off the tibial nerve. This nerve pierces the flexor retinaculum to provide sensory innervations to the medial and posterior heel (Figure 4). Variations include the nerve running superficial to the retinaculum[37] or arising from the lateral plantar nerve.[36]

History and Physical Examination

Patients with TTS typically report burning pain and sometimes paresthesias along the medial and plantar aspects of the foot. Alternatively, radiating, diffuse, or poorly defined pain can be the presenting symptom. Typically, the pain increases with activity and improves with rest. It may also occur at night because of abnormal posture or pressure during sleep. Up to one third of patients also report pain radiating proximally into the midcalf (Valleix phenomenon).[9] Valleix phenomenon is defined as pain that radiates proximal to the tarsal tunnel instead of distal radiation and is sometime seen in double crush syndrome. Valleix phenomenon pain points are seen as tender areas in the course of a nerve, pressure upon which is painful in cases of neuralgia.

Precise and careful questioning is required to evaluate other potential sources of nerve pain. Differential diagnoses include rheumatologic conditions leading to chronic tenosynovitis, lumbar spine issues leading to radicular pain, and double crush syndrome. With double crush syndrome, proximal compression renders the nerve more susceptible for distal entrapment. Diabetes, vitamin deficiency, and alcoholism can also contribute to double crush syndrome.

2: Neuromuscular Disease

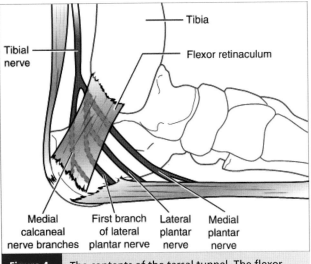

Tibia

Flexor retinaculum

Tibial nerve

Medial calcaneal nerve branches | First branch of lateral plantar nerve | Lateral plantar nerve | Medial plantar nerve

Figure 4 The contents of the tarsal tunnel. The flexor retinaculum passes posteriorly over the tarsal tunnel. The medial calcaneal nerve may originate from the tibial nerve proximal to the tarsal tunnel and may have multiple branches. The first branch of the lateral plantar nerve may originate within the tarsal tunnel. The medial plantar nerve frequently provides one or more calcaneal branches. (Reproduced from Hill KJ: Peripheral nerve disorders, in Pinzur MS, ed: *Orthopaedic Knowledge Update Foot and Ankle,* ed 4. Rosemont, IL, American Academy of Orthopaedic Surgeons, 2008, pp 307-327.)

Physical examination may also provide insight into TTS etiology. The patient should be examined standing to assess hindfoot alignment. Heel valgus puts the nerve under tension, whereas varus may result in nerve compression. While the patient is seated, the medial aspect of the leg, ankle, and foot is examined for any masses, inflammation or swelling. Evaluation of a Tinel sign should be performed in both heel neutral and heel valgus position to assess sensitivity of the tibial nerve. Percussion along the course of the nerve may produce paresthesias. Inversion and eversion of the hindfoot in relation to the ankle can influence tarsal canal pressure and affect symptoms.[38] Another provocative maneuver is a dorsiflexion eversion test, which can induce symptoms in just a few seconds.[39] Sensory testing to touch and use of a Semmes Weinstein monofilament may help to isolate terminal branches responsible for creating symptoms. Demonstration of plantar numbness and intrinsic motor weakness can be difficult, but loss of small toe abduction compared to the opposite, normal foot is more easily measurable and indicates loss of innervation of the abductor digiti quinti muscle.

Diagnostic Studies

Routine radiographs of the foot and ankle are obtained to rule out bony abnormalities such as fractures, bone spurs secondary to arthritis, and any other causes. If a space-occupying lesion is suspected, MRI can be performed.

In one study of 35 feet suspected of TTS, MRI showed abnormality in 85%.[40] MRI studies have shown changes in the volume of the tarsal tunnel in inversion and eversion thereby increasing pressure on the nerve.[41] Ultrasonography can be used as an adjunct to diagnose TTS, but is recognized as operator dependent. Electrodiagnostic studies are performed in most patients with suspected TTS, but literature reports differ as to which test is more reliable. One study has reported electrodiagnostic studies as 90% accurate in identifying tarsal tunnel entrapment.[42] Electrodiagnostic studies do play an important role in helping to differentiate TTS from radiculopathy or peripheral neuropathy. A recent analysis evaluated use of nerve conduction velocity (NCV) studies and electromyography (EMG) at the ankle and concluded that NCV may be useful, but the consensus is that there are no reliable studies available to evaluate reliability and reproducibility of electrodiagnostic studies in TTS.[43]

Nonsurgical Treatment

In the absence of a space-occupying lesion, nonsurgical treatment is indicated and includes NSAIDs, oral vitamin B, and tricyclic antidepressants. Temporary immobilization in a cast, walking boot, or an orthotic device to correct any deformity and correct any pronation of the foot may benefit some patients. A steroid injection is indicated in cases of tenosynovitis of the flexor digitorum longus tendon, which is adjacent to the posterior tibial tendon. Modalities such as heat, cold, and vibration are not recommended because they may irritate the sensitive nerves. Instead, physical therapy may incorporate topical anti-inflammatory agents, nerve relievers, and iontophoresis.

Surgical Treatment

For good surgical results, appropriate patient selection is important. A positive physical examination with appropriate studies such as NCV, EMG, and/or MRI is helpful in making the decision for surgical intervention.

Surgical intervention has been advocated when nonsurgical modalities fail. Space-occupying lesions in TTS, including lipoma, ganglion, and varicose veins, should be removed to reduce pressure on the nerve. If there is an underlying cause of TTS such as hindfoot instability, or calcaneal malunion with bone spurs, these need to be addressed during surgery.

Four separate medial ankle tunnels have been described.[44] Careful anatomic analysis demonstrates that

2: Neuromuscular Disease

the tarsal tunnel is not the equivalent of the carpal tunnel; rather, it is more closely the equivalent of the forearm. Hence, the flexor retinaculum is equivalent to distal forearm fascia. The medial plantar nerve tunnel, lateral plantar tunnel, and the calcaneal tunnel have been described as three additional tunnels within the tarsal tunnel. In a recent cadaver study, pressure changes in the medial and lateral plantar and tarsal tunnels were measured in different ankle positions.[45] This study concluded that pressures within the medial and lateral plantar and the tarsal tunnels increased substantially with changes in the ankle and subtalar position. This increased pressure could be substantially reduced by surgical release of each of these three tunnels, including excision of the septum between medial and lateral plantar tunnels.

In one study of 10 patients with TTS, the authors intraoperatively measured pressures in the tarsal, medial, and lateral plantar tunnels in multiple foot positions before and after excising the tunnel roofs and the intermuscular septum.[46] They also hypothesized that pressures in symptomatic patients would be substantially higher than those in an analogous cadaver study. They found that pronation and plantar flexion significantly increased pressures in the medial and lateral plantar tunnels causing nerve compression. Tunnel release and septum excision greatly reduced those pressures. Intraoperatively measured pressures were similar to cadaver pressures except for higher lateral plantar tunnel pressures noted in some positions. The greater effect on the lateral plantar tunnel could be the result of greater angularity of the passage from the medial ankle to beneath the foot.

In another large study, results of four medial ankle tunnel decompressions in 87 legs were reported.[47] The study included neurolysis of the tibial nerve within the tarsal tunnel with release of the medial plantar tunnel, lateral plantar tunnel, and calcaneal tunnel. Postoperatively, immediate weight bearing and ambulation were permitted in a bulky cotton dressing, which was removed at 1 week. Mean follow-up was 3.6 years. Using the traditional postoperative assessment, there were 82% excellent, 11% good, 5% fair, and 2% poor results.

Endoscopic tarsal tunnel release has been described. A report with short-term follow-up on a small number of patients has shown good results.[48]

Clinical Outcomes

Surgical treatment is generally successful when a space-occupying lesion is identified in the tarsal tunnel. A short-term outcome study reported on a series of patients who underwent tarsal tunnel release for benign space-occupying lesions. Only 13 of 20 patients were available for follow-up. Average age was 51.3 years. Symptom duration averaged 16.5 months. The most common lesion identified was ganglion in 10 patients, but other identified lesions included synovial chondromatosis, Schwannoma, and tarsal coalition.[49] Visual analog scales and American Orthopaedic Foot and Ankle Society (AOFAS) scores were measured in the preoperative and postoperative periods. Seven patients were satisfied, three had fair results, and three were dissatisfied.

Even in the absence of space-occupying lesions, tunnel decompression may provide relief of symptoms in up to 75% of patients.[9] Another study reported that patients with symptoms for less than one year had higher AOFAS score at 12 months after surgery.[50]

In a prospective evaluation of 46 patients (56 feet) who underwent nonsurgical and surgical treatment of TTS, pain intensity was documented before and after treatment with the Wong-Baker FACES Pain Rating Scale applied to anatomic regions of the plantar aspect of the foot. The results of the study showed that pretreatment motor nerve conduction latency was substantially greater in patients who needed surgical treatment than those receiving nonsurgical treatment. It was concluded that anatomic pain intensity rating models may be useful in the pretreatment and follow-up evaluation of TTS. Predictors of failed nonsurgical treatment included longer motor nerve conduction latency (7.4 ms or greater) and greater predominance of foot comorbidities.[51]

Overall, patients who are suspected to have TTS have higher tunnel pressures. Some patients have had recurrences even up to 5 years after index surgery, and a small number have reported increase in symptoms after the release. It is difficult to assess outcomes because some patients perceive no significant improvement even after successful tunnel release. Inadequate release technique has been criticized as one of the main reasons for poor outcome in the past. Studies support decreased nerve pressure with release of individual tunnels and excision of the septum, and with more aggressive tunnel release outcomes may improve with future studies.

Recurrence and Revision

Generally, outcomes for revision surgeries are worse than primary procedures. The most common causes of failure of surgical release are inadequate release because of lack of understanding of the anatomy, failure to properly execute the release, bleeding with scarring, damage to nerve or its branches during release, persistent hypersensitivity of the nerve, and initial intrinsic damage to the nerve. Each cause of failure should be evaluated and treated accordingly.[52] The concept of barrier wrapping of nerves to prevent adhesions to surrounding tissue has also been recommended. Autogenous vein grafts, free fat grafts, and collagen tubes have been used. If the nerve has intrinsic damage, sural nerve grafts and collagen conduits

2: Neuromuscular Disease

or wandering vein conduits have been suggested. Finally, complex regional pain syndrome (CRPS) type 2 should be considered for intractable pain with recurring or persistent symptoms.

MPN Entrapment

MPN entrapment, or jogger's foot, was first described in 1978.[53] The condition is thought to be secondary to local entrapment of the MPN at the fibromuscular tunnel formed by the abductor hallucis muscle and its border with the navicular tuberosity. It is often associated with a valgus foot deformity and long-distance running, and is characterized by neuritic pain at the medial arch radiating into the toes along the distribution of the medial plantar nerve. Rarely, a crush injury or transection of the nerve may occur, leading to severe symptoms.

Anatomy
The MPN branches typically from the tibial nerve under the abductor hallucis muscle and travels under the muscle with the medial plantar artery and veins. It innervates the abductor hallucis and terminates under the plantar fascia into the intermetatarsal nerves to the first and second, second and third, and third and fourth intermetatarsal spaces. It also provides motor branches to the intrinsic muscles of the foot. In the longitudinal arch, the nerve lies medial and adjacent to the flexor digitorum and flexor hallucis longus tendons close to the knot of Henry.

Etiology
MPN entrapment is seen in joggers with a history of repetitive impact and trauma during running, which leads to inflammation of the nerve. This clinical presentation is more common in planovalgus feet, whereby more pressure and stretch are placed on the nerve. An excessively high arch insert may also put pressure on this nerve. MPN entrapment has also been seen as an unusual presentation in ballet dancers.

Clinical Symptoms and Diagnosis
A high index of suspicion and awareness is required for diagnosing MPN entrapment. In many cases, symptoms may be present for more than 1 year before diagnosis. The runner often describes chronic pain on the inside of the middle portion of the foot. In addition, pain, aching, or a burning sensation over the arch of the foot is described and a giving-away sensation in the foot may occur while running. Rarely, the pain may radiate proximally into the ankle.

A detailed foot examination should be performed, specifically looking for hindfoot valgus. Shoes and orthotics should be examined. A stress test can be done by asking the patient to go for a run before the clinical examination. With MPN entrapment, tenderness is noted posterior to the navicular bone on the medial surface of the arch. A Tinel sign may be elicited to indicate the hypersensitive nerve. Local injection of lidocaine with subsequent relief of symptoms can also be a diagnostic tool.

Treatment
Initial treatment involves rest and shoe modifications including inserts. Oral anti-inflammatories and a trial of Cortisone injection may be considered. If conservative measures fail, then surgical decompression is indicated. Decompression of the MPN is done by releasing the fascia over the abductor hallucis and around the Knot of Henry. In addition, part of the naviculocalcaneal ligament is released to provide more space for the MPN. The majority of runners with MPN entrapment improve without surgery. Due to the rarity of this condition, large-scale reporting in the literature is not seen.

LPN Entrapment

Entrapment of the first branch of the LPN (Baxter nerve) can present as plantar heel pain. Because this nerve is in close vicinity to the inflammation associated with plantar fasciitis, it is thought that some degree of nerve entrapment may be a contributing factor in up to 20% of patients with chronic heel pain. Hence, accurate diagnosis is difficult with overlap of symptoms.

Anatomy
The first branch of the LPN is given off posteriorly just under the upper edge of the abductor hallucis. Rarely, it may branch directly from the lateral portion of the main tibial nerve. The first branch travels under the abductor hallucis and its deep fascia and over the medial fascia of the quadratus plantae. It then passes over the quadratus fascia and under the medial edge of the plantar fascia, then continues transversely across the heel under the flexor digitorum brevis muscle and sends a sensory branch to the central heel. It then terminates in the muscle of abductor digiti quinti.

Etiology
Entrapment of the first branch occurs between the abductor hallucis and quadratus plantae muscle. Direct heel trauma and calcaneal fractures can lead to symptoms. More typically, it is a traction neuritis of the LPN and its first branch. Other causes of LPN entrapment include hypertrophy of the abductor hallucis or quadratus plantae, the presence of accessory muscles or bursae, and phlebitis

in the calcaneal venous plexus. In addition, hypermobile flat feet can also put traction on the nerve causing pain.

Clinical Symptoms
This condition occurs in men 88% of the time and in patients between 26 to 28 years old. Patients present with chronic heel pain that is increased on walking or running. Pain can radiate proximally to the medial ankle or to the lateral aspect of the foot. It is worse when the patient takes his or her first step in the morning and may not remit with continued walking or rest.

Diagnosis
Classically, there is distinct tenderness at the origin of abductor hallucis that can radiate both proximally and distally with paresthesias. Pain often exacerbates with hyperpronation or Phalen maneuver (forced inversion and plantar flexion). In advanced cases, patients may lose the ability to abduct the fifth toe when compared with the opposite foot. Potential proximal nerve lesions should be excluded by palpating the nerve proximally. It is equally important to exclude other sources of heel pain. Injury or entrapment of the superficial calcaneal sensory nerve branches may also produce similar symptoms. This can be distinguished clinically by sensory loss that would be atypical of entrapment of the nerve to the abductor digiti quinti, which has no cutaneous sensory function.

Treatment
Nonsurgical treatment includes orthoses limiting pronation and local corticosteroid injection. A custom total contact orthosis with a posteromedial nerve relief channel may be helpful.[54] The channel is placed in the medial wall of the heel component and to the midline in the plantar area corresponding with the anatomy of the LPN and its first branch. Surgical treatment should be considered if nonsurgical treatment fails. The nerve is typically decompressed by releasing the deep fascia beneath the abductor hallucis and a portion of the plantar fascia.

Deep Peroneal Nerve Entrapment (Anterior Tarsal Tunnel Syndrome)

This entity was first described in 1960 and later referred to as anterior tarsal tunnel syndrome in 1968.[55] It is a rare condition, with patients reporting a burning sensation across the dorsum of the foot with paresthesia in the first web space. There may be wasting and weakness of the extensor digitorum brevis muscle.

Anatomy
The deep peroneal nerve in the proximal one third of the leg is a mixed motor and sensory nerve located between tibialis anterior and extensor digitorum longus. It travels with the anterior tibial artery and descends into the leg between the extensor digitorum and hallucis longus 5 cm proximal to the ankle joint. At approximately 1 cm above the ankle joint, the nerve branches to form a mixed branch that courses laterally to innervate extensor digitorum brevis and provide sensation to the lateral tarsal joints. The other branch is sensory only and runs distally with the dorsalis pedis artery between the extensor hallucis longus and brevis tendons to innervate the skin in the first web space.

The extensor retinaculum has a superior band located 5 cm above the ankle joint. The inferior Y-shaped band splits into two bands: the superomedial and inferomedial. The anterior tarsal tunnel is a fibro-osseous canal located just distal to the inferior medial band. The canal is in a 1.5-cm confined space formed superficially by the inferior extensor retinaculum, deep by the capsule of the talonavicular joint, laterally by the lateral malleolus and medially by the medial malleolus. It contains the dorsalis pedis artery and vein, deep peroneal nerve, tendons of extensor hallucis longus, extensor digitorum longus, tibialis anterior, peroneus tertius.

Etiology and Physical Examination
There are several potential sites of deep peroneal nerve entrapment that result in slightly different clinical presentations. The causes are varied and can be because of intrinsic or extrinsic mechanisms. Causes of intrinsic compression include space-occupying lesions, osteophytes, bony fragments, hypertrophic muscle bellies, and peripheral edema. Extrinsic compression can be associated with tight shoelaces and trauma, including single or repetitive events such as multiple ankle sprains.

A rare and very proximal entrapment can occur under the superior extensor retinaculum and involves the motor branch to the extensor digitorum brevis muscle. Referred pain to the sinus tarsi or atrophy and weakness of short toe extensors may develop. The most common site of entrapment occurs at the inferior edge of the extensor retinaculum. This results in sensory deficit only as the motor portion of the nerve has already branched out. These patients have deep, aching pain in the dorsal midfoot along with tingling, numbness, and burning in the area between the first and second toes. The pain is worse with activity and better with rest. Patients may be awakened at night by increased nerve pressure as the foot goes into plantar flexion. Tight-fitting or high lace-up shoes worsen the pain, which improves after removal of the shoes. Hypertrophy of the extensor digitorum brevis muscle may lead to more distal and sensory symptoms only.

2: Neuromuscular Disease

Clinical examination should begin with palpation of the deep peroneal nerve along its entire course. The proximal course of the nerve near the fibular neck is examined for tenderness, Tinel sign, and percussion. Forceful plantar flexion and inversion of the ankle puts the nerve under stretch and reduces available space in the anterior tarsal tunnel compressing the nerve against its floor. This maneuver may clinically produce the symptoms of nerve compression.[56]

Diagnosis

Plain radiographs may play an important role. A lateral foot and ankle radiograph may reveal osteophytes, particularly near the talonavicular joint, and old fractures with bone fragments. CT could be used for detailed bony anatomy of the tarsal canal, whereas an MRI is important if a mass is suspected of causing compression. Electrodiagnostic studies may show a proximal source of nerve compression such as lumbar radiculopathy. It also determines if there is involvement of the extensor digitorum brevis muscle suggesting a lesion proximal to the inferior retinaculum. The results should be correlated with clinical findings because abnormal fasciculations have been found in up to 76% of normal subjects and decreased motor recruitment in 38% of normal adults.[57] Electrodiagnostic data are technically difficult to obtain, and anatomic variations further complicate interpretation.

Treatment

Nonsurgical treatment begins with identification of the source of compression. Shoe wear accommodations may decrease the pressure over the nerve. Orthotics may improve biomechanical alignment and help reduce symptoms.[56] Physical therapy is helpful in patients with ankle instability. NSAIDs and other anti-inflammatory agents can also be used. Local injection of anesthetic and corticosteroid is a useful technique for evaluating and treating many patients. Resolution of pain and paresthesias may be obtained with serial injections into the anterior tarsal tunnel.[56]

When nonsurgical treatment fails, surgery should be considered. A slightly curved S-shaped incision is made over the dorsum of the foot, starting at the bases of the first and second metatarsals and extending proximally to the ankle joint. Care is taken to preserve branches of the superficial peroneal nerve. The extensor retinaculum is released enough to free up the deep peroneal nerve. Any osteophytes or other structures present on the dorsal edge of the talonavicular joint are removed. A hypertrophied extensor hallucis brevis may be resected. Simple closure and soft dressings are used. Noncompressive shoe wear is encouraged before gradual resumption of activity over 4 to 6 weeks.

Superficial Peroneal Nerve

Entrapment of the superficial peroneal nerve (SPN) is a relatively uncommon finding and is referred as mononeuralgia of the peroneal nerve. In a study of 480 patients with chronic leg pain, only 3.5% had pain attributable to SPN entrapment.[58]

Anatomy

The SPN branches off the common peroneal nerve laterally at the level of the neck of fibula. It supplies motor innervations to the lateral compartment of the leg including peroneus longus and brevis, and then continues as a sensory nerve. It passes deep to the peroneus longus, traveling between this muscle and the fibula in the lateral compartment. It becomes superficial as it courses distally between the peroneus longus and brevis piercing the deep fascia approximately 10 to 12 cm proximal to the tip of lateral malleolus as it leaves the lateral compartment. There is significant variation in the course of this nerve. In one anatomic study, the SPN was identified in the lateral compartment immediately adjacent to the fascial septum in 72% of specimens, with a branch in the anterior and lateral compartment in 5% of specimens and located in the anterior compartment only in 23% of specimens. The clinical implications of this study is that the surgeon must be aware that the SPN may be located in the lateral compartment and may also exhibit branches in both the anterior and lateral compartment.[59] Approximately 6 cm proximal to the lateral malleolus the nerve divides into the intermediate dorsal cutaneous nerve (IDCN) and the medial dorsal cutaneous nerve (MDCN). Variation has also been described in the sensory branches of SPN. In one cadaver dissection study, three distinct branching patterns were identified. In type I (63.3%), the SPN penetrated the crural fascia 8.1 cm +/– 1.78 cm proximal to the intermalleolar line and then divided into the IDCN and MDCN (classic type). In type II (26.7%), the IDCN and MDCN arose independently from the SPN. In type III (10%), the SPN penetrated the crural fascia 10.1 cm +/– 7 cm proximal to the intermalleolar line as a single branch. This single branch had a course similar to the MDCN.[60]

Etiology

The most common site of entrapment is usually 8 to 12 cm proximal to the tip of the fibula where the nerve exits from the deep fascia of the lateral compartment. The sharp fascial edge entraps the nerve as it pierces through the lateral fascia. This impingement could also be part of chronic exertional compartment syndrome of the leg. The classically described SPN injury occurs in the setting of repeated ankle inversion sprains resulting in traction on the nerve. This injury is also described in dancers and other athletes with lateral ligament deficiency. These individuals are also at increased risk secondary to their often hypertrophied peroneal musculature that can result in entrapment of the nerve in its short fibrous tunnel as it pierces the fascia.[61] Iatrogenic injuries can occur as a consequence of procedures approaching the ankle anteriorly. Ankle arthroscopy is a common foot and ankle surgical procedure. In one study of 294 cases reporting on complications of ankle arthroscopy using contemporary noninvasive distraction technique, 6 cases (2%) had neurologic complications related to the anterolateral portal. This study suggested an injury to the IDCN branch of the SPN.[62]

One of the most common causes of SPN injury is direct trauma. Compartment fasciotomy with resultant shifting of the peroneal tunnel can result in stretching and impingement of the nerve. Other causes include ganglion, fibular fracture, syndesmotic sprains, and chemotherapy causing neuropathy and edema.

Incidence and Clinical Presentation

SPN entrapment was reported in 17 of 480 patients (3.5%) with chronic leg pain.[58] It occurs equally in men and women, usually between 28 and 36 years old. It is frequent in runners; however, hockey, soccer, and racquetball players also report SPN symptoms.[9]

Clinical presentation can be variable. Classically, pain is located over the middle to distal third of the leg often intense over the anterior aspect with radiation to the dorsal aspect of the foot. Patients also describe numbness or tingling from the lateral side of the ankle extending into the sinus tarsi or dorsum of the foot. Night pain and rest pain are rare and symptoms are usually aggravated with activity. Examination of the foot reveals no specific motor weakness, and approximately two thirds will have no sensory loss in the foot.

Diagnosis

Low back pathology and common peroneal nerve impingement should be evaluated to rule out a proximal etiology for symptoms. SPN irritability is identified by percussion testing along the course of the nerve 8 to 12 cm above the tip of the fibula. Three provocative maneuvers designed to place the nerve on stretch can be used to assist in the diagnosis. First, the foot is palpated and pressure held over the site of entrapment while the patient actively dorsiflexes and everts the foot against resistance. Second, the patient's foot is passively plantar flexed and the ankle inverted without pressure on the nerve. Third, the examiner percusses the foot while passively maintaining stretch with the ankle inverted. A positive result is pain/paresthesia in 2 of 3 maneuvers.[63] Recently, a

fourth toe flexion sign has been described accentuating the subcutaneous course of the SPN.[64]

Imaging/Tests

Standard weight-bearing radiographs of the ankle are obtained to rule out bony impingement by fibular fracture callus, exostoses, or osteochondromas. CT and MRI are used only if specifically indicated. NCV studies are used as adjuncts for diagnosis. One study found an insignificant decrease in conduction velocity from 49 m/s in unaffected nerves to 28 m/s on average on the affected side.[58] It is important to remember that normal NCV studies do not rule out SPN entrapment and thus must be used only as a tool to assist in diagnosis.

Nonsurgical Treatment

Localized injection of anesthetic at the site of maximal tenderness can serve as both a diagnostic and therapeutic intervention. SPN impingement is thought to respond less well to nonsurgical treatment than impingement of the DPN. Lateral shoe wedges may help reduce varus stress on the ankle and the nerve. Use of NSAIDs, neuropathic drugs such as gabapentin and serotonin reuptake inhibitors, relative rest, and physical therapy for ankle strengthening may all be helpful.

Surgical Treatment

After nonsurgical treatment has been tried and failed, surgical intervention may be indicated. If ankle instability coexists, then lateral ligament reconstruction should be done. The SPN is released from the surrounding fascia at the point where it exits the crural fascia. Before surgery, the site of nerve compression is identified and marked. The SPN is decompressed at its entrance into the peroneal fibrous tunnel which varies from 3 to 11 cm in length. If exertional compartment syndrome coexists, the fascia of the lateral compartment should be released completely. Complete opening of the peroneal tunnel close to the anterior intermuscular septum is advocated. In one study, 80% of patients reported relief of symptoms with this approach.[58] Other recent studies support more limited decompression centered 5 to 8 cm proximal to the lateral malleolus.[65] Specific recommendations for limited release will depend on clinical symptoms, sites of compression, and the presence or absence of exertional compartment syndrome. More research is needed for long-term outcomes after various types of release or decompression are performed.

Sural Nerve

Entrapment of the sural nerve is rare but has been extensively studied in humans because of its status as a purely sensory nerve. This nerve is frequently used as a nerve graft.

Anatomy

The sural nerve is a pure sensory nerve derived from the S1 and S2 nerve roots. It has been studied extensively and various terms in regard to its branches have been used interchangeably. This has been confusing because it impedes comparisons and biases statistical data. A recent cadaver study and literature review details the various branches and the names given to them.[66] The sural nerve anatomy adheres to basic principles: it is typically made up of two components merging: a medial component from the tibial nerve (medial sural cutaneous nerve—MSCN or tibial nerve component) and a lateral component from the lateral sural cutaneous nerve (LSCN or common peroneal nerve component). However, it may consist of just a single component, either tibial or common peroneal nerve. In 73% of subjects studied, tibial and peroneal nerve components merge to form the sural nerve (pattern I). The peroneal communicating branch may branch off the LSCN (pattern Ia) or directly originate from the common peroneal nerve (pattern Ib).

In 24%, MSCN alone represented the sural nerve, whereas LSCN coursed independently (pattern II) or the LSCN was absent (pattern III).

In 3%, the LSCN represented the sural nerve, whereas MSCN terminated distally in the calf (pattern IV) or is absent (pattern V).

A peroneal communicating branch (PCB) was present in 63% with three types of origin, including type A: 74% PCB branches off LSCN; type B: 16% PCB and LSCN originate as a common trunk from common peroneal nerve (CPN); type C: 10% PCB and LSCN originate independently from CPN, with the peroneal communicating branch always medial and proximal to LSCN.

In general, the sural nerve begins distal to the popliteal fossa traveling between the two heads of the gastrocnemius and pierces the deep fascia in the middle third of the posterior surface of the leg. At this point it is typically joined by the peroneal communicating branch. Approximately 10 cm from the calcaneus, the sural nerve passes over the lateral edge of the Achilles tendon and continues distally posterior and then inferior to the lateral malleolus. It then passes plantar to the lateral malleolus and posterior to the peroneal tendons, curving anteriorly traveling on the lateral border of the foot where it becomes the lateral dorsal cutaneous nerve. It then divides at the base of the fifth metatarsal to form dorsal and plantar branches. The dorsal branch gives rise to the dorsal digital nerve to the lateral side of the fifth toe and may communicate with other digital branches of the fourth and fifth toe. The plantar branch provides

sensibility along the lateral border distally and may join distal branches of lateral plantar nerve. The sural nerve supplies sensation to the posterior lateral lower leg and ankle, the lateral heel and foot and the fifth toe with or without the fourth toe.

Etiology

Entrapment of the sural nerve in trauma situations can result from direct traumatic contusions, or from fractures of the calcaneus, fifth metatarsal, posterolateral process of the talus, or os peroneum. Traction injury can occur with ankle sprains. Rarely, posterolateral or hindfoot arthroscopy portals are associated with nerve injury.

Clinical Presentation

The clinical findings of sural nerve entrapment are similar to those encountered with entrapment at other sites in the foot. Patients often report chronic burning, numbness or aching along the posterolateral aspect of the leg which frequently becomes worse at night and with physical exertion. Often, there is mild to moderate tenderness to palpation posterior and lateral to the myotendinous junction of the Achilles tendon, which represents the location of the fibrous arcade and the most common site of sural nerve entrapment. Some patients may report recurrent ankle sprains or instability. Percussion may elicit a Tinel sign along the nerve course. Pain can be poorly localized but a focal area of tenderness is occasionally noted along the course of the nerve.[9] Provocative maneuvers such as plantar flexion of the foot and inversion may reproduce symptoms.

A history of direct injury, Achilles tendon surgery, ankle arthroscopy, or calcaneal fracture surgery suggests that the sural nerve may be involved. Concerns about possible referral pain caused by S1 nerve root radiculopathy must be assessed. Reflex and motor function in the leg should be normal if only the sural nerve is involved.

Diagnostic Studies

The diagnosis is primarily based on history, symptoms, and physical examination. Plain radiographs are done to rule out fractures, callus, subtalar arthritis, and other abnormalities. Stress views of the ankle should be obtained if underlying ankle instability is suspected. Electrodiagnostic and NCV studies may be useful but have limited benefit because of difficulty in interpretation of the study and anatomic variations in the nerve. MRI may be helpful to identify space-occupying lesions compressing the nerve. CT can be done if bony compression of the nerve is suspected. Diagnostic injection of local lidocaine in specific areas may assist in isolating the origin of symptoms.

Treatment

Nonsurgical treatment may be tried if ankle instability is the cause. An ankle brace for support and physical therapy to improve strength and proprioception may help relieve some of the symptoms. Treatment of underlying conditions like edema may alleviate symptoms. Topical medication with capsaicin or lidocaine patches can also be helpful along with oral tricyclic antidepressants.

If nonsurgical treatment has failed and there is well-localized entrapment, surgery should be considered. Nerve compression caused by bony fragments, callus, or ganglion can be managed with surgical excision. A thorough nerve decompression should be done with minimal nerve handling. Other procedures, such as peroneal tendon stabilization, lateral ligament repair, and lateral calcaneal wall decompression, should be done as indicated. Nerve injury resulting in neuromas should either be resected or transposed to an area of less vulnerable injury.

Medial Plantar Proper Digital Nerve Syndrome

Medial plantar proper digital nerve (MPPDN) syndrome was first described in 1971 as a traumatic perineural fibrosis of the medial plantar proper digital nerve.[67] The injury occurs either where the nerve crosses the first metatarsophalangeal joint or on the medial aspect of the great toe. Repetitive trauma is seen as a cause in sports involving repetitive pivoting, impact, and motion such as running, basketball, skiing, and ballet. Chronic compression caused by inadequate or tight footwear also can be a cause.

Anatomy

The MPPDN arises from the medial plantar nerve, which is the medial branch of the posterior tibial nerve. The MPPDN bifurcates into two terminal branches at the base of the first metatarsal bone: the medial branch, which forms the first common digital nerve, and the lateral branch, which forms the second and third common digital nerves. As the MPPDN courses distally through the subcutaneous tissue, it supplies sensation to the skin on the medial plantar aspect of the first metatarsophalangeal joint, hallux, and the tip of the toe.

Clinical Presentation

Typically, the patient reports pain and paresthesia on the medial side of the big toe when walking and wearing tight footwear. There can be an area of local sensory disturbance on the toe or an enlarged cordlike nerve immediately proximal to the interphalangeal joint, which is painful to touch. Hypoesthesia or hyperesthesia can be present with a positive Tinel sign in some cases. Forefoot valgus or a plantar-flexed first ray can be a contributing

factor. Abnormal pronation of the great toe leads to increased shearing forces between soft tissue and bones leading to symptoms.

Diagnosis

A thorough history and clinical examination is important in diagnosing MPPDN compression. Recently, a new method to perform MPPDN NCV studies has been described.[68] A technique that records the sensory nerve action potential of the MPPDN was evaluated. It concluded that antidromic stimulation of the MPPDN at a distance of 8 to 10 cm from the medial side of the first metatarsal head of the great toe yields reliable sensory nerve action potential (SNAP) responses. This type of NCV study is done to evaluate impulse along sensory nerve fibers. It is also useful in localizing a nerve lesion in relation to dorsal root ganglion (DRG). The DRG is located in the neural foramen and contains the sensory cell body. Lesions proximal to it (root, spinal cord) preserve the SNAP despite clinical sensory abnormalities. This is because axonal transport from the cell body to the axon continues to remain intact. SNAPs are typically considered more sensitive than compound motor action potential in the detection of an incomplete peripheral nerve injury.

Treatment

Initial treatment should be nonsurgical with footwear modification, protective or accommodative padding, and orthotics. Local corticosteroid injection can be helpful but because the site is very superficial, subcutaneous atrophy and increased symptoms can occur. Surgical treatment may involve surgical neurolysis and transposition of the nerve away from the sesamoid, or shaving a portion of the sesamoid to assist in decompressing the nerve.

Complex Regional Pain Syndrome

CRPS is a neuropathic pain disorder with important autonomic features. It is one of the most difficult and challenging conditions for the physician and patient alike. It can lead to significant disability with chronicity and relapses. In 1864, a civil war surgeon coined the condition as causalgia. Since then it has been known by different names including Sudeck dystrophy, reflex sympathetic dystrophy, posttraumatic dystrophy, painful osteoporosis, and sympathalgia. In an attempt to reduce confusion over naming the condition, the International Association for the Study of Pain (IASP) prefers the phrase "Complex Regional Pain Syndrome." The word "complex" describes the various clinical presentations and "regional" describes the distribution of different symptoms and findings.

Early diagnosis and treatment is required to prevent long-standing or permanent disability. Few treatments

2: Neuromuscular Disease

have proven effective, in part because of the historically poor understanding of the mechanisms underlying the disorder. Research conducted largely in the past 10 years has substantially increased knowledge regarding its pathophysiologic mechanisms, indicating that they are multifactorial. Both the peripheral and central nervous system mechanisms are involved. Relative contributions of the mechanisms underlying CRPS may differ across patients and even an individual patient over time, particularly in the transition from "warm" or acute CRPS to "cold" or chronic CRPS.

CRPS typically develops after acute tissue trauma. It is an exaggerated response with classic neuropathic pain characteristics including intense burning pain, hyperalgesia, and allodynia. It is also associated with autonomic changes including altered sweating and skin color and skin temperature changes. Trophic changes of the skin, hair, and nails are seen. Altered function, including loss of strength, decreased active range of motion, and tremor, also may occur. If central nervous mechanisms are affected because of repeated stimuli, neuronal pathways undergo plastic modification and acute pain is converted to chronic pain.

Classification
The IASP classification system divides CRPS into two types. The clinical presentation is similar in both with two exceptions: type I may have an orthostatic component that worsens with pain with limb dependency, whereas type II is associated with nerve injury.

CRPS Type I
1 After the inciting event, sensory, motor, and autonomic responses occur throughout the extremity.
2 Spontaneous pain, allodynia (perception of pain from a nonpainful stimulus), or hyperalgesia (an exaggerated sense of pain) occur throughout the entire extremity and are not limited to the territory of a single peripheral nerve.
3 Sudomotor activity (abnormal blood flow of the skin) leads to extremity swelling, vasodilation, and skin warming in the area of pain.
4 There are no other coexisting conditions accounting for these changes.

CRPS Type II
1 A peripheral nerve injury is present and is often the trigger.
2 The sensory, motor, and autonomic changes may or may not be limited in the specific distribution of the peripheral nerve.
3 Motor changes, including deficits, are caused by direct injury to motor axons.

4 Swelling and trophic changes are discrete.

Epidemiology
CRPS can affect all ages but diagnosis in the pediatric population is often delayed in comparison with that in adults. In one population-based study, the incidence was found to be 5.46 per 100,000 person-years. The female-to-male ratio was 4:1, with median age of 46 years at onset. The upper limb was affected twice as commonly as lower limb. In almost 46% of cases, fracture was the trigger event.[69] At least, 50,000 new cases of CRPS type I occur annually in the United States alone.[70] Occurrence is strongly associated with cigarette smoking.

Pathophysiology
The factors leading to CRPS are multifactorial. Although pathogenesis remains unclear, various hypotheses have been put forward. It has now been accepted that different mechanisms are involved simultaneously. CRPS is not only sympathetically mediated but also a disease of the central nervous system.[71]

Various mechanisms include central and peripheral sensitization, impaired sympathetic function, inflammatory factors, genetic factors, brain plasticity, and psychological factors.[72]

History and Clinical Examination
The patient may recall specific trauma, but in other cases with no history of trauma the patient may be viewed with suspicion as they report continuing pain. The typical features of spontaneous pain, hyperalgesia, allodynia, and abnormal vasomotor and motor activity may remain beyond the normal time of expected healing. These findings may also get worse and psychological changes may occur in the patient during the course of CRPS development.

The patient may guard and protect the extremity with overzealous care and attention. They may adopt a protective posture and in some cases the patient may not allow anyone to touch or examine the affected extremity.

Skin changes will vary from dry, warm, and erythematous to cold, blue, and mottled. The skin temperature difference usually exceeds 1°C. Motor dysfunction includes tremors, dystonia, and spasms with loss of strength and endurance. Muscle wasting and joint contractures may be seen at later stages. Exaggerated tendon reflexes may be present. In addition, there may be trophic changes in the skin with loss of subcutaneous fat, and nails may become hypertrophic.

Diagnosis
CRPS cannot be proven by any diagnostic test and is essentially a clinical diagnosis. Differential diagnostic tools may help eliminate other possible causes. Infection

and other systemic conditions can be evaluated with CBC, C-reactive protein level, erythrocyte sedimentation rate, antinuclear antibodies, serum calcium and alkaline phosphatase levels, and thyroid function tests.

Plain radiographs of the foot, ankle, and lower extremity typically show spotty osteoporotic changes after 4 to 8 weeks.[73] Disuse osteopenia develops secondary to decreased use and mobility of the affected extremity. Other tests that may be helpful include sweat test, thermography, and electromyography. Diagnostic sympathetic blocks with local anesthetics may help if vasomotor or sudomotor dysfunction is present. A block is considered successful if there is more than 50% pain reduction.

A three-phase bone scan with technetium Tc 99m is used to confirm CRPS. It is usually helpful in early stages where increased uptake in the delayed phase 3 is seen. In later stages the accuracy of the scan is variable. In early stages, 44% to 96% sensitivity and 75% to 98% specificity has been reported[74] (**Figure 5**).

Treatment

A multidisciplinary approach is used to treat CRPS. Both the physical and psychological elements need to be addressed. Patients may present to the orthopaedic surgeon, neurologist, or primary care provider. In some cases, the physical therapist treating the patient may make the diagnosis. The main goals of treatment are pain control, restoration of limb function, and physical and psychological rehabilitation. The treatment is focused on the severity of pain and presentation. Psychiatric evaluation is helpful to address anxiety, depression, and sleep disturbances.

Physical therapy is an important part of the treatment because it can help in edema reduction, avoiding joint contractures and muscle wasting, maintaining limb function, and desensitization of the limb. In a systematic review of physiotherapy management in patients with CRPS, there was good quality level II evidence supporting pain management physiotherapy/medical management.[75]

Various pharmacologic agents have been tried in the treatment of CRPS. Gabapentin and pregabalin are commonly prescribed. Antidepressants, NSAIDs, opioids, and corticosteroids are used by the pain management and psychiatric teams. Newer drugs include bisphosphonates to inhibit bone resorption. Free radical scavengers such as dimethyl sulfoxide, N-acetylcysteine, and mannitol have been tried with limited benefits.

The beneficial effect of vitamin C to prevent CRPS in wrist fractures has already been noted. In a recent study, the effect of 1 g vitamin C daily on prevention of CRPS type I in elective foot and ankle surgery was evaluated. The study demonstrated that vitamin C is effective in preventing CRPS type I of the foot and ankle, and

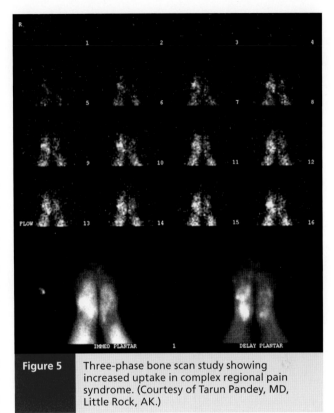

Figure 5 Three-phase bone scan study showing increased uptake in complex regional pain syndrome. (Courtesy of Tarun Pandey, MD, Little Rock, AK.)

the authors recommend use of vitamin C for preventive management.[76]

Topical agents such as lidocaine patch, fentanyl patch, transdermal clonidine, and capsaicin have been used increasingly by the pain management team.

Pain control is essential for management of CRPS. If pain is not adequately controlled by medications, then regional anesthetic blocks can be considered. Sympathetic blocks have been used for many years and are effective if performed early, before central pathways are set.[77] Spinal cord and peripheral nerve stimulation have been used with limited benefits.

Surgical intervention is needed only if there are pain generators such as tarsal tunnel syndrome or fractures. Surgery can also exacerbate CRPS and hence should be done sparingly. Amputation of the limb has been tried, but CRPS can recur in the stump especially if the amputation level was symptomatic at the time of surgery.

Summary

Interdigital plantar neuralgias commonly respond to footwear modifications and local injections. Surgical excision can lead to significant pain relief with the dorsal approach most commonly used. Peripheral nerve entrapments in the foot and ankle are relatively uncommon. Physician knowledge of specific nerve anatomy aids in diagnosis as can the judicial use of imaging modalities and electrodiagnostic tests. Nerve entrapment usually responds to nonsurgical management, but for patients who do not respond and in whom a proper diagnosis has been made surgical intervention has shown good success in relieving symptoms. CRPS remains a difficult condition to diagnose and treat, although significant advances have recently been made in diagnosis and treatment.

Annotated References

1. Giannini S, Bacchini P, Ceccarelli F, Vannini F: Interdigital neuroma: Clinical examination and histopathologic results in 63 cases treated with excision. *Foot Ankle Int* 2004;25(2):79-84.

2. Graham CE, Graham DM: Morton's neuroma: A microscopic evaluation. *Foot Ankle* 1984;5(3):150-153.

3. Kim JY, Choi JH, Park J, Wang J, Lee I: An anatomical study of Morton's interdigital neuroma: The relationship between the occurring site and the deep transverse metatarsal ligament (DTML). *Foot Ankle Int* 2007;28(9):1007-1010.

4. Morscher E, Ulrich J, Dick W: Morton's intermetatarsal neuroma: Morphology and histological substrate. *Foot Ankle Int* 2000;21(7):558-562.

5. Jones JR, Klenerman L: A study of the communicating branch between the medial and lateral plantar nerves. *Foot Ankle* 1984;4(6):313-315.

6. Levitsky KA, Alman BA, Jevsevar DS, Morehead J: Digital nerves of the foot: Anatomic variations and implications regarding the pathogenesis of interdigital neuroma. *Foot Ankle* 1993;14(4):208-214.

7. Govsa F, Bilge O, Ozer MA: Anatomical study of the communicating branches between the medial and lateral plantar nerves. *Surg Radiol Anat* 2005;27(5):377-381.

8. Mann RA, Reynolds JC: Interdigital neuroma: A critical clinical analysis. *Foot Ankle* 1983;3(4):238-243.

9. Schon LC, Mann RA: Diseases of the nerves, in Coughlin MM, Mann RA, Saltzmann C, eds: *Surgery of the Foot and Ankle,* ed 8. Philadelphia, PA, Mosby, 2007, pp 613-686.

10. Bradley NM, Miller WA, Evans JP: Plantar neuroma: Analysis of results following surgical excision in 145 patients. *South Med J* 1976;69(7):853-854.

11. Thompson FM, Deland JT: Occurrence of two interdigital neuromas in one foot. *Foot Ankle* 1993;14(1):15-17.

12. Owens R, Gougoulias N, Guthrie H, Sakellariou A: Morton's neuroma: Clinical testing and imaging in 76 feet, compared to a control group. *Foot Ankle Surg* 2011;17(3):197-200.

    Clinical and MRI findings in 76 surgically treated feet with neuroma and 40 feet with different pathologies (controls) are presented. Positive clinical test results were more frequent in the surgical group than the control group. Level of evidence: III.

13. Cloke DJ, Greiss ME: The digital nerve stretch test: A sensitive indicator of Morton's neuroma and neuritis. *Foot Ankle Surg* 2006;17:201-203.

14. Mulder JD: The causative mechanism in morton's metatarsalgia. *J Bone Joint Surg Br* 1951;33-B(1):94-95.

15. Sharp RJ, Wade CM, Hennessy MS, Saxby TS: The role of MRI and ultrasound imaging in Morton's neuroma and the effect of size of lesion on symptoms. *J Bone Joint Surg Br* 2003;85(7):999-1005.

16. Oliver TB, Beggs I: Ultrasound in the assessment of metatarsalgia: A surgical and histological correlation. *Clin Radiol* 1998;53(4):287-289.

17. Almeida DF, Kurokawa K, Hatanaka Y, Hemmi S, Claussen GC, Oh SJ: Abnormal dip phenomenon: A characteristic electrophysiological marker in interdigital neuropathy of the foot. *Arq Neuropsiquiatr* 2007;65(3B):771-778.

18. Greenfield J, Rea J Jr, Ilfeld FW: Morton's interdigital neuroma: Indications for treatment by local injections versus surgery. *Clin Orthop Relat Res* 1984;185:142-144.

19. Thomson CE, Beggs I, Martin DJ, et al: Methylprednisolone injections for the treatment of Morton neuroma: A patient-blinded randomized trial. *J Bone Joint Surg Am* 2013;95(9):790-798, S1.

    The authors reported on level I patient-blinded randomized trial with 131 patients randomized to receive cortisone and anesthetic or anesthetic alone for Morton neuroma under ultrasonographic control. Corticosteroid injection provide symptomatic benefit for at least 3 months. Level of evidence: I.

20. Mozena JD, Clifford JT: Efficacy of chemical neurolysis for the treatment of interdigital nerve compression of the foot: A retrospective study. *J Am Podiatr Med Assoc* 2007;97(3):203-206.

21. Hughes RJ, Ali K, Jones H, Kendall S, Connell DA: Treatment of Morton's neuroma with alcohol injection under sonographic guidance: Follow-up of 101 cases. *AJR Am J Roentgenol* 2007;188(6):1535-1539.

22. Gurdezi S, White T, Ramesh P: Alcohol injection for Morton's neuroma: A five-year follow-up. *Foot Ankle Int* 2013;34(8):1064-1067.

The authors found that alcohol injection does not permanently resolve symptoms of Morton neuroma in most patients and can be associated with substantial morbidity. Level of evidence: II.

23. Coughlin MJ, Pinsonneault T: Operative treatment of interdigital neuroma: A long-term follow-up study. *J Bone Joint Surg Am* 2001;83-A(9):1321-1328.

24. Coughlin MJ, Schenck RC Jr, Shurnas PS, Bloome DM: Concurrent interdigital neuroma and MTP joint instability: Long-term results of treatment. *Foot Ankle Int* 2002;23(11):1018-1025.

25. Stamatis ED, Myerson MS: Treatment of recurrence of symptoms after excision of an interdigital neuroma: A retrospective review. *J Bone Joint Surg Br* 2004;86(1):48-53.

26. Womack JW, Richardson DR, Murphy GA, Richardson EG, Ishikawa SN: Long-term evaluation of interdigital neuroma treated by surgical excision. *Foot Ankle Int* 2008;29(6):574-577.

A retrospective review of 232 patients who underwent neuroma excision identified location of neuromas in the second web space as a possible prognostic indicator of poor outcome. Neuroma and visual analog scale score showed that long-term outcomes of neuroma excision were not as successful as had previously been reported. Level of evidence: III.

27. Shapiro SL: Endoscopic decompression of the intermetatarsal nerve for Morton's neuroma. *Foot Ankle Clin* 2004;9(2):297-304.

28. Zelent ME, Kane RM, Neese DJ, Lockner WB: Minimally invasive Morton's intermetatarsal neuroma decompression. *Foot Ankle Int* 2007;28(2):263-265.

29. Akermark C, Crone H, Skoog A, Weidenhielm L: A prospective randomized controlled trial of plantar versus dorsal incisions for operative treatment of primary Morton's neuroma. *Foot Ankle Int* 2013;34(9):1198-1204.

The authors present a level I prospective randomized trial of 76 patients who underwent surgery through either a plantar or a dorsal incision. At average follow-up of 34 months with 93% follow-up rate, no significant difference was found regarding pain, restriction of activities, and scar tenderness. Level of evidence: I.

30. Benedetti RS, Baxter DE, Davis PF: Clinical results of simultaneous adjacent interdigital neurectomy in the foot. *Foot Ankle Int* 1996;17(5):264-268.

31. Su E, Di Carlo E, O'Malley M, Bohne WH, Deland JT, Kennedy JG: The frequency of digital artery resection in Morton interdigital neurectomy. *Foot Ankle Int* 2006;27(10):801-803.

32. Amis JA, Siverhus SW, Liwnicz BH: An anatomic basis for recurrence after Morton's neuroma excision. *Foot Ankle* 1992;13(3):153-156.

33. Johnson JE, Johnson KA, Unni KK: Persistent pain after excision of an interdigital neuroma: Results of reoperation. *J Bone Joint Surg Am* 1988;70(5):651-657.

34. Wolfort SF, Dellon AL: Treatment of recurrent neuroma of the interdigital nerve by implantation of the proximal nerve into muscle in the arch of the foot. *J Foot Ankle Surg* 2001;40(6):404-410.

35. Keck C: The tarsal tunnel syndrome. *J Bone Joint Surg Am* 1962;44:180-182.

36. Havel PE, Ebraheim NA, Clark SE, Jackson WT, DiDio L: Tibial nerve branching in the tarsal tunnel. *Foot Ankle* 1988;9(3):117-119.

37. Park TA, Del Toro DR: The medial calcaneal nerve: Anatomy and nerve conduction technique. *Muscle Nerve* 1995;18(1):32-38.

38. Trepman E, Kadel NJ, Chisholm K, Razzano L: Effect of foot and ankle position on tarsal tunnel compartment pressure. *Foot Ankle Int* 1999;20(11):721-726.

39. Kinoshita M, Okuda R, Morikawa J, Jotoku T, Abe M: The dorsiflexion-eversion test for diagnosis of tarsal tunnel syndrome. *J Bone Joint Surg Am* 2001;83(12):1835-1839.

40. Frey C, Kerr R: Magnetic resonance imaging and the evaluation of tarsal tunnel syndrome. *Foot Ankle* 1993;14(3):159-164.

41. Bracilovic A, Nihal A, Houston VL, Beattie AC, Rosenberg ZS, Trepman E: Effect of foot and ankle position on tarsal tunnel compartment volume. *Foot Ankle Int* 2006;27(6):431-437.

42. Galardi G, Amadio S, Maderna L, et al: Electrophysiologic studies in tarsal tunnel syndrome: Diagnostic reliability of motor distal latency, mixed nerve and sensory nerve conduction studies. *Am J Phys Med Rehabil* 1994;73(3):193-198.

43. Patel AT, Gaines K, Malamut R, Park TA, Toro DR, Holland N; American Association of Neuromuscular and Electrodiagnostic Medicine: Usefulness of electrodiagnostic techniques in the evaluation of suspected tarsal tunnel syndrome: An evidence-based review. *Muscle Nerve* 2005;32(2):236-240.

44. Dellon AL: The four medial ankle tunnels: A critical review of perceptions of tarsal tunnel syndrome and neuropathy. *Neurosurg Clin N Am* 2008;19(4):629-648, vii.

The author reviewed the anatomy and mechanism of compression in tarsal tunnel syndrome. Details of the four tarsal tunnels and the perceptions are discussed.

45. Barker AR, Rosson GD, Dellon AL: Pressure changes in the medial and lateral plantar and tarsal tunnels

related to ankle position: A cadaver study. *Foot Ankle Int* 2007;28(2):250-254.

In this cadaver study, pressure measurements were obtained in various ankle positions in tarsal and medial and lateral plantar tunnels. Pressures were increased in all tunnels with ankle pronation and reduced with surgical release, including the septum between medial and lateral plantar tunnels.

46. Rosson GD, Larson AR, Williams EH, Dellon AL: Tibial nerve decompression in patients with tarsal tunnel syndrome: Pressures in the tarsal, medial plantar, and lateral plantar tunnels. *Plast Reconstr Surg* 2009;124(4):1202-1210.

In 10 patients with TTS, intraoperative pressures in tarsal, medial plantar, and lateral plantar tunnels in multiple foot positions were measured before and after excision of tunnel roof and septum. Pronation and plantar flexion of foot increased the pressure; tunnel release and excision of septum relieved these pressures. The lateral plantar tunnel has higher pressures. Level of evidence: IV.

47. Mullick T, Dellon AL: Results of decompression of four medial ankle tunnels in the treatment of tarsal tunnels syndrome. *J Reconstr Microsurg* 2008;24(2):119-126.

The authors discussed results of 77 patients treated with decompression of four medial ankle tunnels. Immediate postoperative ambulation and weight bearing in bulky dressing was allowed. Follow-up at 3.6 years showed 82% excellent results. Level of evidence: III.

48. Krishnan KG, Pinzer T, Schackert G: A novel endoscopic technique in treating single nerve entrapment syndromes with special attention to ulnar nerve transposition and tarsal tunnel release: Clinical application. *Neurosurgery* 2006;59(1, suppl 1):ONS89-ONS100, discussion ONS89-ONS100.

49. Sung KS, Park SJ: Short-term operative outcome of tarsal tunnel syndrome due to benign space-occupying lesions. *Foot Ankle Int* 2009;30(8):741-745.

In this study, 20 patients underwent tarsal decompression, and 13 had space-occupying lesions. Although substantial improvement on AOFAS and visual analog scale scores was noted, subjective satisfaction was only 54%. The authors suggest that expectations be cautiously discussed with the patient. Level of evidence: IV.

50. Sammarco GJ, Chang L: Outcome of surgical treatment of tarsal tunnel syndrome. *Foot Ankle Int* 2003;24(2):125-131.

51. Gondring WH, Trepman E, Shields B: Tarsal tunnel syndrome: Assessment of treatment outcome with an anatomic pain intensity scale. *Foot Ankle Surg* 2009;15(3):133-138.

In this study of 46 patients, pain intensity was documented. Surgical treatment resulted in substantial pain improvement in the medial plantar and medial calcaneal regions but not the lateral plantar nerve regions. Predictors of failed nonsurgical treatment included longer motor nerve conduction latency and foot comorbidities. Level of evidence: II.

52. Gould JS, DiGiovanni BF: Plantar fascia release in combination with proximal and distal tarsal tunnel release, in Wiesel SW ed: *Operative Techniques in Orthopedic Surgery.* Philadelphia, PA, Wolters Kluwer/Lippincott Williams and Wilkins, 2011, pp 3911-3919.

This chapter discusses the importance of surgical technique of combined release of proximal and distal tarsal tunnels.

53. Rask MR: Medial plantar neurapraxia (jogger's foot): Report of 3 cases. *Clin Orthop Relat Res* 1978;134:193-195.

54. Gould JS, Ford D: Orthoses and insert management of common foot and ankle problems, in Schon LC, Porter DA, eds: *Baxter's The Foot and Ankle in Sport.* Philadelphia, PA, Mosby Elsevier; 2008, pp 585-593.

The chapter discusses various orthoses and inserts used in foot and ankle conditions.

55. Marinacci AA: Neurological syndromes of the tarsal tunnels. *Bull Los Angeles Neurol Soc* 1968;33(2):90-100.

56. Gessini L, Jandolo B, Pietrangeli A: The anterior tarsal syndrome: Report of four cases. *J Bone Joint Surg Am* 1984;66(5):786-787.

57. Roselle N, Stevens A: Unexpected incidence of neurogenic atrophy of the extensor digitorum brevis muscle in young adults, in Desmedt JE, ed: *New Developments in Electromyography and Clinical Neurophysiology.* Basel, Switzerland, Karger, 1973, vol 1, pp 69-70.

58. Styf J, Morberg P: The superficial peroneal tunnel syndrome: Results of treatment by decompression. *J Bone Joint Surg Br* 1997;79(5):801-803.

59. Barrett SL, Dellon AL, Rosson GD, Walters L: Superficial peroneal nerve (superficial fibularis nerve): The clinical implications of anatomic variability. *J Foot Ankle Surg* 2006;45(3):174-176.

60. Ucerler H, Ikiz A: The variations of the sensory branches of the superficial peroneal nerve course and its clinical importance. *Foot Ankle Int* 2005;26(11):942-946.

61. Kennedy JG, Baxter DE: Nerve disorders in dancers. *Clin Sports Med* 2008;27(2):329-334.

This article discusses various nerve disorders specific to dancers. Foot and ankle conditions specific to this group are discussed in detail.

62. Young BH, Flanigan RM, DiGiovanni BF: Complications of ankle arthroscopy utilizing a contemporary

noninvasive distraction technique. *J Bone Joint Surg Am* 2011;93(10):963-968.

In this retrospective study of 294 ankle arthroscopic procedures with noninvasive distraction, 20 patients (6.8%) experienced complications. Specifically, anterolateral portal–related superficial peroneal nerve injury was seen in six patients. Level of evidence: IV.

63. Styf J: Entrapment of the superficial peroneal nerve: Diagnosis and results of decompression. *J Bone Joint Surg Br* 1989;71(1):131-135.

64. Stephens MM, Kelly PM: Fourth toe flexion sign: A new clinical sign for identification of the superficial peroneal nerve. *Foot Ankle Int* 2000;21(10):860-863.

65. Yang LJ, Gala VC, McGillicuddy JE: Superficial peroneal nerve syndrome: An unusual nerve entrapment. Case report. *J Neurosurg* 2006;104(5):820-823.

66. Riedl O, Frey M: Anatomy of the sural nerve: Cadaver study and literature review. *Plast Reconstr Surg* 2013;131(4):802-810.

This is detailed cadaver study reviewed more than 220 sural nerve reports. The confusing nomenclature for sural nerve formation and its branches is discussed and resolved.

67. Joplin RJ: The proper digital nerve, vitallium stem arthroplasty, and some thoughts about foot surgery in general. *Clin Orthop Relat Res* 1971;76:199-212.

68. Im S, Park JH, Kim HW, Yoo SH, Kim HS, Park GY: New method to perform medial plantar proper digital nerve conduction studies. *Clin Neurophysiol* 2010;121(7):1059-1065.

This study describes a new technique that records sensory nerve action potential of the medial plantar proper digital nerve. Antidromic nerve responses from 118 volunteers were recorded. The authors concluded that the test nerve should be stimulated at a distance of 8 to 10 cm from the medial side of the first metatarsal head of the big toe to obtain reliable responses. Level of evidence: III.

69. Sandroni P, Benrud-Larson LM, McClelland RL, Low PA: Complex regional pain syndrome type I: Incidence and prevalence in Olmsted county, a population-based study. *Pain* 2003;103(1-2):199-207.

70. Bruehl S, Chung OY: How common is complex regional pain syndrome-type I? *Pain* 2007;129(1-2):1-2.

71. Jänig W, Baron R: Complex regional pain syndrome is a disease of the central nervous system. *Clin Auton Res* 2002;12(3):150-164.

72. Bruehl S: An update on the pathophysiology of complex regional pain syndrome. *Anesthesiology* 2010;113(3):713-725.

73. Genant HK, Kozin F, Bekerman C, McCarty DJ, Sims J: The reflex sympathetic dystrophy syndrome: A comprehensive analysis using fine-detail radiography, photon absorptiometry, and bone and joint scintigraphy. *Radiology* 1975;117(1):21-32.

74. Hogan CJ, Hurwitz SR: Treatment of complex regional pain syndrome of the lower extremity. *J Am Acad Orthop Surg* 2002;10(4):281-289.

75. Daly AE, Bialocerkowski AE: Does evidence support physiotherapy management of adult complex regional pain syndrome type one? A systematic review. *Eur J Pain* 2009;13(4):339-353.

The authors evaluated the effectiveness of physical therapy in managing adult CRPS type I.

76. Besse JL, Gadeyne S, Galand-Desmé S, Lerat JL, Moyen B: Effect of vitamin C on prevention of complex regional pain syndrome type I in foot and ankle surgery. *Foot Ankle Surg* 2009;15(4):179-182.

This chronologic study reviewed two successive groups without and with preventive 1 g of vitamin C daily treatment in patients undergoing foot and ankle surgery. The study demonstrates the effectiveness of vitamin C in preventing CRPS type I of the foot and ankle. Level of evidence: IV.

77. AbuRahma AF, Robinson PA, Powell M, Bastug D, Boland JP: Sympathectomy for reflex sympathetic dystrophy: Factors affecting outcome. *Ann Vasc Surg* 1994;8(4):372-379.

2: Neuromuscular Disease

Arthritis of the Foot and Ankle

SECTION EDITOR:

BRUCE E. COHEN, MD

Chapter 8

Ankle Arthritis: Part 1. Joint Preservation Techniques and Arthrodesis

David N. Garras, MD   Simon Lee, MD

Introduction

The ankle joint is unusual relative to other weight-bearing joints in the body. For example, the ankle joint is much less likely to develop primary osteoarthritis (OA) and is more able to resist degradation than the knee or hip joints.[1,2] Most arthritis seen in the ankle is posttraumatic in nature.[3-5] This posttraumatic arthritis is typically attributed to the severity of the initial injury and the reduction quality of original fractures.[6] Inflammatory arthropathies, neuroarthropathies, primary OA, and hemochromatosis account for the remainder of ankle arthritis cases.[4] Most of those with posttraumatic ankle arthritis are relatively young, active, high-demand patients. They may have multiple previous incisions about the ankle, which creates a difficult treatment situation. Patients with posttraumatic OA are an average of 7 years younger (58 versus 65 years) than those with primary OA, with the condition occurring at a 78% versus 9% rate (compared with primary OA).[5]

Initial treatment of ankle arthritis is nonsurgical. Anti-inflammatory and analgesic medications, variable levels of immobilization, intra-articular injections (corticosteroids, viscosupplementation, and platelet-rich plasma), dietary supplementation, and orthotic devices are the most commonly used nonsurgical treatment options. If a patient's nonsurgical management fails, surgical intervention is indicated. Surgical treatment includes a wide variety of procedures and can be subdivided into

---

Table 1

Joint-Sparing Procedures

Arthroscopic or open débridement

Subchondral drilling

Osteochondral allografts for defects

Chondrocyte transplantation (autologous, juvenile particulate)

Periarticular osteotomy

Distraction arthroplasty

Interposition arthroplasty

---

joint-sparing and joint-sacrificing options based on the amount of arthrosis and deformity present. Joint-sparing procedures are listed in **Table 1**. Joint-sacrificing procedures such as allograft transplantation, ankle arthrodesis, or arthroplasty are usually reserved as the last line of treatment.

Anatomy and Biomechanics

The ankle is a constrained joint that gains most of its stability from the bony anatomy of the medial malleolus, the distal fibula, and the configuration of the tibiotalar articulation. Additional stability is gained through static ligamentous structures, including the interosseous membrane, tibiofibular and collateral ligaments, and dynamic musculotendinous units. The medial ligamentous structures are the primary stabilizers of the ankle.[4]

The ankle joint is directly perpendicular to the mechanical axis of the lower extremity. Both the anatomic and mechanical axis are the same in the tibia and should pass through the midpoint of the ankle articulation in the coronal and sagittal planes. In the coronal plane, the tibial plafond forms an angle with the mechanical axis,

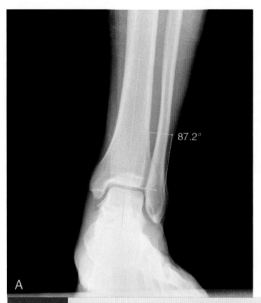
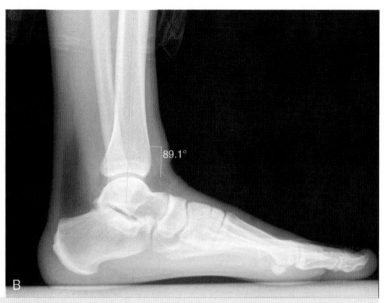

Figure 1   **A,** The tibial plafond makes an angle with the mechanical axis that is referred to as the distal tibial articular surface (TAS) angle. **B,** The tibial lateral surface (TLS) angle is the same measurement in the sagittal plane. The normal TAS angle is 88° to 93°, and the TLS angle is 80° to 81°.

which is referred to as the distal tibial articular surface (TAS) angle. The tibial lateral surface (TLS) angle is the same measurement in the sagittal plane. The normal TAS angle is 88° to 93° and a normal TLS angle is 80° to 81°[7-9] (**Figure 1**).

The ankle joint is mainly a rolling joint with highly congruent surfaces, particularly during weight bearing.[4,5] It is smaller than the knee or hip in surface area and consequently experiences a much higher force per area.[4,5,10] When the ankle is not bearing weight, the joint is incongruent. However, when weight bearing, the ankle joint becomes more congruent and allows for more joint surface area contact.[4] During normal activities, forces in excess of 3.5 times body weight are transmitted across the ankle. The primary motion of the tibiotalar joint is in the sagittal plane and averages a 43° to 63° arc in dorsiflexion and plantar flexion, with only 30° required for steady-state walking. There is an average of 10° of rotational movement of the talus within the mortise.[4]

In contrast to other weight-bearing joints of the lower extremity, the ankle joint is much more resistant to the development of primary OA but is more susceptible to posttraumatic arthritis.[4] Joint motion, cartilage thickness, and metabolic and mechanical factors differ between the knee and ankle and help explain the difference in incidence of primary OA and posttraumatic arthritis.[2,4,5,10] Whereas knee OA affects more women than men, ankle OA affects more men than women.[2] Unlike the knee, the articular cartilage of the ankle is uniform in thickness, measuring 1 mm to 1.7 mm, and displays much higher compressive stiffness than hip or knee cartilage.[2,4,5,10] Although ankle cartilage may develop fissures or fibrillations attributable to aging and wear, these conditions do not progress to OA as they would in the knee or hip.[2,4,5,10] Ankle cartilage also does not decrease in tensile strength with age.[2,4,5,10,11]

Chondrocytes in the ankle respond differently (versus those in the knee or hip) to biochemical and biologic factors and resist degradation. Ankle chondrocytes are less responsive to inflammatory mediators such as interleukin-1 (IL-1) and synthesize much less matrix metalloproteases (MMP) (specifically MMP-8, which is elevated in OA) in response to IL-1 than chondrocytes in the hip or knee.[2,4,5,10] This decreased sensitivity is likely attributable to a smaller number of differing types of IL-1 receptors on ankle chondrocytes. As a result, the ankle is much more refractory to damage by inflammatory mediators.

Primary ankle OA is uncommon because of the protective nature of metabolic factors, biomechanical stability, and the congruent and uniform nature of the joint. However, the overall relative lower thickness of the ankle's cartilage layer and the high stress per surface area can lead to rapid degeneration in posttraumatic settings.

Incidence and Etiology

Ankle arthritis is estimated to occur in 1% of the population.[5] Unlike in the hip or knee, the primary cause of arthritis in the ankle is trauma, accounting for 76% to 78% of all cases, whereas primary OA accounts for 7% to 9% of cases.[4,5,10] The remainder of ankle arthritis cases (12% to 13%) are attributable to secondary arthritis

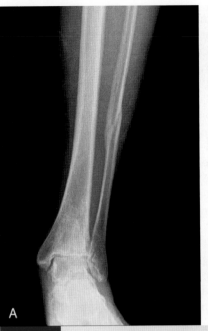 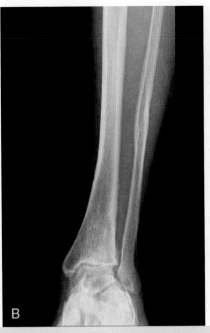 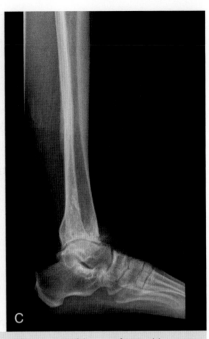

Figure 2 AP (**A**), mortise (**B**), and lateral (**C**) views of the ankle of a 43-year-old man with a 10-year history of an ankle fracture treated nonsurgically. Radiographs show evidence of a midfibular shaft fracture with malunion and unstable syndesmosis with substantial joint space narrowing.

as a result of rheumatoid arthritis, neuroarthropathy, hemochromatosis, and postinfectious degeneration.[4,5,10]

Fractures of the malleoli, tibial plafond, talar dome or neck, and isolated osteochondral injuries all contribute to the development of arthritis.[4,5] Fibular shortening or malrotation can lead to lateral tilt of the talus and instability.[1,4] A 1-mm lateral shift of the tibiotalar articulation causes reduction in the contact area and increased pressures.[4,12] In addition, lateral ankle ligamentous instability may lead to medial ankle overload and degeneration.[4,5]

The overall rate of posttraumatic arthritis is 14% in all ankle fractures; however, arthritis developed in as many as 33% of patients with Weber C fractures in some studies.[4,13] Large posterior malleolar fractures with displacement are associated with a higher incidence of arthritis.[4,13] Arthritis has been estimated to occur in 13% to 54% of tibial plafond fractures, 40% of bimalleolar fractures, and up to 71% of trimalleolar fractures.[8] The adequacy of reduction is believed to be a strong predictor of outcomes[4,13] (**Figure 2**). However, this line of thinking has been disputed in the literature, with different conclusions appearing in various studies.[4,13,14] Chondral injury and extent of damage as well as development of osteonecrosis of the subchondral bone increase the probability for the development of arthritis.[14]

Intra-articular deformities with varus tilting as a result of impaction, distal tibial osteonecrosis, or chronic cavovarus or flatfoot deformity may develop in patients with chronic ankle instability, hindfoot varus, and peroneal tendon dysfunction.[7] This could lead to asymmetric wear and/or progression of degeneration (**Figure 3**). Primary OA is rare but has been described in up to 20% of patients with arthritis in the Japanese population; the practice of sitting cross-legged or with legs tucked beneath is believed to cause this condition.[15,16]

Clinical Presentation

Patients with ankle arthritis usually present with reports of pain, dysfunction, activity restrictions, and swelling. Patients often note pain with any weight-bearing activity such as prolonged standing, walking, running, and stair climbing. Most patients also have reduced self-perceived function as determined by functional assessments and questionnaires.[11]

Ankle motion primarily occurs in the sagittal plane, with an arc of 30° required for normal walking.[4] In the setting of end-stage ankle arthritis (and also with arthrodesis), motion is limited.[4] As a result, compensation by the hindfoot and forefoot is necessary, which increases the shear forces at the midtarsal joints.[4] Patients often have decreased sagittal plane motion, plantar flexion moment and power.[11] Ankle arthritis affects various gait pattern parameters such as walking speed, cadence, and stride length.[4,11] Patients with arthritis also exhibit antalgic gait patterns with abnormal plantar pressures. Those with ankle arthritis also exhibit increased oxygen consumption and decreased gait efficiency.[4] Consequently,

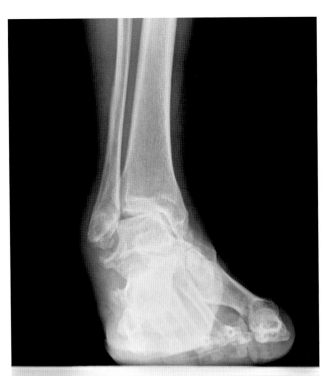

Figure 3 AP radiograph of the ankle of a 54-year-old man with a history of chronic ankle instability with multiple ankle inversion injuries reveals substantial varus deformity with medial tibiotalar joint space loss and chronic spurring of the ankle joint.

prolonged ambulation, fast walking, and running are difficult.[4]

The first step in the treatment of ankle arthritis is to obtain a thorough history and physical examination. The history should ascertain the etiology of the disease, timing of onset of symptoms, current and prior symptoms, history of traumatic events or recurrent injuries, current level of function, treatment to date, and the desired level of function. Confounding factors, including systemic diseases, current medications (including current narcotic use), prior surgeries, history or suspicion of infections or wound healing problems, and a social history that includes drug abuse and smoking history should be investigated in depth. A referral to a primary care physician or rheumatologist may help delineate the etiology of arthritis in patients with no history of mechanical causes or trauma. A neurology consultation may be required for patients with atypical pain, numbness, burning, or nonactivity-related pain to rule out spinal or neuropathic etiology.

Potential complications must be addressed at the initial visit and before surgical intervention. Indolent infections and traumatized soft tissues can pose risks for any surgical intervention. Any patient with a history of infection or nonunion should be considered for a preoperative biopsy or cultures and inflammatory markers (complete blood count with differential, erythrocyte sedimentation rate, and C-reactive protein level) to rule out any indolent infections. Patients with circulatory dysfunction, diabetes mellitus, smoking history, and those with a history of osteonecrosis are at much higher risk for wound complications, infections, and nonunions. Smoking is a well-documented cause of postoperative complications in foot and ankle surgery, increasing risk for nonunion by 16 times versus nonsmokers.[17] Smokers should be encouraged to quit smoking; surgeons have advocated withholding surgical intervention until patients are nicotine free in elective cases. There is no consensus as to the required length of time required for the complications of smoking to dissipate to the level experienced by nonsmokers, or if the variance ever completely normalizes. Patients with diabetes or peripheral neuropathy will require more rigid fixation and longer periods of immobilization.[18]

The physical examination should begin with a gait analysis and evaluation of the alignment of the entire extremity to include the hip and knee. Proximal deformities should be addressed before any treatment of the ankle is considered. A complete examination of a patient's neurovascular status is essential. A patient with any changes in skin color, weak pulses, differences in vascularity compared with the contralateral side, or lymphedema should have a complete vascular workup or referral to a vascular surgeon. The location and condition of all prior incisions and scars should be noted. Range of motion of the ankle, subtalar joint, and transverse tarsal joints should be examined and recorded. Care should be taken to isolate motion to the responsible joints because Chopart joint motion (talonavicular and calcaneocuboid joints) often complicates the examination.

Radiographic assessment should include three views of the weight-bearing ankle (AP, mortise, and lateral) and limb alignment films (full-length mechanical axis) if necessary. The location and degree of deformity are the most important factors in the decision-making process for surgical treatment. The presence of arthritis in the subtalar joint or the transverse tarsal joints may alter treatment algorithms. If radiographs do not correlate with a patient's symptoms or examination, MRI or CT may be indicted. CT may identify adjacent joint arthritis and any specific bony deformities, whereas MRI may be indicated to evaluate for suspected osteonecrosis or associated soft-tissue pathology.

Nonsurgical Treatment

Although the literature is limited regarding the success rate of nonsurgical treatment, all patients with ankle arthritis should undergo a trial of nonsurgical management before proceeding with surgical intervention. However, some authors advocate early surgical intervention for patients with congenital or posttraumatic deformity rather than waiting for symptoms to worsen.[19] Nonsurgical treatments are aimed at relieving symptoms and prolonging the life and function of the native ankle. Rest and activity modification may help relieve the initial inflammation, but these interventions generally are not acceptable long-term solutions for active patients.[19] Walking aids such as canes or walkers are also helpful, but usually are tolerated only by elderly patients. For patients with reports of instability or weakness, a course of physical therapy that includes strength training, proprioceptive training, stretching, and aerobic nonimpact exercise may be beneficial.[1,19]

Oral NSAIDs and, on occasion, a short course of oral steroids may be beneficial, especially for patients with inflammatory arthropathies (but also are useful for all etiologies).[1] NSAIDs exert their function by inhibiting cyclooxygenase and reducing prostaglandins, which are inflammatory mediators that protect gastric mucosa.[20] Corticosteroids also function by inhibiting several inflammatory pathways.[20] Care should be taken in long-term use of NSAIDs because they can have deleterious effects on liver and kidney function, which necessitates monitoring. NSAIDs can also lead to gastric or enteric ulcers and carry an increased risk for bleeding. Analgesic medications, whether topical compounding creams or oral acetaminophen or tramadol, may be useful in controlling pain and increasing function and have a safer side effect profile than NSAIDs.[20]

Intra-articular corticosteroid injections may limit pain and inflammation and can be safely used sparingly. Repeated injections carry risk for skin discoloration, fat necrosis, and soft-tissue destruction and pose increased risk for infection.[1,19] There has been no evidence to indicate destructive effects to cartilage resulting from these injections. Oral and injectable corticosteroids should be used with caution in patients with diabetes because they can lead to alterations in blood glucose levels.

Hyaluronans have been used with success in the knee as well as in other joints. However, scant literature exists to support their use in the ankle. Hyaluronic acid has been shown to inhibit phagocytosis, decrease synovial fluid inflammatory mediators, and stimulate production of hyaluronic acid by chondrocytes.[21] Salk et al[22] performed a randomized controlled, double-blinded study on 20 patients using sodium hyaluronate over five weekly

injections. At 6-month follow-up, there was a decrease in pain and disability and a trend toward better symptomatic relief in the hyaluronate group. It was also found to be as safe as saline.[21,22] This finding was confirmed in other studies that showed a significant decrease in pain and improvement in function with hyaluronate use.[23,24]

Glucosamine is thought to inhibit IL-1 production, prostaglandins, and MMPs and may increase the native production of hyaluronic acid.[21] Chondroitin sulfate inhibits leukocyte elastase and the migration of polymorphonuclear leukocytes and may also increase hyaluronic acid production.[21] There is no research on the use of glucosamine or chondroitin sulfate in the ankle. Most of the current literature suggests that glucosamine and chondroitin sulfate may provide symptomatic relief of moderate to severe arthritis of the knee with minimal side effects.[21]

Although platelet-rich plasma has been used in an expanding number of musculoskeletal disorders, there have been no published studies evaluating its effectiveness in ankle arthritis (anecdotal cases only). The mechanism of action of platelet-rich plasma is thought to involve platelet degranulation with the subsequent release of various growth factors and the stimulation of stem cell lines involved in the healing and reparative process.

Patients with rheumatoid arthritis and other secondary causes of ankle arthrosis would benefit from treating the underlying condition. Disease-modifying antirheumatic drugs (DMARDs) are medications that halt the progression of the rheumatoid destructive process. These include both biologic (IL-1 and tumor necrosis factor antagonists) and nonbiologic (methotrexate and sulfasalazine) options.[20] However, these drugs typically take months to exert their action and should be managed by a rheumatologist.

Bracing is a valuable option with which to control pain and improve function in ankle arthrosis. Ankle motion occurs mainly in the sagittal plane; however, there is coronal plane motion as well. Therefore, brace options must be able to control both sagittal and frontal plane motion to effectively alleviate symptoms.[25] A custom-made ankle-foot orthosis (AFO) will help decrease symptoms and increase endurance.[19] A leather gauntlet (Arizona type) brace has similar properties as the AFO but is usually much better tolerated.[25] When all weight-bearing activities cause pain, a patella tendon-bearing AFO may be used to immobilize and offload the forces across the ankle. Shoe modifications such as a heel lift, solid ankle cushioned heel, and stiff rocker-bottom sole are also useful (Figure 4). Heel lifts will limit dorsiflexion and anterior impingement.[19,25] A stiff-shank, rocker-bottom sole limits ankle motion and normalizes gait.[19] A solid ankle cushioned heel dampens heel strike and lessens

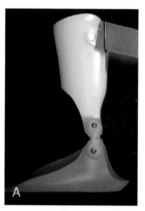
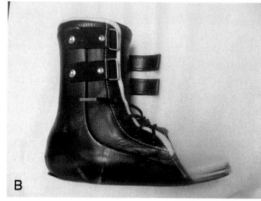
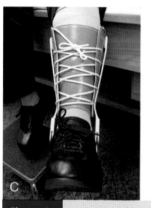
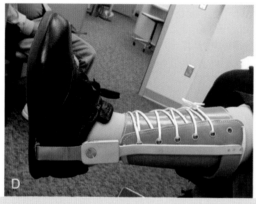
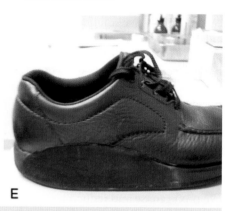

| Figure 4 | Examples of braces and shoe modifications typically used in patients with ankle arthritis. **A,** Hinged ankle-foot orthosis, which allows some sagittal plane motion. **B,** Leather ankle gauntlet (Arizona). **C** and **D,** Double upright metal brace with custom-molded calf lacer with built-in shoe and insert (Charcot arthropathy). **E,** Solid ankle cushioned heel with rocker-bottom shoe modifications. |

rapid ankle plantar flexion during heel strike. Additionally, all of these modifications can be combined, such as a heel lift or a solid ankle cushioned heel and an Arizona or AFO brace.[25]

Surgical Treatment

When obtaining a patient's history, information about their current symptoms and level of function, their desired level of function, and current radiographic studies may help direct treatment. Decisions regarding joint preservation or sacrifice are dependent on many factors, including the patient's age, predisease functional status, current and desired functional level, history of infections, osteonecrosis, systemic diseases such as diabetes or rheumatoid arthritis, vascular status, and radiographic findings. There should be an individualized plan that is agreeable to both the patient and surgeon that provides maximal relief and function from a single procedure and does not preclude salvage options.

Joint Preservation Surgery
Synovectomy and Débridement

Patients recalcitrant to nonsurgical treatment who have localized anterior ankle pain and painful dorsiflexion are defined as having anterior ankle impingement. Patients can present with radiographic evidence of a distal anterior tibial osteophyte and a bony block or limited ankle range of motion (ROM), or they may have anterior ankle pain with terminal dorsiflexion and may benefit from a simple arthroscopic or open anterior decompression. Débridement for mild to moderate arthrosis with osteophytes, synovitis, loose bodies, and mechanical impingement is effective for pain relief and improvements in terminal dorsiflexion ROM[1,19] (**Figure 5**). Patients with rheumatoid arthritis, hemophilia, pigmented villonodular synovitis, and other soft-tissue pathologies may benefit from a simple synovectomy.[19] However, a 5-year survival analysis indicates that débridement is most effective in patients with predominately anterior ankle impingement and minimal global arthritic changes.[26] In a 2007 study of outcomes after anterior débridement, investigators found that none of the patients treated for anterior impingement required

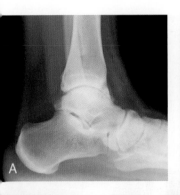
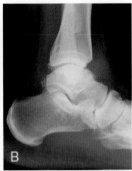
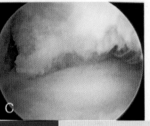
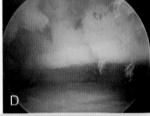

Figure 5 Preoperative (**A**) and postoperative (**B**) lateral radiographs of anterior ankle impingement after an ankle arthroscopy and resection of the distal tibial anterior osteophyte. Arthroscopic views showing preresection (**C**) and postresection (**D**) of the anterior distal tibia.

further surgery at 5-year follow-up compared with 28% of those with degenerative changes.[26] This finding was independent of patient age.

Distraction Arthroplasty
Background
Ankle distraction arthroplasty was first popularized in 1995.[27] Distraction has been used in other joints with relative success.[28-30] This technique uses an Ilizarov-type external fixator to distract the ankle joint and relies on ligamentotaxis to restore normal joint space, offload the joint, and allow cartilage to recover.[28-30] The exact mechanism of its action is not clearly understood. Theories involve mechanical stress relief, continued intermittent intra-articular fluid pressure changes, and increased synovial fluid (believed to enhance chondrocyte reparative activity).[27,29-31] Other theories include a positive stretch effect on nerve endings, decreased synovial inflammation, intra-articular fibrous tissue formation, stretching of the joint capsule, and decreased joint reactive forces.[29,30,32] Maintenance in the fixator for 3 months allows for a reduction of subchondral bone sclerosis, which has been linked to improved clinical outcomes.[28-30] Distraction likely allows for fibrocartilage formation, which may seal cartilage defects and decrease pain from hydrostatic pressure on the subchondral bone.[27-29,33]

In vitro and animal studies have supported distraction for the arthritic ankle. It has been shown that chondrocytes have morphologic and biochemical changes when off loaded and when exposed to intermittent hydrostatic pressure changes.[27] Distraction has been shown to increase proteoglycan content in cartilage to near-normal states.[27,30,34] A 2000 study showed a change and normalization of proteoglycan turnover, but failed to demonstrate actual cartilage repair in the short duration of the experiment.[34]

Indications for ankle distraction are a congruent joint, pain, joint mobility, and moderate to severe arthritis.[28,29] Some authors also have included osteonecrosis of the talus as an indication.[29] Ankle distraction is used when patients are too young for arthroplasty and have no significant angular deformity that necessitate correction. Contraindications for distraction include active infection, coronal plane deformity exceeding 10°, and substantial loss of bone stock.[29,30,32]

Technique
Controversy exists regarding the proper amount of distraction and the need for articulation to allow motion.[27,29,35] A 2012 study showed early and sustained improvement in patient outcomes with the addition of ankle motion.[35] Some authors have advocated adjunctive procedures to increase motion such as elimination of impingement and bony realignment to correct deformity.[29] Others have recommended arthroscopic or open débridement of the joint with synovectomy, loose body removal, and microfracture of exposed bone at the time of external fixator placement.[30,32]

The original distraction frame was described with the use of two tibial rings. The proximal ring was 5 cm below the knee and the distal ring was 5 cm above the ankle. Each ring was fixed with two 1.5-mm Kirschner wires (K-wires) through the tibia placed at 90° to each other. The rings were connected with four screw-threaded rods. Two additional pins were then inserted into the calcaneus at 45° to each other. The K-wires were tensioned and fixed to a U-shaped foot ring. Two additional wires were placed into the metatarsals and fixed to a half ring over the forefoot after tensioning. The forefoot and U-shaped rings were then connected to make the foot plate. This foot plate must be dorsal to the equator of the foot to allow for weight bearing. The foot and tibia are then connected with four Ilizarov distraction rods. Distraction started on day 1 at the rate of 0.5 mm twice a day for 5 days, for a total of 5 mm of distraction. Weight bearing was encouraged within a few days of surgery.[27] Between 6 and 12 weeks, previously incorporated hinges were loosened to start motion (**Figure 6**). Later descriptions of the frame added a talar neck pin attached to the foot plate to avoid distraction through the subtalar joint.[29]

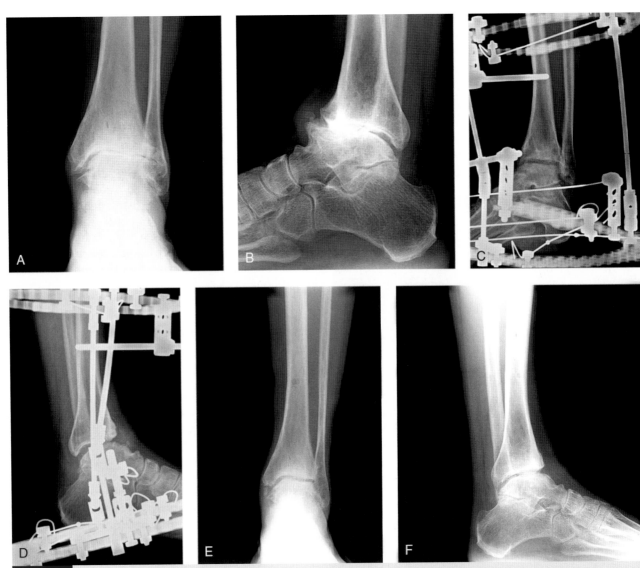

Figure 6   A 33-year-old woman with a history of ankle pilon fracture who underwent distraction arthroplasty. AP (**A**) and lateral (**B**) radiographs preoperatively. Note the substantial joint space narrowing and osteophyte formation. **C** and **D,** Perioperative radiographs showing the hinged external fixator in place; note the joint space created with maximal distraction. One year postoperative AP (**E**) and lateral (**F**) radiographs showing preservation of joint space and improvement of the tibial sclerosis.

A variation on this technique that used a hinged external fixator that permitted ROM exercise was introduced in 2005.[28,29] The authors also advocated the use of concomitant adjunctive procedures to increase the success rate of the procedure, such as removal of impinging osteophytes, release of joint contractures, correction of equinus deformity, and osseous alignment of the ankle. After application of the two tibial rings, a wire is inserted through the Inman ankle axis of rotation from the tip of the lateral malleolus to the tip of the medial malleolus. This is the most important step in the procedure because placement of the hinges can substantially affect resistance to motion. Malposition of the hinges by 10 mm can increase resistance to motion more than fivefold.[36] Threaded rods with hinges are then applied medially and laterally from the distal tibial ring to intersect the axis wire. The medial hinge should be more proximal and anterior to the lateral hinge. The hinge is then connected to the foot ring that is parallel to the sole of the foot. A posterior distraction rod is then added, which can be removed for ROM exercises.

Pin care is performed twice daily with a 50% solution of hydrogen peroxide and saline.[30] Patients should be followed weekly or biweekly until removal of the fixator. The addition of a weight-bearing foot plate or fashioning of accommodative footwear is necessary to ensure compliance with weight bearing.

Results

Results in studies using static ankle distraction showed that 70% of patients demonstrated significant improvement in their pain with increased function.[27,31,37-40] Although joint motion was maintained, it was still considerably diminished when compared with the unaffected ankle.[27,31,37-40] There was also a progressive increase in joint mobility, widening of the joint, and diminished subchondral sclerosis during the first 5 years after the procedure.[27,30,31,37-40]

With the addition of an anatomically located hinge to allow for ROM exercises, one study reported that 78% of a cohort had only occasional mild to moderate pain.[29,33] However, these investigators noted that after 5 years, the outcome scores significantly decreased; they concluded that the benefits of distraction treatment decrease after 5 years.[29] They did not note an increase in joint space narrowing. Whether there is an increase in measured joint space and if this increase correlates to clinical outcomes remains unclear.[27-29,31,37-40] In the largest cohort published to date, investigators in 2002 reported on a prospective study of 57 patients (mean age of 44 years and mean follow-up of 2.8 years); 35 underwent arthroscopic débridement before application of the fixator, and 25 patients had a significant decrease in pain and increase in function.[38] These improvements increased with time. Investigators noted both an increase in joint space and a decrease in subchondral sclerosis.[38] In the same study, the authors conducted a randomized controlled trial in which 17 patients either received distraction arthroplasty or arthroscopic débridement, with the distraction group showing more improvement in pain and function.

In the longest follow-up study on patients undergoing distraction, investigators found that 73% of their patients continued to benefit from distraction at an average 10-year follow-up (range, 7 to 15 years).[41]

In addition to the usual risk factors associated with any foot and ankle procedures, risk factors unique to distraction arthroplasty include pin tract infections, failure of hardware (wires), patient inconvenience, need for frequent follow-up, and a steep learning curve for surgeons. The success rate varies in the literature, ranging between 65% and 78%.[27,29,33,38,40,41] These results mean that one third of patients undergoing this laborious and time-consuming procedure will fail to see any benefits. Further research is needed to more accurately predict which patients are most likely to benefit from distraction arthroplasty. Pin tract infections have been reported to occur in as many as one third of patients, most of whom required treatment with localized wound care and oral antibiotics.[38]

A 2012 review of the literature found insufficient evidence for the use of distraction arthroplasty,[42] yet, in the face of a difficult problem, there remains abundant support for its use.[28-30,32]

Periarticular Osteotomies

Background

Patients with fairly well-preserved joints with substantial varus or valgus deformity may benefit from a periarticular osteotomy with an adjuvant ligamentous reconstruction for chronic ligament instability with mild to moderate degenerative changes.[1] Nonunions and malunions of previous fractures can lead to increased articular loads and pain. These patients may simply benefit from revision of their fixation and realignment if their ankle joint remains salvageable.

Any deformity of the ankle joint, whether single, multiplanar, or rotational, leads to abnormal mechanical loads and is believed to affect joint function and cartilage nutrition and lead to further degeneration.[7,8,15,16] Deformity in any plane exceeding 10° should be corrected.[7] Supramalleolar distal tibial osteotomies are performed to restore anatomic alignment and improve biomechanics by redistributing the joint load onto intact articular cartilage.[7,30]

With a flexible hindfoot, the ankle is able to tolerate certain amounts of deformity. The subtalar joint is crucial in compensating for any coronal plane deformity. Because there is approximately 20° of inversion versus 5° of eversion allowed through the subtalar complex, a valgus ankle deformity is much better tolerated than a varus deformity.[43] Consequently, it is critical that any patient being evaluated for a realignment osteotomy be examined for subtalar joint and hindfoot motion, which helps to assess his or her ability to compensate for the osteotomy. Patients with a stiff hindfoot should undergo hindfoot realignment concomitantly with the supramalleolar osteotomy.[7]

The goals of periarticular osteotomies are to restore normal TAS and TLS angles. Slight overcorrection is recommended at the time of surgery to allow for some collapse.[7] The center of rotation and angulation can easily be determined by intersecting the mechanical axis of the proximal and distal segments of the tibia. If the osteotomy is performed at the center of rotation and angulation, then the deformity can be corrected without any translation of the distal fragment. However, if the osteotomy needs to be above or below the center of rotation and angulation (as in an intra-articular deformity), the distal fragment must be translated relative to the mechanical axis to avoid a secondary translational deformity.

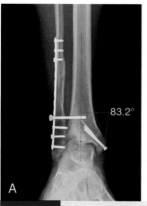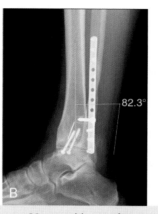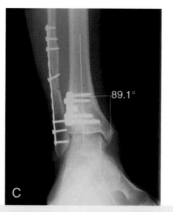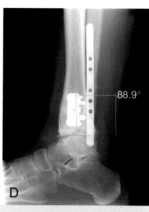

Figure 7 Imaging studies from a 38-year-old man after sustaining an ankle fracture-dislocation with open reduction and internal fixation. Note that this patient appears to have continued shortening of the fibula and collapse of the lateral aspect of the tibial plafond. AP (**A**) and lateral (**B**) radiographs before revision surgery showing the tibial articular surface (TAS) angle and tibial lateral surface (TLS) angle. AP (**C**) and lateral (**D**) radiographs after fibular osteotomy and lengthening through his existing fibular plate. The same lateral incision was used to approach the lateral aspect of the tibia to perform the opening wedge osteotomy with an opening wedge plate. Note the normalization of the TAS and TLS angles.

Multiple osteotomies, fixation methods, and approaches have been described, including opening and closing wedge osteotomies, dome osteotomies, and plafondoplasty.[9,15,16,44-46] Each of these interventions has associated advantages and disadvantages. For example, closing wedge osteotomies do not necessitate an interposition graft, and faster time to union is expected. However, they cause shortening, which can be a problem in a traumatized and already shortened leg. In the same regard, traumatized tissue will be less tolerant of stretching with an opening wedge osteotomy. Dome osteotomies cannot correct multiplanar or sagittal deformities and cannot be translated. The choice of osteotomy, graft, and fixation should be individualized based on the condition of the soft tissues, history or suspicion of infection, and limb-length discrepancy.

Technique
Patients are positioned supine with an ipsilateral hip bump. If a fibular osteotomy is required, it is performed at the level of the planned tibial osteotomy through a lateral incision. This technique was described in detail in 2009 and 2012.[44,47] A medial osteotomy is usually performed through a medial longitudinal incision, and a lateral osteotomy is typically performed through the same incision as the fibular osteotomy. Care is taken to avoid excessive stripping and soft-tissue tension.

For opening wedge osteotomies, whether medial or lateral, a K-wire is inserted parallel to the ankle joint as a cutting guide. The osteotomy is performed using a sagittal saw with irrigation to avoid thermal injury to the bone. The opposite cortex is left intact. An osteotome is used to greenstick the osteotomy, and a laminar spreader is used to spread the osteotomy until the distal tibial articular surface is parallel to the floor or slightly overcorrected. An iliac crest structural autograft or tricortical allograft is then inserted and fixation is obtained (**Figure 7**).

A closing osteotomy is performed by inserting two converging K-wires that meet at the opposite cortex, with one parallel to the ankle joint and the other perpendicular to the mechanical axis of the proximal tibia. The osteotomy is then performed along the K-wires. The wedge of bone created is removed and the osteotomy compressed and fixed.

A dome osteotomy is performed through an anterolateral incision. A K-wire is used to mark the plane of the ankle joint. A drill is then used to make multiple holes in the metaphyseal bone in a dome pattern with the dome height at 1 cm to 1.5 cm. Two 4-mm pins are inserted into each fragment, with the distal pin being parallel to the ankle joint and the proximal pin perpendicular to the proximal mechanical axis. The osteotomy is then completed with a sagittal saw or osteotome and the pins are made parallel before fixation.

Results
Multiple studies have shown that periarticular osteotomies are a viable option for treating various types of ankle arthritis when various osteotomy techniques are used.[8,9,15,16,45,46,48,49] In 1995 and 1998, investigators showed their use in both primary and posttraumatic arthritis with favorable results.[15,16] The authors attributed their few unsatisfied patients to undercorrection of the deformity and noted stiffness and decreased ROM in the posttraumatic group. A 2003 study compared medial

opening and closing wedge osteotomies and showed faster time to union with closing wedge osteotomies as well as halted progression of arthritic changes during their 33-month follow-up.[9] Another group of 2003 investigators reported on the use of external fixation and a percutaneous drilling osteotomy with good results, although the external fixator was used for an average of 5 months.[48] In 2006, researchers used a medial opening wedge osteotomy for varus primary ankle arthritis and reported good or excellent results in 20 of 26 ankles at a mean follow-up longer than 8 years.[49] They compared patients with and without involvement of the talar medial dome and found worse outcomes in ankles with talar involvement.

Osteotomy complications are infrequent, with stiffness being the most commonly reported complication.[9,15] Delayed unions, nonunions, pin site infections, wound breakdown, and superficial or deep infections have also been reported.[9,15,16,45,48,49] Hardware-related complications that necessitated removal were more problematic with use of medial hardware.[8,46,49]

Joint-Sacrificing Surgery
Allograft Arthroplasty
Background

Allografts have been used successfully in the knee, and there is increasing use of allografts in tibiotalar arthritis. Good outcomes have been reported with osteochondral allografts for small- to medium-sized talar defects in the form of single plugs or mosaicplasty.[50] Osteochondral joint allografts are fairly new in the treatment of end-stage ankle arthritis. Although this approach was first described in 1913,[51] it was popularized during the past two decades.[52-54] The major advantages of allograft arthroplasty are maintenance of bone (as opposed to a traditional arthroplasty, which sacrifices bone), chondrocyte survival, and decreased ipsilateral hindfoot degeneration.

The most important concern in allograft transplantation is chondrocyte survival, particularly during the cold storage process.[55,56] More than 80% of transplanted chondrocytes can survive in recovered cartilage.[56] The mechanical properties of the matrix are also maintained.[56] Chondrocytes have been shown to survive the transplantation process primarily because cartilage is avascular and predominately is dependent on synovial fluid for nourishment.[55] Transplanted chondrocytes are not replaced by host chondrocytes. In a long-term retrieval case report in which female donor cartilage was implanted into a male recipient, the retrieved cartilage at 29 years continued to express female chromosomes.[57]

It is not entirely clear if the time from death to harvest of the allograft affects viability of the chondrocytes; however, it has been shown that the time from harvest to implantation is critical in the survival of donor chondrocytes.[55] In one study of specimens stored fewer than 14 days, there was no decrease in chondrocyte viability or density; when tested beyond 28 days, specimens showed significant loss of chondrocytes.[56] These losses were most notable in the important superficial zone of the cartilage.[55] Cold storage in fetal bovine serum and gradual rewarming in a nitric oxide synthase inhibitor also help to increase chondrocyte viability and proteoglycan synthesis and reverse the metabolic suppression of cold storage.[55] On the other hand, the bone in allografts is replaced by host bone through creeping substitution.[55] During the revascularization period, there is increased risk for graft collapse.

Although cartilage was thought to be safe from the host's immune response because of its relative avascularity, recent reports have changed this traditional view.[53,55] A 2005 study reported that 91% of patients had cytotoxic serum human leukocyte antigen antibodies at 6 months.[53] This has been correlated with greater bony edema and wider graft host interface on MRI in antibody-positive patients.[55] In light of these findings, there appears to be some relationship between immune sensitization and graft survival. Yet, there are no reports in the literature that use immune suppressive therapy in allograft transplantation. There have been no cases of disease transmission from allograft arthroplasty; regardless, this risk should be discussed with patients.

Technique

The patient is placed supine with an ipsilateral hip bump. An anterior approach to the ankle is performed through a midline incision using the interval between the tibialis anterior and the extensor hallucis longus. The neurovascular bundle is identified and retracted laterally, and synovectomy and anterior osteophyte débridement is performed. A unilateral external fixator is applied to correct deformity, tension the stabilizing ligaments, and distract the joint 4 to 8 mm.

A total ankle arthroplasty (TAA) tibial cutting block is applied and fluoroscopically confirmed to ensure appropriate positioning and then fixed to the tibia. The distal tibia and medial malleolus are cut using a sagittal saw. To avoid overheating and thermal necrosis, the saw blade should be constantly irrigated. The surgeon must avoid fracturing the medial malleolus and neurovascular bundle injury. The talar cut is then made with or without the aid of a cutting jig, depending on the thickness of the planned cut. The resection from each side of the joint should be between 4 mm to 10 mm, depending on the amount of bone loss. Any cystic lesions are filled with autograft from the resected plafond and talar dome.

The donor allograft is cut in the same manner using a guide one size larger than that used for the host. This

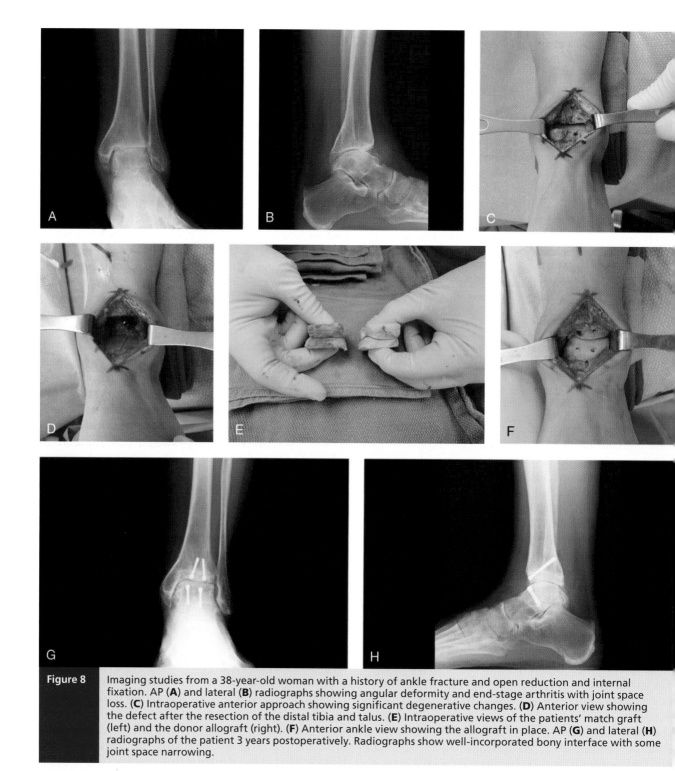

Figure 8 Imaging studies from a 38-year-old woman with a history of ankle fracture and open reduction and internal fixation. AP (**A**) and lateral (**B**) radiographs showing angular deformity and end-stage arthritis with joint space loss. (**C**) Intraoperative anterior approach showing significant degenerative changes. (**D**) Anterior view showing the defect after the resection of the distal tibia and talus. (**E**) Intraoperative views of the patients' match graft (left) and the donor allograft (right). (**F**) Anterior ankle view showing the allograft in place. AP (**G**) and lateral (**H**) radiographs of the patient 3 years postoperatively. Radiographs show well-incorporated bony interface with some joint space narrowing.

ensures that the tibial graft is not too thin and does not lead to fracture. The donor talus cut is done freehand. Each graft then undergoes pulsed lavage to remove any marrow elements and debris. The graft is then placed into the host and verified fluoroscopically and the external fixator is removed and the ankle is ranged to ensure the grafts find their preferred position. The grafts are fixed with two headless or countersunk screws each (**Figure 8**).

Postoperatively, patients are in a non–weight-bearing splint until suture removal at 2 weeks. They are then transitioned to a controlled ankle motion boot and allowed to work on ROM but do not bear weight. At 6 weeks,

3: Arthritis of the Foot and Ankle

patients are allowed to begin partial weight bearing until 12 weeks or until the graft is incorporated, at which time they are allowed full weight bearing. High-impact activities are prohibited during the first year.

Results

Kim et al[58] reported a 42% failure rate at 148 months in seven patients with posttraumatic ankle arthritis that underwent allograft replacement. However, they noted that radiographic and clinical results may not correlate. They attributed the failures to graft fragmentation, subluxation, poor graft fit, and nonunions. These procedures were performed with freehand cuts. A 2003 study reported on nine patients with bipolar allografts with no failures at 21 months using the Agility (DePuy) total ankle cutting guides.[54] They had one allograft failure in a partial unipolar lateral talar dome. In another study by the same group,[53] only 6 of 11 allografts survived at 33 months. Three failures were revised to a repeat allograft, one to a TAA, and one had not yet been revised. Investigators also showed a correlation between graft thickness and survival, with grafts smaller than 7 mm showing poorer results. Six failures at a 2-year follow-up were reported in a cohort of 32 patients.[59]

The results of a retrospective series of patients showed a high failure rate.[55,60] The authors concluded that this procedure should be reserved for patients who are too young to be candidates for arthroplasty and refuse to have an arthrodesis. They found that ideal candidates for this procedure should have good ROM, tend to be older, and have a low body mass index and minimal coronal alignment deformities.[55,60] Their technique varied in that they did not use an external fixator, used the same size jig for host and donor cuts, and used allografts with average time from death to implantation of 23 days.

One of the largest populations and longest follow-up studies of patients who underwent ankle allografting was conducted in 2013, although it is unclear how many of these patients were included in previous studies by the same group.[52] At a mean follow-up of 5.3 years on 86 ankles (82 patients), there was a reoperation rate of 42% and a failure rate of 29%, with a mean time to failure of 3.7 years. The authors defined failure as any reoperation in which the graft was replaced; however, some patients underwent distraction arthrodiastasis for arthritic changes in the grafts and these patients were not considered part of the failure group. The failure group included 10 patients who underwent revision allografting, 7 who were revised to arthrodesis, 6 who had TAAs, and 2 who underwent transtibial amputations. Survivorship of the allograft was reported as 76% at 5 years and 44% at 10 years. However, 92% of the patients reported satisfaction

with the procedure, 85% reported improvement in their pain, and 83% reported improved function.

Although these results reflect a higher failure rate than those of arthrodesis or arthroplasty,[61] allograft arthroplasty remains a viable alternative for the treatment of end-stage ankle arthritis. Further studies are needed to establish the ideal patient for allograft arthroplasty, although general recommendations include patients who are too young for a traditional arthroplasty or an ankle arthrodesis because of long-term complications and those with contralateral ankle arthritis or hindfoot arthrosis. The major deterring factors of this procedure are its total cost and the unpredictability of available fresh matched allografts.[52]

Arthrodesis

Ankle arthrodesis was first described in 1879 and is still considered by many authors as the preferred treatment to alleviate pain and improve function.[3,19,62,63] However, many surgeons have argued that with more recent improvements in TAA materials, techniques, instrumentation, and implants, a paradigm shift of this standard is imminent.

Dissatisfaction with arthrodesis stems from its limitations. Although it is the most reliable and reproducible form of pain relief in end-stage ankle arthritis, it leads to substantial loss of motion, gait alterations, and arthritis in adjacent joints.[3,63-65] The development of arthritis in adjacent joints in the hindfoot was estimated to occur in as many as 50% of patients within 7 to 8 years and 100% of patients within 22 years.[7] Patients who undergo arthrodesis often experience difficulty navigating uneven terrain and inclines, pain with rigorous activities, and increased contact stress at the talonavicular and calcaneocuboid joints.[63,66] Loss of up to 74% of sagittal, 70% of inversion, and 77% of eversion motion has been noted after successful arthrodesis.[67] Additionally, patients with an arthrodesis experience a 16% decrease in gait velocity, a 3% increase in oxygen consumption, and a 10% decrease in gait efficiency. However, clinical results of ankle arthrodesis have been favorable overall. Symptom relief is highly reliable and more than 90% of patients are satisfied with their outcomes.[61,62,65,67,68]

The exact technique and surgical approach are variable throughout the literature. There are abundant preferences regarding the method of fixation, joint preparation, retention or sacrifice of the malleoli, and postoperative care.[19] However, most authors agree that the optimal position for arthrodesis of the ankle is in 5° to 8° of valgus, 5° to 10° of external rotation, neutral dorsiflexion, and about 5 mm of posterior offset to improve the lever arm of the calcaneus.[19,69]

3: Arthritis of the Foot and Ankle

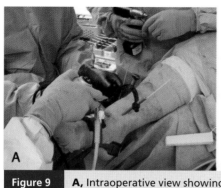 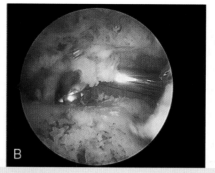 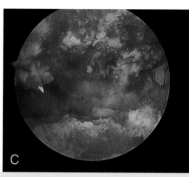

Figure 9 **A,** Intraoperative view showing noninvasive ankle distraction; also note the intra-articular targeting system with guidewires in place before fixation. **B,** Intra-articular view showing curettage of the joint space. **C,** Intra-articular view after complete preparation; note the guide pin for fixation in the upper left corner.

Internal and external fixation techniques have been described. In the absence of open wounds or infections, internal fixation is typically preferred. Compression screws and lateral, anterior, or posterior plating are all options for fixation. Crossed screws form a stronger construct than parallel screws but may prevent compression if not done sequentially.[70,71] Some authors have advocated that the most important screw is one that is placed from the posterior malleolus into the talar neck and head and is referred to as the "home-run" screw.[72] Additional screws can be placed through the medial or lateral malleoli or both.

Complications following arthrodesis involve wound healing, infection, neurovascular injuries, complex regional pain syndrome, venous thromboembolic events, nonunion, malunion, and adjacent joint arthrosis. Most early-onset complications can be avoided with careful patient selection, recognition of high-risk patients, careful dissection, and respecting the soft tissues. Aggressive early treatment is necessary for any suspected infection or wound complication.

Nonunion rates have been reported to be as high as 60%, but it is important to note that most of these nonunions were early reports with no fixation, wire fixation, and no risk stratification or bone grafting. For certain patients such as those with osteonecrosis, sensory neuropathy, and infections, nonunion rates can be as high as 100%.[73] More recent reports show more favorable results,[61,65,74] but further research is needed to evaluate the use of advanced plating systems, bone marrow aspiration concentrates, and newer techniques. Patients with peripheral neuropathy, osteonecrosis of the talus, prior or current deep infections, open injuries, talar dome or pilon fractures, prior subtalar arthrodesis, spasticity, smoking history, and various medical problems are at higher risk for nonunion.[19,74]

Malunions can be quite problematic. Plantar flexion malunions can lead to a vaulting gait pattern and a recurvatum thrust at the knee. This may eventually lead to medial collateral ligament failure attributable to an externally rotated gait resulting from attempts to place the foot flat on the ground. Furthermore, stress fractures and metatarsalgia may develop. Dorsiflexion malunions lead to increased pressure on the heel pad and ulcers or a flexed knee gait. Coronal plane deformities usually lead to ligamentous laxity and added stress on the nearby joints and musculotendinous units leading to early degeneration. Malunion can also affect the knee, as well as the medial or lateral columns of the foot. Valgus malunions are more tolerated than varus malunions because the subtalar joint can compensate for the valgus position of the talus.

Arthroscopic Technique

Arthroscopic ankle arthrodesis is a minimally invasive technique for patients with minimal deformity.[68,75,76] It has been shown to lead to faster fusion rates than open procedures, likely because of decreased tissue stripping and retention of the blood supply.[68,75-77] Fixation is usually obtained with crossing screws. During arthroscopic débridement, a noninvasive distractor can be used instead of an external fixator, which has been shown to be associated with more complications.[78] Positioning and fixation are performed under fluoroscopic guidance. With the advent of newer arthroscopic débridement instruments, arthroscopic ankle arthrodesis has become easier and less time consuming (**Figure 9**).

The major advantages of the arthroscopic technique are significantly less morbidity, shorter surgical and tourniquet times, less blood loss, shorter hospital stays, and better improvement in outcome scores for up to 2 years postoperatively.[75-77] The technique produces similar fusion rates compared to open techniques with minimal complications.[72,76-79] Although experienced surgeons may be able to perform this procedure in less than 1 hour, the learning curve for surgeons may lead them to abandon

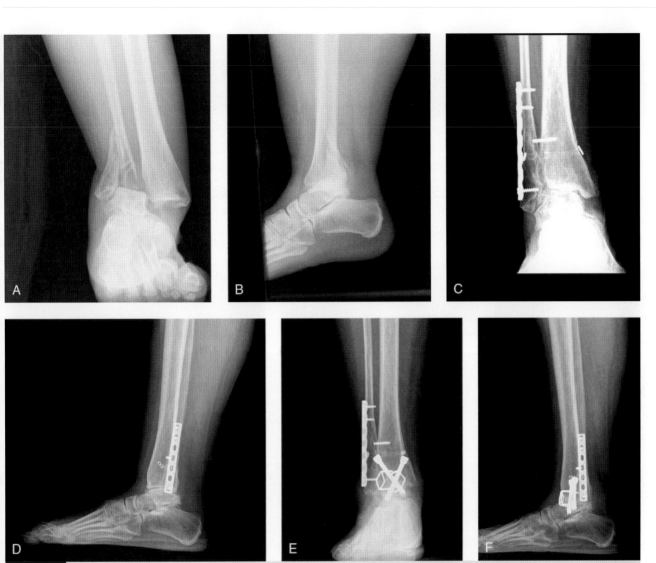

Figure 10   Imaging studies from a 56-year-old woman with history of ankle fracture and open reduction and internal fixation with end-stage ankle arthritis. AP (**A**) and lateral (**B**) radiographs at the time of her original fracture-dislocation. AP (**C**) and lateral (**D**) radiographs 3 years postinjury showing significant posttraumatic arthritis. AP (**E**) and lateral (**F**) radiographs after an ankle arthrodesis. Crossed headless screws from the medial and lateral malleolus with supplemental anterior ankle staples through an anterior approach.

this technique. A contraindication to this procedure may be substantial preoperative deformity, which may make final positioning extremely difficult and limit the use of this technique; guidelines for the amount of deformity that is tolerated for arthroscopic arthrodesis have not been established.[68]

Open Technique
Various approaches have been described for arthrodesis of the ankle, including anterior, lateral transfibular with or without an accessory medial incision, and posterior. The anterior approach is through the interval between the anterior tibialis tendon and extensor hallucis longus. The neurovascular bundle is retracted laterally. The technique allows use of a single incision to approach both the medial and lateral gutter, preserves the fibula, and makes use of the same incision used for most TAAs for possible later conversion. However, this approach places the neurovascular bundle and the superficial peroneal nerve at risk. It has also been associated with neuromas and tendon adhesions. Although it is difficult to reach the posterior aspect of the joint for débridement and it also may be difficult to reduce the talus under the tibia, these challenges have not been known to affect the excellent results achieved with this approach (**Figure 10**).

The lateral approach necessitates a fibular osteotomy to access the ankle joint. The fibula may be morcellized using an acetabular reamer and then used as graft. Or

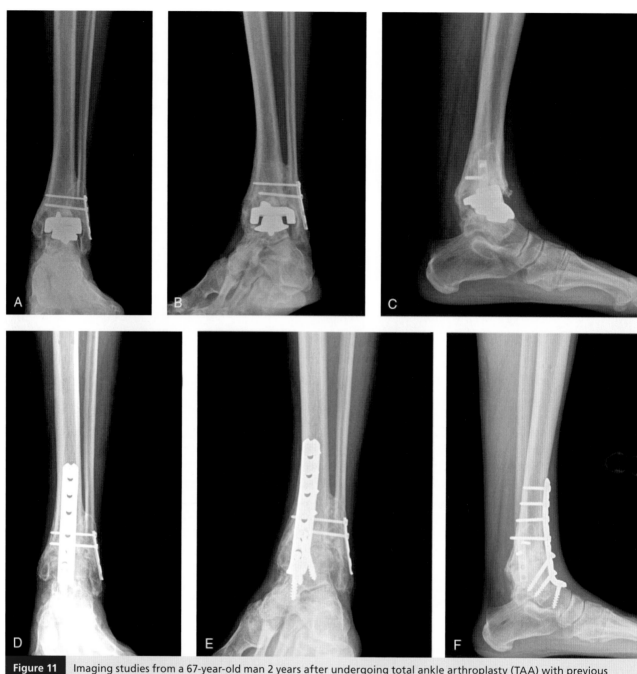

Figure 11   Imaging studies from a 67-year-old man 2 years after undergoing total ankle arthroplasty (TAA) with previous attempted bone grafting and revision who continues to have pain and significant functional limitations. AP (**A**), mortise (**B**), and lateral (**C**) radiographs showing the substantial subsidence and lucency of both the tibial and talar components. The lateral radiograph shows the substantial anterior distal tibial bone loss and subsidence. Mortise (**D**), AP (**E**), and lateral (**F**) radiographs 18 months after surgery. The patient underwent removal of the TAA with aggressive débridement. The defect was filled with a femoral head allograft and an ankle arthrodesis was performed with an anterior arthrodesis plate. Currently, the patient is ambulating with a rocker-bottom shoe without pain.

it may be reattached to the tibia and talus as an onlay graft. Preserving the fibula allows larger bony surfaces for arthrodesis, a lateral strut for more stability, preservation of the peroneal groove, a guide to proper rotation

and alignment of the talus within the mortise, and the possibility for future TAA. A medial incision may be necessary to reduce and débride the medial gutter. The posterior approach may be performed by splitting the

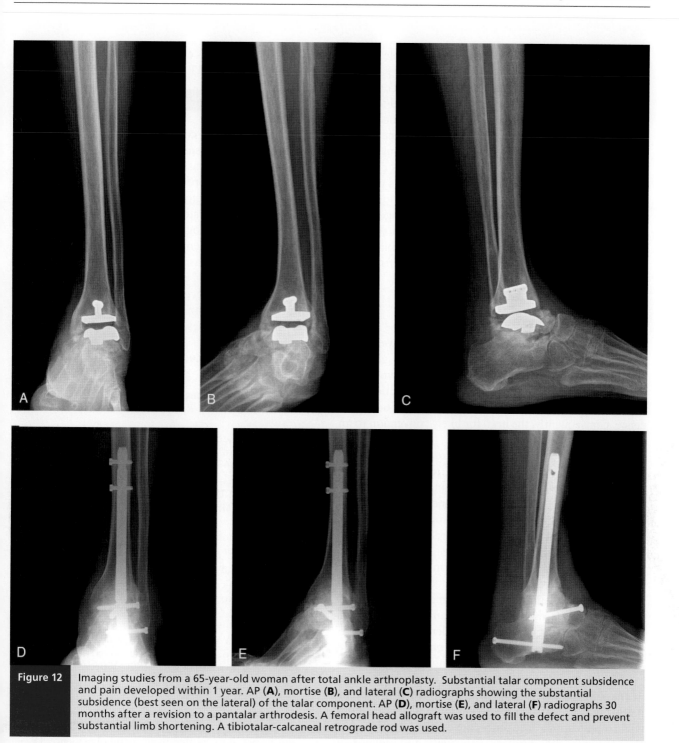

Figure 12 Imaging studies from a 65-year-old woman after total ankle arthroplasty. Substantial talar component subsidence and pain developed within 1 year. AP (**A**), mortise (**B**), and lateral (**C**) radiographs showing the substantial subsidence (best seen on the lateral) of the talar component. AP (**D**), mortise (**E**), and lateral (**F**) radiographs 30 months after a revision to a pantalar arthrodesis. A femoral head allograft was used to fill the defect and prevent substantial limb shortening. A tibiotalar-calcaneal retrograde rod was used.

Achilles, performing a long Z-shaped tenotomy of the Achilles, or performing a calcaneal osteotomy of the insertion of the Achilles and reflecting it superiorly. Although used primarily for tibiotalocalcaneal (TTC) arthrodesis, the posterior approach can be used for an isolated ankle arthrodesis if needed.

The mini-open approach was developed to provide the same advantages as an arthroscopic technique, which involves less soft-tissue stripping and quicker time to fusion.[79] It is performed through anteromedial and anterolateral incisions, which are essentially extended arthroscopic portals and are in the same intervals. The superficial peroneal nerve is at risk with an anterolateral incision. The joint can then be débrided with osteotomes and curettes.

3: Arthritis of the Foot and Ankle

The ankle joint can be prepared in multiple configurations, including simple denuding of the cartilage and subchondral plate while maintaining the congruent curved surfaces, which is the current preferred method. Alternatively, parallel flat cuts can be performed at the apex of the tibia and 5 mm below the apex of the talus.[80] This leads to slight shortening of the limb but is usually well tolerated. Technically, however, this can lead to difficulty determining the exact arthrodesis position rotationally and anterior or posterior translation of the talus relative to the tibia. To avoid this challenge, use of matching chevron cuts has been described in the tibia and talus.[81] An anterior or posterior sliding tibial onlay graft, medial, and/or lateral malleoli onlay grafting have also been reported.[19]

Salvage Failed TAA

With the rising number of TAAs performed, the number of failed arthroplasties will also increase. Ten-year TAA survival ranges between 63% and 91%.[61] Although newer implants and techniques may improve the survival rate, the expanding indications for deformity correction with TAA may lead to an increase in instability and subsidence. Consequently, the need for likely conversion to an arthrodesis will remain.

When a TAA becomes infected, treatment should be staged with the first stage including removal of all implants, irrigation and débridement, an antibiotic spacer if needed, temporary stabilization, and long-term intravenous antibiotic use based on intraoperative cultures. This is followed by arthrodesis, preferably using external fixation and bone grafting.

In noninfectious failed TAA with minimal bone loss, a single-stage procedure is recommended. With minimal bone loss, a revision arthroplasty may be attempted. However, if unsalvageable, isolated ankle fusion should be attempted. Multiple studies have demonstrated favorable results with high fusion rates for primary conversion arthrodesis after failed TAA with minimal bone loss.[82,83]

When significant bone loss is present after removal of the TAA, a TTC fusion with bulk grafting may be performed. TTC fusion following failed TAA is fraught with complications. The procedure carries a much higher nonunion rate than primary arthrodesis and higher risk for complications. With the use of autograft bone, fusion rates of 20% to 93% have been reported.[83] The use of an intramedullary TTC nail was shown to increase the union rate over compression screws in one 2006 study.[83] However, a 2013 study showed that TTC fusions that necessitate bulk allograft such as a femoral head allograft are associated with nonunion rates as high as 50%; nonunions developed in all of the patients with diabetes,

and 19% of nonunions eventually resulted in transtibial amputation[84] (**Figure 11** and **Figure 12**).

Summary

The ankle is a highly congruent joint that experiences large forces through a small surface area. Ankle arthritis is predominantly a disease of young and active individuals and is a challenging problem. The treatment algorithm should consider all factors including age, activity level, etiology, alignment, history, comorbidities, and physical examination and radiographic findings. Surgical treatments include débridement, distraction arthroplasty, interposition arthroplasty, osteotomies, reconstruction, allograft arthroplasty, arthrodesis, and arthroplasty. Further research is necessary to elucidate the optimal treatments and best candidates and to advance current implants and techniques.

Annotated References

1. Demetriades L, Strauss E, Gallina J: Osteoarthritis of the ankle. *Clin Orthop Relat Res* 1998;349:28-42.

2. Huch K, Kuettner KE, Dieppe P: Osteoarthritis in ankle and knee joints. *Semin Arthritis Rheum* 1997;26(4):667-674.

3. Thomas RH, Daniels TR: Ankle arthritis. *J Bone Joint Surg Am* 2003;85(5):923-936.

4. Daniels T, Thomas R: Etiology and biomechanics of ankle arthritis. *Foot Ankle Clin* 2008;13(3):341-352, vii.

   In this review article, authors outline the mechanical and biochemical properties of the ankle joint and how these relate to the etiology of ankle arthritis. Level of evidence: V.

5. Valderrabano V, Horisberger M, Russell I, Dougall H, Hintermann B: Etiology of ankle osteoarthritis. *Clin Orthop Relat Res* 2009;467(7):1800-1806.

   This retrospective review of 390 patients (406 ankles) with end-stage ankle arthritis revealed that 78% of patients had posttraumatic arthritis (compared with 9% having primary OA). Posttraumatic patients were younger, and most were in varus alignment. Level of evidence: IV.

6. Curtis MJ, Michelson JD, Urquhart MW, Byank RP, Jinnah RH: Tibiotalar contact and fibular malunion in ankle fractures. A cadaver study. *Acta Orthop Scand* 1992;63(3):326-329.

7. Garras DN, Raikin SM: Supramalleolar osteotomies as joint sparing management of ankle arthritis. *Semin Arthroplasty* 2010;21(4):230-239.

This is a review article of the indications, types, techniques, and outcomes of periarticular osteotomies in the treatment of ankle arthritis. Level of evidence: V.

8. Harstall R, Lehmann O, Krause F, Weber M: Supramalleolar lateral closing wedge osteotomy for the treatment of varus ankle arthrosis. *Foot Ankle Int* 2007;28(5):542-548.

9. Stamatis ED, Cooper PS, Myerson MS: Supramalleolar osteotomy for the treatment of distal tibial angular deformities and arthritis of the ankle joint. *Foot Ankle Int* 2003;24(10):754-764.

10. Saltzman CL, Salamon ML, Blanchard GM, et al: Epidemiology of ankle arthritis: Report of a consecutive series of 639 patients from a tertiary orthopaedic center. *Iowa Orthop J* 2005;25:44-46.

11. Segal AD, Shofer J, Hahn ME, Orendurff MS, Ledoux WR, Sangeorzan BJ: Functional limitations associated with end-stage ankle arthritis. *J Bone Joint Surg Am* 2012;94(9):777-783.

    Gait analysis, demographics, self-assessed function, and activity monitoring of patients with end-stage ankle arthritis demonstrated that they had decreased physical and perceived function as well as altered gait parameters. Level of evidence: II.

12. Ramsey PL, Hamilton W: Changes in tibiotalar area of contact caused by lateral talar shift. *J Bone Joint Surg Am* 1976;58(3):356-357.

13. Lindsjö U: Operative treatment of ankle fracture-dislocations. A follow-up study of 306/321 consecutive cases. *Clin Orthop Relat Res* 1985;199:28-38.

14. Marsh JL, Buckwalter J, Gelberman R, et al: Articular fractures: Does an anatomic reduction really change the result? *J Bone Joint Surg Am* 2002;84(7):1259-1271.

15. Takakura Y, Takaoka T, Tanaka Y, Yajima H, Tamai S: Results of opening-wedge osteotomy for the treatment of a post-traumatic varus deformity of the ankle. *J Bone Joint Surg Am* 1998;80(2):213-218.

16. Takakura Y, Tanaka Y, Kumai T, Tamai S: Low tibial osteotomy for osteoarthritis of the ankle: Results of a new operation in 18 patients. *J Bone Joint Surg Br* 1995;77(1):50-54.

17. Thevendran G, Younger A, Pinney S: Current concepts review: Risk factors for nonunions in foot and ankle arthrodeses. *Foot Ankle Int* 2012;33(11):1031-1040.

    This is a review article about known risk factors for nonunion. The authors discuss each risk factor and review available literature pertaining to the risk or procedure being performed. They conclude that smoking, diabetes, and soft-tissue injuries are contributing factors. Level of evidence: V.

18. Stuart MJ, Morrey BF: Arthrodesis of the diabetic neuropathic ankle joint. *Clin Orthop Relat Res* 1990;253:209-211.

19. Katcherian DA: Treatment of ankle arthrosis. *Clin Orthop Relat Res* 1998;349:48-57.

20. Anain JM Jr, Bojrab AR, Rhinehart FC: Conservative treatments for rheumatoid arthritis in the foot and ankle. *Clin Podiatr Med Surg* 2010;27(2):193-207.

    A review of nonsurgical, pharmacologic, and physical treatments for rheumatoid disease of the foot and ankle is presented. The authors review NSAIDs, injections, DMARDs, therapy, and bracing. Level of evidence: V.

21. Khosla SK, Baumhauer JF: Dietary and viscosupplementation in ankle arthritis. *Foot Ankle Clin* 2008;13(3):353-361, vii.

    The authors review the literature on the use of glucosamine, chondroitin sulfate, and viscosupplements in other joints and their possible application in ankle arthritis. They conclude that these supplements have promise but lack evidence. Level of evidence: V.

22. Salk RS, Chang TJ, D'Costa WF, Soomekh DJ, Grogan KA: Sodium hyaluronate in the treatment of osteoarthritis of the ankle: A controlled, randomized, double-blind pilot study. *J Bone Joint Surg Am* 2006;88(2):295-302.

23. Sun SF, Chou YJ, Hsu CW, et al: Efficacy of intra-articular hyaluronic acid in patients with osteoarthritis of the ankle: A prospective study. *Osteoarthritis Cartilage* 2006;14(9):867-874.

24. Sun SF, Hsu CW, Sun HP, Chou YJ, Li HJ, Wang JL: The effect of three weekly intra-articular injections of hyaluronate on pain, function, and balance in patients with unilateral ankle arthritis. *J Bone Joint Surg Am* 2011;93(18):1720-1726.

    A prospective study of 46 patients undergoing three weekly injections showed a significant reduction in Ankle Osteoarthritis Scale score, improvement in American Orthopaedic Foot and Ankle Society (AOFAS) hindfoot scores, improved balance, decreased acetaminophen intake, and high satisfaction rates with no adverse events at 6-month follow-up. Level of evidence: II.

25. John S, Bongiovanni F: Brace management for ankle arthritis. *Clin Podiatr Med Surg* 2009;26(2):193-197.

    This is a review of current braces available for ankle arthritis and the rationale behind use of each. Level of evidence: V.

26. Hassouna H, Kumar S, Bendall S: Arthroscopic ankle debridement: 5-year survival analysis. *Acta Orthop Belg* 2007;73(6):737-740.

27. van Valburg AA, van Roermund PM, Lammens J, et al: Can Ilizarov joint distraction delay the need for an

3: Arthritis of the Foot and Ankle

arthrodesis of the ankle? A preliminary report. *J Bone Joint Surg Br* 1995;77(5):720-725.

28. Paley D, Lamm BM: Ankle joint distraction. *Foot Ankle Clin* 2005;10(4):685-698, ix.

29. Paley D, Lamm BM, Purohit RM, Specht SC: Distraction arthroplasty of the ankle: How far can you stretch the indications? *Foot Ankle Clin* 2008;13(3):471-484, ix.

    This review article describes the Baltimore method of distraction arthroplasty. Authors present results of a cohort treated with their method. They demonstrate good results in 14 of 18 patients, but note decreased benefit after 5 years. Level of evidence: V.

30. Morse KR, Flemister AS, Baumhauer JF, DiGiovanni BF: Distraction arthroplasty. *Foot Ankle Clin* 2007;12(1):29-39.

31. van Roermund PM, Lafeber FP: Joint distraction as treatment for ankle osteoarthritis. *Instr Course Lect* 1999;48:249-254.

32. Chiodo CP, McGarvey W: Joint distraction for the treatment of ankle osteoarthritis. *Foot Ankle Clin* 2004;9(3):541-553, ix.

33. Tellisi N, Fragomen AT, Kleinman D, O'Malley MJ, Rozbruch SR: Joint preservation of the osteoarthritic ankle using distraction arthroplasty. *Foot Ankle Int* 2009;30(4):318-325.

    This is a retrospective review of 25 patients who underwent distraction arthroplasty. At a mean follow-up of 30 months, there was significant improvement in AOFAS scores and pain but modest improvement in Medical Outcome Study 36-Item Short Form health survey scores. Two patients required fusion. Level of evidence: VI.

34. van Valburg AA, van Roermund PM, Marijnissen AC, et al: Joint distraction in treatment of osteoarthritis (II): Effects on cartilage in a canine model. *Osteoarthritis Cartilage* 2000;8(1):1-8.

35. Saltzman CL, Hillis SL, Stolley MP, Anderson DD, Amendola A: Motion versus fixed distraction of the joint in the treatment of ankle osteoarthritis: A prospective randomized controlled trial. *J Bone Joint Surg Am* 2012;94(11):961-970.

    This prospective randomized controlled trial compares fixed with motion distraction arthroplasty on 36 patients. Both groups showed significant improvement on the Ankle Osteoarthritis Scale, but the motion group had significant improvement compared with the static distraction group. Level of evidence: I.

36. Bottlang M, Marsh JL, Brown TD: Articulated external fixation of the ankle: Minimizing motion resistance by accurate axis alignment. *J Biomech* 1999;32(1):63-70.

37. Marijnissen AC, van Roermund PM, van Melkebeek J, Lafeber FP: Clinical benefit of joint distraction in the treatment of ankle osteoarthritis. *Foot Ankle Clin* 2003;8(2):335-346.

38. Marijnissen AC, Van Roermund PM, Van Melkebeek J, et al: Clinical benefit of joint distraction in the treatment of severe ankle OA: Proof of concept in an open prospective study and in a randomized controlled study. *Arthritis Rheum* 2002;46(11):2893-2902.

39. van Roermund PM, Marijnissen AC, Lafeber FP: Joint distraction as an alternative for the treatment of osteoarthritis. *Foot Ankle Clin* 2002;7(3):515-527.

40. van Valburg AA, van Roermund PM, Marijnissen AC, et al: Joint distraction in treatment of osteoarthritis: A two-year follow-up of the ankle. *Osteoarthritis Cartilage* 1999;7(5):474-479.

41. Ploegmakers JJ, van Roermund PM, van Melkebeek J, et al: Prolonged clinical benefit from joint distraction in the treatment of ankle osteoarthritis. *Osteoarthritis Cartilage* 2005;13(7):582-588.

42. Smith NC, Beaman D, Rozbruch SR, Glazebrook MA: Evidence-based indications for distraction ankle arthroplasty. *Foot Ankle Int* 2012;33(8):632-636.

    A systematic review of the literature found insufficient evidence to support or refute the use of distraction arthroplasty for many causes of ankle arthritis. The authors encourage further higher-level research on this topic. Level of evidence: III.

43. Heywood AW: Supramalleolar osteotomy in the management of the rheumatoid hindfoot. *Clin Orthop Relat Res* 1983;177:76-81.

44. Becker AS, Myerson MS: The indications and technique of supramalleolar osteotomy. *Foot Ankle Clin* 2009;14(3):549-561.

    This is a review article on the various types, advantages and disadvantages, indications, and techniques of periarticular osteotomies for treating deformities about the ankle. Level of evidence: V.

45. Pagenstert G, Knupp M, Valderrabano V, Hintermann B: Realignment surgery for valgus ankle osteoarthritis. *Oper Orthop Traumatol* 2009;21(1):77-87.

    The authors report their treatment algorithm and the outcomes of 22 patients who underwent realignment osteotomies for valgus ankle degeneration based on the cause of their deformity. Among patients, 20 had significant improvement in pain and AOFAS scores at 4.5 years. Level of evidence: IV.

46. Pagenstert GI, Hintermann B, Barg A, Leumann A, Valderrabano V: Realignment surgery as alternative treatment of varus and valgus ankle osteoarthritis. *Clin Orthop Relat Res* 2007;462(462):156-168.

47. Mann HA, Filippi J, Myerson MS: Intra-articular opening medial tibial wedge osteotomy (plafond-plasty) for the treatment of intra-articular varus ankle arthritis and instability. *Foot Ankle Int* 2012;33(4):255-261.

This is a retrospective review of 19 patients with varus arthritis and instability who had medial intra-articular defects treated with plafondplasty. At 59 months, significant improvements in alignment, pain, and AOFAS scores were noted. Four patients had arthroplasty or arthrodesis. Level of evidence: IV.

48. Sen C, Kocaoglu M, Eralp L, Cinar M: Correction of ankle and hindfoot deformities by supramalleolar osteotomy. *Foot Ankle Int* 2003;24(1):22-28.

49. Tanaka Y, Takakura Y, Hayashi K, Taniguchi A, Kumai T, Sugimoto K: Low tibial osteotomy for varus-type ankle OA. *J Bone Joint Surg Br* 2006;88(7):909-913.

50. Raikin SM: Fresh osteochondral allografts for large-volume cystic osteochondral defects of the talus. *J Bone Joint Surg Am* 2009;91(12):2818-2826.

Authors present a prospective series of 15 patients who received matched bulk osteochondral allograft transplantation for large talar defects. The mean pain score decreased and mean AOFAS scores increased significantly at an average 54 months' follow-up. Two patients required arthrodesis. Level of evidence: II.

51. Eloesser L: Implantation of Joints. *Cal State J Med* 1913;11(12):485-491.

52. Bugbee WD, Khanna G, Cavallo M, McCauley JC, Görtz S, Brage ME: Bipolar fresh osteochondral allografting of the tibiotalar joint. *J Bone Joint Surg Am* 2013;95(5):426-432.

This is a retrospective review of 88 allograft ankle arthroplasties at a mean follow-up of 5.3 years. The authors show a failure rate of 29%, a 5-year survival of 76%, and 10-year survival of 44%. Level of evidence: IV.

53. Meehan R, McFarlin S, Bugbee W, Brage M: Fresh ankle osteochondral allograft transplantation for tibiotalar joint arthritis. *Foot Ankle Int* 2005;26(10):793-802.

54. Tontz WL Jr, Bugbee WD, Brage ME: Use of allografts in the management of ankle arthritis. *Foot Ankle Clin* 2003;8(2):361-373, xi.

55. Jeng CL, Myerson MS: Allograft total ankle replacement: A dead ringer to the natural joint. *Foot Ankle Clin* 2008;13(3):539-547, x.

This is a review of current literature and surgical technique and a presentation of a cohort of patients undergoing allograft TAA. The authors report a 51.7% survival rate. Level of evidence: V.

56. Williams SK, Amiel D, Ball ST, et al: Prolonged storage effects on the articular cartilage of fresh human osteochondral allografts. *J Bone Joint Surg Am* 2003;85-A(11):2111-2120.

57. Jamali AA, Hatcher SL, You Z: Donor cell survival in a fresh osteochondral allograft at twenty-nine years. A case report. *J Bone Joint Surg Am* 2007;89(1):166-169.

58. Kim CW, Jamali A, Tontz W Jr, Convery FR, Brage ME, Bugbee W: Treatment of post-traumatic ankle arthrosis with bipolar tibiotalar osteochondral shell allografts. *Foot Ankle Int* 2002;23(12):1091-1102.

59. Giannini S, Buda R, Grigolo B, et al: Bipolar fresh osteochondral allograft of the ankle. *Foot Ankle Int* 2010;31(1):38-46.

The authors report on 32 allograft arthroplasties using custom jigs and a lateral approach. At a mean of 31 months, there was drastic improvement in AOFAS scores but six failures. Histology showed MMPs in retrieved samples. Level of evidence: III.

60. Jeng CL, Kadakia A, White KL, Myerson MS: Fresh osteochondral total ankle allograft transplantation for the treatment of ankle arthritis. *Foot Ankle Int* 2008;29(6):554-560.

This retrospective review of 29 allograft transplants shows a failure rate of 69% at a mean follow-up of 2 years. Level of evidence: IV.

61. Haddad SL, Coetzee JC, Estok R, Fahrbach K, Banel D, Nalysnyk L: Intermediate and long-term outcomes of total ankle arthroplasty and ankle arthrodesis: A systematic review of the literature. *J Bone Joint Surg Am* 2007;89(9):1899-1905.

62. Ahmad J, Raikin SM: Ankle arthrodesis: The simple and the complex. *Foot Ankle Clin* 2008;13(3):381-400, viii.

This is a review of ankle fusions, revisions, and conversions from failed arthroplasties. Level of evidence: V.

63. Thomas R, Daniels TR, Parker K: Gait analysis and functional outcomes following ankle arthrodesis for isolated ankle arthritis. *J Bone Joint Surg Am* 2006;88(3):526-535.

64. Buchner M, Sabo D: Ankle fusion attributable to post-traumatic arthrosis: A long-term followup of 48 patients. *Clin Orthop Relat Res* 2003;406:155-164.

65. Coester LM, Saltzman CL, Leupold J, Pontarelli W: Long-term results following ankle arthrodesis for post-traumatic arthritis. *J Bone Joint Surg Am* 2001;83(2):219-228.

66. Jung HG, Parks BG, Nguyen A, Schon LC: Effect of tibiotalar joint arthrodesis on adjacent tarsal joint pressure in a cadaver model. *Foot Ankle Int* 2007;28(1):103-108.

67. Mann RA, Rongstad KM: Arthrodesis of the ankle: A critical analysis. *Foot Ankle Int* 1998;19(1):3-9.

3: Arthritis of the Foot and Ankle

68. Myerson MS, Quill G: Ankle arthrodesis. A comparison of an arthroscopic and an open method of treatment. *Clin Orthop Relat Res* 1991;268:84-95.

69. Buck P, Morrey BF, Chao EY: The optimum position of arthrodesis of the ankle. A gait study of the knee and ankle. *J Bone Joint Surg Am* 1987;69(7):1052-1062.

70. Dohm MP, Benjamin JB, Harrison J, Szivek JA: A biomechanical evaluation of three forms of internal fixation used in ankle arthrodesis. *Foot Ankle Int* 1994;15(6):297-300.

71. Ogilvie-Harris DJ, Fitsialos D, Hedman TP: Arthrodesis of the ankle: A comparison of two versus three screw fixation in a crossed configuration. *Clin Orthop Relat Res* 1994;304:195-199.

72. Raikin SM: Arthrodesis of the ankle: Arthroscopic, mini-open, and open techniques. *Foot Ankle Clin* 2003;8(2):347-359.

73. Frey C, Halikus NM, Vu-Rose T, Ebramzadeh E: A review of ankle arthrodesis: Predisposing factors to nonunion. *Foot Ankle Int* 1994;15(11):581-584.

74. Raikin SM, Rampuri V: An approach to the failed ankle arthrodesis. *Foot Ankle Clin* 2008;13(3):401-416, viii.

    This is a review article of ankle fusions, complications, reasons for failures, and salvage approaches.

75. Glick JM, Morgan CD, Myerson MS, Sampson TG, Mann JA: Ankle arthrodesis using an arthroscopic method: Long-term follow-up of 34 cases. *Arthroscopy* 1996;12(4):428-434.

76. Townshend D, Di Silvestro M, Krause F, et al: Arthroscopic versus open ankle arthrodesis: A multicenter comparative case series. *J Bone Joint Surg Am* 2013;95(2):98-102.

    This is a multicenter comparative study of open versus arthroscopic arthrodesis of the ankle. The arthroscopic group had significantly better improvement on the Ankle Osteoarthritis Scale and shorter hospital stays. No differences were found in complications, surgical times, or alignment. Level of evidence: II.

77. O'Brien TS, Hart TS, Shereff MJ, Stone J, Johnson J: Open versus arthroscopic ankle arthrodesis: A comparative study. *Foot Ankle Int* 1999;20(6):368-374.

78. Crosby LA, Yee TC, Formanek TS, Fitzgibbons TC: Complications following arthroscopic ankle arthrodesis. *Foot Ankle Int* 1996;17(6):340-342.

79. Paremain GD, Miller SD, Myerson MS: Ankle arthrodesis: Results after the miniarthrotomy technique. *Foot Ankle Int* 1996;17(5):247-252.

80. Mann RA, Van Manen JW, Wapner K, Martin J: Ankle fusion. *Clin Orthop Relat Res* 1991;268:49-55.

81. Marcus RE, Balourdas GM, Heiple KG: Ankle arthrodesis by chevron fusion with internal fixation and bone-grafting. *J Bone Joint Surg Am* 1983;65(6):833-838.

82. Culpan P, Le Strat V, Piriou P, Judet T: Arthrodesis after failed total ankle replacement. *J Bone Joint Surg Br* 2007;89(9):1178-1183.

83. Hopgood P, Kumar R, Wood PL: Ankle arthrodesis for failed total ankle replacement. *J Bone Joint Surg Br* 2006;88(8):1032-1038.

84. Jeng CL, Campbell JT, Tang EY, Cerrato RA, Myerson MS: Tibiotalocalcaneal arthrodesis with bulk femoral head allograft for salvage of large defects in the ankle. *Foot Ankle Int* 2013;34(9):1256-1266.

    This retrospective review of 32 patients undergoing TTC fusion with bulk femoral head allograft shows only a 50% fusion rate. Nonunion developed in all of the patients with diabetes, and 19% of patients required a transtibial amputation. Level of evidence: IV.

Chapter 9

Ankle Arthritis: Part II. Total Ankle Arthroplasty

W. Bret Smith, DO   Gregory C. Berlet, MD

Introduction

The evolution of total ankle arthroplasty (TAA) has been a story of interesting fits and starts. The first reported ankle arthroplasty was in 1970, with the authors publishing their initial results of 12 patients in 1973.[1] The implant was very simplistic, consisting of a long tibial stem and polyethylene talar-replacing component that necessitated a subtalar fusion. This hinge-type design was modeled after hip implant design; unfortunately, complex motion and stress across the ankle joint did not allow for predictable outcomes.

Early studies of first-generation ankle arthroplasty generated initial promising results, but midterm follow-up revealed evidence of substantial radiographic loosening and high failure rates.[2] Many initial ankle prostheses were designed on a simple hinge axis. Motion was allowed only in the sagittal plane. Examples of early constrained-hinge designs included the Imperial College of London Hospital Prosthesis, TPR prosthesis (Smith

and Richards), Oregon prosthesis (Zimmer), and the Mayo Total Ankle (Mayo Clinic). These early implants necessitated substantial bone resection and were often placed with cement. This resulted in the implants being placed mostly into softer metaphyseal bone. Prosthesis constraint, which transmitted excessive stress to the softer bone, likely caused early loosening and subsequent failures.[2]

Other early ankle implants involved the unconstrained concept. These implants included the New Jersey Low-Contact Stress prosthesis (DePuy), Newton prosthesis (Howmedica), and Smith prosthesis (Dow Corning Wright). These implants were designed to rely on the stability of the ligamentous envelope of the ankle joint. However, as the soft-tissue constraints loosened, outcomes worsened. Because of the unconstrained nature of the implants, multiaxial motion resulted in significant issues with impingement pain.[2]

By this time, hip and knee arthroplasties were producing successful outcomes for patients with advanced arthritis. However, after witnessing the less-promising results of early ankle arthroplasty, enthusiasm quickly diminished.

There is a current resurgence of interest in TAA. In the United States, there are six FDA-approved TAA systems: the Agility Total Ankle Replacement System (DePuy) (**Figure 1**), the Scandinavian Total Ankle Replacement ([STAR] Small Bone Innovations) (**Figure 2**), the Salto-Talaris Total Ankle (TornierTX) (**Figure 3**), the INBONE II Ankle Arthroplasty (Wright Medical Technology) (**Figure 4**), the Eclipse Total Ankle (Integra Life Sciences), and the Trabecular Metal Total Ankle (Zimmer) (**Figure 5**). Limited information is available for two of these implants, however. The Eclipse Total Ankle currently is not in use in the United States, and the experience with the Trabecular Metal Total Ankle is limited because the release date was in 2013. No data are available on outcomes related to these two prostheses.

In markets outside the United States, more than 20 total ankle systems are used. This chapter focuses on current FDA-approved implants, but it is important to

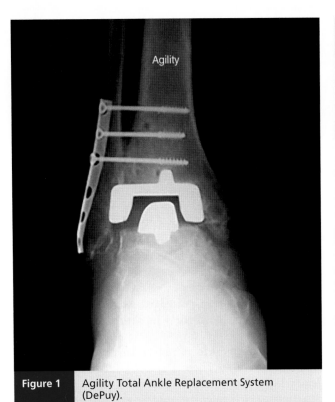

Figure 1 Agility Total Ankle Replacement System (DePuy).

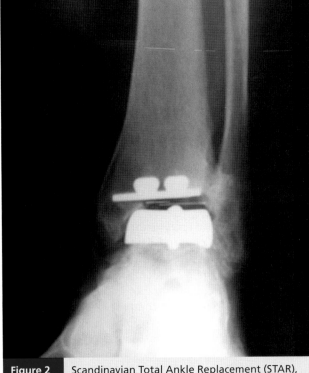

Figure 2 Scandinavian Total Ankle Replacement (STAR), Small Bone Innovations.

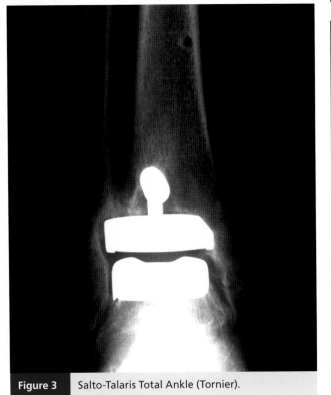

Figure 3 Salto-Talaris Total Ankle (Tornier).

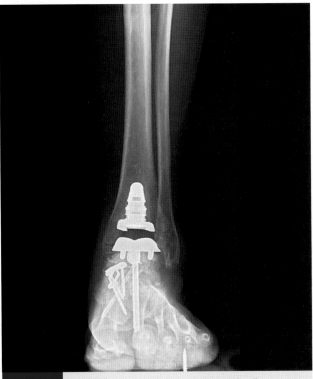

Figure 4 INBONE II total ankle (Wright Medical).

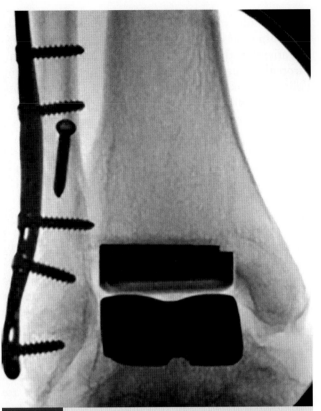

Figure 5 The Trabecular Metal Total Ankle (Zimmer).

understand that much of the available literature is generated outside of the United States; consequently, much of this literature may discuss implants not available to surgeons practicing in this country.

Design Issues and Rationale

Anatomy and Biomechanics

Early ankle prosthesis designers failed to appreciate the complexity of ankle joint motion. The ankle joint consists of three bony interactions: the tibia, fibula, and talus. The morphology of each bone affects the function and relationship of the ankle joint.

Ankle stiffness has been shown to substantially influence the surrounding joints, especially the subtalar joint. Adjacent joint arthritis is an accepted and known complication of ankle stiffness and ankle fusion. The biomechanical rationale for increased wear in adjacent joints was elucidated in a 2009 study, which showed that motion in the subtalar joint in the sagittal, coronal, and transverse planes changes to move in the opposite direction when compared to healthy ankles.[3] The complication of adjacent joint arthritis has fueled the search for ankle fusion alternatives.

Total ankle prosthesis design rapidly evolved over the past decade, and there is a renewed focus on ankle

arthroplasty as outcomes associated with arthroplasty of the hip, knee, and shoulder continue to improve. As the second generation of ankle arthroplasty implants became available, interest increased. The initial wave of second-generation implants, which became available in the 1980s and early 1990s, included the Buechel-Pappas Total Ankle Replacement (Endotec), the STAR, and the Agility Total Ankle Replacement System.[4] The Agility was the first TAA system to receive FDA approval.[5]

The newer generation of implants addressed several shortcomings of the initial implants. Improved materials and fixation techniques were implemented. These implant designs were semi-constrained and used a porous coating, which eliminated the need for cement. Bone resection also was reduced considerably.[2] Most important, understanding of the anatomy and mechanics of the ankle joint became more sophisticated.

The ankle does not act as a simple hinge, and the complex combination of both sliding and rolling is now better understood. Additionally, as earlier designs were reviewed, their indications and contraindications were reconsidered.

Current implants are made of three components. The tibial component is flat and incorporates the ability to stabilize or fixate into the tibia. The talar component is usually anatomically curved in the sagittal plane. The bearing component is composed of a polyethylene material (usually ultra-high–molecular-weight-polyethylene), and, depending on design, either fixed or mobile. Only one mobile-bearing device, the STAR, is approved for use in the United States.

Because the ankle allows for both gliding and rolling motion, implants are designed to accommodate complex three-dimensional ankle motions. Implant use entails a balance of compromises. Fixed-bearing devices offer inherent stability but sacrifice certain planes of motion, particularly rotational. Mobile bearing devices allow for more rotational motion, thus decreasing stress to the implant, but they also can reduce stability, allow for possible bearing impingement, and create the potential for backside polyethylene wear.

Current ankle prosthesis can strike the necessary balance between providing implant stability and decreasing stress transfer to bone. Overly constrained designs allow for too much stress transfer to the bone and create osteolysis, which can cause stability issues associated with implant wear and bearing dislocation.

Because the tibial side of the ankle joint appears to be less complex, most implants of the current generation emphasize a similar approach of minimizing the amount of bone resection to allow for stable fixation on the cortical rim of the distal tibia. Additional stability of the tibial component can be achieved with either the addition of fins, keels, screws, or stems.

The complex anatomy of the talus poses challenges to both implant designers and surgeons. Talar anatomy features complex three-dimensional conical wedges. The radius of curvatures on each side of the talus (medial, lateral, anterior, and posterior) all differ. The axis of rotation of the talus has been described as having a changing instant center of rotation,[6] with the primary axis of rotation correlated with the transmalleolar plane and externally rotated 23°.[7] To further confound the mechanism, the ankle also rotates about 5° in the transverse plane.[8]

Additionally, surgeons continue to debate whether only the superior portion of the talus needs to be resurfaced or if the medial and lateral articulations are also in need of attention. The argument is that when more areas need to be resurfaced, this leads to increased bone removal and possible weakening of the surface for implantation. Further review of implants and their outcomes is needed to improve implant design.

The blood supply of the talus is known to be sensitive to injury and surgical manipulation. Each technique puts different vascular structures at risk. It is not known if the surgical approach to the talus (including bone resection) correlates with talar subsidence or loosening because of compromised talar blood supply.

Indications

An unprecedented amount of data on ankle arthroplasty are becoming available. As this information is reviewed, indications will evolve as well. A common indication for TAA is end-stage ankle arthritis that has failed nonsurgical management. Posttraumatic arthritis, primary osteoarthritis, and rheumatoid arthritis are the most commonly cited reasons for ankle arthroplasty. TAA also may be considered for patients with severe adjacent joint arthritis that may necessitate a pantalar arthrodesis. In these settings, a patient may be offered a triple arthrodesis procedure along with TAA as either a single procedure or staged procedures.

Patient age is a subjective matter in terms of indications for TAA. Traditionally it was thought that only elderly patients with low physical demands should be offered TAA. Data support better outcomes in certain age groups; it has been shown in several reports that implant survivorship and functional outcomes are decreased in younger patients undergoing TAA.[9-12] Several studies have shown equivalent survivorship outcomes among younger and older patients.[13] Because there are no hard and fast rules, it is important that patients understand

the risks inherent to TAA and determine if those risks fit within their expectations for demand and lifestyle.

Patients with rheumatoid or other inflammatory arthropathies may have foot and ankle joint involvement. Following ankle fusion, the forces across midfoot joints increase, which may precipitate additional problems. Ankle arthroplasty may be considered in these patients to help decrease forces across the hindfoot and midfoot.[14-16]

Patient expectations for return to activity must be discussed. A patient should be counseled that return to activities is encouraged, but that lower-impact activities should be considered. Return to impact activities presents a challenge; several studies that have looked at return to sport activity after ankle arthroplasty have shown that lower-impact activities are safe and may be encouraged.[17,18]

In addition to age and activity issues, patients must have sufficient bone stock to allow for implantation of the prosthesis. They must also have a healthy soft-tissue envelope that allows for adequate coverage after procedure completion. Soft-tissue compromise or significant vascular disease may prompt discussion of alternative options. The topic of whether alternative approaches may offer improved results when soft-tissue issues are encountered warrants further discussion.

Contraindications

Contraindications to TAA include active ankle sepsis, osteomyelitis, Charcot or neuropathic joint involvement, complete paralysis of the affected limb, large area of osteonecrosis of the talus or distal tibia, vascular insufficiency, inappropriate soft-tissue coverage, severe deformities that cannot be corrected, and skeletal immaturity.

An MRI should be considered for patients considering ankle arthroplasty who have a history of talar osteonecrosis or infection. The findings will likely provide additional information about the viability of the bone and whether joint arthroplasty should be considered. Partial osteonecrosis in a section that will be removed with the bone cut is not a strict contraindication to TAA. More extensive bone involvement should be considered a contraindication.

Relative contraindications include ligament instability, history of infection, diabetes, morbid obesity, osteoporosis, malalignment, poor soft-tissue quality, smoking, and neuropathy. Patients who have high-demand employment or activity requirements may require an ankle arthrodesis, but those who cannot comply with postoperative protocols may pose their own relative contraindication.

An extensive preoperative consultation is essential to help patients understand if TAA is an option. During an in-depth conversation with a patient, numerous topics may present themselves that will help to introduce possible treatment options. Not all patients with ankle arthritis should receive a TAA option.

Surgical Treatment

Techniques

The authors use two different techniques at their facilities. One option is to use a femoral sciatic peripheral nerve block that is completed before a patient is taken to the surgical suite. An alternative is a popliteal block with intravenous sedation. The patient is then positioned supine on a radiolucent surgical table. The surgical hip is bumped to allow for the foot to be positioned straight. A thigh tourniquet is applied and the surgical limb is prepped and draped to knee level.

An anterior approach is the most commonly used incision for TAA. The incision should start approximately 10 to 15 cm proximal to the ankle joint and proceed distal in a curvilinear fashion to end distal to the talonavicular joint. An adequate incision should be used to decrease tension on the skin during retraction and allow for good visualization. The interval between the anterior tibialis and extensor hallucis longus is developed. Attention is given to the anterior neurovascular bundle, which should be mobilized and protected. Minimal handling of the tissue and judicious use of retractors is warranted to limit undue pressure in the soft tissue because wound complications have been reported to be as high as 28%.[19-21]

After the approach has been developed to the level of the ankle, a complete débridement is done to expose the osseous architecture. Based on the system used, osteophytes may be débrided at this time to allow better visualization of the joint. Prior to beginning the bone cuts to prepare the joint for implant, this chapter's authors prefer to release the tourniquet and confirm hemostasis. At this time, the cuts are completed per the manufacturer-suggested techniques based on the implant being placed.

Key areas of concern outside of the limited soft-tissue envelope include the anterior tendons, which must be protected judiciously during the cutting of the bone. They are at risk for damage by the sagittal saw and must be repaired if accidentally injured. Also, special attention must be given to the posterior medial corner because the posterior neurovascular bundle, posterior tibialis, and flexor hallucis longus are at risk. If any of these posterior medial structures are damaged, every attempt should be made to repair them.

After the prosthesis has been implanted, a meticulous layered closure is completed. The patient is then placed into a well-padded Jones dressing and awakened from anesthesia. Care should be taken to avoid applying undue pressure on the incision line after the dressing is applied.

Approaches

Currently, the anterior approach to the ankle is the only approach for which there is relevant literature for evaluation. A newer implant that has received FDA approval and was released in 2013 (the Trabecular Metal Total Ankle) uses a lateral transfibular approach to gain access for implantation. Data are not available at this time on this particular implant. The posterior approach for TAA is another option. Because the posterior soft tissue of the ankle is often more robust, it seems to be an attractive alternative. A limited number of anecdotal and case reports mention the posterior approach for the current generation of implants.[22] Because the current implant systems are not well designed to handle application via the posterior approach, this approach has limited appeal at this time.

Concomitant Procedures

Ankle arthritis usually does not exist as a lone pathology. Additional issues typically affect patients with this condition, some of which may be related to the underlying arthritis. Retained hardware may need to be addressed when posttraumatic arthritis exists, for example. Adjacent joint arthritis, deformities, equinus contractures, and bone stock issues all may need to be considered when thinking about TAA.

Hardware removal is a common additional procedure when TAA is performed. The anticipated removal instruments must be available during these procedures. After joint preparation, all appropriate hardware will be removed. Based on the implant being used, more or less hardware may be removed. Residual bone defects from hardware removal must be considered stress risers. If the surgeon concludes that risk exists for a periprosthetic fracture, prophylactic stabilization must be placed, or, in some cases, a stemmed implant can bypass the anatomy at risk.

After the ankle joint is prepared for the implant, any equinus contractures should be addressed. Strayer or Baumann procedures to release the gastrocnemius fascia can be used as adjunct procedures. Alternatively, an Achilles tendon lengthening can be performed. This chapter's authors prefer to implant the prosthesis and then reassess whether the equinus contracture still needs attention. This step may not be a possibility if waiting to complete the release would compromise other concomitant procedures.

In regard to adjacent joint arthritis, it is useful to ascertain preoperatively whether the adjacent joints are a significant source of pain. Often, fluoroscopic-guided injections can assist in determining if adjacent joints may be contributing to pain. Patients should be counseled that ankle range of motion likely will not return to normal.[19] It is possible that TAA alone may offer relief to adjacent joints with degenerative changes. Several studies have shown progression in adjacent joint arthritis after TAA.[23,24] Literature also suggests that compared to ankle arthrodesis, TAA is associated with a lower rate of subtalar fusions[25] (**Figure 6**). Adjacent joint arthrodesis procedures can be done in conjunction with ankle arthroplasty or as staged procedures. Subtalar, talonavicular, and triple arthrodesis procedures are commonly performed in coordination with TAA. Additional joint fusions may address other sources of pain or may add bone stock to help stabilize the implant. With potential complications in mind, subsequent joint arthrodesis should be carefully considered during the planning phase to allow for placement of incisions and soft-tissue management. It is considered safe to perform these corrective procedures without increasing risk for complications.[26]

A thorough limb alignment evaluation and deformity analysis is critical when planning TAA surgery. In addition to obtaining standard three-view radiographs of the foot and ankle long-leg and hindfoot alignment views may also be needed. CT images also can be beneficial when ascertaining the extent of deformities before surgery.

Traditionally, it was believed that coronal plane deformities exceeding 10° to 15° should be treated with ankle arthrodesis instead of TAA secondary to increased failure rates.[27-29] More recent literature has refuted these claims. Numerous studies have shown equivalent outcomes for deformities of between 15° and 30°.[7,9,30-32] All authors stressed the importance of complete correction of the coronal plane deformity before placing an ankle implant.

It has been shown that preoperative deformity, especially varus malalignment not corrected at the time of TAA, may cause increased rates of wear and recurrence of deformity.[30-34] Therefore, careful planning is needed to help increase the chance for success. When evaluating an ankle with a coronal misalignment, it is critical to determine what must be done to provide a plantigrade foot.[31] Interventions may include soft-tissue releases, ligament reconstruction, or osseous procedures.

For treatment of varus ankle deformities, the most common adjunctive procedures are lateral displacing calcaneal osteotomy, deltoid ligament release, medial malleolar osteotomy, and lateral ligament reconstruction.[7,30-34] Deformities noted in the foot can be treated with osteotomies and/or fusion procedures. It is essential to achieve a plantigrade foot when planning TAA.

Soft-tissue reconstruction also can be considered either in conjunction with osseous procedures or in isolation. Medial or lateral ligament reconstructions are most commonly encountered. Lateral ligament reconstruction using either locally available tissue (Broström

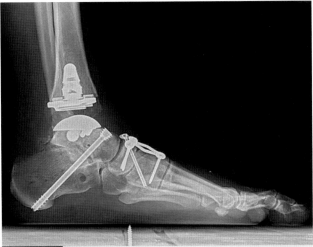

Figure 6 Lateral radiograph of total ankle arthroplasty; this example shows an adjunct procedure (a subtalar fusion) done as a single stage.

imbrication) or augmented nonanatomic reconstruction can be performed at the same surgical time as an index TAA. This chapter's authors prefer to perform medial ligament reconstruction as a staged procedure, with allograft augmented medial reconstruction done several months before the planned ankle joint arthroplasty.

If deformities are noted in an area proximal to the implant, these will need to be treated. Supramalleolar osteotomies offer the opportunity to correct numerous deformities that occur proximal to TAA. These procedures can be done before implantation of the TAA or concomitantly, based on surgeon preference.

Most valgus deformities are a result of posterior tibial tendon dysfunction. The need for a plantigrade foot when placing an ankle arthroplasty has been established; therefore, the same attention to detail must be maintained when evaluating a valgus deformity. If the deltoid complex is intact and the foot holds significant deformity, then the flatfoot deformity (which has been well described) should be treated. When the deltoid ligament is compromised, reconstruction of the ligament with allograft must be completed along with correction of the planus foot.[35] This chapter's authors prefer to perform these steps during a separate surgical session (not during ankle joint arthroplasty).

Complications

A spectrum of TAA-related complications may be encountered. Complications may be short term, last for less than 1 year, or occur over the long term.

Wound dehiscence, acute infections, malleolar fractures, and hardware complications are considered

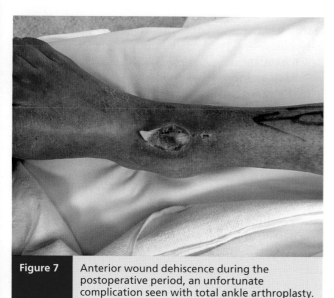

Figure 7 Anterior wound dehiscence during the postoperative period, an unfortunate complication seen with total ankle arthroplasty.

short-term complications if detected early (**Figure 7**). Careful intraoperative inspection may help to identify medial or lateral malleolar fractures. These should be addressed immediately while in the surgical suite, usually with internal fixation. If fractures are diagnosed with early postoperative radiographs, treatment may involve cast immobilization or open reduction and internal fixation.[36]

Wound-healing problems should be treated aggressively. Wound complication rates have been reported as high as 28%.[19-21] Patients with diabetes and inflammatory arthritis can experience increased incision-healing issues.[37] Patients with these associated comorbidities should be counseled accordingly.

If a wound shows signs of drainage or if concern arises at the initial postoperative evaluation, oral antibiotics and local wound care should be considered and close follow-up is recommended. If symptoms worsen or a wound begins to break down, an immediate return to the surgical suite should be discussed. Intravenous antibiotics and negative pressure wound therapy should be considered. If wound-healing problems occur during the first 4 to 6 weeks and the wound is deep enough to necessitate return to the surgical suite, a polyethylene component exchange may be appropriate.

Hardware implanted during TAA (such as implants for associated procedures or hardware used to address intraoperative problems such as a malleolar fracture) may cause complications that should be treated as needed.

To avoid complications that occur in the longer term, the follow-up period may necessitate more critical investigation. Heterotopic ossification (HO) and gutter impingement have been reported.[38-41] Aggressive resection of the medial and lateral gutters should be considered

during the primary procedure. One article has suggested that initial gutter resection may lead to fewer revision procedures for gutter débridement.[41]

Late infections of a TAA may occur as a result of hematogenous seeding. Aggressive irrigation and débridement with or without removal of the prosthesis will need to be completed. If an infection represents long-term involvement, the prosthesis usually needs to be removed. An antibiotic-impregnated cement spacer should be placed and the patient started on long-term culture-specific antibiotic therapy.

Salvage after infection should prompt a detailed discussion with the patient. The potential for amputation must be covered in any discussion about revision and salvage after a TAA becomes infected. Numerous options exist in salvage situations. Replantation of a new prosthesis can be considered if bone stock is available and the infection appears to have been eradicated. Intraoperative biopsy to evaluate white blood cells per high-powered field may be considered. When replantation is planned, an alternative prosthesis may be required or a revision version of the former implant may be needed.

When a failed TAA is not amenable to revision prosthesis, an arthrodesis procedure likely is needed. Hindfoot nail systems, plate-and-screw fixation options, or ring and wire fixation devices could all be considered as options for salvage procedures. Surgeon experience and preference will likely determine the path for treatment. Acceptable fusion rates have been shown with both local bone grafting and structural bone grafting techniques.[42,43] Among patients with underlying inflammatory arthritis, careful evaluation and follow-up is important because there appears to be a higher rate of nonunion in this population.[42]

Amputation may also be considered in certain situations when a prostheses fails. Rates of amputation after attempted salvage of failed total ankle implants have been reported at 19%.[44] Diabetes and the presence of preoperative ulcers appear to increase risk for amputation after salvage procedures.[44,45] Counseling is warranted for patients at increased risk for amputation. Some patients may elect amputation versus a salvage procedure, which may be reasonable in some cases. Every attempt should be made to give a patient the most acceptable residual limb to allow for prosthesis wear. It is advisable to send patients for a preoperative consultation with a prosthetist to discuss future needs after surgery.

Radiolucencies that appear in postoperative follow-up radiographs warrant evaluation. Although the presence of lucency does not dictate pending failure of an implant, it is prudent to follow TAA with yearly radiographs to monitor for changes.[16,24,29,46-48] If lucencies are progressive and the implant appears stable, bone grafting should

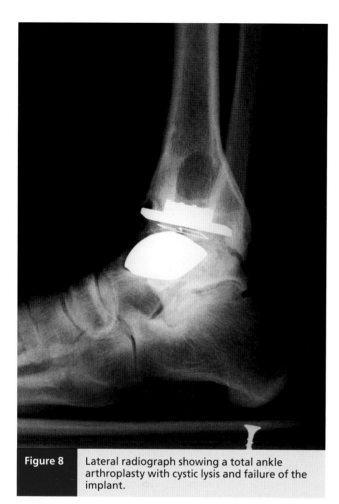

Figure 8 Lateral radiograph showing a total ankle arthroplasty with cystic lysis and failure of the implant.

be considered with maintenance of the implant.[11,24,47] A minor amount of implant shifting may be related to an implant settling in a more appropriate position[16,27,46,48,49] (Figure 8).

Outcomes

TAA has grown in popularity over the past two decades. Within that time, a focused effort on improving implant design and surgical technique has raised the level of TAA sophistication. Along with improvements in the actual implants and techniques, there has been a tremendous increase in the collection and analysis of data associated with TAA.

Several studies demonstrate a surgical learning curve associated with TAA. These studies have shown that perioperative complications and outcomes were worse for the initial group of people undergoing TAA versus patients who had implants placed later by the same surgeon.[20,46,50] This is important to bear in mind for surgeons who are considering adding TAA to their practice. Despite the

learning curve associated with TAA, low-volume centers can achieve good results and outcomes.[51]

Current survivorship for TAA ranges between 70% and 98% at 3 to 6 years and between 80% and 95% at 8 to 12 years.[10] A meta-analysis showed the adjusted failure rate at 5 years to be 10%.[19] These data represent multiple prostheses and protocols for ankle implants. As such, superiority could not be identified between the different prostheses.[19] Because no clear superiority has been established in regard to specific implants, surgeons must evaluate the available literature on the specific implants they are considering.

Several implants have a longer history and multiple associated publications written by their developers; consequently, it is often challenging to interpret outcomes data. Several attempts have been made to look at information from national registries to more clearly identify actual rates of revision. One report shows that based on national registry results, the actual rate of revision was 21.8% at 5 years and 43.5% at 10 years.[52] Several other national registries have shown 5-year survivorship to be between 78% and 86%.[12,53,54] Because it is not possible to know how a case was coded, less involved procedures such as exchange of a polyethylene spacer may be considered the same as complete revision of an entire implant. Overall, registry databases likely provide a more realistic account of implant survivorship.

The most common reasons for revision of an ankle implant are aseptic loosening and instability.[12,53,54] The information gained from registry databases can be helpful in decreasing some of the biases found in implant studies. Because implant developers at high-volume centers account for a disproportionate number of papers, their works may not reflect average experience with certain implants.[52] When considering TAA, the physician should recall that individual results may vary from the published data.

Revision TAA

A TAA revision may be the best alternative when an index arthroplasty has failed. Failure can be characterized by pain, recurrent deformity, progressive bone loss compromising implant stability, or polyethylene failure by wear or fracture.

Revision TAA involves challenges including the soft-tissue envelope, the bone defect, and any mechanical problems that may have predisposed the previous implant to failure. The soft-tissue envelope around the human ankle is fragile, and surgical manipulation outcomes can be considered predictable a finite number of times. The anterior approach allows for the best visualization of the ankle joint for arthroplasty and balancing, but wound complication rates pose a challenge. Inflammatory disease poses the highest risk for major wound complications.[37] Alternatives to the anterior approach include the lateral and posterior approaches. There are published case reports regarding the posterior approach, but no reports on the lateral approach for revision TAA.[22]

Bone defects are variable and influence implant type. The original bone resection amount correlates poorly with the residual preserved bone facing the revision arthroplasty. On the tibial side, the challenge is rotational control because there are usually compromised malleoli; as such, some proximal rotational control built into the revision prosthesis is desirable. Fixation into the tibia is challenging because there is little distal bone and this favors vertical fixation with stems. Ideally, further osteotomy of the tibia is avoided to maximize stem and implant stability. The joint line can be reestablished by using an augmented base plate, allograft prosthetic composites, or large polyethylene spacers.

Talus bone defects pose the biggest challenge during revision TAA. Although the etiology of cystic disease of the talus is not clear (osteolysis or blood supply compromise and subsequent osteonecrosis), the end situation is a loose talar component that migrates. This migration often occurs inferiorly until the keel rests on the subtalar joint, creating pain and swelling. Reconstruction options include a subtalar joint fusion to reestablish a stable base for the prosthesis. In the event of a contained talar defect, impaction grafting is effective. Experience treating contained defects with cement has been limited, with only case reports to date.[55] In the event of an uncontained defect, bulk allograft reconstruction with extensive biologic augments has demonstrated short-term success.

When performing revision arthroplasty, the surgeon has the responsibility to evaluate the mechanical alignment and provide periarticular osteotomies to reestablish the mechanical axis if necessary.

Published case series on revision arthroplasty with implants currently available in the United States are limited. Level V evidence (only) supports revision TAA.[56,57]

Arthrodesis Versus Arthroplasty

Ankle arthrodesis has been considered the standard for treatment of end-stage ankle arthritis for well over a century. In the last several decades, TAA has been gaining popularity as an alternative to fusion.

Ankle arthritis has been shown to create as much disability—both mentally and physically—as end-stage hip arthrosis.[58] Ankle arthritis can substantially influence quality of life; as a result, treatment options include both ankle arthrodesis and TAA.

Topics that have been evaluated regarding ankle arthrodesis versus arthroplasty are gait, pain relief, functional outcome, range of motion, and cost effectiveness. Complications associated with both procedures have also been evaluated on multiple occasions.

Both ankle arthrodesis and TAA can offer pain relief.[46,59,60] Because pain reduction is a criterion when evaluating options, both interventions may be considered equivalent.[46] Of course, the potential to decrease pain is among the most important considerations when discussing ankle arthritis treatment.

Complications such as infections, wound issues, and neurovascular injuries can occur with both ankle arthrodesis and TAA. However, each procedure involves unique potential complications. Unique to ankle arthrodesis is nonunion. The rate of nonunion commonly suggested is around 10%.[11] Malunion, limb shortening and atrophy, and adjacent joint arthritis may also be seen over time after ankle arthrodesis.

TAA also presents unique complications for surgeons and patients. Because it is a mobile structure, wear on the prosthesis over time becomes an issue. Loosening of the implant and instability also can occur following TAA, and these are the most common causes for revision.[12,53,54]

For many patients, gait issues and return of function are vital. Antalgic gait issues and loss of ability to participate in activities will often carry substantial weight when patients make decisions about surgical intervention. It has been shown in several studies that gait parameters are affected differently by arthrodesis versus arthroplasty.[61,62] Studies have compared patients who have undergone ankle fusion and TAA and used age-adjusted norms in regard to gait.[62-64] Patients with ankle arthritis have a shorter stride length, reduced walking speed, and shorter duration of the stance phase in the affected limb during a gait cycle.[61,65,66]

Ankle arthritis significantly influences quality of life indicators and overall well-being.[67] Both arthrodesis and TAA have been shown to improve patient quality of life.[67] There are significant differences in postoperative gait for people undergoing both arthrodesis and arthroplasty. Debate is ongoing as to whether gait velocity is increased with arthrodesis or with TAA.[61,62] It has been noted, however, that neither arthrodesis nor arthroplasty returns the gait cycle to within normal parameters.[61,62]

Ankle arthrodesis groups exhibit more asymmetry in gait and increased hip range of motion.[63,64] In contrast, patients who undergo TAA demonstrate increased ankle and knee range of motion, reduced limp, and a more normal gait cycle.[61-64,68]

Conversion of Arthrodesis to Arthroplasty

There are limited situations in which a conversion from arthrodesis to arthroplasty is appropriate. A malunited ankle fusion with symptomatic adjacent joint arthritis could prompt consideration of TAA to create a mobile segment along with fusion of the adjacent joint arthritis. A persistent nonunion of an ankle fusion at which the anatomy has been preserved may be another appropriate indication.

Motion following an ankle arthrodesis conversion to TAA is restricted because of the stiff soft-tissue envelope. There are limited published outcomes on these conversions.[69,70] Conversion of a well-positioned and healed arthrodesis with minimal adjacent joint arthritis should be discouraged.

Summary

TAA has evolved into a treatment option that should be discussed with patients with end-stage arthritis of the ankle. The contrasts and similarities between ankle arthrodesis and TAA should be part of a comprehensive preoperative consultation. The decision algorithm should emphasize the discussion points of motion, activity expectation, pain improvement, implant longevity, and adjacent joint arthritis.

Annotated References

1. Lord G, Marotte JH: Total ankle prosthesis: Technic and 1st results. Apropos of 12 cases[French]. *Rev Chir Orthop Reparatrice Appar Mot* 1973;59(2):139-151.

2. Vickerstaff JA, Miles AW, Cunningham JL: A brief history of total ankle replacement and a review of the current status. *Med Eng Phys* 2007;29(10):1056-1064.

3. Kozanek M, Rubash HE, Li G, de Asla RJ: Effect of post-traumatic tibiotalar osteoarthritis on kinematics of the ankle joint complex. *Foot Ankle Int* 2009;30(8):734-740 .

4. Bonasia DE, Dettoni F, Femino JE, Phisitkul P, Germano M, Amendola A: Total ankle replacement: Why, when and how? *Iowa Orthop J* 2010;30:119-130.

    The authors review the current state of TAA and discuss the rationale for current implant designs. A concise review of ankle biomechanics and preoperative planning is included. An excellent review of more recent results and comparison to historical outcomes is featured. Level of evidence: IV.

5. Chou LB, Coughlin MT, Hansen S Jr, et al: Osteoarthritis of the ankle: The role of arthroplasty. *J Am Acad Orthop Surg* 2008;16(5):249-259.

    This is a review article on the current aspects of TAA through the first half of the 2000s. The authors encourage long-term outcome studies and state that patient selection and surgical experience are paramount for success. Level of evidence: IV.

6. Buechel FF, Pappas MJ, Iorio LJ: New Jersey low contact stress total ankle replacement: Biomechanical rationale and review of 23 cementless cases. *Foot Ankle* 1988;8(6):279-290.

7. Kim BS, Choi WJ, Kim YS, Lee JW: Total ankle replacement in moderate to severe varus deformity of the ankle. *J Bone Joint Surg Br* 2009;91(9):1183-1190.

    Investigators review clinical and radiographic outcomes in two TAA populations with a mean follow-up of 27 months. One group with 23 patients had preoperative varus deformities exceeding 10°. The other group of 24 patients had neutral alignment. The Hintegra implant was used in all cases by a single surgeon. Equivalent outcomes were seen in both groups; the group with preoperative deformity required more concomitant procedures to achieve alignment. Level of evidence: III.

8. Michael JM, Golshani A, Gargac S, Goswami T: Biomechanics of the ankle joint and clinical outcomes of total ankle replacement. *J Mech Behav Biomed Mater* 2008;1(4):276-294.

    A thorough and in-depth evaluation of ankle anatomy, mechanics, gait cycle, and force distribution is presented. These variables are then correlated with outcomes of multiple studies on TAA results. The authors suggest that redesign of ankle implants is needed to address numerous shortcomings and to help decrease failure rates. Level of evidence: IV.

9. Spirt AA, Assal M, Hansen ST Jr: Complications and failure after total ankle arthroplasty. *J Bone Joint Surg Am* 2004;86-A(6):1172-1178.

10. Fevang BT, Lie SA, Havelin LI, Brun JG, Skredderstuen A, Furnes O: 257 ankle arthroplasties performed in Norway between 1994 and 2005. *Acta Orthop* 2007;78(5):575-583.

11. Haddad SL, Coetzee JC, Estok R, Fahrbach K, Banel D, Nalysnyk L: Intermediate and long-term outcomes of TAA and ankle arthrodesis. A systematic review of the literature. *J Bone Joint Surg Am* 2007;89(9):1899-1905.

12. Henricson A, Skoog A, Carlsson A: The Swedish Ankle Arthroplasty Register: An analysis of 531 arthroplasties between 1993 and 2005. *Acta Orthop* 2007;78(5):569-574.

13. Kofoed H, Lundberg-Jensen A: Ankle arthroplasty in patients younger and older than 50 years: A

prospective series with long-term follow-up. *Foot Ankle Int* 1999;20(8):501-506.

14. Hurowitz EJ, Gould JS, Fleisig GS, Fowler R: Outcome analysis of agility total ankle replacement with prior adjunctive procedures: Two to six year followup. *Foot Ankle Int* 2007;28(3):308-312.

15. van der Heide HJ, Schutte B, Louwerens JW, van den Hoogen FH, Malefijt MC: Total ankle prostheses in rheumatoid arthropathy: Outcome in 52 patients followed for 1-9 years. *Acta Orthop* 2009;80(4):440-444.

    There are concerns about TAA in patients with rheumatoid arthropathy because early implants were associated with high failure rates. The investigators review outcomes and survivorship data on 52 patients who received the Buechal-Pappas or STAR ankle implants. Results with a mean follow-up of 2.7 years showed satisfactory outcomes in this population, and the authors suggest that TAA may be considered for these patients. Level of evidence: II.

16. Mann JA, Mann RA, Horton E: STAR™ ankle: Long-term results. *Foot Ankle Int* 2011;32(5):S473-S484.

    This study is a prospective cohort investigation reviewing the results of a surgery involving a STAR design performed by two senior surgeons. Eighty patients were followed for an average of 9.1 years. The authors show a probability of survivorship of 96% at 5 years and 90% at 10 years. Among patients, 92% were satisfied with their outcomes and showed improvement in pain scales. Level of evidence: IV.

17. Bonnin MP, Laurent JR, Casillas M: Ankle function and sports activity after total ankle arthroplasty. *Foot Ankle Int* 2009;30(10):933-944.

    This study looks at return to sport activity after TAA. Return to sport activity is rarely looked at when discussing TAA. Return to low-impact activity was significantly higher then return to high-impact activity. Return to high-impact activity is limited, as noted by the authors, and should be discussed with patients to temper expectations. Authors did not note any increase in loosening in the population pursing high-impact activities, although this was not a definitive conclusion. Level of evidence: III.

18. Naal FD, Impellizzeri FM, Loibl M, Huber M, Rippstein PF: Habitual physical activity and sports participation after total ankle arthroplasty. *Am J Sports Med* 2009;37(1):95-102.

    The study suggests that return to low-impact sports activity is possible after TAA; at 3.7-year follow-up after TAA, there was no increased evidence of periprosthetic lucencies with sports activity. Discussion with patients is warranted to manage expectations about return to sport activity, especially for patients who have experienced trauma. Level of evidence: IV.

19. Gougoulias N, Khanna A, Maffulli N: How successful are current ankle replacements? A systematic review of the literature. *Clin Orthop Relat Res* 2010;468(1):199-208.

    This is a well-done review of current ankle implants based on an analysis of relevant literature. The authors suggest an overall failure rate of 10% at 5 years. Seven different implants were included in the review. No one implant was associated with superior results or survivorship. Level of evidence: IV.

20. Lee KT, Lee YK, Young KW, Kim JB, Seo YS: Perioperative complications and learning curve of the Mobility Total Ankle System. *Foot Ankle Int* 2013;34(2):210-214.

    This is an interesting article that looks at complications related to the learning curve associated with a single TAA. Among 60 patients, 30 received initial implants and 30 received subsequent implants. There was a higher incidence of perioperative complications in the initial group versus the second group, but statistical significance was not established. The authors suggest that a learning curve exists for TAA procedures. Level of evidence: III.

21. Whalen JL, Spelsberg SC, Murray P: Wound breakdown after total ankle arthroplasty. *Foot Ankle Int* 2010;31(4):301-305.

    Wound issues after TAA are the most common surgical complication. Fifty-seven patients who underwent TAA were reviewed in a single-surgeon study. A 28% wound complication rate (16 of 57 patients) was observed. All wounds were managed successfully with retention of implants in all but four patients. Wound breakdown was more common in patients with one or more cardiovascular issues or those who had smoked more than 12 pack years. Caution is recommended when preforming TAA in patients with cardiovascular disease and a heavy smoking history. Level of evidence: IV.

22. Bibbo C: Posterior approach for total ankle arthroplasty. *J Foot Ankle Surg* 2013;52(1):132-135.

    TAA is a technically challenging reconstruction, with soft-tissue complications posing potential significant morbidity, especially when the anterior ankle soft-tissue envelope is not pristine. Alternate approaches to the ankle may need to be sought in unique cases. The author describes a posterior surgical approach for TAA. Level of evidence: IV.

23. Knecht SI, Estin M, Callaghan JJ, et al: The Agility total ankle arthroplasty: Seven to sixteen-year follow-up. *J Bone Joint Surg Am* 2004;86-A(6):1161-1171.

24. Wood PL, Prem H, Sutton C: Total ankle replacement: Medium-term results in 200 Scandinavian total ankle replacements. *J Bone Joint Surg Br* 2008;90(5):605-609.

    This is a single-center review of the STAR implant. Patients were followed for a minimum of 5 years and survivorship was 93.3% at 5 years. Emphasis was placed on correction of anterior subluxation of the talus to restore the anatomic axis of rotation. Level of evidence: III.

25. SooHoo NF, Zingmond DS, Ko CY: Comparison of reoperation rates following ankle arthrodesis and total ankle arthroplasty. *J Bone Joint Surg Am* 2007;89(10):2143-2149.

3: Arthritis of the Foot and Ankle

26. Schuberth JM, Patel S, Zarutsky E: Perioperative complications of the Agility total ankle replacement in 50 initial, consecutive cases. *J Foot Ankle Surg* 2006;45(3):139-146.

27. Wood PL, Deakin S: Total ankle replacement. The results in 200 ankles. *J Bone Joint Surg Br* 2003;85(3):334-341.

28. Nagashima M, Takahashi H, Kakumoto S, Miyamoto Y, Yoshino S: Total ankle arthroplasty for deformity of the foot in patients with rheumatoid arthritis using the TNK ankle system: Clinical results of 21 cases. *Mod Rheumatol* 2004;14(1):48-53.

29. Wood PL, Sutton C, Mishra V, Suneja R: A randomised, controlled trial of two mobile-bearing total ankle replacements. *J Bone Joint Surg Br* 2009;91(1):69-74.

This is a review of 200 ankle replacements that compares the STAR with the Buechel-Pappas ankle replacement. Both groups were followed for a minimum of 3 years. Survivorship was not statistically significant between the two implant designs, but hazard rates for failure suggest the STAR implant may result in better survivorship at a longer-term follow-up. The authors caution against TAA for ankles with preoperative varus or valgus exceeding 15°. Level of evidence: I.

30. Hobson SA, Karantana A, Dhar S: Total ankle replacement in patients with significant pre-operative deformity of the hindfoot. *J Bone Joint Surg Br* 2009;91(4):481-486.

Preoperative deformities of the hindfoot often complicate TAA. The authors of this study review 123 consecutive patients with hindfoot deformities who underwent TAA who were divided into two groups: those with deformity up to 10° and those with deformity between 11° and 30°. They suggest that as long as a deformity is corrected appropriately, there is no increased failure in the group with more serious deformities. Level of evidence: III.

31. Reddy SC, Mann JA, Mann RA, Mangold DR: Correction of moderate to severe coronal plane deformity with the STAR ankle prosthesis. *Foot Ankle Int* 2011;32(7):659-664.

The authors review a case series of STAR ankle replacements over a 9-year period. They had 130 ankle replacements available for review, with 43 included in the study. All patients included had a preoperative coronal deformity of at least 10°. The patients were placed in two groups: 10° to 19° of deformity and those with greater then 20°. Results suggest that deformities up to 25° can be managed with appropriate soft-tissue releases and balancing.

32. Trincat S, Kouyoumdjian P, Asencio G: Total ankle arthroplasty and coronal plane deformities. *Orthop Traumatol Surg Res* 2012;98(1):75-84.

The authors suggest that coronal plane deformity exceeding 10° is not a contraindication for TAA if the deformity is correctable. This is a relatively short-term follow-up study of an average of 38 months. Often, multiple adjunct procedures are required to balance the ankle in the coronal plane during TAA. A combination of soft tissue and osseous procedures may be needed. Correction must be obtained to allow for durable outcomes. Level of evidence: IV.

33. Cornelis Doets H, van der Plaat LW, Klein JP: Medial malleolar osteotomy for the correction of varus deformity during total ankle arthroplasty: Results in 15 ankles. *Foot Ankle Int* 2008;29(2):171-177.

Several options exist for treating ankle varus during TAA. A medial malleolar osteotomy is used in this study to correct this deformity. After an ankle was prepared for placement, an osteotomy of the medial malleolus was completed if required for coronal plane balancing. Correction was possible with up to 30° of varus, with good outcomes reported out to 5 years on average. Level of evidence: IV.

34. Daniels TR, Cadden AR, Lim K: Correction of varus talar deformities in ankle joint replacement. *Oper Tech Orthop* 2008;18(4):282-286.

The article discusses arthroplasty in ankles with a varus deformity of up to 15°. The authors suggest that ankle varus deformity is associated with external rotation of the mortise. This rotational deformity should be addressed at the time of correction. Among TAAs, 75% necessitated ancillary procedures to assist in correction. Level of evidence: IV.

35. Coetzee JC: Management of varus or valgus ankle deformity with ankle replacement. *Foot Ankle Clin* 2008;13(3):509-520, x.

This review article discusses the systematic management of varus and valgus ankle deformity. A discussion of Alvine's classification is helpful in defining potential adjunct procedures that may be required during TAA surgery when deformity is present. Level of evidence: IV.

36. Manegold S, Haas NP, Tsitsilonis S, Springer A, Märdian S, Schaser KD: Periprosthetic fractures in total ankle replacement: Classification system and treatment algorithm. *J Bone Joint Surg Am* 2013;95(9):815-820, S1-S3.

This article presents a thorough systematic algorithm for treatment of periprosthetic fractures associated with TAA. Two implants were included in the study: the STAR and Hintegra. Good outcomes can be achieved with appropriate management and stable fixation when needed. Level of evidence: IV.

37. Raikin SM, Kane J, Ciminiello ME: Risk factors for incision-healing complications following total ankle arthroplasty. *J Bone Joint Surg Am* 2010;92(12):2150-2155.

This study suggests that patients with a history of diabetes and inflammatory arthritis should be counseled on the possibility of increased wound complications following TAA. Minor complications were noted in the diabetes group, and major wound complications were noted in the inflammatory arthritis groups. It is recommended that additional effort be made to educate patients about their risk profile when undergoing TAA. Level of evidence: IV.

38. Kurup HV, Taylor GR: Medial impingement after ankle replacement. *Int Orthop* 2008;32(2):243-246.

The authors present a case review of a single-center experience with the Buechel-Pappas TAA. They discuss medial impingement as a potential complication after TAA. Medial impingement may be a source of continued pain after TAA. They suggest that implant design may be a factor with this problem. Level of evidence: IV.

39. Choi WJ, Lee JW: Heterotopic ossification after total ankle arthroplasty. *J Bone Joint Surg Br* 2011;93(11):1508-1512.

The authors suggest that HO after TAA may occur in as many as 34% of patients. Radiographic evidence and clinical outcomes were examined. The authors conclude that HO is not significantly detrimental to outcomes after TAA despite radiographic evidence of bone growth. Level of evidence: IV.

40. Lee KB, Cho YJ, Park JK, Song EK, Yoon TR, Seon JK: Heterotopic ossification after primary total ankle arthroplasty. *J Bone Joint Surg Am* 2011;93(8):751-758.

A 25% rate of HO was shown in this study, with 10% of patients being symptomatic. The authors suggest that more challenging cases and longer surgical time may increase HO. They do not recommend prophylactic treatment with radiation or nonsteroidal anti-inflammatory drugs for HO. Decreasing surgical time, meticulous soft-tissue dissection, and appropriate implant size are suggested to decrease HO issues. Level of evidence: IV.

41. Schuberth JM, Babu NS, Richey JM, Christensen JC: Gutter impingement after total ankle arthroplasty. *Foot Ankle Int* 2013;34(3):329-337.

These authors recommend complete full-gutter resections at the time of implantation. The four current implant designs available in the United States are described. Aggressive gutter resection at the time of implantation benefited all designs. The Agility implant showed the least benefit among implants. Level of evidence: IV.

42. Doets HC, Zürcher AW: Salvage arthrodesis for failed total ankle arthroplasty. *Acta Orthop* 2010;81(1):142-147.

This article presents a case series of 18 salvage arthrodesis procedures after failed TAA. The authors suggest that blade plate fixation can be successful in these cases. They do highlight the fact that they had more non-unions in the subset of patients that had underlying inflammatory joint disease. Level of evidence: IV.

43. Berkowitz MJ, Clare MP, Walling AK, Sanders R: Salvage of failed total ankle arthroplasty with fusion using structural allograft and internal fixation. *Foot Ankle Int* 2011;32(5):S493-S502.

As TAA becomes more popular, failure of implants will increase. The authors present their data on salvage arthrodesis following failed TAA. They suggest that good clinical outcomes can be expected after successful fusion. They caution that the subtalar joint should be approached via a separate incision and that the joint should be fully prepared to help decrease nonunion in the subtalar component of a tibiotalocalcaneal fusion. Level of evidence: IV.

44. Jeng CL, Campbell JT, Tang EY, Cerrato RA, Myerson MS: Tibiotalocalcaneal arthrodesis with bulk femoral head allograft for salvage of large defects in the ankle. *Foot Ankle Int* 2013;34(9):1256-1266.

Bulk allograft salvage arthrodesis is a technically demanding procedure that is associated with a significant complication rate. The authors show a nonunion rate of 50% in their study, but also demonstrate that 7 of 16 nonunions did not cause symptoms. They also showed a below-knee amputation rate of 19%, underscoring the complex nature of these salvage cases. Level of evidence: IV.

45. DeVries JG, Berlet GC, Hyer CF: Predictive risk assessment for major amputation after tibiotalocalcaneal arthrodesis. *Foot Ankle Int* 2013;34(6):846-850.

Risk for amputation must be considered when discussing a plan for a tibiotalocalcaneal arthrodesis. The authors created a large database looking at risk factors when performing TTC fusions. Diabetes and age of the patient carried the highest risk for amputation in the group. Overall salvage rate was 88.2% in the study. Level of evidence: II.

46. Saltzman CL, Mann RA, Ahrens JE, et al: Prospective controlled trial of STAR total ankle replacement versus ankle fusion: Initial results. *Foot Ankle Int* 2009;30(7):579-596.

This article reviews the initial results of a large multicenter study looking at the STAR ankle replacement. This study was a noninferiority study using ankle fusion and the control. The initial group consisted of 416 STAR ankles that were followed for 24 months. The authors conclude that the STAR group and ankle fusion group were equivalent in pain relief and the STAR group had better function. Level of evidence: II.

47. Bonnin M, Gaudot F, Laurent JR, Ellis S, Colombier JA, Judet T: The Salto total ankle arthroplasty: Survivorship and analysis of failures at 7 to 11 years. *Clin Orthop Relat Res* 2011;469(1):225-236.

This is a long-term follow-up study of a single implant from a prior cohort studied at an earlier time point. Average follow-up was 8.9 years. The authors show an overall survival rate of 65% with any revision surgery on the ankle and an 85% survivorship when only revision of the components was considered as the end point. Minimal subsidence or loosening was noted in the study group. Level of evidence: IV.

48. Rippstein PF, Huber M, Coetzee JC, Naal FD: Total ankle replacement with use of a new three-component implant. *J Bone Joint Surg Am* 2011;93(15):1426-1435.

This is a large short-term study of a single three-component implant (Mobility) with a mean follow-up of 15.3 months. Authors show a revision surgery rate of 7.7%, with 2.1% of the implants failing. Nonprogressive

3: Arthritis of the Foot and Ankle

radiolucency was shown in as many as 37.3% of implants. The authors are encouraged by the short-term findings, but suggest that longer-term follow-up is needed to confirm their current findings. Level of evidence: IV.

49. Nelissen RG, Doets HC, Valstar ER: Early migration of the tibial component of the buechel-pappas total ankle prosthesis. *Clin Orthop Relat Res* 2006;448(448):146-151.

50. Rippstein PF, Huber M, Naal FD: Management of specific complications related to total ankle arthroplasty. *Foot Ankle Clin* 2012;17(4):707-717.

    This is a well-compiled review of complications related to TAA surgery. Despite advancements, complications remain a significant issue. The authors suggest that surgeon experience may play an important role in decreasing complications. Level of evidence: IV.

51. Reuver JM, Dayerizadeh N, Burger B, Elmans L, Hoelen M, Tulp N: Total ankle replacement outcome in low volume centers: Short-term followup. *Foot Ankle Int* 2010;31(12):1064-1068.

    This is a report of a study done at four low-volume TAA centers (three TAAs per year per center) that looked at outcomes compared to those achieved at high-volume TAA centers. Two implants were included in the study (STAR and Salto). Mean follow-up was 36 months. The authors showed an 86% survival rate at low-volume centers and suggest that functional outcomes at lower-volume centers can be comparable to those at higher-volume centers, but survivorship results may not be as positive. Level of evidence: III.

52. Labek G, Klaus H, Schlichtherle R, Williams A, Agreiter M: Revision rates after total ankle arthroplasty in sample-based clinical studies and national registries. *Foot Ankle Int* 2011;32(8):740-745.

    This is a meta-analysis of current studies and national registries related to TAA outcomes. The authors show that implant developers represented more than 50% of all publications, and results often significantly differed from those published by nondevelopers. Authors showed outcome deviations between 300% and 500% among developer versus nondeveloper groups and suggested that literature must be reviewed critically and inherent study biases must be understood. Level of evidence: II.

53. Hosman AH, Mason RB, Hobbs T, Rothwell AG: A New Zealand national joint registry review of 202 total ankle replacements followed for up to 6 years. *Acta Orthop* 2007;78(5):584-591.

54. Skyttä ET, Koivu H, Eskelinen A, Ikävalko M, Paavolainen P, Remes V: Total ankle replacement: A population-based study of 515 cases from the Finnish Arthroplasty Register. *Acta Orthop* 2010;81(1):114-118.

    This study reviewed results of two implants (STAR and Ankle Evolutive System (AES)) from a national database to assess outcomes and survivorship. Authors showed a rate of 1.5 implants per 105 inhabitants. Five-year survivorship was 83% overall. No significant difference was shown to demonstrate superiority in either implant. Hospital volume also did not significantly influence outcomes. Level of evidence: III.

55. Prissel MA, Roukis TS: Management of extensive tibial osteolysis with the Agility™ total ankle replacement systems using geometric metal-reinforced polymethylmethacrylate cement augmentation. *J Foot Ankle Surg* 2014;53(1):101-107.

    The authors describe a novel approach to treating extensive areas of osteolysis for a failed TAA. They suggest that using a metal reinforced cement augmentation can be an effective salvage technique compared with impaction bone grafting. Level of evidence: IV.

56. Devries JG, Berlet GC, Lee TH, Hyer CF, Deorio JK: Revision total ankle replacement: An early look at agility to INBONE. *Foot Ankle Spec* 2011;4(4):235-244.

    A two-center study looking at a retrospective review of revision TAA from one specific implant (Agility) to the revision implant (INBONE). Five patients were included in the study with at least 12 months follow-up. The authors note a high complication rate and caution against revision procedures in the face of previous infection or nonreconstructible deformities. Level of evidence: IV.

57. Ellington JK, Gupta S, Myerson MS: Management of failures of total ankle replacement with the agility total ankle arthroplasty. *J Bone Joint Surg Am* 2013;95(23):2112-2118.

    Retrospective review of 53 patients with failed TAA that underwent revision at a single institution. Minimum follow-up after revision was 2 years. The author note that average time from primary TAA to revision was 51 months. The authors suggest that outcomes were reasonable for the revision patients and that revision may be considered an alternative to arthrodesis in the setting of a failed TAA. Level of evidence: IV.

58. Glazebrook M, Daniels T, Younger A, et al: Comparison of health-related quality of life between patients with end-stage ankle and hip arthrosis. *J Bone Joint Surg Am* 2008;90(3):499-505.

    The authors present a multicenter study that compared health-related quality-of-life questionnaires between two groups with end-stage arthritis. One group had ankle arthritis and the other group hip arthritis. Both groups showed significant effect on quality of life because of the arthritis. The authors conclude that end-stage ankle arthritis has as severe an effect on health-related quality of life as end-stage hip arthritis. Level of evidence: II.

59. Easley ME, Adams SB Jr, Hembree WC, DeOrio JK: Results of total ankle arthroplasty. *J Bone Joint Surg Am* 2011;93(15):1455-1468.

    The results of total ankle arthroplasty and overall survivorship are reviewed. Survivorship was shown to be 70% to 98% at 3 to 6 years and 80% to 95% at 8 to 12 years. The authors suggest that there may be a need for obligatory reoperation during the lifetime of the implant that is not complete revisions. Level of evidence: III.

60. Queen RM, De Biassio JC, Butler RJ, DeOrio JK, Easley ME, Nunley JA: J. Leonard Goldner Award 2011: Changes in pain, function, and gait mechanics two years following total ankle arthroplasty performed with two modern fixed-bearing prostheses. *Foot Ankle Int* 2012;33(7):535-542.

This is a kinematic study looking at gait function and pain at a 2-year follow-up after TAA. Two fixed-bearing implants were included in the study (Salto and In Bone). Significant improvement was seen in hindfoot score and all parameters of kinematic evaluation. The authors propose that a fixed-bearing prosthesis can be considered as an alternative to mobile-bearing implants. Level of evidence: II.

61. Valderrabano V, Nigg BM, von Tscharner V, Stefanyshyn DJ, Goepfert B, Hintermann B: Gait analysis in ankle osteoarthritis and total ankle replacement. *Clin Biomech (Bristol, Avon)* 2007;22(8):894-904.

62. Flavin R, Coleman SC, Tenenbaum S, Brodsky JW: Comparison of gait after total ankle arthroplasty and ankle arthrodesis. *Foot Ankle Int* 2013;34(10):1340-1348.

This is a prospective study of 28 patients in two groups. Among patients, 14 underwent TAA and 14 underwent arthrodesis. Gait analysis was completed preoperatively and at 1 year postoperatively. Each group demonstrated significant differences in gait parameters. The authors show that gait in neither group returned to normal, and nonsuperiority was demonstrated between the two groups. Level of evidence: III.

63. Piriou P, Culpan P, Mullins M, Cardon JN, Pozzi D, Judet T: Ankle replacement versus arthrodesis: A comparative gait analysis study. *Foot Ankle Int* 2008;29(1):3-9.

Gait analysis was performed before and after ankle arthroplasty in a small group of patients and compared to a similar-sized group that had undergone ankle arthrodesis. The authors suggest that neither group resumed normal gait patterns. The ankle fusion group had a faster gait but more asymmetry. The replacement group had a slower gait but more symmetrical timing of their gate. Level of evidence: III.

64. Hahn ME, Wright ES, Segal AD, Orendurff MS, Ledoux WR, Sangeorzan BJ: Comparative gait analysis of ankle arthrodesis and arthroplasty: Initial findings of a prospective study. *Foot Ankle Int* 2012;33(4):282-289.

This is a longitudinal study of 18 patients who underwent TAA or ankle fusion (9 patients each). Gait analysis was completed preoperatively and at 1 year postoperatively.

Pain reduction and improvements in gait parameters were seen in both groups. The authors suggest that the population that underwent TAA regained more natural ankle motion. Level of evidence: IV.

65. Stauffer RN, Chao EY, Brewster RC: Force and motion analysis of the normal, diseased, and prosthetic ankle joint. *Clin Orthop Relat Res* 1977;127:189-196.

66. Khazzam M, Long JT, Marks RM, Harris GF: Preoperative gait characterization of patients with ankle arthrosis. *Gait Posture* 2006;24(1):85-93.

67. Slobogean GP, Younger A, Apostle KL, et al: Preference-based quality of life of end-stage ankle arthritis treated with arthroplasty or arthrodesis. *Foot Ankle Int* 2010;31(7):563-566.

This is a multicenter prospective cohort study comparing quality of life indicators for TAA versus ankle arthrodesis. The groups were evaluated preoperatively and at 1 year postoperatively. The study suggests that ankle arthritis significantly affects quality-of-life measures. Ankle arthroplasty and arthrodesis both resulted in significant improvement in quality of life indicators after surgical intervention. Level of evidence: II.

68. Brodsky JW, Polo FE, Coleman SC, Bruck N: Changes in gait following the Scandinavian Total Ankle Replacement. *J Bone Joint Surg Am* 2011;93(20):1890-1896.

This is a prospective single-center study of 50 consecutive STAR TAAs. The patients had a mean follow-up at 49 months after TAA. Three-dimensional gait analysis was completed using a motion capture system. The authors concluded that at midterm follow-up, those who underwent TAA had a more normal gait than those who underwent ankle arthrodesis. Level of evidence: III.

69. Greisberg J, Assal M, Flueckiger G, Hansen ST Jr: Takedown of ankle fusion and conversion to total ankle replacement. *Clin Orthop Relat Res* 2004;424:80-88.

70. Hintermann B, Barg A, Knupp M, Valderrabano V: Conversion of painful ankle arthrodesis to total ankle arthroplasty. *J Bone Joint Surg Am* 2009;91(4):850-858.

Thirty painful ankles in 28 patients (average age 58.2 years) who were treated with takedown of a fusion and TAA were followed for a minimum of 36 months (average 55.6 months). The outcome was assessed on the basis of clinical and radiographic evaluations. For patients who had pain at the site of a failed ankle arthrodesis, conversion to TAA with the use of a three-component ankle implant was a viable treatment option that provided reliable intermediate-term results. Key factors contributing to the success of this procedure may be intrinsic coronal plane stability provided by ankle implants and the use of wider talar implants. Level of evidence: IV.

3: Arthritis of the Foot and Ankle

Chapter 10

Hindfoot Arthritis

Tobin T. Eckel, MD   Scott B. Shawen, MD

Introduction

Hindfoot arthritis is a painful and debilitating condition that is experienced by an unknown number of people. Although it most commonly results from traumatic injury, it also can occur secondary to inflammatory or degenerative arthritis or result from a multitude of foot deformities. Joint disease and clinical disability progress in tandem and result in increasing difficulty with shoe wear and ambulation. Nonsurgical measures are the first line of treatment; when these fail, the preferred surgical procedure is arthrodesis.

Anatomy and Biomechanics

The hindfoot consists of the calcaneus, talus, cuboid, and navicular bones, which articulate through the subtalar (ST), calcaneocuboid (CC), and talonavicular (TN) joints. The ST joint consists of posterior, middle, and anterior facets. The TN and CC joints are referred to as the transverse tarsal joint. The spring ligament, an important stabilizer of the medial arch, supports the TN joint plantarly.[1] These joints work synchronously and are mainly responsible for inversion and eversion of the hindfoot to accommodate ambulation on uneven ground. Coupled movements of these joints allow the foot to act as a shock absorber at heel strike and become a rigid lever at push-off. The ST joint everts at heel strike, which aligns the TN and CC joints parallel to each other. This effectively "unlocks" the transverse tarsal joint and midfoot, allowing motion and flexibility to absorb impact and balance the foot on the ground. As the foot progresses through the stance phase, the ST joint inverts, causing the TN and

Dr. Shawen or an immediate family member serves as a board member, owner, officer, or committee member of the American Orthopaedic Foot and Ankle Society and the American Orthopaedic Foot and Ankle Society Humanitarian Aid Committee. Neither Dr. Eckel nor any immediate family member has received anything of value from or has stock or stock options held in a commercial company or institution related directly or indirectly to the subject of this chapter.

CC joint axes to diverge, now "locking" the midfoot to create a rigid lever for push-off.[2]

Considering this complex motion coupling, it can be difficult to measure individual motion of each joint. Although the entire hindfoot joint complex is involved in inversion and eversion, the transverse tarsal joint is responsible for 26% of foot dorsiflexion and plantar flexion.[3] Cadaver studies of residual joint motion after selective arthrodeses have helped to increase understanding of the complexity of hindfoot motion. Isolated CC arthrodesis had little effect on ST motion, but decreased TN motion to 67% of its normal value. ST arthrodesis limited CC and TN motion to 56% and 46% of their normal values, respectively. Isolated TN arthrodesis had the most substantial effect, reducing both ST and CC motion to less than 8% of normal values.[2,4,5]

Pathophysiology and Etiology

Hindfoot arthritis develops much in the same way as arthritis affecting other joints. It is the result of direct cartilage or chondrocyte damage from acute macrotrauma, repetitive microtrauma, abnormal weight-bearing stress from articular incongruity, joint malalignment, adjacent joint arthrodesis, or increased shear stress from ligamentous instability.[6]

The calcaneus is the most commonly fractured bone in the foot, and posttraumatic arthritis most commonly occurs secondary to intra-articular calcaneal fractures. When these injuries are managed nonsurgically, there may be as much as a fivefold increase in the incidence of late ST arthrodesis.[7] Damage to the articular surface can occur at the initial injury and over time as a result of a malreduced joint causing uneven loading patterns and progressive cartilage wear.[1]

Inflammatory arthritis also commonly affects the hindfoot. Foot and ankle pain will develop in more than 90% of patients with rheumatoid arthritis (RA). Joint destruction is the result of synovial inflammation leading to cartilage erosion and periarticular bony resorption. This is exacerbated by subsequent ligamentous laxity and possible tendon rupture. Substantial deformity can lead to increased stress on the cartilage and accelerated wear.[8,9]

The hindfoot is also the second most common site of Charcot arthropathy in the foot, occurring in 10% to 30% of all cases. Neurotraumatic and neurovascular theories describe the pathophysiology of neuropathic arthropathy. The neurotraumatic theory implicates loss of protective sensation and proprioception, which leads to repetitive microtrauma. Continued weight bearing prevents healing and leads to rapid joint destruction. The neurovascular theory attributes hyperemia and autonomic nervous system dysfunction to increased osteoclastic resorption and fracture.[10]

Any soft-tissue or bony pathology that causes hindfoot deformity can lead to degenerative changes. These changes most commonly are seen during the late stages of posterior tibial tendon deficiency when abnormal load distribution secondary to chronic planovalgus deformity results in hindfoot arthritis.[11] Another less common example is spontaneous osteonecrosis of the navicular, known as Müller-Weiss disease, which leads to hindfoot deformity and arthrosis.[12]

Iatrogenic hindfoot arthritis occurs when foot or ankle surgery leads to increased loads on adjacent joints with subsequent adjacent joint degeneration. One noteworthy example is hindfoot arthritis that develops after ankle arthrodesis. In one study, investigators noted a 90% incidence of adjacent hindfoot arthritis after ankle arthrodesis with a mean follow-up of 22 years.[13] This concept has led to increased popularity of selective single- and double-hindfoot arthrodesis procedures over standard triple arthrodesis as surgeons attempt to preserve hindfoot motion and diminish loading on adjacent joints.[4,14,15]

Clinical Presentation

Patients with symptomatic hindfoot arthritis report pain, swelling, and stiffness of the foot. The pain is often localized to the sinus tarsi or to areas just distal to the malleoli. Walking on uneven surfaces such as grass, gravel, or sand exacerbates the pain associated with hindfoot arthritis. It is important to obtain a patient's history of previous trauma or surgeries of the foot.

With the patient standing and undressed from the knees down, overall alignment should be assessed and any deformities noted and determined to be flexible or rigid. The Coleman block test can be used to establish the flexibility of a varus hindfoot deformity and guide treatment.[16] Similarly, the flexibility of the hindfoot in long-standing planovalgus deformity is also critical in guiding treatment.[17] The hindfoot joints should be assessed for motion as well as point tenderness. Any pain

with motion or limited motion may indicate joint degeneration and should be compared with the contralateral side. Diagnostic injections of local anesthetic may aid in identifying specific joint involvement. The ST joint can typically be injected in the office setting, whereas injections of the TN and CC joints often necessitate fluoroscopic guidance. Fluoroscopy remains the preferred method for intra-articular injections in the foot and ankle, yet there has been a recent surge in the use of ultrasound guidance for diagnostic injections with comparable accuracy without radiation exposure. Although these injections may help to localize pathology, communications can exist between these joints and should be considered before relying solely on these diagnostic injections to guide treatment.[18,19] It is also important to assess ankle motion to determine if there is an Achilles contracture because this will also need to be addressed in treatment. A Silfverskiöld test can further help to determine if the contracture is in the gastrocnemius or the tendon proper.[20] A detailed neurovascular examination is also critical. Any motor weakness or sensory loss should be noted because this may indicate a neuromuscular or neuropathic disorder. Patients without palpable pulses should be further evaluated with vascular studies, especially if surgery is being considered.

Imaging

AP, lateral, and oblique standing radiographs are routinely performed to evaluate the hindfoot. Weight-bearing radiographs accurately assess alignment and the degree of degenerative joint changes. The AP view will reveal any arthritic change at the TN joint. Additionally, forefoot adduction or abduction can be determined as well as talar head uncovering, which indicates valgus hindfoot deformity. Arthritis of the CC joint is best seen on an oblique radiograph. The ST and TN joints are well visualized on lateral radiograph, along with any pes planus or cavus deformities.[1] Hindfoot alignment and axillary views are also useful to assess varus or valgus hindfoot deformity[21] (**Figure 1**).

Although not a weight-bearing study, CT scans provide the most accurate assessment of the hindfoot joints and may be useful in surgical planning. Ultrasound effectively identifies cortical erosions and synovitis in inflammatory arthritides at low cost and without radiation exposure. However, ultrasound's effectiveness is operator-dependent, and this technology is not routinely used in the workup for arthritis. MRI has high sensitivity for detecting arthritic changes in joints, but is currently used more as a research tool and not part of routine imaging. Nuclear medicine studies, CT, and magnetic resonance arthrography also can be used to

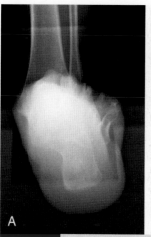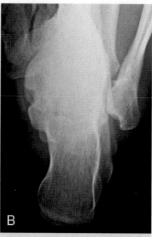

Figure 1 | Hindfoot alignment view (**A**) and axillary heel view (**B**) demonstrating valgus and varus malalignment, respectively.

evaluate arthritis but are cost-prohibitive and rarely used clinically.[22]

Nonsurgical Treatment

The first step in managing hindfoot arthritis is activity modification and a trial of nonsteroidal anti-inflammatory medication. High-impact activity such as running should be avoided and substituted with low-impact activities that involve elliptical trainers, stationary bicycles, and swimming. Avoiding uneven terrain (not walking barefoot on sand, for example) and wearing appropriate shoes may also provide substantial relief of symptoms. The next step in management includes the use of orthotic devices. A variety of orthotic devices, braces, and shoe modifications exist for the treatment of hindfoot arthritis.[23] These orthotic devices may provide temporary pain relief for patients who want to delay or avoid surgical procedures or are poor surgical candidates. Although these devices cannot correct existing deformities or existing degenerative joint surfaces, they may facilitate healing through soft-tissue rest. Orthotic devices can reduce pain, prevent deformity progression, and slow the development of arthritis, perhaps eliminating the need for surgical intervention altogether.[24]

The extent of hindfoot joint disease and the presence of deformity will determine the appropriate orthotic device. A simple shoe modification to include a rocker-bottom sole may be sufficient to offload the hindfoot and decrease pain. When degenerative disease and/or deformity is more advanced, the addition of an orthotic device can be added to relieve pressure, correct flexible deformities, limit motion, and accommodate fixed deformities. Flexible deformities may be stabilized or corrected by adding a post to an orthotic device; fixed

deformities may be accommodated using soft, moldable contours to protect against skin breakdown and ulceration.[23] The University of California Biomechanics Laboratory (UCBL) orthotic device can be used to limit painful hindfoot motion and correct flexible hindfoot deformity. An advantage of the UCBL device is that it will fit inside of a regular shoe; however, it is rigid and may be poorly tolerated by some patients.[25] More severe deformity or advanced arthrosis cannot be managed with a foot orthotic device alone, and an orthotic device that goes above the ankle joint to more effectively offload arthritic joints and correct or accommodate deformity is necessary. One common ankle-foot orthosis is the Arizona brace, which is a custom-molded leather brace that limits ankle and hindfoot motion and decreases pain at these arthritic joints.[24]

Corticosteroid injections have been used to reduce inflammation and provide temporary pain relief for foot arthritis. In one study, 38 children with juvenile idiopathic arthritis were treated with ST steroid injection.[26] The mean duration of pain relief was 1.2 years ±0.9 years]. Of note, 53% of these patients experienced either hypopigmentation or subcutaneous atrophy in response to the injection.[26] In an adult population, the benefit of steroid injection tends to be more limited. Investigators in a 2011 study reported on 63 patients who underwent steroid injection for midfoot arthritis.[27] Approximately 60% of patients experienced relief that persisted for up to 3 months after injection; however, fewer than 15% experienced relief beyond 3 months. Considering the lack of long-term efficacy and potential complications, steroid injections likely should be used sparingly to treat hindfoot arthritis.

Surgical Treatment

Arthrodesis of the involved hindfoot joints remains the standard of care after a failed course of nonsurgical treatment. Historically, treatment entailed a triple arthrodesis and involved fusion of the ST, TN, and CC joints. More recently, there has been a trend toward selective one- or two-joint arthrodesis in an attempt to preserve motion and possibly limit adjacent joint degeneration and decrease surgical time and potential complications.[11,15,28]

Active infection is the only absolute contraindication to hindfoot fusion. Caution should be exercised when treating patients with peripheral vascular disease or potential arterial or venous insufficiency. These patients should undergo the appropriate vascular studies and, possibly, a vascular surgery consultation before hindfoot arthrodesis.[29] Tobacco use is another relative contraindication to any foot or ankle arthrodesis, with hindfoot

3: Arthritis of the Foot and Ankle

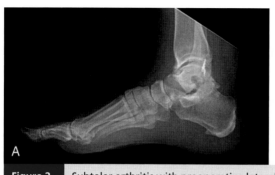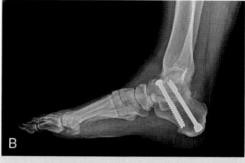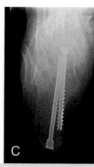

Figure 2   Subtalar arthritis with preoperative lateral (**A**) and postoperative lateral (**B**) and axillary (**C**) radiographic views.

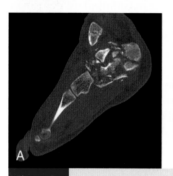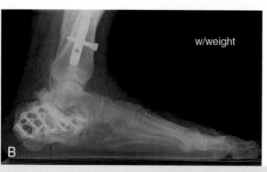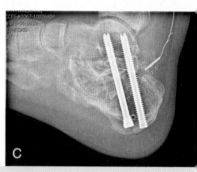

Figure 3   **A**, Preoperative CT scan of a comminuted calcaneal fracture. **B**, Lateral radiograph showing initial treatment with open reduction and internal fixation. **C**, Loss of calcaneal height and subtalar arthritis was then treated with distraction arthrodesis.

nonunion rates approximately three times higher among smokers.[30]

ST Arthrodesis

Isolated ST arthritis commonly occurs after intra-articular calcaneal fractures are sustained, but also can be the result of RA, ST coalition or a long-standing hindfoot deformity.[7] ST arthrodesis is typically performed through a lateral approach. The hindfoot should be positioned in approximately 5° of valgus and fixed with one or two screws. Headless screws are low profile and may be less irritating to the patient. If headed screws are used, it is important that they be placed away from the weight-bearing portion of the calcaneus (**Figure 2**).

Posttraumatic ST arthritis after calcaneal fracture can pose several additional challenges. A lateral calcaneal wall exostectomy may be required to relieve lateral impingement. There may also be anterior impingement because of loss of calcaneal height, which necessitates distraction arthrodesis. This will restore hindfoot height and talar declination, thereby relieving anterior impingement[31] (**Figure 3**). In a 2008 study,[32] investigators described a posterior approach for ST distraction arthrodesis. This approach offers the advantages of avoiding previous surgical incisions, provides excellent ST joint exposure, and is optimal for correcting large varus or valgus deformities in addition to joint distraction. Union

rates for open ST arthrodesis range between 84% and 100%.[33] Controversy exists regarding the optimal time at which to perform a distraction ST arthrodesis and in situ arthrodesis. The only clear indication for distraction arthrodesis remains anterior ankle impingement. Even though a distraction arthrodesis necessitates fusion across two surfaces, union rates have been comparable between the two procedures. Clinical outcomes also have been similar for both techniques, although the complications associated with distraction tend to be more numerous and include wound healing problems, neuralgia, and varus malunion.[31] Despite preservation of the transverse tarsal joints, adjacent joint degeneration still occurs, with one study noting a 10% incidence of adjacent joint arthrosis at 4 years after ST arthrodesis.[34]

Arthroscopic ST Arthrodesis

Arthroscopic ST arthrodesis has been advocated when distraction or large deformity correction is not required. One advantage of arthroscopic arthrodesis is potential preservation of the talar and calcaneal blood supply because the interosseous ligament and its associated vasculature is preserved. This technique can be performed in the supine, lateral, or prone positions with no appreciable difference in outcomes. Fusion rates are reported between 91% and 100%, and time to union ranges between 9 and 12 weeks. Advantages of the arthroscopic technique

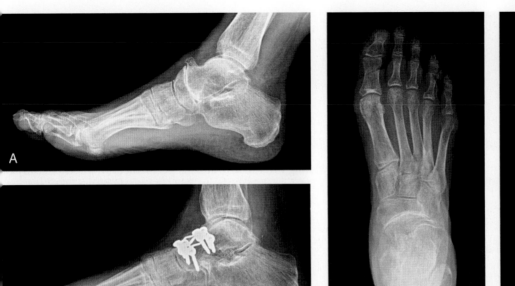
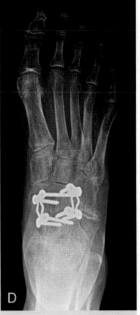

Figure 4 Isolated talonavicular arthrodesis. **A,** Preoperative lateral view. **B,** Postoperative lateral view. **C,** Preoperative AP view. **D,** Postoperative AP view.

include shorter hospitalization and decreased wound complications and sural nerve injuries. Clinical outcomes tend to be similar to those of open arthrodesis.[33,35]

TN Arthrodesis

TN arthritis can develop after traumatic injury, RA, or osteoarthritis (**Figure 4**). Arthrodesis may be necessary to treat all of these conditions, as well as in cases of flatfoot deformity with an unstable TN joint.[9,36] Osteonecrosis of the navicular can also lead to joint degeneration. Navicular osteonecrosis occurs most commonly after fracture but may be idiopathic in nature. Muller-Weiss disease, or idiopathic adult-onset navicular osteonecrosis, is characterized by sclerosis and lateral fragmentation of the navicular. Definitive treatment depends largely on the extent of arthrosis and collapse at presentation. Patients with disease isolated to the TN joint can appropriately undergo TN arthrodesis, but if substantial fragmentation and collapse exist, a bone block graft may be necessary to restore length. If there is substantial adjacent joint breakdown, additional fusion procedures may be necessary, including pantalar arthrodesis.[12]

Fusion of the TN joint greatly reduces motion of the remaining hindfoot joints to less than 8% of prearthrodesis motion. Despite the shear and torsional stresses across the TN joint, and even though this is the most common nonunion site in triple arthrodesis, fusion rates for isolated TN arthrodesis are quite high, ranging between 90% and 97%.[37] Adjacent joint degeneration is still seen with isolated TN arthrodesis, particularly in the ST and naviculocuneiform joints. However, peak pressure load in the ankle joint is lower and more evenly distributed after TN arthrodesis compared with triple arthrodesis.[4]

CC Arthrodesis

The CC joint, which is rarely fused in isolation, is more typically fused in double or triple arthrodesis or to correct planovalgus deformity.[38] Lateral column lengthening is a common procedure performed in planovalgus corrective surgery. It is either performed as an osteotomy 10 mm to 15 mm proximal to the joint or as a distraction arthrodesis through the CC joint (**Figure 5**). Opponents of distraction arthrodesis argue that lengthening the lateral column increases contact pressure at the CC joint, predisposing it to accelerated degeneration. Although multiple studies suggest increased contact pressure at the CC joint following a lengthening procedure, there is no clear correlation between increased pressure and accelerated CC arthrosis. Those in favor of osteotomy point to the increased complications associated with distraction arthrodesis and the equivalent outcomes between the two procedures.[39]

Triple Arthrodesis

Triple arthrodesis consists of fusion of the TN joint through a medial approach and the CC and ST joints through a lateral approach (**Figure 6**). Recent fusion rates are reported at approximately 95%. Adjacent joint degeneration is the major concern, with ankle arthrosis reportedly ranging between 40% and 100% and midfoot

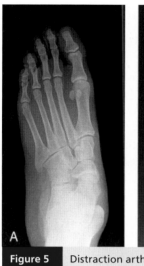 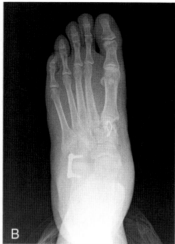

Figure 5 Distraction arthrodesis through the calcaneocuboid joint for pes planus. **A,** Preoperative AP view. **B,** Postoperative AP view.

arthrosis near 50% at follow-up. Nevertheless, clinical outcomes and patient satisfaction remain high after triple arthrodesis.[1] Some concern over lateral wound dehiscence in the presence of valgus deformity and contracted lateral soft tissues has led to the development of a single medial approach to triple arthrodesis. In one study, the authors[40] demonstrated in their series that the degree of radiographic correction in medial triple arthrodesis was similar to results achieved with standard two-incision triple arthrodesis. In a follow-up cadaver study, they were able to prepare 91% of all articular surfaces through the isolated medial approach, compared with 88% of the articular surfaces through the standard two-incision approach.[41] Although a medial-only approach precludes lateral wound complications, there is increased risk for disruption of talar blood supply and a risk to the deltoid ligament that can lead to medial instability.[28,42]

Double Arthrodesis

The term double arthrodesis refers to selective fusion of two of the three hindfoot joints. A double arthrodesis can refer to arthrodesis of the TN and CC joints or the ST and TN joints (**Figure 7**). This concept arose from the idea of fusing only the arthritic joints and preserving the remaining joint in hopes of off-loading the adjacent joints to prevent or delay adjacent joint breakdown. There are potential advantages to double ST/TN arthrodesis. There is one less surgical site at which potential complications can develop. Additionally, although the TN joint remains the most common nonunion site in hindfoot fusion, the CC joint can still account for as many as 20% of all nonunions.[15] After double arthrodesis, there

is only approximately 2° of residual motion at the CC joint, but this may be enough to reduce the forces across the adjacent joints.[15]

Accelerated degeneration of the CC joint in double arthrodesis has been a topic of concern. In one study of 14 feet that underwent double arthrodesis, no foot developed CC arthritis.[28] However, this study had a relatively short follow-up period ranging from 6 months to 4 years, and arthritic symptoms can continue to develop long after arthrodesis is performed. In another study of 16 feet that underwent double arthrodesis, 5 feet developed radiographic evidence of CC arthritis, although no patient was symptomatic.[15] This study had a longer follow-up period ranging from 18 months to 9 years. This study also revealed decreased adjacent joint disease, with 38% and 32% of feet showing degenerative changes in the ankle and the midfoot, respectively, compared with 61% and 73% of feet that underwent conventional triple arthrodesis.[15,28]

Complications

Several potential complications are associated with surgical treatment, none of which are unique to hindfoot arthrodesis. Superficial wound complications reportedly affect between 3% and 30% of patients undergoing foot arthrodesis.[33] For healthy patients having elective hindfoot fusion, the wound complication rate is approximately 3%. Complication rates increase slightly in the case of revision hindfoot surgery. Patients with diabetes have an overall wound complication rate of around 14%, which may increase to as high as 50% for revision or salvage surgeries. Problems involving prominent hardware can occur 20% of the time, and symptoms may necessitate removal in 50% of patients with prominent hardware.[43]

Infection is another potential complication, with superficial infections occurring in 3% of patients who undergo hindfoot fusion; among elderly patients, the infection rate has been reported as high as 11%.[43] Deep infection and osteomyelitis occurs in approximately 2% of cases.[4,43]

Nerve injury is another risk of surgery, and this can present as a neuroma, neuritis, or complex regional pain syndrome. Direct nerve injury is most common with CC arthrodesis, with the incidence of sural nerve injury as high as 32%. Complex regional pain syndrome has been reported in as many as 18% of cases in some studies; however, most literature quotes rates at 2% to 3%.[4,33,43] This can be a particularly difficult entity to treat and often necessitates a multimodal approach that includes physical therapy and pain management.

Nonunion is another potentially devastating complication, and unless a patient is stable and asymptomatic,

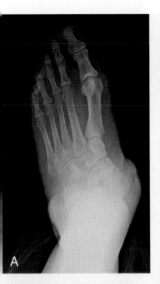
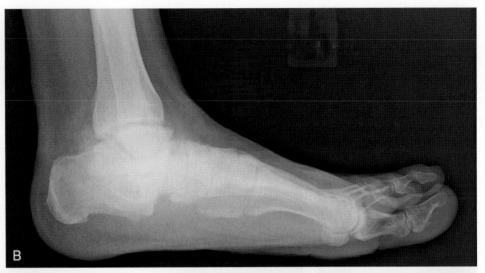
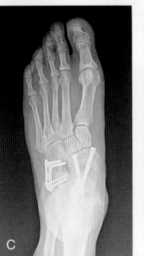
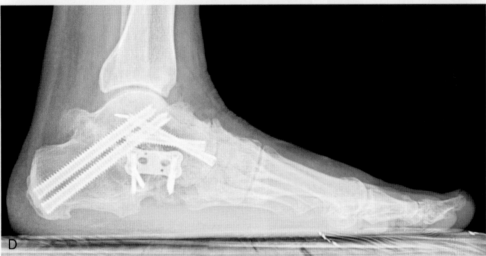

Figure 6   Triple arthrodesis. Preoperative AP (**A**) and lateral (**B**) images of fixed planovalgus deformity. Postoperative AP (**C**) and lateral (**D**) images after triple arthrodesis.

he or she will almost always need revision surgery (**Figure 8**). Rates of nonunion after triple arthrodesis range between 3% and 17%.[43] The fusion rates of double (ST/TN) arthrodesis are higher, with a nonunion rate of approximately 6%.[15,43] The nonunion rates for single-joint arthrodesis are reportedly as high as 35% for isolated TN or CC joint arthrodeses.[4,43]

A 6% malunion rate is associated with midfoot and hindfoot fusion procedures. The malunion rate after triple arthrodesis is 3%, but this rate doubles in revision cases. The most common deformity is equinovarus, followed by hindfoot varus and hindfoot valgus.[43]

Adjacent joint degeneration may be considered a natural progression of the disease process as opposed to a true complication. Nonetheless, it remains a relevant topic when deciding on the most appropriate surgical procedure. After triple arthrodesis, progression of ankle

and midfoot arthritis may develop in 30% to 50% of patients.[43] Arthritis of the transverse tarsal joint will develop in 10% to 30% of patients after isolated ST arthrodesis, with similar results of ST and NC arthritis after isolated TN arthrodesis.[4,43]

Adjuvant Treatment in Hindfoot Arthrodesis

There are three basic requirements for bone healing. An osteoconductive matrix must provide the scaffold upon which new bone can grow. Osteoinductive growth factors that can recruit osteogenic progenitor cells and guide their differentiation into osteoblasts are needed. A local population of theses progenitor cells to respond to the osteoinductive proteins must be present.[44,45]

Iliac crest autograft has long been the preferred procedure because it meets all three requirements and there

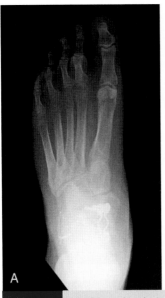
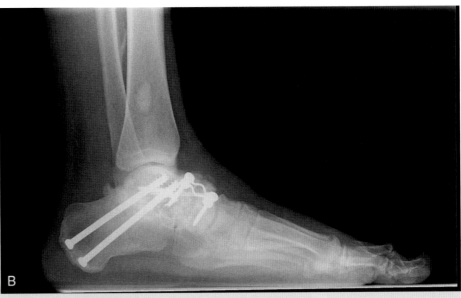

Figure 7 Double arthrodesis. AP (**A**) and lateral (**B**) radiographic views after selective fusion of the subtalar and talonavicular joints, preserving the calcaneocuboid articulation.

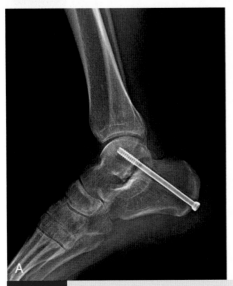
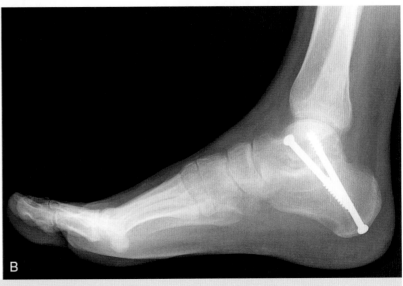

Figure 8 **A**, Subtalar nonunion that underwent revision arthrodesis (**B**).

is no risk for disease transmission. However, several complications are associated with autograft harvest, most commonly, nerve injury, hematoma, and donor site pain. These complications occur in 2.4% to 9.5% of foot and ankle cases.[46] It is not necessary to procure the large quantity of bone graft available in the iliac crest for routine foot procedures. The tibia is another common autograft harvest site and has the advantage of proximity to the primary surgical site. However, the active marrow content in the tibia is substantially lower than in the iliac crest.[46] This has led to the increasing use of allografts, bone graft substitutes, and osteobiologic agents and devices to promote bone healing without the associated morbidity of autograft harvest.

Allograft bone has the advantage of being both osteoconductive and osteoinductive. Although its osteoconductive properties are the same as autograft, its osteoinductive capabilities are reduced. There is also a small risk for disease transmission associated with allograft. Advantages of allograft use include the availability of large quantities (with which to fill a large void or defect) and the structural support provided by cortical or corticocancellous grafts.[44]

Synthetic bone graft substitutes are used mainly for their osteoconductive properties. These materials have a structure and porosity that resembles cancellous bone and they ideally address capillary and bone ingrowth. Calcium-based ceramics, calcium sulfate, calcium phosphate, and tricalcium phosphate are most commonly used. All are osteoconductive, but they vary in their strength and rate of resorption. Calcium sulfate has a rapid resorption period of approximately 6 weeks. Although this may be ideal for early bone formation, it can lead to serous wound drainage and potential wound complications. Calcium phosphate has markedly higher compressive strength than cancellous bone. Studies have shown improved compressive strength and stability and early weight bearing after internal fixation of calcaneal fractures.[47] The resorption rate varies depending on the form, but it generally resorbs over 6 months to 1 year. Tricalcium phosphate has a compressive and tensile strength similar to that of cancellous bone, and it is not suited for load-bearing applications. Resorption occurs at between 6 and 18 months. These grafts commonly are used in combination or along with osteoinductive agents to enhance their efficacy.[44,47]

Osteobiologic agents refer to the osteoinductive proteins and osteogenic cells that are used to promote bone healing. The common agents include demineralized bone matrix, bone morphogenetic protein (BMP), bone marrow, and platelet-rich plasma (PRP). Demineralized bone matrix is allograft that has been processed to remove the mineral phase of bone and leave the proteinaceous growth factors, making it an effective osteoinductive agent. However, the content and activity of these osteoinductive agents varies widely between products and the way in which they are processed, making it difficult to assess efficacy.[44]

BMPs are a family of growth factors, many of which have osteoinductive properties. There are two commercially available recombinant human (rh) BMPs: rhBMP-2 and rhBMP-7. These are currently FDA-approved for use in acute open tibia fractures, lumbar interbody fusion, and tibial nonunions. Although they are often used in foot and ankle surgery to augment fracture fixations, repair nonunions, and aid in arthrodesis, these uses remain off-label.[48-50] There is ample evidence to suggest the efficacy of BMPs in foot and ankle fusion. In one study of 69 high-risk patients (112 fusion sites) undergoing ankle and hindfoot arthrodesis augmented by rhBMP-2, there was a 96% fusion rate at a mean of 11 weeks.[48] Another study of 35 high-risk patients undergoing ankle and hindfoot fusion with the use of rhBMP-2 demonstrated an 84% incidence of union.[49] A 2009 study[50] reported on use of rhBMP-7 as an adjunct to ankle and hindfoot arthrodesis in 19 patients, and successful union in 90%

of patients. These studies were all retrospective, and the determination of "high-risk" varied and included, but was not limited to, patients who were smokers, had peripheral vascular disease and/or diabetes, were having revision surgery, and had a history of nonunion. The data suggest that BMPs are an effective adjunct in these complex cases.

Bone marrow aspirate and PRP have been used extensively to augment bone healing. Bone marrow aspirate is obtained for its osteogenic stem cells and is often harvested from the calcaneus, tibia, and iliac crest, although the iliac crest has the highest concentration of these mesenchymal stem cells. Bone marrow aspirate is commonly mixed with allograft or a synthetic substitute for its osteoconductive properties.[45] PRP is derived from autologous blood and is defined as a volume of plasma with a platelet concentration higher than five times the physiologic level. Platelets contain osteoinductive growth factors, and PRP has a concentration of these growth factors that is 300% to 500% higher than usual levels. In one study of 62 high-risk patients undergoing 123 ankle and foot fusions augmented with PRP, ankle and hindfoot arthrodeses had union rates of 95% and 92%, respectively.[51] In a 2005 study,[52] investigators compared the rates of syndesmotic fusion in Agility (DePuy) total ankle replacement with and without PRP. At 6 months, syndesmotic fusion occurred in 85% of control group patients versus 97% in the PRP group. Fusion at 6 months for smokers was 50% in the control group and 80% in the PRP group.

Osteobiologic "devices" can be used as adjuvants to promote bone healing and arthrodesis. These include electrical and ultrasound bone stimulators and high-energy extracorporeal shock wave therapy (ESWT). The mechanisms of action for these devices are not fully understood and are beyond the scope of this chapter but warrant a brief introduction. The use of electrical current to stimulate bone formation was first reported in 1955. Bone stimulators can be internal or external devices and use either electrical current or low-intensity ultrasound to promote healing. A successful association has been shown between electrical stimulation and bone growth, typically in long bone nonunions or spinal fusion. When an internal bone stimulator was used as an adjunct to hindfoot arthrodesis in high-risk patients in one study,[53] successful arthrodesis was demonstrated in 92% of patients.

ESWT is also being used to treat foot and ankle pathology, typically recalcitrant plantar fasciitis and nonunions. It is believed to induce inflammation, increase microcirculation, and stimulate cell growth that leads to tissue healing. In regard to bone healing, it is thought to induce trabecular microfractures that stimulate fracture healing. However, the mechanism is not fully understood at this time. Metatarsal nonunions treated with ESWT had a 90% success rate at 1 year.[54] There does not seem to be a specific role for ESWT in primary hindfoot arthrodesis at this time.[54]

Summary

Hindfoot arthritis can occur as the result of traumatic, inflammatory, or degenerative processes. Techniques continue to evolve to promote improved wound healing and alignment, increase fusion rates while decreasing time to union, reduce postoperative disability, and contribute to optimal patient outcomes. The role of synthetic and biologic adjuvants in hindfoot arthrodesis continues to expand and will be vital in the treatment of patients at high risk for this condition.

Annotated References

1. Seybold JD, Kadakia AR: Foot arthritis, in Parekh SG, ed: *Foot & Ankle Surgery*. New Delhi, India: Jaypee Brothers Medical Publishers, 2012, pp 175-237.

   This text provides a review of the anatomy and biomechanics of the hindfoot. It also reviews diagnosis and treatment options for hindfoot and midfoot arthritis.

2. Sammarco VJ: The talonavicular and calcaneocuboid joints: Anatomy, biomechanics, and clinical management of the transverse tarsal joint. *Foot Ankle Clin* 2004;9(1):127-145.

3. Thordarson DB: Fusion in posttraumatic foot and ankle reconstruction. *J Am Acad Orthop Surg* 2004;12(5):322-333.

4. Crevoisier X: The isolated talonavicular arthrodesis. *Foot Ankle Clin* 2011;16(1):49-59.

   This article provides an overview of the indications, surgical techniques, biomechanical consequences, and results associated with TN arthrodesis, and discusses the relationship between the pathologic conditions treated and the results obtained. Level of evidence: V.

5. Wülker N, Stukenborg C, Savory KM, Alfke D: Hindfoot motion after isolated and combined arthrodeses: Measurements in anatomic specimens. *Foot Ankle Int* 2000;21(11):921-927.

6. Jagadale VS: Arthritis of the ankle and hindfoot, in Means KW, Kortebein P, eds: *Geriatrics*. New York, NY, Demos Medical, 2013, pp 101-103.

   This text provides an overview of the etiology and pathophysiology of ankle and hindfoot arthritis.

7. Radnay CS, Clare MP, Sanders RW: Subtalar fusion after displaced intra-articular calcaneal fractures: Does initial operative treatment matter? *J Bone Joint Surg Am* 2009;91(3):541-546.

   This article presents a consecutive series of 69 patients who underwent ST fusion after calcaneus fracture. Thirty-four patients had previous open reduction and internal fixation (ORIF) of their calcaneus and the other 35 patients were treated nonsurgically. Better functional outcomes and fewer wound complications occurred in the ORIF group. Level of evidence: III.

8. Jeng C, Campbell J: Current concepts review: The rheumatoid forefoot. *Foot Ankle Int* 2008;29(9):959-968.

   This review discusses the diagnosis and pathophysiology of RA and the current options available to manage the effects of this disease on the forefoot. Level of evidence: V.

9. Popelka S, Hromádka R, Vavrík P, et al: Isolated talonavicular arthrodesis in patients with rheumatoid arthritis of the foot and tibialis posterior tendon dysfunction. *BMC Musculoskelet Disord* 2010;11:38.

   This is a retrospective review of 26 patients with RA and posterior tibial tendon dysfunction who were treated with isolated TN arthrodesis. They demonstrated excellent pain relief and no progression of deformity. Level of evidence: IV.

10. Trepman E, Nihal A, Pinzur MS: Current topics review: Charcot neuroarthropathy of the foot and ankle. *Foot Ankle Int* 2005;26(1):46-63.

11. Saville P, Longman CF, Srinivasan SC, Kothari P: Medial approach for hindfoot arthrodesis with a valgus deformity. *Foot Ankle Int* 2011;32(8):818-821.

    This is a retrospective review of 18 patients with severe valgus deformity who underwent hindfoot arthrodesis through a medial-only approach. They reported excellent deformity correction and only one nonunion and avoided the potential complications associated with the lateral approach. Level of evidence: IV.

12. Doyle T, Napier RJ, Wong-Chung J: Recognition and management of Müller-Weiss disease. *Foot Ankle Int* 2012;33(4):275-281.

    An overview of the diagnosis and management of Müller-Weiss disease is presented. The authors introduce a series of 12 patients treated for this condition over a 10-year period. Level of evidence: IV.

13. Coester LM, Saltzman CL, Leupold J, Pontarelli W: Long-term results following ankle arthrodesis for post-traumatic arthritis. *J Bone Joint Surg Am* 2001;83(2):219-228.

14. Knupp M, Stufkens SA, Hintermann B: Triple arthrodesis. *Foot Ankle Clin* 2011;16(1):61-67.

    The authors describe their surgical technique for double arthrodesis and compare it to a standard triple arthrodesis.

They also discuss the indications for performing a double or triple arthrodesis. Level of evidence: V.

15. Sammarco VJ, Magur EG, Sammarco GJ, Bagwe MR: Arthrodesis of the subtalar and talonavicular joints for correction of symptomatic hindfoot malalignment. *Foot Ankle Int* 2006;27(9):661-666.

16. Ryssman DB, Myerson MS: Tendon transfers for the adult flexible cavovarus foot. *Foot Ankle Clin* 2011;16(3):435-450.

    This article discusses the etiology and evaluation of the adult cavovarus foot. It also covers treatment options for the various tendon transfer and arthrodesis procedures in the management of the cavovarus foot. Level of evidence: V.

17. Gluck GS, Heckman DS, Parekh SG: Tendon disorders of the foot and ankle, part 3: The posterior tibial tendon. *Am J Sports Med* 2010;38(10):2133-2144.

    This article reviews posterior tibial tendon pathology and the authors' preferred management depending on the stage of involvement. Level of evidence: V.

18. Carmont MR, Tomlinson JE, Blundell C, Davies MB, Moore DJ: Variability of joint communications in the foot and ankle demonstrated by contrast-enhanced diagnostic injections. *Foot Ankle Int* 2009;30(5):439-442.

    This study reviews 389 arthrograms of the hindfoot and midfoot and reports on the incidence of various communications between joints in the hindfoot and between the hindfoot and midfoot. Level of evidence: IV.

19. Khosla S, Thiele R, Baumhauer JF: Ultrasound guidance for intra-articular injections of the foot and ankle. *Foot Ankle Int* 2009;30(9):886-890.

    This cadaver study demonstrates how ultrasound guidance significantly increased injection accuracy into tarsometatarsal joints compared with palpation alone. Level of evidence: IV.

20. Chen L, Greisberg J: Achilles lengthening procedures. *Foot Ankle Clin* 2009;14(4):627-637.

    This article reviews the anatomic and evolutionary basis for human foot structure, implications of tight gastrocnemius, and specific disease states. Surgical releases for lengthening, including proximal gastrocnemius recession, Achilles tendon lengthening, and endoscopic recession, are detailed. Level of evidence: V.

21. Saltzman CL, el-Khoury GY: The hindfoot alignment view. *Foot Ankle Int* 1995;16(9):572-576.

22. Guermazi A, Hayashi D, Eckstein F, Hunter DJ, Duryea J, Roemer FW: Imaging of osteoarthritis. *Rheum Dis Clin North Am* 2013;39(1):67-105.

    This article reviews the roles of various imaging modalities including plain radiography, CT, MRI, ultrasound, and nuclear medicine studies as they pertain to evaluation for arthritis. Level of evidence: V.

23. Janisse DJ, Janisse E: Shoe modification and the use of orthoses in the treatment of foot and ankle pathology. *J Am Acad Orthop Surg* 2008;16(3):152-158.

    This article reviews the basic shoe modifications and orthoses for common foot and ankle pathologies. Level of evidence: V.

24. Logue JD: Advances in orthotics and bracing. *Foot Ankle Clin* 2007;12(2):215-232, v.

25. Bono CM, Berberian WS: Orthotic devices. Degenerative disorders of the foot and ankle. *Foot Ankle Clin* 2001;6(2):329-340.

26. Cahill AM, Cho SS, Baskin KM, et al: Benefit of fluoroscopically guided intraarticular, long-acting corticosteroid injection for subtalar arthritis in juvenile idiopathic arthritis. *Pediatr Radiol* 2007;37(6):544-548.

27. Drakonaki EE, Kho JS, Sharp RJ, Ostlere SJ: Efficacy of ultrasound-guided steroid injections for pain management of midfoot joint degenerative disease. *Skeletal Radiol* 2011;40(8):1001-1006.

    This is a review of 63 patients who underwent ultrasound-guided steroid injection for treatment of midfoot arthritis. Among patients, 57% maintained pain relief for up to 3 months, but fewer than 15% experienced pain relief that persisted beyond 3 months. Level of evidence: IV.

28. Brilhault J: Single medial approach to modified double arthrodesis in rigid flatfoot with lateral deficient skin. *Foot Ankle Int* 2009;30(1):21-26.

    This is a retrospective case series of 11 patients (14 feet) with fixed hindfoot valgus who underwent double arthrodesis through a medial incision. They demonstrated adequate deformity correction, successful fusion, no wound complications, and no CC arthrosis. Level of evidence: IV.

29. Sammarco GJ, Conti SF: Surgical treatment of neuroarthropathic foot deformity. *Foot Ankle Int* 1998;19(2):102-109.

30. Ishikawa SN, Murphy GA, Richardson EG: The effect of cigarette smoking on hindfoot fusions. *Foot Ankle Int* 2002;23(11):996-998.

31. Trnka HJ, Easley ME, Lam PW, Anderson CD, Schon LC, Myerson MS: Subtalar distraction bone block arthrodesis. *J Bone Joint Surg Br* 2001;83(6):849-854.

32. Deorio JK, Leaseburg JT, Shapiro SA: Subtalar distraction arthrodesis through a posterior approach. *Foot Ankle Int* 2008;29(12):1189-1194.

    The authors describe a surgical technique for performing distraction ST arthrodesis through a posterior approach and report the results of a series of six patients treated with this technique. Level of evidence: IV.

33. Muraro GM, Carvajal PF: Arthroscopic arthodesis of subtalar joint. *Foot Ankle Clin* 2011;16(1):83-90.

    This article reviews the indications and contraindications of arthroscopic ST arthrodesis. The surgical techniques are discussed and a literature review is performed to compare open and arthroscopic outcomes. Level of evidence: V.

34. Easley ME, Trnka HJ, Schon LC, Myerson MS: Isolated subtalar arthrodesis. *J Bone Joint Surg Am* 2000;82(5):613-624.

35. Lee KB, Park CH, Seon JK, Kim MS: Arthroscopic subtalar arthrodesis using a posterior 2-portal approach in the prone position. *Arthroscopy* 2010;26(2):230-238.

    This is a retrospective review of 16 patients who underwent posterior ST arthroscopy after intra-articular calcaneus fracture. The purpose of this study was to evaluate the results of the posterior arthroscopic approach. Level of evidence: IV.

36. Lechler P, Graf S, Köck FX, Schaumburger J, Grifka J, Handel M: Arthrodesis of the talonavicular joint using angle-stable mini-plates: A prospective study. *Int Orthop* 2012;36(12):2491-2494.

    This is a prospective study of 30 patients who underwent TN fusion with locking plate fixation. Outcomes were assessed based on radiographic fusion and American Orthopaedic Foot and Ankle Society score and visual analog scale scores. Level of evidence: IV.

37. Jarrell SE III, Owen JR, Wayne JS, Adelaar RS: Biomechanical comparison of screw versus plate/screw construct for talonavicular fusion. *Foot Ankle Int* 2009;30(2):150-156.

    This biomechanical cadaver study compares the strengths of three different TN fusion constructs. No significant differences were demonstrated between plate, plate and cancellous screw, and three screws with regard to bending stiffness or failure.

38. Barmada M, Shapiro HS, Boc SF: Calcaneocuboid arthrodesis. *Clin Podiatr Med Surg* 2012;29(1):77-89.

    This article reviews the main conditions of the lateral column and CC joint in particular. The surgical technique for isolated CC arthrodesis is discussed. Level of evidence: V.

39. Grunander TR, Thordarson DB: Results of calcaneocuboid distraction arthrodesis. *Foot Ankle Surg* 2012;18(1):15-18.

    This is a retrospective case series of 16 feet that underwent CC distraction arthrodesis. The authors report a high nonunion rate of 44% and recommend against this procedure for lateral column lengthening. Level of evidence: IV.

40. Jeng CL, Vora AM, Myerson MS: The medial approach to triple arthrodesis: Indications and technique for management of rigid valgus deformities in high-risk patients. *Foot Ankle Clin* 2005;10(3):515-521, vi-vii.

41. Jeng CL, Tankson CJ, Myerson MS: The single medial approach to triple arthrodesis: A cadaver study. *Foot Ankle Int* 2006;27(12):1122-1125.

42. Phisitkul P, Haugsdal J, Vaseenon T, Pizzimenti MA: Vascular disruption of the talus: Comparison of two approaches for triple arthrodesis. *Foot Ankle Int* 2013;34(4):568-574.

    This cadaver study demonstrates more disruption of talar blood supply with the isolated medial versus two-incision approach to triple arthrodesis.

43. Bibbo C, Anderson RB, Davis WH: Complications of midfoot and hindfoot arthrodesis. *Clin Orthop Relat Res* 2001;391:45-58.

44. Sammarco VJ, Chang L: Modern issues in bone graft substitutes and advances in bone tissue technology. *Foot Ankle Clin* 2002;7(1):19-41.

45. Guyton GP, Miller SD: Stem cells in bone grafting: Trinity allograft with stem cells and collagen/beta-tricalcium phosphate with concentrated bone marrow aspirate. *Foot Ankle Clin* 2010;15(4):611-619.

    This article provides a review of two bone graft options. Trinity (Osiris) is a combination of allograft bone and allograft stem cells and offers osteoconductive and osteoinductive as well as osteogenerative sources for new bone formation.

46. Winson IG, Higgs A: The use of proximal and distal tibial bone graft in foot and ankle procedures. *Foot Ankle Clin* 2010;15(4):553-558.

    This article provides a review of the indications, techniques, and outcomes related to autograft bone harvest in the proximal and distal tibia for procedures about the foot and ankle. Level of evidence: V.

47. Panchbhavi VK: Synthetic bone grafting in foot and ankle surgery. *Foot Ankle Clin* 2010;15(4):559-576.

    This article reviews the basic science and use of synthetic bone graft materials in foot and ankle surgery for conditions related to trauma, tumors, and infection. Level of evidence: V.

48. Bibbo C, Patel DV, Haskell MD: Recombinant bone morphogenetic protein-2 (rhBMP-2) in high-risk ankle and hindfoot fusions. *Foot Ankle Int* 2009;30(7):597-603.

    This is a retrospective review of the effect of rhBMP-2 on bone healing in patients undergoing high-risk ankle and hindfoot fusions. A total of 69 patients with 112 fusion sites were included in this review, and they demonstrated a 96% fusion rate. Level of evidence: IV.

49. El-Amin SF, Hogan MV, Allen AA, Hinds J, Laurencin CT: The indications and use of bone morphogenetic proteins in foot, ankle, and tibia surgery. *Foot Ankle Clin* 2010;15(4):543-551.

A review of strategies in tissue engineering and current applications and results of BMP use in tibia, foot, and ankle surgery are provided. Future applications of BMP and novel materials in foot and ankle surgery are also reviewed. Level of evidence: V.

50. Kanakaris NK, Mallina R, Calori GM, Kontakis G, Giannoudis PV: Use of bone morphogenetic proteins in arthrodesis: Clinical results. *Injury* 2009;40(suppl 3):S62-S66.

This is a review of 19 patients who underwent an arthrodesis procedure augmented by rhBMP-7. The authors noted a 90% fusion rate in the study population. Level of evidence: IV.

51. Bibbo C, Hatfield PS: Platelet-rich plasma concentrate to augment bone fusion. *Foot Ankle Clin* 2010;15(4):641-649.

This article provides a review of the basic science and clinical applications of PRP for the augmentation of bone healing in foot and ankle surgery. A classification system that assesses relative risks for poor bone healing and the need for orthobiologic augmentation is presented. Level of evidence: V.

52. Coetzee JC, Pomeroy GC, Watts JD, Barrow C: The use of autologous concentrated growth factors to promote syndesmosis fusion in the Agility total ankle replacement: A preliminary study. *Foot Ankle Int* 2005;26(10):840-846.

53. Donley BG, Ward DM: Implantable electrical stimulation in high-risk hindfoot fusions. *Foot Ankle Int* 2002;23(1):13-18.

54. Alvarez RG, Cincere B, Channappa C, et al: Extracorporeal shock wave treatment of non- or delayed union of proximal metatarsal fractures. *Foot Ankle Int* 2011;32(8):746-754.

This is a retrospective case series of 32 patients undergoing ESWT for metatarsal stress fractures. The treatment success rate was 89% at 6 months. Level of evidence: IV.

3: Arthritis of the Foot and Ankle

Chapter 11
Midfoot Arthritis

Kathryn L. Williams, MD

Introduction

Foot and ankle specialists routinely encounter patients with arthritis of the midfoot, which is a common cause of pain and disability. Its numerous etiologies include primary and inflammatory processes, but posttraumatic degeneration also is common. Mild to moderate symptoms can usually be managed with shoe modifications, orthotic devices, and joint injections. As the condition progresses, deformity and disabling pain can necessitate surgical treatment.

Anatomy and Biomechanics

The bones and ligaments of the midfoot have a complex relationship and varying degrees of stability. The midfoot is divided into three distinct longitudinal columns: middle, medial, and lateral. The medial column consists of the medial cuneiform-first metatarsal articulation. The central column includes the middle cuneiform-second metatarsal joint and the lateral cuneiform-third metatarsal joint and the intercuneiform joints. The lateral column is composed of the cuboid-fourth and cuboid-fifth metatarsal articulations (**Figure 1**). The bones of the midfoot joint complex form a Roman arch configuration with the apex at the second metatarsal, which is recessed 1 to 4 mm between the medial and lateral cuneiforms.

In addition to the bony arrangement, complex ligamentous connections consisting of dorsal, plantar, and intercuneiform ligaments provide increased stability to the midfoot. The plantar and intercuneiform ligaments are more important to stability than the dorsal ligaments. The Lisfranc ligament, which runs obliquely between the medial cuneiform and the base of the second metatarsal, is the largest in the complex, and a separate plantar ligament that connects the second and third metatarsals to the medial cuneiform is the strongest.

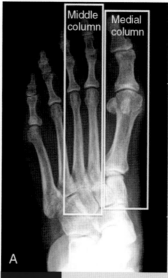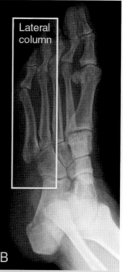

Figure 1 AP (**A**) and oblique (**B**) weight-bearing radiographs of the left foot with the medial, middle, and lateral columns marked. Note the primary middle column midfoot arthrosis.

Midfoot motion varies at each joint, with the lateral column having considerably more motion than the medial and middle columns. In the sagittal plane and supination-pronation, the cuboid-metatarsal joints have approximately 10° of motion, whereas cuneiform-metatarsal joint motion ranges between 0.6° and 3.5°, with the second metatarsal-middle cuneiform having the least motion.[1] Because of this rigidity, the second and third metatarsal cuneiform are likely sources of symptomatic arthritis. In conjunction with the Chopart joint, the midfoot complex allows the center of the load to be effectively transferred from the hindfoot and ankle through the midfoot to the forefoot.

Pathophysiology

Whether the cause of midfoot arthritis is primary osteoarthritis, traumatic degeneration, or inflammatory disorders such as gout or rheumatoid arthritis, articular cartilage damage is usually progressive. As the disease process advances, continued stress is placed across the metatarsal-cuneiform and intercuneiform joints, which leads to further deterioration of these joints. The destruction of the articular cartilage, periarticular osteophytes, and joint surface erosions commonly seen in osteoarthritis can disrupt the complex relationships of the articulations and small joints in the foot and can lead to instability and pain. With weight bearing, the loss of midfoot stability can lead to collapse of the longitudinal arch and a pes planus deformity. Patients with painful midfoot arthritis may adopt a stiffening strategy by allowing for less motion through the first metatarsal during normal walking. This results in an increase in calcaneal eversion and first metatarsal range of motion when compared with matched controls.[2] This condition reflects the loss of stability that occurs as a result of joint destruction. The degenerative process can also result in osteophytes over the dorsal aspect of the midfoot that make shoe wear difficult. With further deterioration of the midfoot and worsening instability of the joint complex, a progressive deformity of pronation, dorsiflexion, and/or abduction can develop.

Incidence and Etiology

The multiple etiologies of midfoot arthritis include inflammatory disorders such as rheumatoid arthritis and gout, neuropathic degeneration, degenerative joint disease or osteoarthritis, and trauma to the midfoot joint complex. Although posttraumatic midfoot arthritis can occur at any age with a history of trauma, patients with primary osteoarthritis of the midfoot tend to be older and may have a wide spectrum of deformity and a number of affected joints. Anatomic and/or mechanical factors may be involved in the development of primary degenerative arthritis, such as a short first metatarsal or a long second metatarsal. Advanced adult-acquired flatfoot, especially in the setting of a hypermobile first ray, can also be a predisposing factor for midfoot arthritis. The typical deformity is hindfoot valgus, midfoot abduction, and collapse of the longitudinal arch.

Trauma is likely the leading cause of midfoot arthritis. Cartilage damage at the time of injury, whether the injury involves a fracture or is purely ligamentous, can lead to posttraumatic arthrosis of the tarsometatarsal (TMT) joint complex. This can occur despite advances in diagnosis of these injuries and aggressive surgical treatment to anatomically restore the relationships within the TMT joint complex. Persistent malalignment, collapse of the medial or lateral column of the foot, and significant articular injury can be seen with posttraumatic arthrosis.

Clinical Presentation

Pain is the most commonly reported symptom among patients with midfoot arthritis. Pain usually increases with weight bearing, and a deep, aching pain is often present at rest. Patients may also report bony prominences dorsally and associated swelling that can be worse when closed shoes are worn. The bony prominences can cause inflammation of the extensor tendons and pain with extension of the toes or nerve irritation against the osteophytes, which may lead to radiating pain to the big toe and first web space. Severe deformities such as arch collapse can develop as the condition progresses and cause difficulty with shoe wear. Ganglion cysts may be noted secondary to small rents in the TMT joint capsule and can present as soft-tissue masses that may change in size with activity.

A standing examination of the feet is initially performed to determine the amount of deformity. The examiner should then perform a systematic seated examination of both feet, evaluating range of motion of the ankle, hindfoot, and midfoot, taking care to identify a tight gastrocnemius muscle or Achilles tendon contracture. Each TMT joint should be palpated and tenderness noted, and a pronation-abduction midfoot stress maneuver can be performed. A skin and neurovascular examination should always be performed, especially when neuroarthropathy is suspected.

Standing AP, lateral, and oblique radiographs of the affected foot or feet are performed as part of the initial evaluation to identify the location and extent of the disease and determine the amount and focus of any deformity (Figure 2). It is important to note the apex of any collapse of the midfoot both in the coronal and sagittal planes so that reconstruction can focus on correction through the affected joints. For example, treatment of primary degenerative arthritis secondary to pes planovalgus deformity should focus on improvement of the abduction deformity as opposed to midfoot arthritis with rocker-bottom deformity and correction of the sagittal plane deformity.[3] CT with three-dimensional reconstruction can be helpful in the setting of severe deformity or if the amount of arthritis is not easily determined with radiographs, but this is not a weight-bearing study. MRI or bone scans may be of use if chronic osteomyelitis is suspected, but these studies rarely are needed.

Often, the physical examination and radiographs may yield insufficient information and further diagnostic studies will be indicated. Selective injections of lidocaine under ultrasound or fluoroscopic guidance into joints under clinical suspicion of involvement can indicate a patient's potential positive response to surgery.

Nonsurgical Treatment

Symptoms of midfoot arthritis are likely secondary to lack of stability, altered midfoot mechanics, and loading on the inflamed joints. Therefore, the goal of nonsurgical

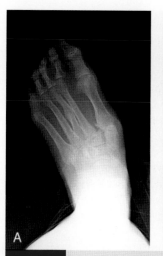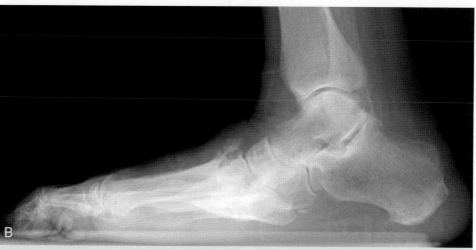

Figure 2 AP (**A**) and lateral (**B**) radiographs showing medial and middle column midfoot arthrosis with dorsal osteophytes and sagittal and coronal deformity. (Courtesy of Bruce E. Cohen, MD, Charlotte, NC.)

treatment is to employ methods that stabilize the joints and improve their mechanics.

NSAIDs and/or acetaminophen are commonly recommended as first-line pharmaceutical treatment. Selective injections into affected joints with local anesthetic with or without cortisone can help to determine which joints are symptomatic and their potential response to surgical treatment, although scientific evidence of their effectiveness is minimal, demonstrating short-term results. Published results on 59 patients who underwent ultrasound-guided steroid injections for midfoot arthritis showed a positive response for up to 3 months after injection, with 57.5% of patients still experiencing relief at 3 months.[4,5]

Shoe modifications and orthotic devices can help minimize motion and modify the load allowed through the midfoot and play a substantial role in nonsurgical management of midfoot arthritis. Rocker-bottom shoes or stiff-soled shoes with or without a steel shank modification are commonly used, but the addition of a stiff orthotic device may be adequate to simulate a stiff-soled shoe. A 2009 study demonstrated that a full-length carbon graphite insert reduced the magnitude and duration of plantar loading of the medial midfoot and offered symptomatic relief.[6] For more severe deformities, a brace extending more proximally, such as a patellar tendon-bearing brace, can restrict ankle motion and off-load the plantar foot by as much as 30%.[7]

Surgical Treatment

Medial Midfoot Joints
When nonsurgical methods have failed for treatment of midfoot arthritis, surgery is often a consideration. The extent of the surgical treatment is determined by the degree of deformity and symptoms. Simple resection of prominent bony prominences may improve symptoms with shoe wear but likely will not relieve all pain. Arthrodesis of the medial and middle columns of the midfoot is considered the preferred treatment for most surgical approaches targeting arthritis of the TMT joint and naviculocuneiform joint. In situ arthrodesis is acceptable only for patients who have normal weight-bearing radiographic findings; often, a deformity correction is necessary with or without osteotomies. The goal of arthrodesis is to achieve stability, and this often requires involvement of the first, second, and potentially third TMT joints. The intercuneiform joints often are included as well. The naviculocuneiform joint also is included if a sag is present on the lateral weight-bearing radiographs.

A variety of methods of internal fixation have been proposed and used. These include Kirschner wires and screws (both cannulated and noncannulated [2.7 to 4.5 mm in diameter]). More recently, plating (dorsal, medial, and/or plantar) has been used, often in combination with transarticular screws (the goal being to provide rigid internal fixation to facilitate successful fusion after appropriate joint preparation). Many different plate designs facilitate fusion of multiple joints with a single plate to obtain a stable construct (**Figure 3**). Authors of a 2012 study reported on 72 patients undergoing multijoint arthrodesis using a novel hybrid plate consisting of locking and nonlocking screws; healing rate and time compared favorably to other reported results, with a union rate of 93% by 16 weeks.[8]

Many patients will also have some degree of deformity in the sagittal, coronal, and/or transverse planes that must be addressed at the time of fusion; often there is a need for corrective osteotomies. An abduction and plantar flexion deformity can be corrected by medial

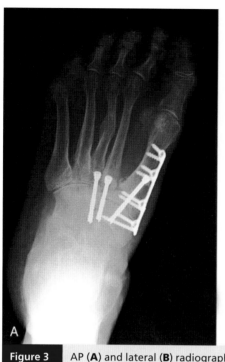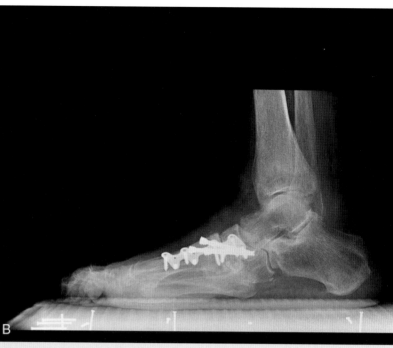

Figure 3 AP (**A**) and lateral (**B**) radiographs after medial and middle column arthrodesis for abduction deformity, sagittal midfoot collapse, and midfoot arthritis. (Courtesy of Bruce E. Cohen, MD, Charlotte, NC.)

and plantar closing wedge osteotomies, respectively. Concomitant procedures such as peroneus brevis release or lengthening, peroneus longus to brevis transfer, and Achilles or gastrocnemius lengthening can aid in correction and maintenance of deformity. The addition of autograft or allograft including demineralized bone matrix can be used to fill any defects at the fusion site and to aid healing, but no randomized controlled trials exist to support use in all midfoot arthrodesis.

Authors of a 2011 study reported on 95 patients (104 feet) who underwent midfoot arthrodesis and deformity correction with or without gastrocnemius recession for primary midfoot arthritis with a mean age at surgery of 62.[9] Of the 68 patients (74 feet) available for analysis, there was a mean follow-up of 56 months; in 62 of those feet, multiple joints were fused, involving only the medial and middle columns. The overall union rate was 92%. Revision arthrodesis was required in seven of eight nonunions. The four major complications included three deep infections and one case of complex regional pain syndrome (CRPS). Minor complications including delayed wound healing and union, stress fracture, and failed hardware occurred at a rate of 11%. The pain score improved from a mean of 6.9 preoperatively to 2.3 postoperatively, with a mean increase in American Orthopaedic Foot & Ankle Society (AOFAS) score of 46.7.[9]

Lateral Column

Regardless of the etiology, treatment of lateral TMT joint arthrosis remains challenging. Often, there is radiographic evidence of arthritis with minimal or no symptoms. However, when symptoms are present and nonsurgical measures have failed, surgical options continue to be a subject of controversy. Because of the increased mobility of the lateral column relative to the medial and middle, arthrodesis usually is not recommended. Arthrodesis of the lateral column may lead to complications such as nonunion, chronic lateral foot pain, or an increased rate of chronic stress fractures. In the setting of neuroarthropathic rocker-bottom deformity, arthrodesis of the lateral column can provide improvement in pain and functional capacity, but lateral foot stiffness and prominence of the lateral midfoot continue to be of concern.[10]

Other surgical techniques have focused on maintaining motion across the fourth and fifth TMT joints with interpositional arthroplasty to avoid arthrodesis of the lateral column. Resection of the lateral TMT joints with soft-tissue interposition using a peroneus tertius tendon showed a 35% decrease in pain and subjective maintenance of lateral column motion in a small series of patients.[11] A ceramic spherical interpositional arthroplasty has been developed as an alternative motion-preserving procedure (**Figure 4**). Authors of a 2007 study reported on 11 patients who underwent placement of a ceramic spherical implant into the resected fourth and/or fifth

TMT joint with an average AOFAS score improvement of 87%, and all patients reported satisfaction with their surgery at 34 months' follow-up.[12] There was one patient with asymptomatic implant subsidence. Authors of a 2012 study presented a case series reporting on five patients with an average follow-up of 18 months who underwent ceramic interpositional arthroplasty for osteoarthritis and posttraumatic arthritis.[13] All patients had subjective improvements in pain and maintained some motion of the lateral column, and there were no implant failures. Ceramic spherical interpositional arthroplasty may be a viable surgical option for lateral column arthritis, but long-term studies are currently lacking.

Other Osteotomies

Concomitant procedures including osteotomies may be required to correct coexisting deformity of the ankle, hindfoot, or forefoot. Symptomatic hallux valgus and second hammer toe can often be corrected by a first TMT joint fusion, but a hallux proximal phalanx medial closing wedge also may be needed. Hindfoot valgus or varus may necessitate a medial displacement calcaneal osteotomy or lateral closing wedge calcaneal osteotomy, respectively, and a lateral column lengthening may be needed with associated severe pes planovalgus. Ankle varus or valgus deformity without severe degenerative radiographic changes may necessitate a distal tibial osteotomy. It is important to evaluate the alignment of the entire lower leg, foot, and ankle when determining surgical treatment to avoid complications related to underappreciated coexisting deformities.

Complications

There are several types of complications related to midfoot arthrodesis.[14] Complications are associated with wound healing, infection (3%, both deep and superficial), peripheral nerve injury (9%), painful neuroma formation (7%), and nonunion of midfoot arthrodesis (3% to 8%, with a higher likelihood in elderly patients). Implant complications include screw irritation or breakage (9%). Long-term complications include development of secondary arthritis in adjacent joints (4.5%), and rare complications involve asymptomatic nonunion, wound slough, superficial infections, CRPS, and stress fractures.[3,9,15] Painful conditions including sesamoid pain, lateral foot pain, and metatarsalgia have been reported in up to nearly 40% of patients after midfoot fusion.[3,15]

Wound-healing complications can affect 3% to 50% of patients with diabetes who undergo revision surgery. Appropriate patient selection and assessment of comorbid conditions can help to minimize wound-healing complications. A patient's vascular status can be evaluated

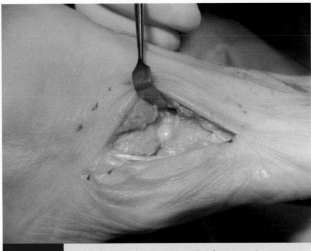

Figure 4 Intraoperative photograph of a ceramic interpositional arthroplasty at the fifth tarsometatarsal joint. (Courtesy of Bruce E. Cohen, MD, Charlotte, NC.)

with a physical examination and/or noninvasive arterial studies. Transcutaneous oxygen measurements can be helpful, with pressures higher than 40 mm Hg predictive of wound healing. For patients with chronic disease, nutritional status should be evaluated, and, if poor, improved upon before elective surgery. Minor wound complications can usually be managed with local wound care, but when wound problems are more severe, débridement with placement of a negative-pressure dressing or skin graft may be required.

Nonunion rates for midfoot arthrodesis range from 3% to 8%.[3,9,14] There has been no substantial difference between nonunion rates when arthrodesis is performed for posttraumatic versus primary midfoot arthritis.[9,13] A nonunion of an isolated or limited joint fusion often is symptomatic versus a nonunion associated with a larger fusion procedure.

Primary Arthrodesis for Trauma

Because of the high incidence of painful posttraumatic midfoot arthritis despite anatomic reduction and stable internal fixation, the ideal surgical treatment for TMT joint fracture-dislocations has become a topic of debate. These injuries are uncommon but have a high potential to cause chronic disability. Open anatomic reduction with internal fixation traditionally was the initial treatment for these injuries, with arthrodesis reserved as a salvage procedure for those who developed painful posttraumatic arthritis and/or deformity. Some authors, however, have advocated primary arthrodesis as a favorable treatment option for TMT joint injuries.

Authors of a 2006 study performed a prospective randomized controlled study comparing primary arthrodesis with open reduction internal fixation (ORIF) for initial treatment of primary ligamentous Lisfranc joint injuries with an average follow-up of 42 months.[16] Two years after surgery, AOFAS scores and the percentage of patients who had returned to a preinjury level of activity were both statistically significantly higher in the arthrodesis group.[16] The subsequent surgery rate was four times higher in the ORIF group, and 75% of ORIF-group patients showed loss of correction, increasing deformity, and degenerative joint disease on follow-up radiographs.[16] The authors suggest that primary stable arthrodesis may be a better alternative, primarily for ligamentous Lisfranc joint injuries.

A prospective randomized study of 32 patients at an average follow-up of 53 months was performed in which primary ORIF was compared to primary arthrodesis for acute TMT joint fractures and fracture-dislocations.[17] There were no statistically significant differences in the two groups with regard to Short Form 36 (SF-36) or Short Musculoskeletal Function Assessment (SMFA) scores, but the revision surgery rate in the ORIF group was nearly five times higher. A retrospective comparative study conducted in 2012 looked at partial primary arthrodesis for purely ligamentous injuries compared to combined osseous and ligamentous injuries and found no difference in AOFAS scores, visual analog scale (VAS) pain scores, or return to preinjury level of activity between the two groups.[18] Primary arthrodesis for high-energy injuries of the TMT joint complex is emerging as an encouraging option for primary treatment.

Malunion

Malunions following midfoot fusions can usually be avoided by having thorough knowledge of foot and ankle anatomy and a detailed preoperative examination and surgical planning. When they do occur, malunions can be categorized as varus or valgus, dorsiflexion or plantar flexion, or abduction or adduction deformities. If attempts at nonsurgical management with modified shoe wear and orthotic devices fail, these deformities are addressed surgically by an osteotomy and rigid fixation through the apex of the deformity. The position and motion of the ankle, hindfoot, and forefoot must also be assessed and necessary corrections made as needed.

Nonunion

Treatment of a nonunion depends mainly on a patient's symptoms and any mechanical instability. Isolated or limited joint fusions tend to be more symptomatic than those that are performed as part of a larger joint complex fusion. If a painless nonunion without mechanical

instability of the limb is present, shoe modifications such as an extended steel shank, rocker-bottom, or offset soles may be tried. Other alternatives to revision surgery include a trial of bracing or casting and external bone stimulators. If progressive pain and/or deformity are present, revision surgical treatment is indicated.

As with any nonunion, a workup should include assessment of a patient's history (tobacco use), nutritional and metabolic status, signs of infection, and any pharmaceutical agents that may hinder healing. The use of allograft and/or autograft with or without bone matrix protein derivatives should be considered. Compression fixation techniques with rigid internal fixation should be used, and internal or external bone stimulators should be considered for patients at exceptionally high risk for wound-healing complications.

Functional Outcomes Following Midfoot Arthrodesis

Because midfoot arthritis can be debilitating, a successful arthrodesis can result in a substantial improvement in pain, and, often, function. Authors of a 2007 study reported a postoperative AOFAS score of 83.9, an improvement from 34.1 preoperatively, as well as significant improvements in the pain, disability, and activity limitation categories.[3] Midfoot arthrodesis for primary arthritis as reported by authors of a 2011 study was associated with a nearly 90% satisfaction rate as well as similar improvements in AOFAS score. Nonunion was the most common complication associated with patient dissatisfaction and poor outcomes.[9]

Summary

Midfoot arthritis has many etiologies and can be very debilitating. If nonsurgical treatment fails, surgical treatment should focus on identifying and treating symptomatic joints and correcting underlying deformity. Primary fusion for trauma to the TMT joint complex is a reasonable option for treatment of these severe injuries.

Annotated References

1. Ouzounian TJ, Shereff MJ: In vitro determination of midfoot motion. *Foot Ankle* 1989;10(3):140-146.

2. Rao S, Baumhauer JF, Tome J, Nawoczenski DA: Comparison of in vivo segmental foot motion during walking and step descent in patients with midfoot arthritis and matched asymptomatic control subjects. *J Biomech* 2009;42(8):1054-1060.

   In this study, the authors compared in vivo segmental foot motion during walking and step descent in patients with and without midfoot arthritis. With step descent, there was increased first metatarsal plantar flexion and calcaneal eversion in the midfoot arthritis group, which may have caused increased articular stresses and helps to explain evolution of symptoms in patients with midfoot arthritis. Level of evidence: V.

3. Jung HG, Myerson MS, Schon LC: Spectrum of operative treatments and clinical outcomes for atraumatic osteoarthritis of the tarsometatarsal joints. *Foot Ankle Int* 2007;28(4):482-489.

4. Drakonaki EE, Kho JS, Sharp RJ, Ostlere SJ: Efficacy of ultrasound-guided steroid injections for pain management of midfoot joint degenerative disease. *Skeletal Radiol* 2011;40(8):1001-1006.

    This is a retrospective review of 59 patients with symptomatic midfoot joint degenerative changes who underwent ultrasound-guided steroid injections. Pain relief was seen in the majority of patients at 3 months (57.5%), but after 3 months fewer than 15% reported continued relief.

5. Khosla ST, Thiele R, Baumhauer JF: Ultrasound guidance for intra-articular injections of the foot and ankle. *Foot Ankle Int* 2009;30(9):886-890.

    The authors used a cadaver model to compare the accuracy of intra-articular injections of the foot and ankle using palpation versus dynamic ultrasound. Needle placement into the ankle and the subtalar or first and second TMT joints was confirmed with radiopaque dye/methylene blue mixture. The use of ultrasound significantly improved the accuracy of the injection compared to palpation. Level of evidence: V.

6. Rao S, Baumhauer JF, Becica L, Nawoczenski DA: Shoe inserts alter plantar loading and function in patients with midfoot arthritis. *J Orthop Sports Phys Ther* 2009;39(7):522-531.

    The authors assessed the effectiveness of full-length insert on the function of patients with midfoot arthritis and determined if there was a difference in plantar loading between full-length and three-quarter–length carbon graphite inserts. The full-length insert improved symptoms and reduced the magnitude and duration of loading under the medial midfoot. Level of evidence: IV.

7. Saltzman CL, Johnson KA, Goldstein RH, Donnelly RE: The patellar tendon-bearing brace as treatment for neurotrophic arthropathy: A dynamic force monitoring study. *Foot Ankle* 1992;13(1):14-21.

8. Filippi J, Myerson MS, Scioli MW, et al: Midfoot arthrodesis following multi-joint stabilization with a novel hybrid plating system. *Foot Ankle Int* 2012;33(3):220-225.

    The authors report on a multicenter review of the use of a novel hybrid plating system that incorporates locked and nonlocked compression screw multijoint midfoot arthrodesis. The healing rate and time to fusion compared favorably to other studies, and the described plate was deemed a reasonable alternative in multijoint disease. Level of evidence: IV.

9. Nemec SA, Habbu RA, Anderson JG, Bohay DR: Outcomes following midfoot arthrodesis for primary arthritis. *Foot Ankle Int* 2011;32(4):355-361.

    This is a retrospective case series of 68 patients (74 feet) who underwent midfoot arthrodesis for primary midfoot arthritis (mean age of 62 years and mean follow-up of 56 months). Authors reported a union rate of 92% and a complication rate of 4%, including three deep infections and one CRPS. AOFAS scores improved from a mean of 32 preoperatively to a mean of 79 postoperatively. Level of evidence: IV.

10. Raikin SM, Schon LC: Arthrodesis of the fourth and fifth tarsometatarsal joints of the midfoot. *Foot Ankle Int* 2003;24(8):584-590.

11. Berlet GC, Hodges Davis W, Anderson RB: Tendon arthroplasty for basal fourth and fifth metatarsal arthritis. *Foot Ankle Int* 2002;23(5):440-446.

12. Shawen SB, Anderson RB, Cohen BE, Hammit MD, Davis WH: Spherical ceramic interpositional arthroplasty for basal fourth and fifth metatarsal arthritis. *Foot Ankle Int* 2007;28(8):896-901.

13. Viens NA, Adams SB Jr, Nunley JA II: Ceramic interpositional arthroplasty for fourth and fifth tarsometatarsal joint arthritis. *J Surg Orthop Adv* 2012;21(3):126-131.

    This is a retrospective consecutive case series evaluating the short-term results for five patients who underwent ceramic interpositional arthroplasty of the lateral TMTJs. No implant failures or subsidence were reported at 18 months. Level of evidence: IV.

14. Bibbo C, Anderson RB, Davis WH: Complications of midfoot and hindfoot arthrodesis. *Clin Orthop Relat Res* 2001;391:45-58.

15. Rao S, Nawoczkenski DA, Baumhauer J: Midfoot arthritis: Nonoperative options and decision making for fusion. *Tech Foot Ankle Surg* 2008;7(3):188-195.

    The authors discuss strategies for nonsurgical management and detail surgical techniques for TMT fusion. Outcomes including complication rate details are presented. Level of evidence: IV.

16. Ly TV, Coetzee JC: Treatment of primarily ligamentous Lisfranc joint injuries: Primary arthrodesis compared with open reduction and internal fixation. A prospective, randomized study. *J Bone Joint Surg Am* 2006;88(3):514-520.

17. Henning JA, Jones CB, Sietsema DL, Bohay DR, Anderson JG: Open reduction internal fixation versus primary arthrodesis for lisfranc injuries: A prospective randomized study. *Foot Ankle Int* 2009;30(10):913-922.

3: Arthritis of the Foot and Ankle

This is a prospective randomized trial of 32 patients with a mean follow-up of 53 months who underwent either primary arthrodesis (PA) or primary ORIF for dislocations and fracture-dislocations of the TMT joint. There was no difference in satisfaction rates, SF-36 scores, or SMFA scores between the two groups, but the revision surgery rate was 78.6% in the ORIF group and 16.7% in the PA group. Level of evidence: I.

18. Reinhardt KR, Oh LS, Schottel P, Roberts MM, Levine D: Treatment of Lisfranc fracture-dislocations with primary partial arthrodesis. *Foot Ankle Int* 2012;33(1):50-56.

The authors present their results on 25 patients who underwent primary partial arthrodesis for primarily ligamentous or combined osseus and ligamentous Lisfranc fracture-dislocation in this retrospective comparative study. With a mean follow-up of 42 months, there was an 84% satisfaction rate and an 85% return to preinjury activity level. The mean AOFAS and VAS pain scores were 81 and 1.8, respectively, with no difference between the two groups. Six patients (24%) required further surgeries. Level of evidence: III.

Chapter 12

Adult-Acquired Flatfoot and Posterior Tibial Tendon Dysfunction

J. Kent Ellington, MD, MS

Introduction

Adult-acquired flatfoot deformity (AAFD) is a common problem. The most common etiology of AAFD is posterior tibial tendon dysfunction (PTTD). Other causes of AAFD include osteoarthritis, inflammatory arthropathies, posttraumatic deformity, and congenital anomalies. Symptoms usually begin in the fifth and sixth decades of life, and treatment is based on the severity of pain and deformity.

Anatomy and Pathophysiology

The posterior tibial tendon (PTT) is the primary dynamic stabilizer of the arch. It originates from the posterior tibia and fibula and the interosseous membrane. It courses behind and around the medial malleolus and inserts mainly on the navicular, but has attachments to the cuneiforms and metatarsal bases. PTTD is caused by an elongated or degenerative tendon over the course of its watershed area from the tip of the medial malleolus to 2 cm distal.[1] In addition to tendon dysfunction, other structures can be involved and exacerbate pain and deformity. The spring ligament, talonavicular capsule, and deltoid ligament all may contribute to pathology.

The spring ligament has two components: the superior medial and the inferior calcaneonavicular ligament. AAFD may compromise the superior portion, which combines with the deltoid ligament.[2] In rare instances, isolated spring ligament rupture may be the etiology of AAFD.

Dr. Ellington or an immediate family member is a member of a speakers' bureau or has made paid presentations on behalf of Arthrex and BME; serves as a paid consultant to or is an employee of Amniox, Arthrex, BME, Conventusortho, Pacira, and Zimmer; and has received research or institutional support from Amniox.

The PTT adducts and inverts the foot and plantarflexes the ankle. Adduction of the midfoot provides a rigid lever as a person progresses through the gait cycle during midstance and push-off. The antagonist to the posterior tibialis is the peroneus brevis. As PTTD progresses, the unopposed peroneus brevis causes attenuation of the spring ligament.[3] With further progression, the talar head falls into plantar flexion and the Achilles or gastrocnemius-soleus complex develops a contracture. The forefoot then abducts, creating talonavicular uncoverage. With advanced disease, flexible deformities can become rigid, limiting treatment options.

Etiology

Among AAFD's multiple etiologies, PTTD is the most common; consequently, AAFD treatment is directed toward this cause. AAFD also may develop after midfoot trauma, specifically resulting from an untreated Lisfranc injury. This untreated Lisfranc injury leads to arch collapse and forefoot abduction, often with associated arthritis. Inflammatory arthropathy such as rheumatoid arthritis may lead to AAFD, with midfoot arthritis leading to joint degeneration and deformity. Affected patients may also have simultaneous PTTD. Idiopathic osteoarthritis may lead to AAFD, but this is not as common. Congenital anomalies such as tarsal coalitions and accessory navicular also can be underlying causes of AAFD.

Although a PTT rupture may occur, the most common cause of PTTD is slow degeneration/elongation of the tendon, which decreases its elastic properties and ability to support the foot's medial column. This process has been confirmed histologically, demonstrating myxoid and mucinous degeneration in PTT samples taken from patients during reconstruction.[4] Visual inspection of the PTT during surgery confirms degenerative tendon with longitudinal tearing, disorganized collagen, tendinosis, and decreased excursion. This degenerative process may be painful, and resection of the diseased tendon is considered a useful adjunct during reconstruction to alleviate pain.

Classification

PTTD staging was first described in 1989[5] was later modified in 1996, and refined in 2007[6,7] (**Tables 1** and **2**). Other classification systems have been described.[8,9] Stage 1 PTTD is defined as tenosynovitis with retained strength (the patient can still perform a single-limb heel rise). No alteration of foot alignment is noted. Stage II PTTD is characterized by progressive deformity, which remains flexible, and decreased strength, demonstrated by the inability to perform a single-limb heel rise. Stage III PTTD is defined by a rigid planovalgus deformity, and stage IV involves changes to the ankle joint with deltoid laxity, resulting in ankle valgus deformity.

Stage I PTTD is attributable to tenosynovitis of the PTT. Patients report medial ankle and hindfoot pain. Their foot remains flexible and they are able to perform a single-heel rise; however, a patient may have pain with repetitive rising. The tendon has normal function and length.

Stage II PTTD is the most common presentation of AAFD. Affected patients have increased pain, progressive deformity in most cases, and cannot perform single-limb heel rise. However, they usually can perform a double-limb heel rise. Swelling is common and recently has been shown to be an excellent predictor of PTTD confirmed with MRI. Swelling in the distal PTT area, when correlated with MRI, had a sensitivity of 86% and specificity of 100% for PTT degeneration.[10] These patients continue to have a flexible deformity and, as deformity progresses, they may report lateral foot pain attributable to subtalar or subfibular impingement or peroneal tendinitis. Fibular stress fractures also can occur with severe deformity because of calcaneofibular abutment.

Stage III PPTD is characterized by a rigid deformity. The hindfoot is fixed in valgus and patients cannot perform a single-heel rise. Often, the subtalar joint is arthritic. Varying degrees of talonavicular and calcaneocuboid arthrosis may also be present. With advanced disease, deformity may develop further down the medial column, extending to the naviculocuneiform joints and the first tarsometatarsal (TMT) joint. This can be observed on a lateral radiograph with collapse at the naviculocuneiform joint and plantar gapping at the first TMT joint (**Figure 1**).

Stage IV PTTD is based on deformity located in the ankle joint (**Figure 2**). With prolonged AAFD, the deltoid is attenuated and its laxity contributes to ankle valgus. Patients can have either a stage II (flexible) or stage III

(rigid) deformity of the foot. All patients with an AAFD should obtain AP ankle radiographs to ensure ankle congruity.

Table 1

Clinical Staging of Posterior Tibial Tendon Dysfunction

Stage I	Pain over the posterior tibialis with no deformity
Stage II	Deformity is flexible A. Medial pain only B. Lateral pain
Stage III	Deformity is not flexible
Stage IV	Deformity is not flexible and changes at the ankle

(Reproduced from Alvarez RG, Price J, Marini A, Turner NS, Kitaoka HB: Adult acquired flatfoot deformity and posterior tibial tendon dysfunction, in Pinzur MS, ed: *Orthopaedic Knowledge Update Foot and Ankle*, ed 4. Rosemont, IL, American Academy of Orthopaedic Surgeons, 2008, pp 215–229.)

Clinical Presentation

Patients present with medial and, sometimes, lateral foot pain. Medial swelling is common, and prolonged ambulation and uneven terrain aggravate symptoms. Patients may report uneven shoe wear, with the medial aspect of the heel wearing out faster. Some patients report a prior injury, and many have been treated by their primary physicians for an "ankle sprain." Some patients state that they have had a flatfoot their entire life, which should raise suspicion for a tarsal coalition or accessory navicular. Comorbidities, specifically inflammatory conditions, should be documented.

Examination

The physical examination includes both standing and seated positions. In a standing position, a patient with AAFD will have a decreased arch, increased hindfoot valgus (**Figure 3**), and the "too many toes sign" (attributable to forefoot abduction) when viewed from behind. In the seated position, the flexibility of the hindfoot, Chopart joints, and the gastrocnemius-soleus complex are assessed. Findings should be compared to the opposite foot/ankle. A flexible deformity allows for osteotomies and tendon transfers, whereas rigid deformities are usually treated with arthrodesis procedures. Tightness of the heel cord is divided into a contracture of the Achilles tendon or gastrocnemius-soleus complex and is assessed

Table 2

Clinical Classification System for Posterior Tibial Tendon

Stage	Substage	Characteristic Clinical Findings	Radiographic Findings	Treatment
I	A: Inflammatory disease	Normal anatomy, tender PTT	Normal	NSAIDs, immobilization, ice, orthoses, tenosynovectomy, treat specific systemic disease
	B: Partial tear	Normal anatomy, tender PTT	Normal	Same as for substage A
	C: Partial tear with mild HF valgus	Slight HF valgus, tender PTT	Slight HF valgus	Same as for substage A
II	A1: HF valgus with flexible FF varus	Flexible HF valgus, flexible FF varus ± tender PTT	HF valgus, Meary angle disrupted, calcaneal pitch lost	Orthoses, medial slide calcaneal osteotomy, Strayer or Achilles tendon lengthening, FDL transfer (if deformity corrects only with ankle PF)
	A2: HF valgus with rigid FF varus	Flexible HF valgus, rigid FF varus ± tender PTT	Same as A1	Same as for substage A1, Cotton osteotomy
	B: FF abduction	Same as for substages A1 and A2 with FF abduction	HF valgus, talonavicular uncovering, FF abduction	Medial slide calcaneal osteotomy, lateral column lengthening, Strayer or Achilles tendon lengthening, FDL transfer
	C: Medial ray instability	Flexible HF valgus, fixed FF varus, medial column instability, first ray dorsiflexion with HF correction, sinus tarsi pain	HF valgus, first TMT joint plantar gaping	Medial slide calcaneal osteotomy, FDL transfer, Cotton osteotomy, or first TMT joint fusion
III	A: Rigid HF valgus	Rigid HF valgus, sinus tarsi pain	Decreased subtalar joint space, angle of Gissane sclerosis	Triple arthrodesis, custom AFO if not a surgical candidate
	B: FF abduction	Same as for substage IIIA, FF abduction	Same as for substage IIIA, FF abduction	Triple arthrodesis with lateral column lengthening, custom AFO if not a surgical candidate
IV	A: Rigid HF valgus, flexible ankle valgus, deltoid ligament insufficiency, minimal ankle arthritis	Flexible tibiotalar valgus	Tibiotalar valgus, HF valgus	Correct HF valgus, reconstruct deltoid ligament
	B: Significant ankle arthritis, with or without rigid ankle valgus	Rigid tibiotalar valgus	Tibiotalar valgus, HF valgus	Pantalar fusion or TTC fusion

AFO = ankle-foot orthosis, FDL = flexor digitorum longus, FF = forefoot, HF = hindfoot, NSAIDs = nonsteroidal anti-inflammatory drugs, PF = plantar flexion, PTT = posterior tibial tendon, TMT = tarsometatarsal, TTC = tibiotalocalcaneal.

(Adapted with permission from Bluman EM, Title CI, Myerson MS: Posterior tibial tendon rupture: A refined classification system. *Foot Ankle Clin* 2007;12:233–249.)

3: Arthritis of the Foot and Ankle

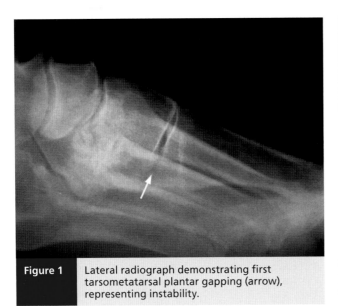

Figure 1 Lateral radiograph demonstrating first tarsometatarsal plantar gapping (arrow), representing instability.

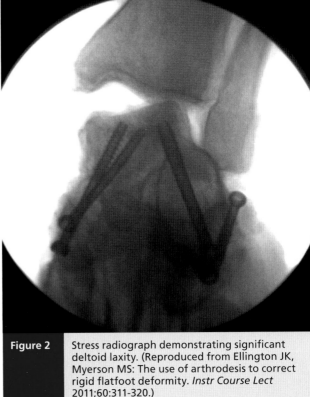

Figure 2 Stress radiograph demonstrating significant deltoid laxity. (Reproduced from Ellington JK, Myerson MS: The use of arthrodesis to correct rigid flatfoot deformity. *Instr Course Lect* 2011;60:311-320.)

by performing the Silfverskiold test. A patient performs this test by dorsiflexing the ankle with the knee flexed in the extended position. If ankle dorsiflexion increases above neutral only with knee flexion, then only the gastrocnemius is contracted (this is dependent on the location of the gastrocnemius origin). If ankle dorsiflexion does not increase with knee flexion, then the entire gastrocnemius-soleus complex is contracted. This detail is important for surgical planning. If the gastrocnemius is contracted, then it is lengthened, also known as a Strayer recession. If the entire complex is contracted, then Achilles tendon lengthening is performed. This procedure often involves a percutaneous triple-cut hemisection of the Achilles tendon. Swelling and pain with palpation over the course of the tendon and its insertion on the navicular are documented. An accessory navicular may become obvious when a painful prominence is present at the PTT insertion. Additional signs include a callus that may develop under the medial column with advancing deformity and possibly a medial rocker-bottom deformity. Patients may also experience tenderness in the sinus tarsi, subfibular area, and peroneal tendons. Finally, forefoot supination, also referred to as varus, is assessed in the seated position. With the hindfoot corrected to neutral, residual forefoot deformity may be apparent (**Figure 4**). It is important to ascertain if the forefoot supination is flexible (ie, the physician can manipulate the medial column back to a plantigrade position) because it is also involved in surgical planning.

One of the most sensitive tests for PTTD is the single-heel rise. The patient must elevate the unaffected limb from the floor. The physician views the patient from behind and asks him or her to rise up on their toes. An insufficient tendon is demonstrated by either the inability

to perform the rise because of weakness or pain or weak plantar flexion without evidence of hindfoot inversion as the patient rises onto the ball of the foot.

Imaging

Weight-bearing foot and ankle radiographs are necessary when evaluating patients with AAFD. The hindfoot alignment view can be useful as well, and is performed in the following manner: The gantry is placed behind the standing patient and raised 20° from the floor. The radiograph cassette is placed in front of the patient and positioned perpendicular to the x-ray beam. These radiographs will reveal the extent and location of deformity and the presence of arthritis or other conditions. An AP foot radiograph shows the extent of talonavicular uncoverage. A lateral foot radiograph is useful in measuring the Meary angle and medial cuneiform height (**Figure 5**). Lateral and oblique foot and axial heel radiographs may also demonstrate a tarsal coalition. A tarsal coalition (middle facet) is present when the C sign is on the lateral radiograph (this can also be observed on the axial view). The oblique foot radiograph will show a coalition at the calcaneonavicular joint. A weight-bearing AP radiograph of the ankle evaluates for stage IV PTTD and subfibular impingement (**Figure 3**).

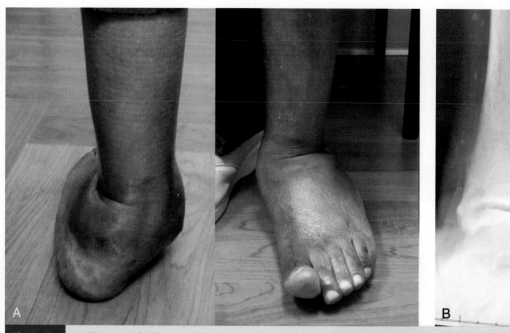
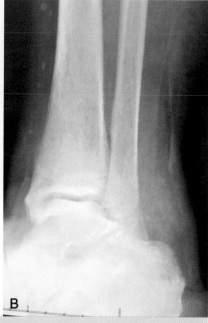

Figure 3   **A**, Photographs demonstrating substantial AAFD. **B**, Corresponding radiograph showing subfibular impingement.

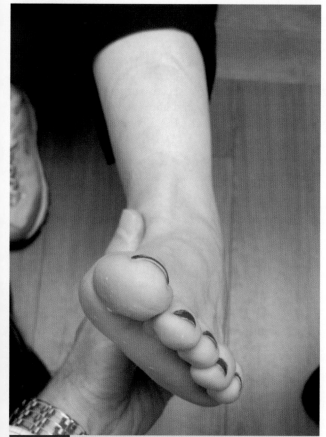

Figure 4   Photograph demonstrating residual forefoot varus after the hindfoot has been corrected to neutral.

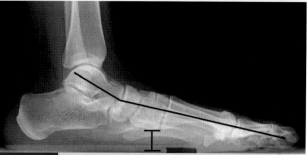

Figure 5   Radiograph showing the Meary angle (the line down the axis of the talus and first metatarsal; normal is 0 (± 10°). Medial cuneiform height is measured from the floor to the plantar aspect of the medial cuneiform (normal 15–25 mm).

Ultrasound can be used to evaluate the PTT, but its usefulness is user-dependent and no studies have provided prognostic information based on ultrasound studies. Ultrasound can also be used to evaluate the peroneal tendons.

MRI is the next-most-common imaging method after weight-bearing films. MRI is important in that it not only confirms PTTD, but also can help to evaluate the entire ankle and hindfoot. This additional information can be used to tailor a treatment plan. MRI can describe the degree of PTTD. For example, in **Figure 6**, the patient had stage I PTTD clinically, and the MRI demonstrates substantial tenosynovitis without tendinopathy.

CT traditionally has not been used for PTTD diagnosis because MRI is much more sensitive and accurate. However, certain centers have the ability to obtain

3: Arthritis of the Foot and Ankle

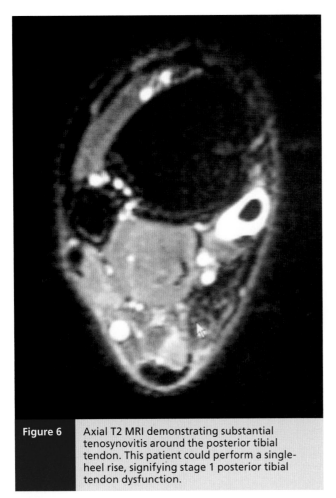

| Figure 6 | Axial T2 MRI demonstrating substantial tenosynovitis around the posterior tibial tendon. This patient could perform a single-heel rise, signifying stage 1 posterior tibial tendon dysfunction. |

weight-bearing CT scans. This novel technology, which is still in its infancy, can better detail deformity, presence of coalitions, associated arthritic joints, cystic development, and, to some degree, tendon degeneration. CT scans are mostly helpful in assessing hindfoot and transverse tarsal joints for arthritis. The presence of arthritis may lead a surgeon to consider an arthrodesis procedure instead of a joint-sparing reconstruction.

Nonsurgical Treatment

The goal of nonsurgical treatment is to decrease pain, improve function, protect the PTT, and prevent further deformity. A variety of modalities are available, ranging from custom braces or orthotics to off-the-shelf devices. Flexible deformities are treated with supportive devices and rigid deformities are treated with accommodative devices. Corticosteroid injections should never be administered around the PTT, but may be useful if administered intra-articularly.

Off-the-shelf options include orthotic devices with a longitudinal arch support, a variety of lace-up ankle braces (specifically, the PTTD brace), medial heel posting, and walker boots. Short leg casting is another strategy. Short leg casting and removable boots are an effective means with which to immobilize an inflamed foot. These devices are great options in the clinic setting for patients who are limping and/or experiencing pain or swelling. After the acute inflammatory symptoms resolve with immobilization, physical therapy can be initiated. Home exercises or supervised therapy has been shown to be equally effective in relieving pain and improving functional outcome in patients with stage 1 to 3 PTTD.[11]

Customized options include custom-molded orthotic devices and articulated and nonarticulated ankle-foot orthoses (AFOs). Traditionally, these braces include a full-length short leg molded polypropylene solid AFO. A University of California Biomechanics Laboratory insert is an effective strategy with reported success.[12] A customized leather gauntlet brace can also be used. Recent studies report the successful use of a "shell brace" that conserves hindfoot motion in most of the study patients.[13] Use of a short, customized articulated AFO combined with a physical therapy-directed exercise program has been demonstrated effective for stage II PTTD.[14] In a 2006 study, patients completed high-repetition exercises, aggressive plantar flexion activities, and an aggressive high-repetition home exercise program that included gastrocnemius-soleus complex tendon stretching.[14] Only 11% of patients progressed to surgery, and 89% were satisfied and demonstrated improved strength.[14] A short, customized articulated AFO also is the preferred brace among patients with PTTD.[15]

Surgical Treatment

Surgical treatment is offered to patients in whom nonsurgical treatment strategies fail. There are a variety of surgical procedures, each chosen to meet individual needs. The surgical decision-making process takes into account the stage of PTTD, patient age and activity level/demands, and extent of deformity. The goal is to reduce pain and improve function by obtaining a plantigrade foot. Contraindications include vascular disease or open wounds; these conditions should be treated appropriately before reconstruction.

Stage I PTTD

Surgical treatment is rarely indicated for stage I PTTD. Most patients respond well to immobilization. After symptoms improve, patients benefit from a rehabilitation program and supportive orthotic devices. For patients without deformity, open tenosynovectomy with repair of the PTT can improve symptoms. PTT tendoscopic synovectomy has been described as a minimally invasive and effective surgical procedure to treat patients with stage I PTTD.[16] It offers the advantages of less wound pain and fewer scar and wound complications. The authors advocated that if a tendon tear is observed during tendoscopy, it must be repaired with nonabsorbable sutures using a 3-cm or 4-cm incision.[16] However, tendoscopic procedures are not the standard in treatment of stage I PTTD. This technique can be technically difficult, visualization may be challenging, and there is a significant learning curve. After tenosynovectomy, patients are immobilized for 4 weeks and a rehabilitation program and use of a supportive orthotic device are initiated.

Stage II PTTD
Soft-Tissue Reconstruction Options
Patients with stage II PTTD in whom nonsurgical treatment fails usually undergo a reconstructive procedure consisting of osteotomies and tendon transfers. Soft-tissue repairs are rarely performed in isolation. Direct repair of the PTT is not recommended because the tendon is degenerated and will not heal. The mainstay of treatment is a medial displacement calcaneal osteotomy (MDCO) accompanied by a flexor digitorum longus (FDL) tendon transfer. However, in PTTD stage IIA1, a MDCO may not be required. The flexor hallucis longus has also been described, and some prefer the FHL because it is stronger.[17] The FDL is traced into the arch of the foot and tenotomy is performed with care to avoid injury to the nearby neurovascular bundle. The FDL is then transferred to the PTT stump or, more commonly, to the navicular through a drill hole and secured with a biotenodesis screw. The tendon transfer is tensioned with the ankle in mild plantar flexion and inversion of the foot. Also, the peroneus brevis has been described as an option in the revision setting or to augment a potential weak FDL tendon.[18] The purpose of these procedures is to improve pain and alignment and to avoid arthrodesis. Although clinical and radiographic parameters improve with these treatments, restoration of normal alignment is not the goal and is usually not achievable.

The previously discussed procedures do not address the static medial foot stabilizers. Other soft-tissue considerations include repairing the spring ligament and lengthening the heel cord with either a gastrocnemius or Achilles procedure. The spring ligament can be difficult to repair because it is attenuated and a direct repair is challenging. It can simply be imbricated or also repaired using a portion of the posterior tibial tendon remnant. Recently, a cadaver flatfoot model was used to test a novel reconstruction of the spring ligament.[19] The authors described using a tendon "sling" through the talar neck and into the medial cuneiform secured with a biotenodesis screw.[19] Following reconstruction, all radiographic parameters demonstrated statistically significant improvements. Another technique has also been described; autologous peroneal longus tendon transfer was added intraoperatively to reconstruct the spring ligament following a flatfoot reconstruction with MDCO, lateral column lengthening, and FDL tendon transfer.[20] The spring ligament repair was added when talonavicular uncoverage was believed to be undercorrected. The study involved 13 patients and 8.9-year follow-up demonstrating statistically significant improvements in all radiographic parameters without a compromise in eversion strength.

The gastrocnemius is lengthened by a posteromedial incision over the calf that helps circumvent injury to the posterolateral sural nerve. The fascia is identified and horizontally incised until approximately 10° above neutral ankle dorsiflexion is achieved. The entire complex is released by a triple-cut hemisection of the Achilles tendon, achieving the same goal.

Periarticular Osteotomy Options
Although the MDCO is the workhorse for osseous reconstructive procedures, other osteotomies are used. The standard MDCO is created with an oblique osteotomy, and the posterior tuberosity is then slid medially about 1 cm. This corrects the hindfoot valgus and protects the FDL tendon transfer by restoring foot alignment. This osteotomy can be fixed with headed or headless screws or with newer step plates (Figure 7). A 2013 report demonstrated less frequent screw removal with a headless screw and more wound complications with the plate, likely because of greater need for exposure.[21] However, biomechanical studies have supported the concept that plate fixation is stronger and may allow earlier weight bearing.[22] This osteotomy is commonly combined with medial soft-tissue reconstruction in stage IIA1 PTTD without additional osteotomies. A recent comparative study of 72 feet using different corrective options demonstrated that patients who had both lateral column lengthening and MDCO experienced more improvement in all radiographic parameters (versus MDCO alone).[23] To address stage IIA2, in which fixed forefoot varus/supination exists, a dorsal opening-wedge osteotomy of the medial cuneiform is also added (also known as a Cotton osteotomy) (Figure 8). This plantarflexes the medial column, restoring the plantigrade foot. This forefoot deformity is a compensatory development that occurs with long-standing hindfoot valgus and, as the hindfoot is everted for a prolonged period of time, the forefoot resides in varus to obtain a plantigrade foot. This fixed varus is evident after hindfoot correction, and, if not supple, necessitates the Cotton osteotomy. However, a plantar closing-wedge osteotomy of the medial cuneiform has also

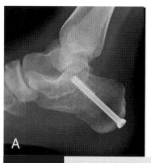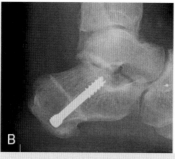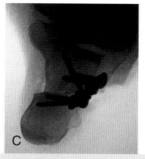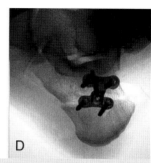

Figure 7 Radiographs showing multiple options for medial displacement calcaneal osteotomy fixation. **A**, A headed screw is used. **B**, A headless screw is used. **C** and **D**, Plate fixation is used.

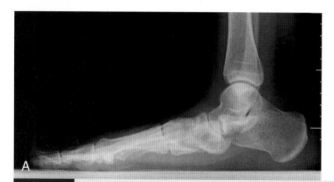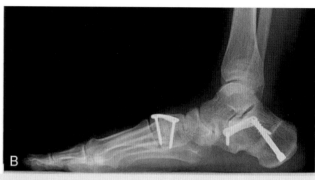

Figure 8 Preoperative (**A**) and postoperative (**B**) radiographs. This patient required a Cotton osteotomy.

been described; the authors advocate its use for simplicity, and a bone graft is not required.[24] One study examines the postoperative correction by describing a new radiographic measurement following a Cotton osteotomy.[25] The angle between the proximal and distal articular surfaces of the medial cuneiform was measured on lateral radiographs preoperatively, postoperatively before weight-bearing, and at the final follow-up visit. The average angle increase was 6.5°, improving the forefoot varus.[25]

Stage IIB PTTD is characterized by significant forefoot abduction that is radiographically appreciated by increased talonavicular uncoverage (**Figure 9**). The foot is corrected as described for stage IIA1/2, but a lateral column calcaneal lengthening osteotomy also added (**Figure 9**). Typically, lateral column lengthening is performed separately from the MDCO through two incisions. Lateral column calcaneal lengthening can also be created by a Z-calcaneal osteotomy, which allows for a shift and lengthening of the calcaneus. This procedure offers increased inherent stability and may allow for better correction of deformity[26,27] (**Figure 10**). Lateral column lengthening poses concern as a cause of calcaneocuboid arthritis attributable to joint overloading. However, a biomechanical study demonstrated that lateral column lengthening to a certain extent will decrease pressure in the calcaneocuboid joint with a flatfoot deformity, with 8 mm being the best option.[28] If calcaneocuboid

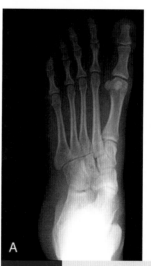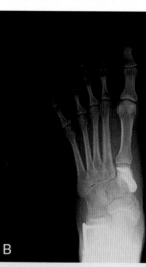

Figure 9 Preoperative (**A**) and postoperative (**B**) radiographs demonstrating significant uncoverage and the need for a lateral column lengthening.

arthritis is already present, lateral column lengthening can be performed through a distraction arthrodesis at this joint. However, this technique must be used with caution because high nonunion rates have been reported. A study demonstrated a nearly 50% nonunion rate

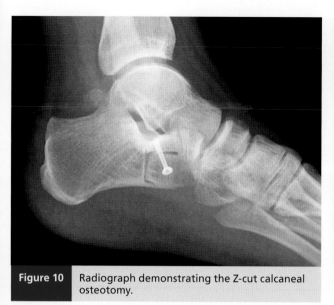

Figure 10 | Radiograph demonstrating the Z-cut calcaneal osteotomy.

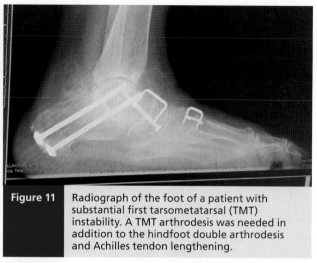

Figure 11 | Radiograph of the foot of a patient with substantial first tarsometatarsal (TMT) instability. A TMT arthrodesis was needed in addition to the hindfoot double arthrodesis and Achilles tendon lengthening.

and advocated locked plate fixation and delayed weight bearing if distraction arthrodesis was to be performed.[29]

Stage IIC PTTD is defined by medial column instability, which is defined subjectively with increased motion at the first TMT joint or by first TMT joint plantar gapping on a lateral radiograph. Medial column instability may also exist at the naviculocuneiform joint, which is seen by the apex of the deformity occurring at this level on a lateral radiograph. This is addressed with either a Cotton osteotomy, a first TMT arthrodesis or naviculocuneiform arthrodesis, or a combination of these procedures[30] (Figure 11).

Finally, subtalar arthroerisis can be performed to help correct hindfoot valgus. There are metallic and bioabsorbable options and removal is debated. Use of this technique has decreased over the years. It can be recommended in conjunction with MDCO and/or FDL transfer and has been proposed for use in elderly patients as a replacement for a full reconstruction because the recovery is easier. Routine use of this procedure should be approached with caution.[31]

Stage III PTTD

Stage III is a rigid flatfoot deformity, so joint-sparing procedures are not an option. Arthrodesis procedures are performed for stage III deformity, patients with stage II PTTD with significant deformity, obese patients, patients with underlying inflammatory arthropathy, and for revision of failed procedures.

A triple arthrodesis is the standard procedure; however, future adjacent joint arthrosis is a concern. A triple arthrodesis should be selected for patients with substantial deformity and underlying arthritis of the three joints (Figure 12). Selective arthrodesis is another

option that has gained recent popularity. This can be an isolated arthrodesis (talonavicular or subtalar) or a "double arthrodesis." Isolated talonavicular arthrodesis is a useful and effective alternative to double arthrodesis. It is less complicated, less invasive, and a functionally equivalent surgical option for arthritic alterations of the hindfoot and transverse tarsal joint.[32]

A double arthrodesis involves the Chopart joint (the talonavicular and calcaneocuboid joints). It also can involve the subtalar and calcaneocuboid joints. A double arthrodesis of the subtalar/talonavicular joints can be performed through an all-medial or combined lateral/medial or lateral/dorsal approach. Usually a surgeon would approach the subtalar joint through the lateral approach and the talonavicular through either a dorsal or medial approach depending on his or her preference. Another option is the all-lateral approach. Accessing the talonavicular joint this way can be challenging, but a cadaver study demonstrated that 90% of the talonavicular joint can be prepared.[33]

For the all-medial approach, the incision extends from the tip of the medial malleolus down the midline of the foot. The PTT can be preserved or removed. The spring ligament can also be repaired if needed. The surgeon must be careful not to violate the deltoid ligament; this could lead to iatrogenic ankle valgus. The medial approach allows access to both the subtalar and talonavicular joints, and has several advantages.[34] When addressing long-standing deformity and contracted lateral skin, the medial approach avoids the lateral foot, which lowers the wound complication rate (specifically, closure difficulty at the time of surgery and wound dehiscence postoperatively). Correction of hindfoot valgus creates lateral tension and yields redundant skin medially, allowing closure without tension. Several authors have reported on the single medial approach.[35] In a series of

3: Arthritis of the Foot and Ankle

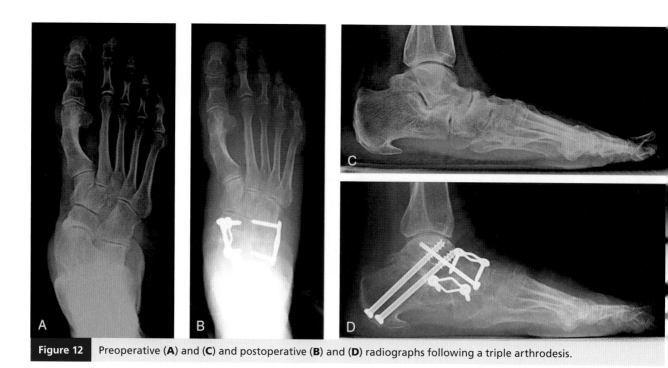

Figure 12 Preoperative (**A**) and (**C**) and postoperative (**B**) and (**D**) radiographs following a triple arthrodesis.

14 feet, arthrodesis of the subtalar and talonavicular joints through a medial approach combined with peroneal lengthening was a reliable procedure for the treatment of rigid flatfoot with deficient lateral skin and no calcaneocuboid joint degeneration.[35] Also, the all-medial approach allows for better visualization of the middle facet, which can be important with subtalar coalitions. In a series of 18 patients, there were no wound-related complications. The union rate was 89% with two malunions, and two feet developed valgus ankle deformity. The overall satisfaction rate among patients was 78%.[36] In another study of 15 feet, outcome scores improved, axis of the hindfoot decreased from 21° to 11° in valgus, and arch foot angle improved.[37] Finally, 32 feet in 30 patients underwent correction with a double arthrodesis through a medial approach. The mean follow-up was 21 months. Fusion was achieved in all feet at a mean of 13 weeks. Apart from the calcaneal pitch angle, all angular measurements improved substantially after surgery. Primary wound healing occurred without complications. The medial approach was associated with fewer problems with wound healing than the standard lateral approach.[38] Gait analysis also improved following double arthrodesis of the subtalar/talonavicular joints.[39]

Stage IV PTTD

Stage IV deformity is associated with ankle valgus attributable to prolonged hindfoot valgus and resultant deltoid incompetence. The ankle can either be flexible (stage IVa) or rigid (stage IVb). The underlying flatfoot also can be rigid or flexible. The flatfoot is corrected depending on the details described earlier. Often, a triple or double arthrodesis is required. Ankle valgus is corrected with deltoid ligament repair in an effort to preserve the ankle joint when appropriate. Recent techniques have been developed; however, no clinical data are available for sufficient follow-up. These techniques vary from tendon allograft weaved through the medial tibia and into the navicular to use of ACL guides to direct tunnel placement and use of synthetic material to augment the repair. These techniques are challenging and studies are pending. When ankle preservation is not possible, a tibiotalocalcaneal arthrodesis or a pantalar arthrodesis may be required. Patients must be counseled on limitations following an extensive arthrodesis. Finally, total ankle replacement, with or without deltoid repair, can be performed. Total ankle replacement can be performed simultaneously with foot correction or in a staged fashion. There are no studies with outcome data evaluating such techniques. These deformities are complex and necessitate detailed preoperative planning to obtain a satisfactory result.

Complications

Patients undergoing reconstruction for PTTD may experience complications. These include, but are not limited to, infection, nerve (specifically sural) and vessel injury, wound complications, malunion, nonunion, failure of tendon transfer incorporation, undercorrection, overcorrection, progression of deformity, pain or arthritis, and medical complications such as deep vein thrombosis. Risks are directly associated with deformity and complexity of each case. Risks can be decreased with careful planning and encouragement of patients with diabetes to closely monitor their serum glucose levels and smokers to discontinue tobacco use. Patients taking corticosteroids and those with preexisting ulcers caused by chronic deformity are at an increased risk for complications. Also, in patients with long-standing deformity, lateral incisions may pose difficulty with closure and healing after hindfoot valgus has been corrected. Hardware-related pain or prominence may necessitate a second procedure to remove the implant. Failures following reconstructions with osteotomies and tendon transfers are salvaged with arthrodesis procedures.

Summary

PTTD is a common problem and should be considered in patients presenting with medial or lateral hindfoot and ankle pain. A thorough history and physical examination is required for diagnosis and to effectively treat these patients. Treatment is individualized to a patient's age, weight, stage of deformity, activity level, and expectations. Many nonsurgical options are available when treating these patients initially. When nonsurgical management is unsuccessful, a surgical procedure can improve pain, alignment, and function. Recovery may take up to 1 year.

Annotated References

1. Frey C, Shereff M, Greenidge N: Vascularity of the posterior tibial tendon. *J Bone Joint Surg Am* 1990;72(6):884-888.

2. Davis WH, Sobel M, DiCarlo EF, et al: Gross, histological, and microvascular anatomy and biomechanical testing of the spring ligament complex. *Foot Ankle Int* 1996;17(2):95-102.

3. Mizel MS, Temple HT, Scranton PE Jr, et al: Role of the peroneal tendons in the production of the deformed foot with posterior tibial tendon deficiency. *Foot Ankle Int* 1999;20(5):285-289.

4. Mosier SM, Lucas DR, Pomeroy G, Manoli A II: Pathology of the posterior tibial tendon in posterior tibial tendon insufficiency. *Foot Ankle Int* 1998;19(8):520-524.

5. Johnson KA, Strom DE: Tibialis posterior tendon dysfunction. *Clin Orthop Relat Res* 1989;239:196-206.

6. Myerson MS: Adult acquired flatfoot deformity: Treatment of dysfunction of the posterior tibial tendon. *Instr Course Lect* 1997;46:393-405.

7. Bluman EM, Title CI, Myerson MS: Posterior tibial tendon rupture: A refined classification system. *Foot Ankle Clin* 2007;12(2):233-249, v.

8. Raikin SM, Winters BS, Daniel JN: The RAM classification: A novel, systematic approach to the adult-acquired flatfoot. *Foot Ankle Clin* 2012;17(2):169-181.

This system classifies adult-acquired flatfoot into three independent levels of involvement: the rearfoot, ankle, and midfoot.

9. Conti S, Michelson J, Jahss M: Clinical significance of magnetic resonance imaging in preoperative planning for reconstruction of posterior tibial tendon ruptures. *Foot Ankle* 1992;13(4):208-214.

10. DeOrio JK, Shapiro SA, McNeil RB, Stansel J: Validity of the posterior tibial edema sign in posterior tibial tendon dysfunction. *Foot Ankle Int* 2011;32(2):189-192.

The authors identify swelling over the PTT as highly sensitive to the presence of a PTT tear. Knowledge of this sign may help lower the cost of diagnosis by eliminating the need for expensive tests that are not always necessary.

11. Bek N, Simşek IE, Erel S, Yakut Y, Uygur F: Home-based general versus center-based selective rehabilitation in patients with posterior tibial tendon dysfunction. *Acta Orthop Traumatol Turc* 2012;46(4):286-292.

This study evaluated effectiveness of home- and center-based therapy for PTTD. Both groups received orthotics. Therapy demonstrated a significant improvement in function and pain (home- or center-based). Also, home- and center-based forms of rehabilitation were equally effective.

12. Chao W, Wapner KL, Lee TH, Adams J, Hecht PJ: Nonoperative management of posterior tibial tendon dysfunction. *Foot Ankle Int* 1996;17(12):736-741.

13. Krause F, Bosshard A, Lehmann O, Weber M: Shell brace for stage II posterior tibial tendon insufficiency. *Foot Ankle Int* 2008;29(11):1095-1100.

The shell brace was highly effective in reducing pain. Patients with a stage III deformity had poorer results with the brace.

14. Alvarez RG, Marini A, Schmitt C, Saltzman CL: Stage I and II posterior tibial tendon dysfunction treated by a structured nonoperative management protocol: An orthosis and exercise program. *Foot Ankle Int* 2006;27(1):2-8.

15. Neville CG, Houck JR: Choosing among 3 ankle-foot orthoses for a patient with stage II posterior tibial tendon dysfunction. *J Orthop Sports Phys Ther* 2009;39(11):816-824.

3: Arthritis of the Foot and Ankle

Based on gait analysis, the higher-cost custom articulated orthosis was chosen as optimal for the patient. It was associated with the most notable change in flatfoot deformity during gait analysis. The patient also reported that the orthoses seemed to better correct the deformity. Level of evidence: IV.

16. Khazen G, Khazen C: Tendoscopy in stage I posterior tibial tendon dysfunction. *Foot Ankle Clin* 2012;17(3):399-406.

This article describes a technique using PTT tendoscopic synovectomy as a minimally invasive and effective surgical procedure with which to treat patients with stage I PTTD. It offers the advantages of less wound pain and fewer scar and wound problems.

17. Sammarco GJ, Hockenbury RT: Treatment of stage II posterior tibial tendon dysfunction with flexor hallucis longus transfer and medial displacement calcaneal osteotomy. *Foot Ankle Int* 2001;22(4):305-312.

18. Song SJ, Deland JT: Outcome following addition of peroneus brevis tendon transfer to treatment of acquired posterior tibial tendon insufficiency. *Foot Ankle Int* 2001;22(4):301-304.

19. Tan GJ, Kadakia AR, Ruberte Thiele RA, Hughes RE: Novel reconstruction of a static medial ligamentous complex in a flatfoot model. *Foot Ankle Int* 2010;31(8):695-700.

A description of this cadaver model demonstrated that reconstruction of the spring ligament with a tendon graft improved the alignment of a severe flatfoot.

20. Williams BR, Ellis SJ, Deyer TW, Pavlov H, Deland JT: Reconstruction of the spring ligament using a peroneus longus autograft tendon transfer. *Foot Ankle Int* 2010;31(7):567-577.

This is a case series of patients who, after flatfoot reconstruction, continued to have persistent forefoot abduction intraoperatively. The treating surgeon added a peroneal longus autograft tendon transfer to reconstruct the spring ligament, with improved alignment and no eversion weakness.

21. Abbasian A, Zaidi R, Guha A, Goldberg A, Cullen N, Singh D: Comparison of three different fixation methods of calcaneal osteotomies. *Foot Ankle Int* 2013;34(3):420-425.

Calcaneal osteotomies have high union. Fixation using a headed screw is associated with a high rate of secondary screw removal. Hardware problems were less common in the headless screw or lateral plate groups; however, the incidence of local wound complications and radiologic delayed union was higher in the group undergoing fixation with lateral plates.

22. Konan S, Meswania J, Blunn GW, Madhav RT, Oddy MJ: Mechanical stability of a locked step-plate versus single compression screw fixation for medial displacement calcaneal osteotomy. *Foot Ankle Int* 2012;33(8):669-674.

Eight matched pairs of cadaver limbs were loaded using a mechanical testing rig. The limbs underwent a 10-mm medial displacement osteotomy stabilized either with a single 7-mm screw or a step plate with four locking screws. In this cadaver model, a locked step plate supported a substantially higher maximum force than a single large cannulated screw.

23. Iossi M, Johnson JE, McCormick JJ, Klein SE: Short-term radiographic analysis of operative correction of adult acquired flatfoot deformity. *Foot Ankle Int* 2013;34(6):781-791.

The 68 patients followed in this study underwent different reconstructions based on their deformity and were divided into three groups. The group that had a lateral column lengthening and MDCO had the best correction based on radiographic findings.

24. Ling JS, Ross KA, Hannon CP, et al: A plantar closing wedge osteotomy of the medial cuneiform for residual forefoot supination in flatfoot reconstruction. *Foot Ankle Int* 2013;34(9):1221-1226.

Ten feet were followed postoperatively in this study, which demonstrated that a plantar osteotomy can be considered an alternative to the Cotton osteotomy for the treatment of forefoot supination deformity in adult flatfoot reconstruction. The main advantage of this technique over the Cotton osteotomy was simplicity.

25. Castaneda D, Thordarson DB, Charlton TP: Radiographic assessment of medial cuneiform opening wedge osteotomy for flatfoot correction. *Foot Ankle Int* 2012;33(6):498-500.

The average angle between the proximal and distal articular surfaces of the medial cuneiform on lateral foot radiographs was 1.0° preoperatively (± 0.8°). The average angle postosteotomy at final follow-up was 7.5° (± 2.9°). All patients achieved bony union.

26. Guha AR, Perera AM: Calcaneal osteotomy in the treatment of adult acquired flatfoot deformity. *Foot Ankle Clin* 2012;17(2):247-258.

This article provides an excellent review of the different calcaneal osteotomies, indications, techniques, complications, strengths, and limitations.

27. Scott RT, Berlet GC: Calcaneal Z osteotomy for extra-articular correction of hindfoot valgus. *J Foot Ankle Surg* 2013;52(3):406-408.

In recognition of the limitations of traditional lateral column lengthening, these authors describe a new technique to obtain correction and reduce complication rates.

28. Xia J, Zhang P, Yang YF, Zhou JQ, Li QM, Yu GR: Biomechanical analysis of the calcaneocuboid joint pressure after sequential lengthening of the lateral column. *Foot Ankle Int* 2013;34(2):261-266.

Six cadaver specimens were physiologically loaded and the peak pressure of the calcaneocuboid joint was measured after lateral column lengthening. The pressure reached its minimum value with 8-mm lengthening of the lateral column. Lateral column lengthening to a certain extent will decrease pressure in the calcaneocuboid joint with a flatfoot deformity.

29. Grunander TR, Thordarson DB: Results of calcaneocuboid distraction arthrodesis. *Foot Ankle Surg* 2012;18(1):15-18.

    Seven of 16 feet developed a nonunion; because of the unacceptably high complication rate associated with this procedure, the authors have abandoned it and strongly recommend using rigid locking fixation and a longer period of protected immobilization.

30. McCormick JJ, Johnson JE: Medial column procedures in the correction of adult acquired flatfoot deformity. *Foot Ankle Clin* 2012;17(2):283-298.

    If the elevation of the medial column is identified to be at the first naviculocuneiform or the first TMT joint, the joint should be carefully examined for evidence of instability, hypermobility, or arthritic change. If these issues are not present, the surgeon can consider use of the joint-sparing Cotton medial cuneiform osteotomy to correct residual forefoot varus. However, if these issues are present, the surgeon should consider an arthrodesis of the involved joint to correct residual forefoot varus.

31. Zaret DI, Myerson MS: Arthroerisis of the subtalar joint. *Foot Ankle Clin* 2003;8(3):605-617.

32. Thelen S, Rütt J, Wild M, Lögters T, Windolf J, Koebke J: The influence of talonavicular versus double arthrodesis on load dependent motion of the midtarsal joint. *Arch Orthop Trauma Surg* 2010;130(1):47-53.

    Ten cadavers were compared following talonavicular arthrodesis or a double arthrodesis. Both fusions lead to equal residual tarsal bone motion postoperatively and provide the midtarsal and subtalar joints with comparable biomechanical stability. Isolated talonavicular arthrodesis is a less complicated, less invasive, and functionally equivalent surgical option for arthritic alterations of the hindfoot and transverse tarsal joint.

33. Jeng CL, Tankson CJ, Myerson MS: The single medial approach to triple arthrodesis: A cadaver study. *Foot Ankle Int* 2006;27(12):1122-1125.

34. Jeng CL, Vora AM, Myerson MS: The medial approach to triple arthrodesis. Indications and technique for management of rigid valgus deformities in high-risk patients. *Foot Ankle Clin* 2005;10(3):515-521, vi-vii.

35. Brilhault J: Single medial approach to modified double arthrodesis in rigid flatfoot with lateral deficient skin. *Foot Ankle Int* 2009;30(1):21-26.

    Fourteen feet with deficient lateral skin and a fixed hindfoot valgus deformity for which adequate correction may have led to lateral wound complications were followed after a single medial approach modified double arthrodesis. There were no wound-healing complications. Arthrodesis of the subtalar and talonavicular joints through a medial approach combined with peroneal lengthening is a reliable procedure for the treatment of rigid flatfoot with deficient lateral skin and no calcaneocuboid joint degeneration.

36. Anand P, Nunley JA, DeOrio JK: Single-incision medial approach for double arthrodesis of hindfoot in posterior tibialis tendon dysfunction. *Foot Ankle Int* 2013;34(3):338-344.

    Eighteen feet were followed after a single-incision medial approach for double arthrodesis. The union rate was 89%. There were two malunions, and two feet developed valgus ankle deformity. The overall satisfaction rate among patients was 78%. There were no wound complications.

37. Philippot R, Wegrzyn J, Besse JL: Arthrodesis of the subtalar and talonavicular joints through a medial surgical approach: A series of 15 cases. *Arch Orthop Trauma Surg* 2010;130(5):599-603.

    Fifteen feet were followed. This medial approach procedure permits fusion without developing nonunion and provides a significant correction of fixed deformities.

38. Knupp M, Schuh R, Stufkens SA, Bolliger L, Hintermann B: Subtalar and talonavicular arthrodesis through a single medial approach for the correction of severe planovalgus deformity. *J Bone Joint Surg Br* 2009;91(5):612-615.

    In this large series, 32 feet were followed after undergoing the single medial approach for double arthrodesis. Apart from the calcaneal pitch angle, all angular measurements improved significantly after surgery. Primary wound healing occurred without complications.

39. Schuh R, Salzberger F, Wanivenhaus AH, Funovics PT, Windhager R, Trnka HJ: Kinematic changes in patients with double arthrodesis of the hindfoot for realignment of planovalgus deformity. *J Orthop Res* 2013;31(4):517-524.

    The load changed after double arthrodesis. The hindfoot and hallux represented decreased load in patients who underwent double arthrodesis, whereas load increased in the midfoot region compared with healthy controls.

3: Arthritis of the Foot and Ankle

Section 4

The Forefoot

SECTION EDITOR:

CLIFFORD L. JENG, MD

Chapter 13

Hallux Valgus and Hallux Varus

Jeremy T. Smith, MD   Eric M. Bluman, MD, PhD

Hallux Valgus

Hallux valgus is a common forefoot deformity in which the first metatarsal deviates medially and the hallux both deviates laterally and pronates, leaving a prominence at the first metatarsal head. The causes of hallux valgus are intrinsic and extrinsic. In an individual patient, the cause of hallux valgus may be multifactorial, involving both intrinsic predisposition and extrinsic factors.

Anatomy and Pathogenesis

The stability of the first ray depends on a balance of static and dynamic structures. Loss of stability anywhere along the length of the first ray can contribute to hallux valgus. In addition to the bony architecture of the first tarsometatarsal (TMT) and first metatarsophalangeal (MTP) joints, several soft-tissue structures contribute to joint stability (**Table 1**). The four requirements for stability of the first ray are a congruent and stable MTP joint, a distal metatarsal articular angle that encourages stability, balanced static and dynamic constraints, and a stable TMT joint.[1]

Hallux valgus typically progresses in a stepwise fashion. The process is believed to begin with attenuation of the medial supporting structures of the MTP joint. Progressive deformity often occurs as the medial supporting structures attenuate further and the lateral structures contract. As the first metatarsal drifts into varus, the

Dr. Bluman or an immediate family member serves as a paid consultant to Biomet, Integra, and Norvartis; serves as an unpaid consultant to SBI; has received nonincome support (such as equipment or services), commercially derived honoraria, or other non–research-related funding (such as paid travel) from Rogerson Orthopaedics; and serves as a board member, owner, officer, or committee member of the American Academy of Orthopaedic Surgeons and the American Orthopaedic Foot and Ankle Society. Neither Dr. Smith nor any immediate family member has received anything of value from or has stock or stock options held in a commercial company or institution related directly or indirectly to the subject of this chapter.

Table 1

Soft-Tissue Stabilizers of the First Tarsometatarsal and First Metatarsophalangeal Joints

First Tarsometatarsal Joint	First Metatarsophalangeal Joint
Flexor hallucis longus	Abductor hallucis
Tibialis anterior	Adductor hallucis
Intrinsic muscles of the foot	Extensor hallucis brevis
Joint capsule	Extensor hallucis longus and extensor hood
	Flexor hallucis brevis
Peroneus longus	Flexor hallucis brevis and sesamoid complex
Plantar fascia	Joint capsule
	Medial and lateral collateral ligaments
	Sesamoid ligaments
	Transverse metatarsal ligament

sesamoids displace into the first intermetatarsal space. In addition, pronation of the hallux may occur, causing loss of the normal physiologic tripod of the foot and transfer of weight from the first MTP joint to the adjacent lesser MTP joints.

Numerous factors are believed to contribute to the development of hallux valgus. The extrinsic factors include poorly fitting shoes and trauma. The possible intrinsic etiologies include metatarsal head morphology, metatarsus primus varus, hypermobility of the first TMT joint, pes planus, general ligamentous laxity, tight heel cord, inflammatory arthropathy, and neuromuscular disorders. Heritable anatomic factors such as hypermobility and arch height are believed to have an important role in the development of hallux valgus. The genetic contribution to deformity is even stronger in children than in adults.

A much higher prevalence of hallux valgus has been observed in women than in men. Wearing shoes with an elevated heel or a narrow toe box, which is more common among women than men, may be responsible for this sexual dimorphism. In addition, fundamental anatomic differences between women and men may predispose women to the development of hallux valgus. In general, women have a smaller and rounder metatarsal head, an adducted first metatarsal, and higher rates of ligamentous laxity than men. A recent study reported a 15 to 1 ratio of women to men among patients undergoing surgical treatment for hallux valgus, thus confirming earlier reports.[2] On average, the men had surgery at a younger age than the women, and 68% of the men had a familial history of hallux valgus, compared with 35% of the women. Radiographic measurements showed a larger deformity in men than in women as well as a higher rate of first MTP joint congruence. The study conclusions were that hallux valgus in men who were surgically treated often was hereditary, was associated with a high distal metatarsal articular angle, and was more severe than in women.

Diagnostic Evaluation

Patients with hallux valgus typically have pain over the medial eminence. The patient also may have generalized pain at the first MTP joint, pain from associated lesser toe abnormalities such as hammer toes, or pain at the lesser metatarsal heads caused by abnormal physiologic loading (transfer metatarsalgia). Skin lesions caused by chafing from shoes is common. Guidance and care should be tailored to the patient's symptoms, limitations, goals, and expectations.

The physical examination should include a standing assessment of alignment and a careful inspection for skin lesions including callosities. The specific location of pain should be determined based on direct palpation as well as history. Joint motion and passive correction of the deformity should be assessed. To evaluate for contractures, it is important to determine the dorsiflexion and plantar flexion of the first MTP joint in a reduced position. Neurologic and vascular status should be evaluated for all patients. Intrinsic causes of hallux valgus should be assessed by examining for hypermobility of the first TMT joint, pes planus, general ligamentous laxity, a tight heel cord, inflammatory arthropathy, and neuromuscular disorders.

Weight-bearing foot radiographs should be obtained. The AP view is used to measure the intermetatarsal angle, hallux valgus angle, and distal metatarsal articular angle (**Figure 1**). Compared with a normal foot, the deformity is classified as mild, moderate, or severe (**Table 2**). The sesamoids should be reduced in the cristae of the first metatarsal head. The first MTP joint should be evaluated radiographically for arthritic changes.

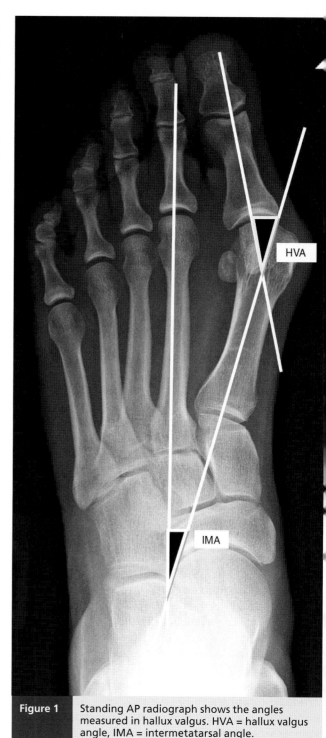

Figure 1 Standing AP radiograph shows the angles measured in hallux valgus. HVA = hallux valgus angle, IMA = intermetatarsal angle.

The surgical correction of hallux valgus is based on whether the first MTP joint is congruent or incongruent. In a congruent deformity, there is a concentric relationship between the first metatarsal head and the base of the proximal phalanx. An incongruent deformity occurs when the hallux is laterally subluxated from the

Table 2

Radiographic Angles Used to Measure the Severity of Deformity in Hallux Valgus

Severity of Deformity	Hallux Valgus Angle	First-Second Intermetatarsal Angle	Distal Metatarsal Articular Angle
None (normal)	<15°	<9°	<10°
Mild	<20°	<11°	—
Moderate	20° to 40°	11° to 16°	—
Severe	>40°	>16°	—

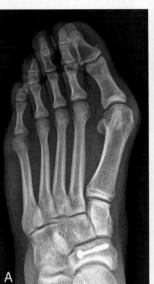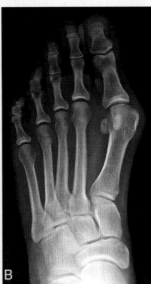

Figure 2 Standing AP radiographs show a congruent (**A**) and an incongruent (**B**) hallux valgus deformity.

metatarsal head (**Figure 2**). Most patients have an incongruent deformity.

Instability of the first TMT joint primarily is diagnosed by clinical assessment, although efforts continue to achieve an objective definition.[3] Several devices can be used to measure sagittal plane motion.[4] A study of a mobile fluoroscopic device used to analyze first ray motion in the sagittal plane found that patients with hallux valgus had increased maximal dorsiflexion of the first TMT joint during gait.[5]

Nonsurgical Treatment

Patient education and shoe modification are the mainstays of nonsurgical hallux valgus management. The patient should understand the importance of shoe modification as a means of minimizing symptoms. Shoes with a wide toe box should be worn to accommodate a wide forefoot, and elevated heels should be avoided to minimize forefoot pressure during gait. Bunion splints, toe spacers, and pads can be used to avoid shoe rubbing on the medial eminence. In-shoe orthotic devices may be useful to treat transfer metatarsalgia, but they are unlikely to relieve symptoms directly related to the hallux valgus deformity.

Surgical Treatment

Surgical reconstruction can be considered if the patient has persistent pain that limits the ability to function, despite nonsurgical management. Cosmesis alone is not an appropriate indication for surgery to treat hallux valgus. More than 100 procedures have been described for treating a hallux valgus deformity. The outcome is assessed by using a functional outcome tool, in addition to radiography. The Foot and Ankle Outcome Score recently was validated in patients with hallux valgus.[6]

Several basic principles of hallux valgus correction are useful for simplifying the choice of reconstruction. The first principle is that in the presence of arthritis, a first MTP joint arthrodesis should be considered. The second principle is that the choice of procedure depends on whether the deformity is classified as congruent or incongruent. A procedure to treat a congruent deformity should not disrupt joint congruency; for example, a procedure that relies on correction through the first MTP joint should be avoided in favor of an extra-articular correction. A procedure to treat an incongruent deformity should gain correction by realigning the first MTP joint through the joint, as in a modified McBride procedure.

The third general principle of hallux valgus correction is that as the severity of the deformity increases, the more proximal the correction needs to be (**Table 2**). For a mild deformity, a procedure that includes a distal soft-tissue release or distal osteotomies often is sufficient. For a moderate deformity, the correction often involves a first metatarsal shaft osteotomy accompanied by a distal soft-tissue release. A severe deformity requires a more proximal osteotomy or a first TMT fusion. The most obvious exception to this rule is that a first MTP joint fusion can be a powerful tool for correcting an advanced arthritic deformity.

Regardless of the choice of technique, several details are paramount to durable surgical success. The first of

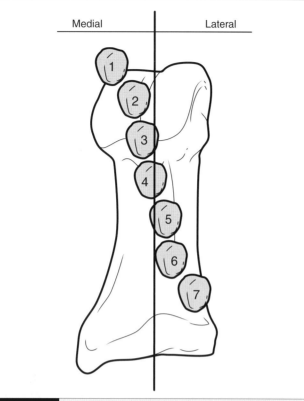

Figure 3 Illustration shows how the severity of sesamoid subluxation or dislocation can be graded using a system created by Hardy and Clapham. The medial-to-lateral position of the medial sesamoid (numbered circles) is determined in relation to the longitudinal axis of the first metatarsal (vertical line).

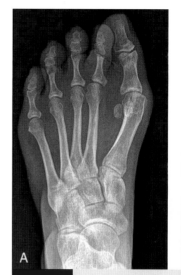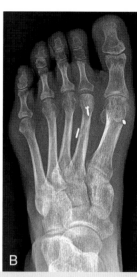

Figure 4 Preoperative (**A**) and postoperative (**B**) standing AP radiographs show hallux valgus deformity corrected with a suture suspensory device and a second metatarsal–shortening osteotomy.

these is that a sesamoid reduction is correlated with maintenance of deformity correction. In a hallux valgus deformity, the sesamoids come to lie laterally relative to their reduced position within the cristae. The severity of the subluxation-dislocation can be graded using the Hardy-Clapham scale for determining the position of the medial sesamoid with respect to the longitudinal axis of the first metatarsal[7] (**Figure 3**). A significant correlation was found between the magnitude of sesamoid displacement at early follow-up and the risk of hallux valgus recurrence. Patients with an abnormal sesamoid position (grades 5 to 7) at the time of early follow-up were found to have a tenfold greater risk of recurrence than those with a normal position (grades 1 to 4).[8]

Release of the soft tissues in the distal first-second intermetatarsal space is necessary for complete and durable correction of most hallux valgus deformities. The adductor hallucis tendon, the sesamoid suspensory ligament, and the lateral first MTP capsule should be released to facilitate the reduction of the proximal phalanx on the metatarsal head as well as the sesamoids within the

cristae. Dorsal, distal, transarticular, and endoscopic approaches have been described to obtain this correction.[9,10]

There has been recent interest in procedures that maintain the length of the first ray and thereby theoretically minimize the development of transfer lesions in the lesser metatarsal heads. Correction procedures using a suture suspension technique or an opening-wedge proximal metatarsal osteotomy avoid fusion. Suture suspensory techniques recently have been introduced as an alternative to metatarsal osteotomy for mild or moderate deformity.[11] The procedure consists of a distal soft-tissue release followed by suture suspension to reduce and hold the first-second intermetatarsal angle (**Figure 4**).

Several recent studies reported success when a suture suspensory device was used to correct a hallux valgus deformity.[11-14] Two of these studies assessed American Orthopaedic Foot and Ankle Society scores preoperatively and postoperatively and reported improved scores. The other studies simply reported postoperative American Orthopaedic Foot and Ankle Society scores, which is not particularly useful. Second metatarsal fracture was reported in patients treated with this technique, most often with the use of a large device designed for syndesmotic reduction and fixation.[13-17] An updated technique that uses a small device and avoids overdrilling appears to carry minimal risk of a second metatarsal fracture.[14,17] This novel technique must be further evaluated in large, long-term studies.

A proximal opening-wedge osteotomy can be used to obtain angular correction without shortening at the first-second intermetatarsal angle. Like other procedures involving proximal first metatarsal osteotomy, this technique avoids obliteration of the first TMT joint. Both a lateral release and medial capsular imbrication are required to obtain and maintain correction at the first MTP joint. The available studies found no shortening and only modest lengthening.[18,19] Greater lengthening is claimed to be an advantage of the scarf osteotomy for correcting hallux valgus. Although few studies have reported on this parameter, lengthening as great as 10 mm was found to be possible.[20-22]

For some patients, arthrodesis has been the preferred treatment for hallux valgus correction. This type of fixation recently has received renewed attention. Fusions of the first TMT and first MTP joints can be powerful tools to correct a hallux valgus deformity. Many surgeons have used two or three crossed screws as the standard fixation for a first TMT joint fusion. Several recent cadaver studies examined the relative benefit (in terms of rigidity) of using a locking-plate construct or crossed screws.[23-25] In general, superior rigidity was found when a locking plate was used rather than crossed screws. A retrospective study found better union and earlier return to full weight bearing when a locking plate was used, compared with crossed screws.[26] A cadaver study of fixation at the first MTP joint found greater stiffness when a locking plate and screw construct was used, compared with a nonlocking plate and screw construct.[27]

Studies have examined whether a proximal corrective procedure should accompany first MTP joint fusion for hallux valgus correction. Good correction was reported after first MTP fusion alone in patients with a mean preoperative 33° hallux valgus angle and 13° intermetatarsal angle.[28] The researchers suggested that tension is pulled through the adductor hallucis with fusion of the first MTP in a reduced position. Because the proximal phalanx is fixed to the metatarsal head, the pull of the adductor hallucis acts to correct the intermetatarsal angle. In others, first MTP fusion coupled with proximal correction has been shown to be a powerful technique for correcting severe deformities.[29]

Hallux Varus

Hallux varus occurs when the great toe is aligned in varus relative to the first metatarsal (**Figure 5**). The severity of hallux varus varies, and the condition can be treated nonsurgically or with surgical reconstruction.

Anatomy and Pathogenesis
The first MTP joint is stabilized by its bony architecture and the surrounding soft-tissue restraints (**Table 1**). Relative laxity of the lateral soft-tissue structures at the first MTP joint, compared with the medial structures, contributes to hallux varus deformity. The lateral capsule, the

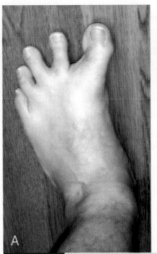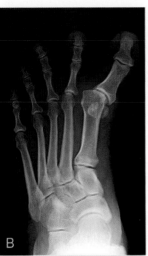

Figure 5 Clinical photograph (**A**) and standing AP radiograph (**B**) show a posttraumatic hallux varus deformity.

lateral ligaments, the adductor hallucis, the lateral aspect of the flexor hallucis brevis, and the fibular sesamoid are important restraints to varus deformity.

The etiology of hallux varus can be congenital, idiopathic, or posttraumatic, but the most common cause is overcorrection during hallux valgus surgery. The reported incidence of hallux varus after hallux valgus surgery is 2% to 15%.[30] Hallux varus can result from excessive release of the lateral soft-tissue structures, excision of the fibular sesamoid, excessive resection of the medial aspect of the first metatarsal head, excessive tightening of the medial capsular structures, or overcorrection with a metatarsal osteotomy or arthrodesis during surgery for hallux valgus. The classic hallux varus deformity after fibular sesamoid excision during the McBride procedure is accompanied by MTP joint hyperextension and interphalangeal (IP) joint flexion.

Diagnostic Evaluation
The evaluation of a patient with hallux varus should begin with an assessment of the symptoms. Patients often report pain with shoe wear, even if the shoes have a wide toe box. As with hallux valgus, the clinical examination should include a standing assessment of alignment, an inspection for callosities, and a determination of the specific site of pain. The motion of the MTP and IP joints should be measured, and the flexibility of the deformity should be assessed. A neurologic and vascular examination should be performed.

An attempt should be made to understand the cause of the deformity. A review of specific features of any earlier procedures may clarify the underlying cause of the deformity. Scars from any hallux valgus surgery should

4: The Forefoot

be taken into consideration if surgical reconstruction is necessary.

The radiographic evaluation of the foot should include weight-bearing AP and lateral views and a non–weight-bearing oblique view. The images should be studied to determine the hallux varus angle, the intermetatarsal angle, the location of the sesamoids relative to the first metatarsal head, and the extent of arthrosis at the first MTP joint (**Figure 6**).

Nonsurgical Treatment

Nonsurgical treatment of a hallux varus deformity consists of patient education and shoe modifications. A shoe with a wide toe box can best accommodate the foot. The hallux sometimes can be taped or splinted to correct the deformity and improve symptoms.

Surgical Treatment

Several surgical techniques have been described for treating hallux varus deformity. It is important to assess the extent of arthrosis of the first MTP joint before surgery. If significant degenerative changes are present, the best treatment option may be arthrodesis of the first MTP joint. In the absence of degenerative changes, joint-sparing realignment procedures may be considered; these include bony as well as soft-tissue procedures such as releases and tendon transfers.

Extensor tendon transfer is a reliable method of correcting a flexible, nonarthritic hallux varus deformity. This technique initially was described as using the entire extensor hallucis longus (EHL) tendon. The tendon is harvested distally, passed deep to the transverse metatarsal ligament, and fixed to the hallux proximal phalanx. A complete EHL tendon transfer typically is coupled with an IP joint arthrodesis, which may become problematic if an MTP arthrodesis subsequently becomes necessary. A popular modification of this procedure uses a split EHL transfer that leaves a portion of the EHL to control the IP joint and thus eliminates the need for an IP joint arthrodesis. The extensor hallucis brevis (EHB) can be used instead of the EHL; the EHB attachment is left in place, and the proximal portion of the tendon is transected, passed deep to the intermetatarsal ligament, and secured to the first metatarsal head to create a static tenodesis that corrects the varus deformity. A small-incision technique for EHL or EHB tendon transfer has been described.[31]

Suture suspension has been proposed for correcting hallux varus as well as hallux valgus.[17,32,33] A suture suspensory device is passed first from medial to lateral through the hallux proximal phalanx and then from lateral to medial through the first metatarsal head to replicate the path of the EHB tendon transfer. As the

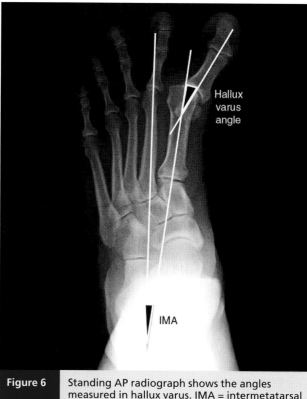

Figure 6 Standing AP radiograph shows the angles measured in hallux varus. IMA = intermetatarsal angle.

suture is tensioned, it becomes a static tether that corrects the varus deformity.

A bony correction often is required if the hallux varus deformity resulted from excessive correction during a first metatarsal osteotomy. A proximal metatarsal osteotomy or a first TMT arthrodesis is a reliable option. A reverse distal chevron osteotomy has been described as an alternative.[34,35] The bony procedure should be combined with distal soft-tissue realignment.

Summary

Hallux valgus is a common disorder that often can be managed nonsurgically. If nonsurgical management is unsuccessful, a large number of procedures can be considered. The decision-making process before surgical treatment of any hallux valgus deformity must consider numerous factors including the presence of arthritis, joint congruency, extent of deformity, presence of articular deformity, soft-tissue balance, and exact location of the deformity. The general principles that guide treatment decisions include treatment of an arthritic joint with fusion, avoidance of procedures that cause incongruence, the choice of a relatively proximal site for correction of a large deformity, and reduction of the sesamoids. Both new and older techniques should be further evaluated to determine their long-term value.

Hallux varus most commonly occurs as a complication of hallux valgus surgery. It is important to understand the etiology of the deformity and to carefully assess the patient's symptoms. Some patients with hallux varus can be treated nonsurgically, but others require surgical reconstruction. The reconstructive options include soft-tissue and bony procedures. The factors affecting the choice of procedure include the patient's symptoms and goals, the specifics of any earlier surgical procedure, the flexibility of the deformity, and the presence of arthrosis.

Annotated References

1. Perera AM, Mason L, Stephens MM: The pathogenesis of hallux valgus. *J Bone Joint Surg Am* 2011;93(17):1650-1661.

   The pathogenesis of hallux valgus was discussed with a focus on the pathoanatomy and anatomy of the deformity. Level of evidence: V.

2. Nery C, Coughlin MJ, Baumfeld D, Ballerini FJ, Kobata S: Hallux valgus in males: Part 1. Demographics, etiology, and comparative radiology. *Foot Ankle Int* 2013;34(5):629-635.

   A study of 31 men with hallux valgus found that, in comparison with women, bunions were more commonly hereditary and had an earlier onset, a greater severity, and a higher distal metatarsal articular angle. Level of evidence: III.

3. Van Beek C, Greisberg J: Mobility of the first ray. *Foot Ankle Int* 2011;32(9):917-922.

   The role of first ray mobility in the development of hallux valgus was reviewed, and techniques for measuring first ray mobility were discussed. Level of evidence: V.

4. Kim JY, Park JS, Hwang SK, Young KW, Sung IH: Mobility changes of the first ray after hallux valgus surgery: Clinical results after proximal metatarsal chevron osteotomy and distal soft tissue procedure. *Foot Ankle Int* 2008;29(5):468-472.

   The change in first ray mobility after hallux valgus surgery was evaluated. There was a significant reduction in dorsiflexion mobility. Level of evidence: IV.

5. Dietze A, Bahlke U, Martin H, Mittlmeier T: First ray instability in hallux valgus deformity: A radiokinematic and pedobarographic analysis. *Foot Ankle Int* 2013;34(1):124-130.

   First ray instability was dynamically evaluated with a mobile fluoroscopic device. Patients with a hallux valgus deformity had increased maximal dorsiflexion of the first ray during gait.

6. Chen L, Lyman S, Do H, et al: Validation of foot and ankle outcome score for hallux valgus. *Foot Ankle Int* 2012;33(12):1145-1155.

   The Foot and Ankle Outcome Score was validated in patients with hallux valgus. Construct validity, reliability, and responsiveness were evaluated.

7. Hardy RH, Clapham JC: Observations on hallux valgus based on a controlled series. *J Bone Joint Surg Br* 1951;3(3):376-391.

8. Okuda R, Kinoshita M, Yasuda T, Jotoku T, Kitano N, Shima H: Postoperative incomplete reduction of the sesamoids as a risk factor for recurrence of hallux valgus. *J Bone Joint Surg Am* 2009;91(7):1637-1645.

   The effect of postoperative sesamoid reduction on hallux valgus recurrence was evaluated. Incomplete reduction of the sesamoids was associated with greater risk of recurrence. Level of evidence: IV.

9. Panchbhavi VK, Rapley J, Trevino SG: First web space soft tissue release in bunion surgery: Functional outcomes of a new technique. *Foot Ankle Int* 2011;32(3):257-261.

   A new technique for first web space soft-tissue release was described, and its results were evaluated. Level of evidence: IV.

10. Choi YR, Lee HS, Jeong JJ, et al: Hallux valgus correction using transarticular lateral release with distal chevron osteotomy. *Foot Ankle Int* 2012;33(10):838-843.

    Outcomes of hallux valgus correction using a transarticular lateral release, distal chevron, and Akin phalangeal osteotomy were reported, and the technique was found to be effective. Level of evidence: IV.

11. Holmes GB: Correction of hallux valgus deformity using the mini TightRope device. *Tech Foot Ankle Surg* 2008;7:(1)9-16.

    Hallux valgus correction using a suture suspensory device was described. Level of evidence: V.

12. Kayiaros S, Blankenhorn BD, Dehaven J, et al: Correction of metatarsus primus varus associated with hallux valgus deformity using the Arthrex mini tightrope: A report of 44 cases. *Foot Ankle Spec* 2011;4(4):212-217.

    A suture suspensory device was used in 44 hallux valgus corrections. Improved functional outcome scores and alignment were reported, with a low rate of recurrence. Level of evidence: IV.

13. Cano-Martínez JA, Picazo-Marín F, Bento-Gerard J, Nicolás-Serrano G: Tratamiento del Hallux valgus moderado con sistema mini TightRope®: Técnica modificada. *Rev Esp Cir Ortop Traumatol* 2011;55(5):358-368.

    A study of 36 hallux valgus corrections using a suture suspensory device found improved angular correction and outcome scores at 24-month follow-up. Level of evidence: IV.

4: The Forefoot

14. Weatherall JM, Chapman CB, Shapiro SL: Postoperative second metatarsal fractures associated with suture-button implant in hallux valgus surgery. *Foot Ankle Int* 2013;34(1):104-110.

    A retrospective review of the outcomes of 25 patients treated with a suture suspensory device for hallux valgus correction found that a satisfactory reduction was achieved, but there was a high rate of second metatarsal stress fracture. Level of evidence: IV.

15. Kemp TJ, Hirose CB, Coughlin MJ: Fracture of the second metatarsal following suture button fixation device in the correction of hallux valgus. *Foot Ankle Int* 2010;31(8):712-716.

    A case report described a second metatarsal fracture after suture suspensory device correction of a hallux valgus deformity. Level of evidence: V.

16. Mader DW, Han NM: Bilateral second metatarsal stress fractures after hallux valgus correction with the use of a tension wire and button fixation system. *J Foot Ankle Surg* 2010;49(5):e15-e19.

    A case report described a bilateral second metatarsal fracture after bilateral hallux valgus correction with a suture suspensory device. Level of evidence: V.

17. Holmes GB Jr, Hsu AR: Correction of intermetatarsal angle in hallux valgus using small suture button device. *Foot Ankle Int* 2013;34(4):543-549.

    The short-term outcomes of hallux valgus correction using a suture suspensory device showed improved alignment. Level of evidence: IV.

18. Shurnas PS, Watson TS, Crislip TW: Proximal first metatarsal opening wedge osteotomy with a low profile plate. *Foot Ankle Int* 2009;30(9):865-872.

    A proximal opening-wedge first metatarsal osteotomy led to improvement in pain and angular deformity. Level of evidence: IV.

19. Saragas NP: Proximal opening-wedge osteotomy of the first metatarsal for hallux valgus using a low profile plate. *Foot Ankle Int* 2009;30(10):976-980.

    A retrospective study examined the results of a proximal opening-wedge first metatarsal osteotomy for hallux valgus correction. Patients had an improved hallux valgus angle and American Orthopaedic Foot and Ankle Society score, but a hallux varus deformity developed in 8%. Level of evidence: IV.

20. Jäger M, Schmidt M, Wild A, et al: Z-osteotomy in hallux valgus: Clinical and radiological outcome after Scarf osteotomy. *Orthop Rev (Pavia)* 2009;1(1):e4.

    At 22-month follow-up after 131 scarf first metatarsal osteotomies for hallux valgus, angular measurements were improved and patient satisfaction was high. Level of evidence: IV.

21. Paczesny L, Kruczyński J, Adamski R: Scarf versus proximal closing wedge osteotomy in hallux valgus treatment. *Arch Orthop Trauma Surg* 2009;129(10):1347-1352.

    The difference in postoperative hallux valgus correction after a proximal closing-wedge osteotomy or a scarf osteotomy was found to be related to the preoperative distal metatarsal articular angle. Level of evidence: III.

22. Singh D, Dudkiewicz I: Lengthening of the shortened first metatarsal after Wilson's osteotomy for hallux valgus. *J Bone Joint Surg Br* 2009;91(12):1583-1586.

    The results of lengthening for iatrogenic first brachymetatarsia in 16 patients were described. Lengthening of as much as 10 mm was achieved with a scarf osteotomy. Level of evidence: IV.

23. Gruber F, Sinkov VS, Bae SY, Parks BG, Schon LC: Crossed screws versus dorsomedial locking plate with compression screw for first metatarsocuneiform arthrodesis: A cadaver study. *Foot Ankle Int* 2008;29(9):927-930.

    A cadaver biomechanical investigation examined stiffness and load to failure in two fixation constructs for first tarsometatarsal joint arthrodesis. The addition of a dorsomedial locking plate did not add rigidity to the construct compared with the use of screws alone.

24. Scranton PE, Coetzee JC, Carreira D: Arthrodesis of the first metatarsocuneiform joint: A comparative study of fixation methods. *Foot Ankle Int* 2009;30(4):341-345.

    A cadaver biomechanical study found that a new locking plate had better load to failure than crossed screws.

25. Klos K, Gueorguiev B, Mückley T, et al: Stability of medial locking plate and compression screw versus two crossed screws for Lapidus arthrodesis. *Foot Ankle Int* 2010;31(2):158-163.

    A cadaver biomechanical investigation of two fixation constructions for first TMT joint arthrodesis found that a medial locking plate with an adjunct compression screw was superior to crossed screws with cyclic loading.

26. DeVries JG, Granata JD, Hyer CF: Fixation of first tarsometatarsal arthrodesis: A retrospective comparative cohort of two techniques. *Foot Ankle Int* 2011;32(2):158-162.

    A clinical study of two fixation techniques for first tarsometatarsal joint arthrodesis found that the use of a locking-plate construct led to a better union rate than crossed screw constructs. Level of evidence: III.

27. Hunt KJ, Barr CR, Lindsey DP, Chou LB: Locked versus nonlocked plate fixation for first metatarsophalangeal arthrodesis: A biomechanical investigation. *Foot Ankle Int* 2012;33(11):984-990.

    A biomechanical study compared locked and nonlocked plates for first metatarsophalangeal fusion strength and stiffness. Locked plates had less plantar gapping after 10,000 cycles of fatigue endurance testing.

28. Pydah SK, Toh EM, Sirikonda SP, Walker CR: Intermetatarsal angular change following fusion of the first metatarsophalangeal joint. *Foot Ankle Int* 2009;30(5):415-418.

    After first metatarsophalangeal fusion without metatarsal osteotomy, the intermetatarsal angle was reliably corrected. Level of evidence: IV.

29. Rippstein PF, Park YU, Naal FD: Combination of first metatarsophalangeal joint arthrodesis and proximal correction for severe hallux valgus deformity. *Foot Ankle Int* 2012;33(5):400-405.

    First metatarsophalangeal fusion with the addition of a proximal osteotomy for severe hallux valgus deformity had a high correction capability. Level of evidence: IV.

30. Devos Bevernage B, Leemrijse T: Hallux varus: Classification and treatment. *Foot Ankle Clin* 2009;14(1):51-65.

    The etiology, classification, and treatment of hallux varus were reviewed. Level of evidence: V.

31. Lui TH: Technique tip: minimally invasive approach of tendon transfer for correction of hallux varus. *Foot Ankle Int* 2009;30(10):1018-1021.

    A minimally invasive technique was described for correction of hallux varus using the extensor hallucis brevis or extensor hallucis longus. Level of evidence: V.

32. Pappas AJ, Anderson RB: Management of acquired hallux varus with an endobutton. *Tech Foot Ankle Surg* 2008;7:(2)134-138.

    A technique for hallux varus correction using a suture suspensory device was described. Level of evidence: V.

33. Gerbert J, Traynor C, Blue K, Kim K: Use of the Mini TightRope® for correction of hallux varus deformity. *J Foot Ankle Surg* 2011;50(2):245-251.

    A second technique for hallux varus correction using a suture suspensory device was described. Level of evidence: V.

34. Lee KT, Park YU, Young KW, Kim JS, Kim KC, Kim JB: Reverse distal chevron osteotomy to treat iatrogenic hallux varus after overcorrection of the intermetatarsal 1-2 angle: Technique tip. *Foot Ankle Int* 2011;32(1):89-91.

    A technique for hallux varus correction using a distal first metatarsal osteotomy was described. Level of evidence: V.

35. Choi KJ, Lee HS, Yoon YS, et al: Distal metatarsal osteotomy for hallux varus following surgery for hallux valgus. *J Bone Joint Surg Br* 2011;93(8):1079-1083.

    The outcomes of 19 patients after distal chevron metatarsal osteotomy for hallux varus correction were described. Level of evidence: IV.

4: The Forefoot

Chapter 14
Hallux Rigidus

John Y. Kwon, MD

Introduction

The term hallux rigidus is used to describe a painful degenerative condition of the hallux metatarsophalangeal (MTP) joint. Hallus rigidus is characterized by progressive loss of joint motion, joint space narrowing, and osteophyte formation, which lead to pain and declining physical function. The condition was first reported in 1887 as a plantarflexed hallux at the first MTP joint with degenerative arthritis.[1,2]

Etiology and Pathophysiology

Hallux rigidus is believed to be incited by a single-episode trauma to the hallux, as in an intra-articular fracture or a turf toe injury, or by repetitive, cumulative microinjury.[3,4] Any loading injury to the hallux can cause compressive or shear forces across the joint and, in association with hyperdorsiflexion or plantar flexion, can cause acute chondral or osteochondral injury. Not all patients recall such an injury. In addition, acute injury to the hallux can lead to detection of long-standing but previously asymptomatic degenerative changes.

After articular cartilage is damaged, loss of articular cartilage and alteration in bony anatomy progress as in other posttraumatic arthritic conditions. An initial softening of articular cartilage is related to depletion of the matrix proteoglycans. Early fibrillation results from a roughening of the articular surface incurred by unmasking and fragmentation of the collagen fibril structure. As the disease progresses, clefts and fissures form, and the eventual result is full-thickness cartilage loss, eburnation of the bony surfaces, formation of subchondral cysts, and osteophyte formation.

Several factors in addition to trauma are believed to be related to the etiology of hallus rigidus or a predisposition to the condition; these include female sex, bilateral symptoms associated with a positive family history, hallux valgus interphalangeus, metatarsus adductus,

and metatarsal head morphology.[4-10] Hallux rigidus has long been associated with metatarsus primus elevatus, although this condition was found to be a compensatory deformity often corrected by surgical treatment of hallux rigidus.[4,10,11] Another study found no relationship between the two conditions.[12] No association has been found between hallux rigidus and hindfoot contracture, abnormal foot posture, first ray hypermobility, metatarsal length, or the patient's occupation or shoe wear.[4,11]

The differential diagnosis includes crystalline disorders such as gout and pseudogout, rheumatoid arthritis, other types of inflammatory arthritis, and septic arthritis. Sesamoiditis, sesamoid fracture, turf toe injury, acute isolated osteochondral injury to the hallux MTP joint, hallux varus, and hallux valgus can cause pain around the joint but typically do not lead to joint space narrowing or other radiographic signs of arthritis of the hallux MTP joint.

Clinical Evaluation

Physical Examination

Patients report pain and physical limitation. Early in the course of hallux rigidus, pain often occurs only during activities requiring an increase in motion or loading of the hallux MTP joint, such as running or wearing high-heeled shoes. The symptoms tend to be intermittent and easily tempered with NSAID use, shoe wear modification, or slight changes in activity. As synovial thickening and inflammation increase with further degeneration of articular cartilage, the symptoms become more consistent. The patient begins to have progressive loss of joint motion, and activities of daily living become more difficult. As joint space narrowing and dorsal osteophyte formation progress, painful impingement causes increasing difficulty with shoe wear. Simple activities such as prolonged walking or standing can elicit symptoms.

An inflamed and tender hallux MTP joint is found on physical examination. Erythema may be present, although typically not the cherry-red hyperemic inflammation characteristic of an acute gout flare-up. Although the dorsal soft-tissue envelope is usually intact, the patient (especially a patient with diabetic neuropathy) may present with skin ulceration. The patient may have a history of wearing ill-fitting shoes. With MTP joint palpation, the patient may experience tenderness secondary to chronic bursitis, synovitis, tenosynovitis of overlying extensor tendons, or painful dorsal spurs. Range-of-motion restriction depends on the stage of the disease; terminal dorsiflexion and plantar flexion elicit pain. The range of motion should be compared with that of the lesser toes and contralateral hallux MTP joints. Typically the hallux and lesser toe MTP joints should have similar dorsiflexion. Pain during midrange motion or gentle loading of the MTP joint (the grind test) indicates a more profound MTP joint cartilage loss. Clicking, catching, or grinding is found in relatively advanced hallux rigidus. Neuritis or loss of sensation to light touch can result from compressive neuropathy of the terminal branch of the superficial peroneal nerve, typically as a result of shoe pressure over the dorsal spur. In the absence of a comorbid condition such as peripheral vascular disease, perfusion of the toe usually is maintained.

Radiographic Examination and Classification

The radiographic examination requires AP, oblique, and lateral weight-bearing views of the affected foot. Plain radiographs reveal joint asymmetry, joint space narrowing, sclerosis, subchondral cyst formation, osteophyte formation, and toe deviation at the MTP joint; the level of severity depends on the stage of disease. Joint space narrowing and toe alignment are best seen in the AP view, and dorsal spur formation is best seen in the lateral view. MRI or CT is rarely required for diagnosis but may be useful if the differential diagnosis is unclear. Similarly, laboratory studies or joint aspiration can be useful to rule out crystalline disorders but typically are not required unless the diagnosis of hallux rigidus is unclear.

The Coughlin grading system is commonly used to guide treatment in conjunction with clinical findings.[10] In grade 0, the patient has mild pain only during recreational activity or while wearing high-heeled shoes. Examination reveals slight tenderness to palpation but no clinical deformity. The range-of-motion loss is minimal; dorsiflexion is approximately 40° to 60°, or 10% to 20% less than in the normal contralateral joint. Radiographic findings are essentially normal. In grade 1, the symptoms are similar, but examination reveals tenderness, a palpable tender dorsal spur, and dorsiflexion of 30° to 40° (20% to 50% less than in the normal contralateral joint). The grind test does not elicit pain. Radiographs reveal a small dorsal spur (mild to moderate osteophyte formation) but minimal joint narrowing, sclerosis, or change to the articular morphology. A patient with grade 2 hallux rigidus reports more consistent pain, pain with activities of daily living, and greater difficulty with shoe

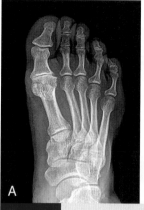
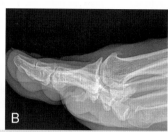

Figure 1 AP (**A**) and lateral (**B**) radiographs showing grade 3 hallux rigidus.

wear than in grade 1. The range of motion is more restricted; dorsiflexion is 10° to 30°, or 50% to 75% less than at the normal contralateral joint. The osteophytes are palpable and tender. Radiographs reveal mild to moderate (less than 50%) joint space narrowing, mild to moderate sclerosis, and osteophyte formation extending medially and laterally with increased dorsal prominence. Typical periarticular arthritic changes of the sesamoids are not profound, although irregularities may appear. At grade 3, the patient has near-constant pain during activities of daily living and increased difficulty with shoe wear. Range of motion is restricted to dorsiflexion of no more than 10°, or 75% to 100% less than at the normal contralateral joint side, with loss of as much as 10° of plantar flexion. Osteophytes are clinically palpable and tender. Patients report pain at the terminal range of motion but may not have increased pain with the grind test. Radiographic findings are similar to those in grade 2, but with more than 50% narrowing of the joint space, greater cystic changes and sclerosis, and greater sesamoid involvement (**Figure 1**). The radiographic and clinical findings in grade 4 are consistent with those of grade 3, but the grind test is positive.

Nonsurgical Treatment

The nonsurgical treatment of hallux rigidus is similar to that of other degenerative arthritides and must be tailored to the individual needs of the patient. The decision to manage hallux rigidus nonsurgically depends on not only the grade but also the patient's symptoms, limitations, and activity level. In general, nonsurgical treatment consists of the use of NSAIDs, injections, immobilization, shoe wear modification, and activity modification.

Hallux rigidus grade 0, 1, or 2 usually can be effectively managed with NSAIDs, toe strapping, and shoe stretching to accommodate early osteophyte formation.

Shoes with a stiff sole or a rocker-bottom sole can reduce the transmission of forces across the MTP joint and limit its motion. The patient is instructed to limit the inciting activities. Grade 3 or 4 is managed with the same modalities. A Morton extension can be used to further reduce MTP joint motion; care is required, however, because a shoe insert reduces the space in the toe box and thereby can increase dorsal spur pressure. The use of shoes with a deep toe box is recommended. A steel shank can be custom inserted into the shoe to further increase rigidity.

Nonsurgical treatment has been found effective. At a mean 14.4-year follow-up of nonsurgical treatment in 22 patients (24 feet), the patient agreed with the earlier decision not to have surgery for 18 of the feet (75%), despite an overall lack of symptom improvement and worsening radiographic findings.[13] These encouraging study findings are somewhat surprising because patients generally report a stepwise decline in function and an increase in symptoms, as in other degenerative arthritic conditions.

Intra-articular cortisone can be used sparingly. Administration into the MTP joint becomes more difficult as the joint space narrows and may require the use of fluoroscopy or consultation with an interventional radiologist. The deleterious effects of cortisone (in particular, thinning of the dorsal soft tissues and impaired wound healing) must be taken into account if surgical intervention is later considered as the disease progresses. Intra-articular steroid injection into the MTP joint and gentle joint manipulation led to clinical improvement of 6 months' duration in patients with mild to moderate hallux rigidus.[14] However, patients with severe hallux rigidus had little symptomatic relief and required surgical treatment.

Surgical Treatment

The decision to undertake surgical treatment is based not only on the disease grade but also on the patient's symptoms and response to nonsurgical treatment. The patient's personal goals and perception of the effect of the disease on quality of life are paramount. The appropriate nonsurgical modalities must be tried before surgical intervention is pursued. Few level I studies have compared the available surgical modalities, and a 2010 Cochrane review identified only one clinical study that met the inclusion criteria.[15] More robust randomized controlled studies are needed to determine the efficacy of interventions for the treatment of hallux rigidus. A review of evidence-based reports found that no definitive conclusions could be drawn from adequately powered studies using appropriate validated outcomes measures.[16] There is a need for high-quality level I studies. Nonetheless, many studies have shown the benefits of surgical intervention. The available procedures are characterized as joint sparing, joint modifying, or joint ablation.

Joint-Sparing Procedures

Joint-sparing procedures typically are used for low-grade (grades 1 and 2) hallux rigidus after unsuccessful nonsurgical treatment. An MTP joint synovectomy can be done as an isolated procedure, but usually a joint-modifying procedure is added. In a retrospective review of surgically treated osteochondral defects of the first metatarsal head, 14 of 24 patients had subchondral drilling and 10 had osteochondral autograft transfer.[17] Patients with a small lesion had a good result with either modality, but those with a larger defect or subchondral cyst were more likely to benefit from osteochondral autograft transfer.

Joint-Modifying Procedures

The joint-modifying procedures include cheilectomy, osteotomy, and MTP joint arthroscopy. Often these procedures are used in combination.

Cheilectomy

The most common joint-modifying procedure is cheilectomy, which is excision of the dorsal osteophytes and the degenerative dorsal portion of the articular surface of the first metatarsal head (**Figure 2**). Cheilectomy is an effective surgical option for relieving symptoms directly over the prominent dorsal spur as well as limitations in motion from a bony block and associated dorsal joint wear pattern. This procedure was first described in 1930.[9] In a review of patients with hallux valgus and hallux rigidus who were treated from 1920 to 1950, 68 patients underwent excision of the dorsal spur alone. Although a large number of these patients required additional surgery and/or nonsurgical treatment, good functional results were achieved.[5] Cheilectomy became popular after a 1959 report of 90% satisfactory results at short-term follow-up.[7] At a mean 9.6-year follow-up of 80 patients (93 feet), the largest study of cheilectomy reported that 86 of the cheilectomies (92%) were considered successful.[10] The mean improvement in dorsiflexion was from 14.5° before surgery to 38.4° after surgery. Of the nine patients who had midrange intra-articular pain before surgery, five later underwent arthrodesis and the remaining four had a self-reported fair or poor outcome. The researchers found that the clinical outcome was not correlated with the radiographic appearance of the joint at final follow-up. A recent gait analysis study of 17 patients found increases in MTP joint range of motion and peak sagittal-plane ankle push-off power at 1-year follow-up.[18]

In general, cheilectomy has been found effective, especially for patients with low-grade hallux rigidus, and

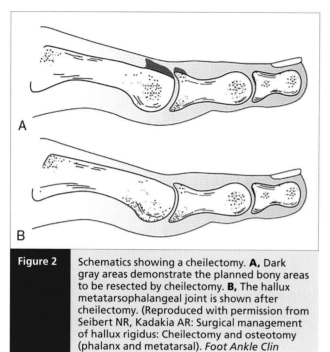

Figure 2 Schematics showing a cheilectomy. **A,** Dark gray areas demonstrate the planned bony areas to be resected by cheilectomy. **B,** The hallux metatarsophalangeal joint is shown after cheilectomy. (Reproduced with permission from Seibert NR, Kadakia AR: Surgical management of hallux rigidus: Cheilectomy and osteotomy (phalanx and metatarsal). *Foot Ankle Clin* 2009;14[1]:9-22.)

some evidence suggests it is effective for higher grade disease. At a mean 56-month follow-up, none of 25 patients had required additional surgical intervention after cheilectomy, and only 3 patients reported minimal discomfort.[8] Of 20 patients treated with isolated cheilectomy over a 6-year period, 18 (90%) reported near-complete pain relief; 16 (74%) had improvement in range of motion, and 13 (68%) had more than 30° of dorsiflexion with minimal progression of the degenerative process.[19] Forty-two patients treated with cheilectomy had subsequent improvement in range of motion, return to previous level of activity, dissipation of pain (within 3 months), and a high level of satisfaction.[20]

Simple cheilectomy appears to be less effective in patients with advancing disease and increasing joint involvement than in patients with lower grade disease. A review of 58 cheilectomies in 53 patients found that 53% of patients had a satisfactory result, 19% had a satisfactory result with reservations, and 28% had an unsatisfactory result.[21] When clinical results were correlated with the radiographic grade of the joint, the researchers found an unsatisfactory result in 15% of patients with grade 1 disease, 31.8% of those with grade 2 disease, and 37.5% of those with grade 3 disease. A study of 52 patients who underwent a dorsal cheilectomy through a medial approach found a 90% satisfaction rate at a mean 63-month follow-up, improved patient-reported outcomes scores, and an increase in dorsiflexion range of motion from 19° to 39°.[22] None of the 82% of feet

with grade 1 or 2 disease required a subsequent procedure, but 67% of the 18% with grade 3 disease had continuing pain and 25% required arthrodesis during the study period.

However, good results have also been reported regardless of the radiographic grade of the joint. Fifty-seven of 67 patients who underwent cheilectomy were available at a mean 65-month follow-up.[23] Radiographic disease grade was not used in the study, but patients with symptoms of advanced disease were excluded. An overall satisfaction rate of 78% was found, with a 91% satisfaction rate in patients older than 60 years, including those requiring a salvage procedure.

An isolated cheilectomy is an excellent treatment option that typically is reserved for lower grade hallux rigidus, although it appears to have some benefit in more advanced disease. Adequate dorsal resection with the goal of 90° intraoperative dorsiflexion is important. Careful patient selection and preoperative counseling as to expectations are even more important.

Osteotomy

Osteotomies have been used to treat hallux rigidus when joint preservation is preferred. These joint-modifying procedures include osteotomies of the proximal phalanx and distal first metatarsal. Proximal osteotomies of the first metatarsal have been described primarily for the treatment of metatarsus primus elevatus.

The Moberg osteotomy, a dorsiflexion osteotomy of the proximal phalanx, is beneficial for patients with hallux rigidus (**Figure 3**). As hallux rigidus advances, dorsiflexion is limited to a greater extent than plantar flexion. The use of a dorsal closing wedge osteotomy of the proximal phalanx repositions the toe into an extended position, thus altering and improving the arc of motion. This procedure typically is done in conjunction with cheilectomy and was first used in pediatric patients with painful hallux rigidus.[5] Ten adolescent patients had improvement in mean dorsiflexion from 5° before surgery to 44° at a mean 28-month follow-up.[24] Nine patients had significant pain relief with a good return to normal activities. Eight patients had a satisfactory result at short-term follow-up.[25] Seventeen patients (24 feet) with grade 1 or 2 disease underwent Moberg osteotomy and cheilectomy.[26] At a mean 5.2-year follow-up, overall satisfaction was high: 96% of the patients said they would undergo the procedure again, 58% reported no pain, and 42% reported only mild pain. A recent study found that all 34 patients who underwent dorsal cheilectomy with a combined Moberg and Akin biplanar osteotomy had radiographic healing at an average 22.5-month follow-up; 90% reported a good or excellent result, with pain relief, improvement in function, and decreased shoe wear limitation.[27] Only one patient required additional surgical intervention, for hardware removal. The role of cheilectomy and proximal phalangeal extension osteotomy in treating advanced disease recently was examined in 81 patients.[28] At a mean 4.3-year follow-up, the mean dorsiflexion of the first MTP joint had improved 27° (from 32.7° before surgery to 59.7°). The average American Orthopaedic Foot and Ankle Society (AOFAS) score had improved from 67.2 points to 88.7 points. Radiographs of the interphalangeal joint showed no evidence of interphalangeal joint arthritis. Sixty-nine patients (85%) were satisfied with the results of treatment; four patients (5%) subsequently underwent arthrodesis to treat persistent symptoms at the first MTP joint.

The effectiveness of distal first metatarsal osteotomy has been examined for the treatment of hallux rigidus and associated conditions such as metatarsus primus elevatus.[29-31] These osteotomies are focused on reorientation of the proximal portion of the first MTP joint to improve the functional range of motion and to treat dorsal articular wear. The goal of a dorsal closing wedge trapezoidal osteotomy of the distal metaphysis of the first metatarsal is to reorient intact articular cartilage on the plantar surface of the metatarsal head into a more functional position.[32] It can be difficult to interpret published studies on the use of distal first metatarsal osteotomies to treat hallux rigidus for two primary reasons: the additional use of cheilectomy in most patients and lack of clarity as to whether patients' symptoms were caused by hallux rigidus, metatarsus primus elevatus, or a combination of the two conditions.

Arthroscopy

Arthroscopy for the treatment of hallux rigidus has been reported, but there are no comparative studies, and the therapeutic benefit is unclear. Arthroscopy has been used for the treatment of an osteochondritis dissecans lesion of the first metatarsal head.[32] Fifteen patients had good results after arthroscopic cheilectomy, with rapid recovery and rehabilitation reported at short-term followup.[33] Arthroscopic treatment of hallux rigidus as well as associated osteochondral lesions and sesamoid conditions in 24 patients led to early rehabilitation and an early return to regular activities; arthroscopic cheilectomy and sesamoidectomy had less favorable results.[34] The indications for arthroscopy and its effectiveness are unclear, and it is not commonly used for the treatment of hallux rigidus.

Joint Ablation Procedures

Resection and Interposition Arthroplasty

Resection arthroplasty was first reported in 1904, and it continues to be a treatment option for end-stage hallux rigidus.[35] Although modifications have been made to the

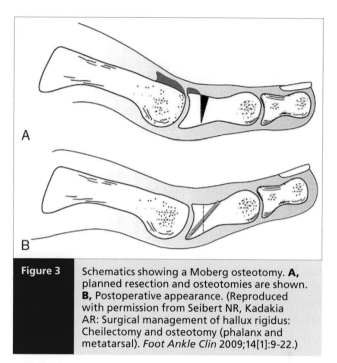

Figure 3 Schematics showing a Moberg osteotomy. **A,** planned resection and osteotomies are shown. **B,** Postoperative appearance. (Reproduced with permission from Seibert NR, Kadakia AR: Surgical management of hallux rigidus: Cheilectomy and osteotomy (phalanx and metatarsal). *Foot Ankle Clin* 2009;14[1]:9-22.)

original procedure and interpositional techniques have been added, the basic procedure still entails resection of the base of the hallux proximal phalanx with an associated cheilectomy and/or medial eminence resection to decompress the joint. Because of the functional sequelae and the difficulty of salvage surgery, Keller resection arthroplasty and the interposition techniques are best reserved for older patients who have low physical demands.[36-38] The loss of intrinsic muscular attachments, alterations in static and dynamic joint constraints, and bone shortening required for this procedure commonly lead to sequelae including a flail hallux, cock-up or deviational deformities, hammer toes, transfer metatarsalgia, toe shortening, push-off weakness, and poor cosmesis.[37-43]

Modifications of the Keller procedure with interposition arthroplasty have improved the results and may represent a viable treatment option for relatively younger patients who want to avoid arthrodesis. The modifications include oblique proximal phalangeal osteotomies to preserve the flexor hallucis brevis insertion and interposition of the extensor hallucis brevis or another autograft or allograft material. Relatively young, active patients with end-stage hallux rigidus underwent both cheilectomy and interposition arthroplasty as part of the Keller procedure, with tenodesis of the extensor hallucis brevis to the flexor hallucis brevis tendon; 94% had a good to excellent result.[44,45] An oblique osteotomy of the base of the proximal phalanx to preserve the flexor hallucis brevis insertion with interposition of the extensor hallucis brevis led to a good to excellent result in all 11 patients, with preserved motion and no instability.[46] At a mean

38-month follow-up after interposition arthroplasty in 18 patients, the hallux MTP joint range of motion had increased a mean of 37°, most patients had substantial pain relief, and 17 patients stated they would choose to have the procedure again.[47] The researchers concluded that interposition arthroplasty was a reasonable treatment option for end-stage hallux rigidus and was associated with fewer complications than previously reported. An excellent functional result was reported in all seven patients who underwent resection and soft-tissue interposition arthroplasty using a gracilis tendon graft, with preserved flexion power and increased hallux MTP joint motion.[11] In a long-term study, 104 patients underwent a Keller resection arthroplasty.[48] Thirty-two patients (42 feet) were available at a mean 7.6-year follow-up. Of the 32 patients, 76% were completely satisfied, 21.5% were satisfied with reservations, and 2.5% were dissatisfied. Ninety-five percent reported improvement in their symptoms, but 9.5% reported transfer metatarsalgia, and 19%, all of whom were women, were not happy with the cosmetic appearance of the foot. At a mean 23-year follow-up of 87 patients who underwent Keller resection arthroplasty, only five feet had required revision surgery.[49] The average AOFAS score was 83 points. Sixty-nine of the 73 patients who had not undergone revision surgery (95%) reported they would choose the same procedure again under the same circumstances.

Arthrodesis

Arthrodesis of the hallux MTP joint is an effective treatment option for patients with high-grade hallux rigidus after unsuccessful nonsurgical management or an unsuccessful joint-sparing procedure. The primary indication for hallux MTP arthrodesis is end-stage arthritis, regardless of whether the cause is severe hallux rigidus, a crystalline disorder, rheumatic or inflammatory disease, or septic arthritis. MTP arthrodesis also is an effective salvage procedure after unsuccessful cheilectomy, resection or interpositional arthroplasty, or prosthetic arthroplasty, and it is appropriate for treating hallux valgus or hallux varus deformity with concomitant arthritis if simple angular correction would lead to continued pain from arthritis.

Arthrodesis has long been considered the gold standard for end-stage disease. Patient variables such as tobacco use, diabetes, immunosuppression, and lack of compliance should be considered before hallux MTP arthrodesis or any other surgical procedure. Although pain relief is the primary objective of arthrodesis, fusion of the first MTP joint has biomechanical and functional consequences. As with any arthrodesis procedure, patients are concerned about the effect on their ability to perform activities of daily living and participate in

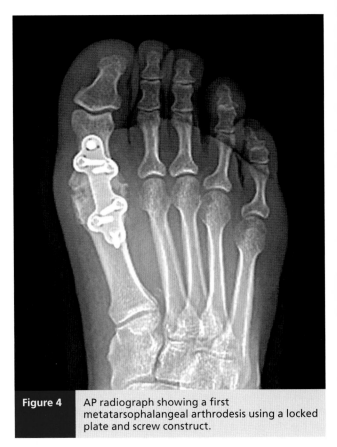

Figure 4 AP radiograph showing a first metatarsophalangeal arthrodesis using a locked plate and screw construct.

recreational activities after surgery. Shoe wear also is an area of concern, particularly in women who wish to wear fashionably high-heeled shoes. In compensation for the loss of first MTP joint motion, one study found a postoperative increase in weight bearing on the hallux and medial column as well as subtle changes in normal ankle kinematics (loss in the ankle plantar flexion moment and ankle power at toe-off).[50] However, other studies found no observable change in the gait pattern of patients who underwent hallux MTP arthrodesis.

The reported means of fixation include Kirschner wires, crossed screws, staples, external fixation devices, locking and nonlocking plates, and screw constructs[51] (Figure 4). Evidence exists to support the effectiveness of each technique, and the choice often is based on surgeon preference. Regardless of fixation technique, proper positioning of the arthrodesis is paramount for restoring function and avoiding compensatory changes.

Typically the hallux is fused in a functional position; the most recommended position approximates 20° to 30° of dorsiflexion in comparison with the long axis of the first metatarsal shaft and 5° to 15° of valgus positioning with neutral rotation.[51-54] Malpositioning of the hallux can lead to significant difficulties. Excessive dorsiflexion can cause irritation of the tip of the hallux during shoe wear, compensatory loading of the interphalangeal joint, and transfer metatarsalgia. In patients who wish to wear high-heeled shoes, a slight increase in dorsiflexion positioning has been recommended but should be considered with caution[51,55] (**Figure 5**). Excessive plantar flexion can lead to gait abnormalities secondary to a stiff toe-off as well as compensatory loading of the interphalangeal joint and plantar distal overloading of the toe. In addition to the ideal position of the hallux, other deformities of the midfoot and hindfoot must be considered when deciding on optimal positioning in the sagittal plane. The first metatarsal declination angle is affected by conditions such as metatarsus primus elevatus, cavovarus deformity, and pes planus deformity.[51] Before surgery, proper positioning of the hallux is best determined by carefully examining lateral weight-bearing radiographs and measuring the first metatarsal–proximal phalangeal angle. The most effective intraoperative method of assessing dorsiflexion of the hallux may be to simulate weight bearing by holding the ankle in neutral dorsiflexion on a flat sterile instrument tray.

The frontal plane alignment should be in 5° to 15° of valgus, although it is important to consider lesser toe alignment, the presence of a condition such as metatarsus adductus, and an increased intermetatarsal angle. Varus malpositioning can lead to painful impingement of the toe against the shoe toe box and can accelerate the progress of interphalangeal joint arthritis. Excessive valgus malpositioning can lead to painful impingement against the second toe. Rotational alignment is best evaluated by observing the position of the hallux nail bed relative to the lesser toes. A neutral alignment is preferred, although any iatrogenic rotational malpositioning in an otherwise well-positioned arthrodesis typically is more a cosmetic than a functional concern.

Rates of fusion after arthrodesis are reported to be 90% to 100%, with excellent overall functional outcomes.[10] A 94% fusion rate and good or excellent results were found in all 34 patients with advanced hallux rigidus at a mean 6.7-year follow-up.[10] A 100% fusion rate was reported at a mean 44-month follow-up after a parallel screw fixation technique was used in 60 feet.[56] Satisfaction rates were uniformly high, and most patients were able to return to their earlier sports activities.

Prosthetic Replacement

The potential benefits of prosthetic replacement of the first MTP joint include pain relief, restoration of joint motion, better function than with arthrodesis, and prevention of adjacent-joint degeneration or transfer loading. The design of prosthetic implants used to treat hallux rigidus, like implants for total knee and hip arthroplasty, has undergone an evolution. Early implant failures and difficult

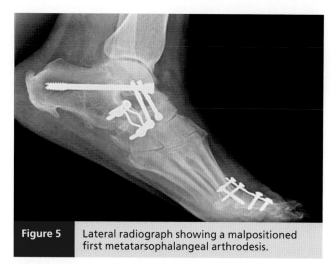

Figure 5 Lateral radiograph showing a malpositioned first metatarsophalangeal arthrodesis.

salvage reconstruction after unsuccessful arthroplasty led to infrequent use of the procedure, but changes in implant design and the theoretic advantages of arthroplasty over arthrodesis have led to renewed enthusiasm. Few studies have compared the benefits of prosthetic replacement to those of arthrodesis, which has long been considered the gold standard.

The first widely used implant designs were intended to preserve length while allowing MTP joint motion through an articulation with a Silastic-based hemiarthroplasty.[57] These designs were abandoned because of high rates of implant failure and osteolysis as well as difficulty in reconstruction. A 10% rate of implant failure was found in 66 patients with rheumatoid arthritis, primary hallux rigidus, or unsuccessful bunion surgery who received a double-stemmed silicone implant. As many as one third of patients had osteolytic changes.[58] A study of 91 patients had similar results, with a high rate of implant mechanical failure; nonetheless, the subjective results were generally satisfactory.[59] In addition to implant fracture and osteolysis, the reported complications included Silastic synovitis, foreign body reactions caused by silicone debris, and systemic infiltration.

Subsequent implant designs used metal as a surface-replacement bearing.[60] The early hemiarthroplasty designs used a cobalt-chromium alloy that allowed resurfacing of the proximal phalanx of the great toe. A study of 279 patients treated for hallux rigidus, rheumatoid arthritis, or unsuccessful bunion surgery found that 95% had a good or excellent clinical result at follow-up of as much as 33 years.[60] Other studies had difficulty replicating these encouraging results, however. In a study of 37 patients who underwent hemiarthroplasty, 5 of the 28 patients available at a mean 33-month follow-up were not completely satisfied with the procedure result.[61] Four patients had malpositioning of the implant, and three patients had evidence of subsidence and loosening, which was attributed to technical errors. A retrospective study of 41 toes over a 6-year period found a high revision rate with only moderate patient satisfaction (67% of patients).[62] Seventeen percent of patients underwent revision surgery an average 29 months after arthroplasty. A comparison of the Townley hemiarthroplasty with arthrodesis concluded that arthrodesis more predictably alleviated symptoms and restored function.[63] A poor result was found in 7 of the 21 patients who underwent hemiarthroplasty but in only 1 of the 27 patients who underwent arthrodesis.

Resurfacing of the metatarsal rather than the proximal phalanx was introduced in 2005, using technology and an implant design similar to those used in procedures for knee and shoulder arthritis. Early results have been promising. Thirty patients treated using the HemiCAP implant (Arthrosurface) had statistically significant improvements in range of motion, AOFAS scores, and Medical Outcomes Study Short Form–36 outcomes scores at a mean 27-month follow-up.[64] All patients reported excellent satisfaction. Implant survivorship was 87% at 5-year follow-up.

The most recent implant designs typically use a metal-on-polyethylene bearing and are press fit or cemented. The available studies primarily focused on specific implant designs, and few comparative or prospective studies have been completed.[65-68] A prospective randomized study compared arthrodesis of the first MTP joint and total joint arthroplasty in 63 patients with symptomatic hallux rigidus.[69] At 2-year follow-up, the patients treated with arthrodesis (38 feet) reported 82% improvement compared with 45% after arthroplasty (39 feet). Six patients in the arthroplasty group had loosening of the phalangeal component and subsequent removal. The remaining patients who underwent arthroplasty had a poor range of motion, with transfer loading to the lateral foot. Forty percent of patients treated with arthroplasty stated they would not undergo the procedure again.

The published studies in general show that the use of prosthetic implants may be a viable option, but there are few comparative studies, and high complication rates were reported in multiple studies (**Figure 6**). As implant designs evolve and high-quality prospective randomized studies are performed, the use of prosthetic implants may appear more promising.

Summary

Hallux rigidus is a painful degenerative condition of the hallux MTP joint characterized by progressive loss of joint motion, joint space narrowing, and osteophyte formation. Nonsurgical modalities are tried before surgery is considered. The choice of surgical option depends on

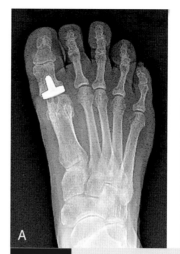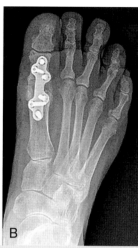

Figure 6 AP radiographs showing an unsuccessful hemiarthroplasty of the first metatarsophalangeal joint (**A**) and conversion to arthrodesis (**B**).

the grade of arthritis and the patient's symptoms. Long-term comparison studies are required to determine the optimal surgical treatment of end-stage hallux rigidus.

Annotated References

1. Davies-Colley M: Contraction of the metatarsophalangeal joint of the great toe. *BMJ* 1887;1:728.

2. Cotterill JM: Stiffness of the great toe in adolescents. *Br Med J* 1887;1(1378):1158.

3. Coughlin MJ: Conditions of the forefoot, in DeLee J, Drez D, eds: *Orthopaedic Sports Medicine: Principles and Practice*. Philadelphia, PA, WB Saunders, 1994, pp 221-244.

4. Coughlin MJ, Shurnas PS: Hallux rigidus: Demographics, etiology, and radiographic assessment. *Foot Ankle Int* 2003;24(10):731-743.

5. Bonney G, Macnab I: Hallux valgus and hallux rigidus: A critical survey of operative results. *J Bone Joint Surg Br* 1952;34-B(3):366-385.

6. Coughlin MJ, Mann RA: Arthrodesis of the first metatarsophalangeal joint as salvage for the failed Keller procedure. *J Bone Joint Surg Am* 1987;69(1):68-75.

7. Yee G, Lau J: Current concepts review: Hallux rigidus. *Foot Ankle Int* 2008;29(6):637-646.

   The etiology, nonsurgical management, and surgical treatment of hallux rigidus were summarized. Studies of cheilectomy, osteotomy, arthrodesis, and arthroplasty were evaluated based on level of evidence. Cheilectomy was supported for grade 1 or 2 hallux rigidus. Arthrodesis was the mainstay treatment for advanced disease. There was inadequate evidence to support osteotomy, interposition arthroplasty, or prosthetic arthroplasty.

8. Mann RA, Clanton TO: Hallux rigidus: Treatment by cheilectomy. *J Bone Joint Surg Am* 1988;70(3):400-406.

9. Nilsonne H: Hallux rigidus and its treatment. *Acta Orthop Scand* 1930;1:295-303.

10. Coughlin MJ, Shurnas PS: Hallux rigidus: Grading and long-term results of operative treatment. *J Bone Joint Surg Am* 2003;85-A(11):2072-2088.

11. Coughlin MJ, Shurnas PJ: Soft-tissue arthroplasty for hallux rigidus. *Foot Ankle Int* 2003;24(9):661-672.

12. Horton GA, Park YW, Myerson MS: Role of metatarsus primus elevatus in the pathogenesis of hallux rigidus. *Foot Ankle Int* 1999;20(12):777-780.

13. Smith RW, Katchis SD, Ayson LC: Outcomes in hallux rigidus patients treated nonoperatively: A long-term follow-up study. *Foot Ankle Int* 2000;21(11):906-913.

14. Solan MC, Calder JD, Bendall SP: Manipulation and injection for hallux rigidus: Is it worthwhile? *J Bone Joint Surg Br* 2001;83(5):706-708.

15. Zammit GV, Menz HB, Munteanu SE, Landorf KB, Gilheany MF: Interventions for treating osteoarthritis of the big toe joint. *Cochrane Database Syst Rev* 2010;9:CD007809.

Only one study of interventions for hallux rigidus fulfilled the inclusion criteria; that study evaluated physical therapy in the treatment of osteoarthritis of the great toe.

16. McNeil DS, Baumhauer JF, Glazebrook MA: Evidence-based analysis of the efficacy for operative treatment of hallux rigidus. *Foot Ankle Int* 2013;34(1):15-32.

An evidence-based literature review of surgical interventions for hallux rigidus found fair evidence to support the use of arthrodesis for hallux rigidus; poor evidence to support cheilectomy, osteotomy, and arthroplasty; and insufficient evidence for cheilectomy with osteotomy.

17. Kim YS, Park EH, Lee HJ, Koh YG, Lee JW: Clinical comparison of the osteochondral autograft transfer system and subchondral drilling in osteochondral defects of the first metatarsal head. *Am J Sports Med* 2012;40(8):1824-1833.

A retrospective review of first metatarsal head osteochondral defects treated with the osteochondral autograft transfer system or subchondral drilling in 24 patients found that defect size greater than 50 mm and presence of subchondral cysts were important predictors of poor outcome in subchondral drilling. There was no between-group difference in visual analog scores, but AOFAS scores were substantially poorer after subchondral drilling.

18. Smith SM, Coleman SC, Bacon SA, Polo FE, Brodsky JW: Improved ankle push-off power following cheilectomy for hallux rigidus: A prospective gait analysis study. *Foot Ankle Int* 2012;33(6):457-461.

Gait analysis 4 weeks before and at least 1 year after cheilectomy in patients with grade 1 or 2 hallux rigidus found substantial postsurgical improvement.

19. Mann RA, Coughlin MJ, DuVries HL: Hallux rigidus: A review of the literature and a method of treatment. *Clin Orthop Relat Res* 1979;142:57-63.

20. Gould N: Hallux rigidus: Cheilotomy or implant? *Foot Ankle* 1981;1(6):315-320.

21. Hattrup SJ, Johnson KA: Subjective results of hallux rigidus following treatment with cheilectomy. *Clin Orthop Relat Res* 1988;226:182-191.

22. Easley ME, Davis WH, Anderson RB: Intermediate to long-term follow-up of medial-approach dorsal cheilectomy for hallux rigidus. *Foot Ankle Int* 1999;20(3):147-152.

23. Feltham GT, Hanks SE, Marcus RE: Age-based outcomes of cheilectomy for the treatment of hallux rigidus. *Foot Ankle Int* 2001;22(3):192-197.

24. Kessel L, Bonney G: Hallux rigidus in the adolescent. *J Bone Joint Surg Br* 1958;40-B(4):669-673.

25. Moberg E: A simple operation for hallux rigidus. *Clin Orthop Relat Res* 1979;142:55-56.

26. Thomas PJ, Smith RW: Proximal phalanx osteotomy for the surgical treatment of hallux rigidus. *Foot Ankle Int* 1999;20(1):3-12.

27. Hunt KJ, Anderson RB: Biplanar proximal phalanx closing wedge osteotomy for hallux rigidus. *Foot Ankle Int* 2012;33(12):1043-1050.

A retrospective review of 34 patients who underwent cheilectomy and biplanar oblique closing-wedge proximal phalanx (Moberg-Akin) osteotomy for hallux rigidus or hallux valgus interphalangeus found that all osteotomies healed and 90% of patients had a good or excellent result. Radiographic angles were improved.

28. O'Malley MJ, Basran HS, Gu Y, Sayres S, Deland JT: Treatment of advanced stages of hallux rigidus with cheilectomy and phalangeal osteotomy. *J Bone Joint Surg Am* 2013;95(7):606-610.

In 81 patients who underwent cheilectomy and proximal phalangeal extension osteotomy for grade 3 hallux rigidus, dorsiflexion improved significantly, and 85% were satisfied at 4.3-year follow-up. AOFAS scores were significantly improved, but 5% later required arthrodesis.

29. Seibert NR, Kadakia AR: Surgical management of hallux rigidus: Cheilectomy and osteotomy (phalanx and metatarsal). *Foot Ankle Clin* 2009;14(1):9-22.

Generally, cheilectomy was found to be indicated for treatment of mild to moderate arthrosis. Metatarsal and phalangeal osteotomies are useful joint-sparing procedures. For severe arthrosis, fusion or joint arthroplasty is appropriate.

30. Malerba F, Milani R, Sartorelli E, Haddo O: Distal oblique first metatarsal osteotomy in grade 3 hallux rigidus: A long-term followup. *Foot Ankle Int* 2008;29(7):677-682.

An oblique distal osteotomy was described for the treatment of hallux rigidus in 20 patients with metatarsus primus elevatus. At a mean 11-year follow-up, AOFAS scores had increased from 44 to 82. The average motion of the first MTP joint increased from 8° to 44°. Patient satisfaction was high, and the complication rate was low.

31. Watermann H: Die arthritis deformans des großzehengrundgelenkes als selbständiges krankheitsbild. *Z Orthop Chir* 1927;48:346-355.

32. Bartlett DH: Arthroscopic management of osteochondritis dissecans of the first metatarsal head. *Arthroscopy* 1988;4(1):51-54.

33. Iqbal MJ, Chana GS: Arthroscopic cheilectomy for hallux rigidus. *Arthroscopy* 1998;14(3):307-310.

34. van Dijk CN, Veenstra KM, Nuesch BC: Arthroscopic surgery of the metatarsophalangeal first joint. *Arthroscopy* 1998;14(8):851-855.

35. Keller WL: The surgical treatment of bunions and hallux valgus. *NY State Med J* 1904;80:741-742.

36. Shereff MJ, Baumhauer JF: Hallux rigidus and osteoarthrosis of the first metatarsophalangeal joint. *J Bone Joint Surg Am* 1998;80(6):898-908.

37. Schenk S, Meizer R, Kramer R, Aigner N, Landsiedl F, Steinboeck G: Resection arthroplasty with and without capsular interposition for treatment of severe hallux rigidus. *Int Orthop* 2009;33(1):145-150.

Patients with grade 2 or 3 hallux rigidus were treated with the Keller procedure with cheilectomy and interposition arthroplasty or the Keller procedure alone. At 15-month follow-up, there were no differences in AOFAS scores, patient satisfaction, or range of motion. The rate of osteonecrosis of the first metatarsal head was high in both patient groups.

38. Keiserman LS, Sammarco VJ, Sammarco GJ: Surgical treatment of the hallux rigidus. *Foot Ankle Clin* 2005;10(1):75-96.

39. Reize P, Schanbacher J, Wülker N: K-wire transfixation or distraction following the Keller-Brandes arthroplasty in Hallux rigidus and Hallux valgus? *Int Orthop* 2007;31(3):325-331.

40. Sizensky JA: Forefoot and midfoot arthritis: What's new in surgical management. *Curr Opin Orthop* 2004;15:55-61.

41. Fuhrmann RA, Anders JO: The long-term results of resection arthroplasties of the first metatarsophalangeal joint in rheumatoid arthritis. *Int Orthop* 2001;25(5):312-316.

42. Altınmakas M, Şarlak O, Gür E, Gültekin N, Kırdemir V, Baydar M: Halluks valgus deformitesinde Keller rezeksiyon artroplastisi. *Acta Orthop Traumatol Turc* 1991;25:4-7.

43. Anderl W, Knahr K, Steinböck G: Long term results of the Keller-Brandes method of hallux rigidus surgery[in German]. *Z Orthop Ihre Grenzgeb* 1991;129(1):42-47.

44. Hamilton WG, O'Malley MJ, Thompson FM, Kovatis PE: Capsular interposition arthroplasty for severe hallux rigidus. *Foot Ankle Int* 1997;18(2):68-70.

45. Hamilton WG, Hubbard CE: Hallux rigidus: Excisional arthroplasty. *Foot Ankle Clin* 2000;5(3):663-671.

46. Can Akgun R, Şahin Ö, Demirörs H, Cengiz Tuncay İ: Analysis of modified oblique Keller procedure for severe hallux rigidus. *Foot Ankle Int* 2008;29(12):1203-1208.

Eleven patients with grade 3 or 4 hallux rigidus were treated with a modified oblique Keller resection with interposition arthroplasty. Range of motion and AOFAS scores were significantly improved at 27-month follow-up.

47. Kennedy JG, Chow FY, Dines J, Gardner M, Bohne WH: Outcomes after interposition arthroplasty for treatment of hallux rigidus. *Clin Orthop Relat Res* 2006;445(445):210-215.

48. Coutts A, Kilmartin TE, Ellis MJ: The long-term patient focused outcomes of the Keller's arthroplasty for the treatment of hallux rigidus. *Foot (Edinb)* 2012;22(3):167-171.

A review of patients who underwent Keller excisional arthroplasty for grade 4 hallux rigidus found that 76% were completely satisfied at a mean 7.6-year follow-up, and 95% reported symptom improvement; 9.5% reported transfer metatarsalgia, and 19% were unhappy with cosmetic appearance of the hallux.

49. Schneider W, Kadnar G, Kranzl A, Knahr K: Long-term results following Keller resection arthroplasty for hallux rigidus. *Foot Ankle Int* 2011;32(10):933-939.

Keller resection arthroplasty for hallux rigidus was reviewed in 87 patients at 23-year follow-up. Only 5% required revision surgery, and 94% stated they would have the surgery again. Pedobarograph studies showed moderate weight-bearing alterations. Outcome scores were comparable to age-matched norms.

50. DeFrino PF, Brodsky JW, Pollo FE, Crenshaw SJ, Beischer AD: First metatarsophalangeal arthrodesis: A clinical, pedobarographic and gait analysis study. *Foot Ankle Int* 2002;23(6):496-502.

51. Kelikian AS: Technical considerations in hallux metatarsalphalangeal arthrodesis. *Foot Ankle Clin* 2005;10(1):167-190.

52. Harper MC: Positioning of the hallux for first metatarsophalangeal joint arthrodesis. *Foot Ankle Int* 1997;18(12):827.

53. Conti SF, Dhawan S: Arthrodesis of the first metatarsophalangeal and interphalangeal joints of the foot. *Foot Ankle Clin* 1996;1:33-53.

54. Fitzgerald JA: A review of long-term results of arthrodesis of the first metatarso-phalangeal joint. *J Bone Joint Surg Br* 1969;51(3):488-493.

55. Esway JE, Conti SF: Joint replacement in the hallux metatarsophalangeal joint. *Foot Ankle Clin* 2005;10(1):97-115.

56. Brodsky JW, Passmore RN, Pollo FE, Shabat S: Functional outcome of arthrodesis of the first metatarsophalangeal joint using parallel screw fixation. *Foot Ankle Int* 2005;26(2):140-146.

57. Wenger RJ, Whalley RC: Total replacement of the first metatarsophalangeal joint. *J Bone Joint Surg Br* 1978;60(1):88-92.

58. Cracchiolo A III, Weltmer JB Jr, Lian G, Dalseth T, Dorey F: Arthroplasty of the first metatarsophalangeal joint with a double-stem silicone implant: Results in patients who have degenerative joint disease failure of previous operations, or rheumatoid arthritis. *J Bone Joint Surg Am* 1992;74(4):552-563.

59. Granberry WM, Noble PC, Bishop JO, Tullos HS: Use of a hinged silicone prosthesis for replacement arthroplasty of the first metatarsophalangeal joint. *J Bone Joint Surg Am* 1991;73(10):1453-1459.

60. Townley CO, Taranow WS: A metallic hemiarthroplasty resurfacing prosthesis for the hallux metatarsophalangeal joint. *Foot Ankle Int* 1994;15(11):575-580.

61. Taranow WS, Moutsatson MJ, Cooper JM: Contemporary approaches to stage II and III hallux rigidus: The role of metallic hemiarthroplasty of the proximal phalanx. *Foot Ankle Clin* 2005;10(4):713-728, ix-x.

62. Jelinek A, Anderson J, Bohay D: Management of hallux rigidus: The metallic hemiarthroplasty resurfacing prosthesis revisited. *Foot Ankle Surg* 2007;13(2):99-106.

63. Raikin SM, Ahmad J, Pour AE, Abidi N: Comparison of arthrodesis and metallic hemiarthroplasty of the hallux metatarsophalangeal joint. *J Bone Joint Surg Am* 2007;89(9):1979-1985.

64. Kline AJ, Hasselman CT: Metatarsal head resurfacing for advanced hallux rigidus. *Foot Ankle Int* 2013;34(5):716-725.

   A prospective study of 26 patients with grade 2 or 3 hallux rigidus treated with HemiCAP metallic resurfacing arthroplasty of the metatarsal head found that active range of motion had increased from 19.7° to 47.9° at 27-month follow-up. Outcome scores had improved significantly. Implant survivorship was 87% at 5-year follow-up.

65. Fuhrmann RA, Wagner A, Anders JO: First metatarsophalangeal joint replacement: The method of choice for end-stage hallux rigidus? *Foot Ankle Clin* 2003;8(4):711-721, vi.

66. Ess P, Hämäläinen M, Leppilahti J: Non-constrained titanium-polyethylene total endoprothesis in the treatment of hallux rigidus: A prospective clinical 2-year follow-up study. *Scand J Surg* 2002;91(2):202-207.

67. Konkel KF, Menger AG: Mid-term results of titanium hemi-great toe implants. *Foot Ankle Int* 2006;27(11):922-929.

68. Pulavarti RS, McVie JL, Tulloch CJ: First metatarsophalangeal joint replacement using the bio-action great toe implant: Intermediate results. *Foot Ankle Int* 2005;26(12):1033-1037.

69. Gibson JN, Thomson CE: Arthrodesis or total replacement arthroplasty for hallux rigidus: A randomized controlled trial. *Foot Ankle Int* 2005;26(9):680-690.

4: The Forefoot

Chapter 15

Lesser Toe Deformities

J. Kent Ellington, MD, MS

Introduction

A lesser toe deformity may appear to be unimportant but it can have a substantial effect on a patient's daily life, regardless of whether a shoe is being worn. A lesser toe deformity can be caused by trauma, intrinsic muscle imbalance, a neurologic disorder, an inflammatory disorder, an ill-fitting shoe, diabetes, hallux valgus, or a congenital etiology. Population-based studies in Australia and Sweden found that surgical management of these deformities accounted for 28% to 46% of all forefoot procedures.[1,2] Multiple nonsurgical and surgical options exist if the presence of symptoms indicates a need for intervention.

Mallet Toe, Hammer Toe, and Claw Toe

Pathoanatomy and Etiology

A basic understanding of the anatomy of the lesser toes is important to appreciate the pathologic changes that occur with deformity. The lesser toes are important for pressure distribution and balance of the foot. Deformities lead to pain, callus formation, transfer lesions, and compensatory gait changes. The deformity initially is flexible, but it may become more rigid as it progresses.

Mallet toe is defined as flexion of the distal interphalangeal (DIP) joint. Hammer toe is flexion of the proximal interphalangeal (PIP) joint, with or without DIP joint involvement. Claw toe is an extension of the metatarsophalangeal (MTP) joint with flexion of the PIP and DIP joints (Figure 1). Claw toes often are associated with a neuromuscular condition, usually involving multiple lesser toes and affecting both feet. A hammer toe, however, can occur in isolation; the second toe is most commonly affected.[3]

Dr. Ellington or an immediate family member is a member of a speakers' bureau or has made paid presentations on behalf of Arthrex and BME; serves as a paid consultant to or is an employee of Amniox, Arthrex, BME, Conventusortho, Pacira, and Zimmer; and has received research or institutional support from Amniox.

The static stabilizers of the lesser toes include the plantar plate, joint capsule, plantar aponeurosis, and collateral ligaments. The dynamic stabilizers include the extrinsic muscles (extensor digitorum longus and flexor digitorum longus [FDL]) and the intrinsic muscles (extensor digitorum brevis and flexor digitorum brevis, lumbricals, and interossei. The FDL tendon inserts on the distal phalanx and flexes the DIP joint. The flexor digitorum brevis tendon inserts on the middle phalanx and flexes the PIP joint. Because there is no direct flexor insertion on the proximal phalanx, the MTP joint in the extended position lacks antagonists, resulting in flexion in the PIP and DIP joints. The extensor digitorum longus tendon divides into three slips over the proximal phalanx (Figure 2); the middle slip inserts onto the base of the middle phalanx, and the medial and lateral slips pass laterally and converge to form the terminal tendon that inserts on the base of the distal phalanx. The transverse metatarsal ligament divides the intrinsic musculature, with the interossei dorsal and the lumbricals plantar to the ligament. Both muscles are plantar to the MTP joint axis and provide flexion of the MTP joint. The intrinsic muscles pass dorsal to the PIP and DIP joint axes to extend these joints.[4] Hammer toe and claw toe deformities occur with simultaneous contracture of the long flexors and extensors of the toe, causing imbalance and overpowering the weaker intrinsic muscles.[5]

The MTP joint often is involved in these deformities. It is stabilized by collateral ligaments and the plantar plate. As the deformity progresses, attenuation of the plantar plate leads to subluxation of the proximal phalanx dorsally onto the metatarsal head. The metatarsal fat pad is pulled distally, and the metatarsal head is depressed plantarly, leading to metatarsalgia.

Clinical Evaluation

Patients commonly report pain that is often associated with footwear, as well as callus formation over the PIP joint, corn formation, and pain at the tip of the toe. In addition, the patient may have pain and callosity under the MTP joint. A standing and seated foot examination is imperative. Many deformities cannot be truly appreciated during the seated examination alone. The position of the

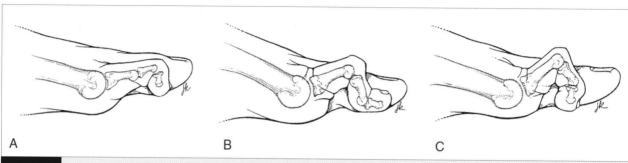

Figure 1 Lateral-view schematics showing a mallet toe (**A**), a hammer toe (**B**), and a claw toe (**C**).

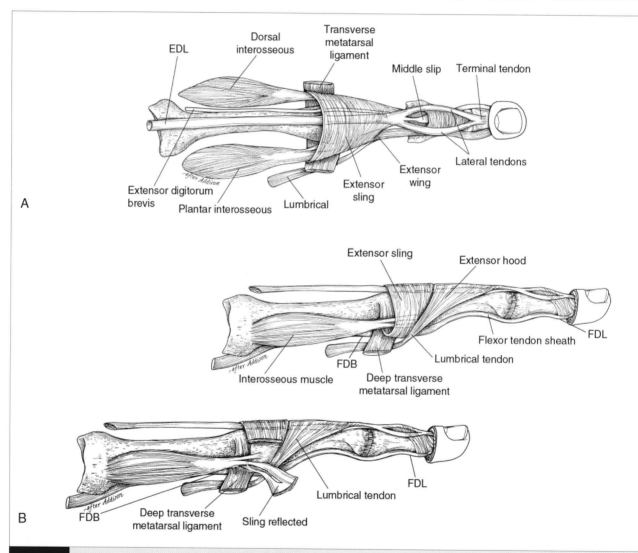

Figure 2 Schematics showing the anatomy of a lesser toe. **A,** The dorsal extrinsic and intrinsic musculature. The extensor digitorum longus (EDL) tendon traverses the metatarsophalangeal joint dorsally and splits into three parts. The middle slip extends the proximal interphalangeal joint. The lateral and medial slips form the terminal tendon and extend the distal interphalangeal joint (DIP). The tendon extends the metatarsophalangeal joint through the extensor sling, which is composed of medial and lateral fibroaponeurotic bands that originate on each side of the EDL tendon. **B,** The lateral extrinsic (top) and intrinsic (bottom) musculature. The flexor digitorum longus (FDL) tendon inserts onto the plantar base of the distal phalanx and flexes the DIP joint. The flexor digitorum brevis (FDB) tendon is split by the central FDL tendon into medial and lateral slips that insert onto the plantar base of the middle phalanx; this tendon is responsible for proximal interphalangeal joint flexion.

hallux should be evaluated as a possible contributor to lesser toe deformity. A careful examination of the patient's neurovascular status is important because a neurologic condition may be the underlying etiology. If surgery is being considered, it is necessary to ensure that tissue perfusion is adequate for successful healing.

The seated examination determines whether the deformity is flexible or rigid. A flexible toe deformity will be corrected when the ankle is passively placed into plantar flexion but a rigid deformity will not be corrected. The stability of the MTP joint should be tested using the vertical drawer test. Standard weight-bearing radiographs of the foot are required to evaluate overall forefoot alignment and identify hallux valgus, metatarsus adductus, and the relative lengths of the lesser metatarsals. Severe flexion deformities of the lesser toes are readily observed on radiographs, often as a so-called gun barrel sign.

Nonsurgical Treatment

In most patients, the initial treatment is nonsurgical. The patient is encouraged to wear shoes with a wide and deep toe box to accommodate the deformity and alleviate impingement of the digits. High-heeled shoes should be avoided because they] transfer pressure to the forefoot. Periodic trimming or shaving of painful calluses may be helpful. If the affected toes are flexible, taping or strapping may improve their alignment, although these techniques do not provide a permanent solution. Padding painful calluses with felt or silicone gel pads can relieve impingement over bony prominences, but often the padding is too cumbersome for routine use.

Surgical Treatment

Several surgical options are available to correct lesser toe deformity, including soft-tissue releases, bony procedures, and a combination of these two options. The decision to undertake surgical intervention is based on a logical, stepwise approach to the deformity. A thorough preoperative discussion with the patient is necessary to explain that a normally functioning toe usually is not achievable. Stiff, short toes with persistent numbness are common after surgery. Floating toes also are common. Recurrent deformity, incomplete correction, or vascular injury requiring amputation can occur.[6]

Mallet Toe

Mallet toe is uncommon but often causes pain at the tip of the affected toe. If the toe is flexible, the condition is easily correctable with a percutaneous flexor tenotomy at the DIP joint. This procedure can be done in the office setting using a digital block. A rigid deformity requires correction of the DIP joint with a DIP arthrodesis or arthroplasty. A central longitudinal incision or a horizontal elliptical

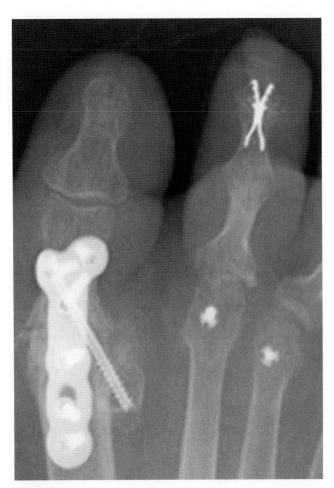

Figure 3   Radiograph showing a mallet toe fixed with an intramedullary distal interphalangeal implant.

incision can be used. The elliptical incision offers the advantage of removing redundant, often callused skin. The extensor, capsule, and collateral ligaments are released. The FDL is released through the incision. The options for fixation range from a simple Kirschner wire (which may require crossing the PIP joint to obtain proximal purchase and must be removed 4 to 6 weeks after surgery) to an intramedullary implant[7-9] (**Figure 3**).

Hammer Toe

Characterization of a hammer toe deformity as flexible or rigid is important in the surgical decision-making process. A flexible deformity is present during the standing examination but is corrected during active manipulation or ankle plantar flexion. A fixed deformity cannot be so corrected. A flexible deformity can be surgically corrected with an FDL tendon transfer, but a fixed deformity requires PIP arthroplasty or arthrodesis.

Many procedures have been described for correcting the PIP joint, including soft-tissue capsulotomy, tendon release or transfer, proximal phalangeal condylectomy, PIP arthroplasty, PIP arthrodesis, diaphysectomy, silicone implant, amputation, and partial proximal phalangectomy. In addition, numerous fixation techniques are available, using pins, wires, screws, bone dowels, bioabsorbable pins, digital implants, or intramedullary implants.[8-20]

For flexible deformities, a split FDL tendon transfer to the extensor hood at the proximal phalanx allows realignment with limited retention of motion.[18] This technique sometimes can be used in combination with a PIP arthroplasty or arthrodesis. The tendon transfer is used to prevent further dorsiflexion of the toe, which is common with hammer toe correction, and is accomplished by exposing the FDL tendon at the plantar base of the toe. The FDL tendon is percutaneously released from the distal phalanx and delivered in the plantar proximal wound. The tendon is split, and its lateral and medial parts are passed up to the corresponding parts of the proximal phalanx base. Care must be taken to ensure that the transfer is deep to the neurovascular bundle but superficial to the extensor hood. A dorsal incision is made, and the limbs of the FDL are sutured to the extensor hood and each other, with the toe in slight plantar flexion to obtain the correct tension.

Fixed deformities require bone removal to obtain correction, using a PIP arthroplasty or arthrodesis. Both procedures are done with a longitudinal incision or a horizontal (elliptical) incision over the PIP joint. The extensor hood is removed, and the proximal phalanx condyle is resected at its base with a cut perpendicular to the shaft and parallel to the joint, using a bone cutter or microsagittal saw.

After joint preparation, the PIP joint is stabilized. Most commonly, a Kirschner wire is driven anterograde out through the tip of the toe, then retrograde across the PIP joint (**Figure 4**). The use of a Kirschner wire has several disadvantages, the most important of which are the inconvenience to the patient and the risk of breakage, migration, accidental removal, or infection associated with the exposed wire. In addition, there is a risk of loss of correction, and the patient experiences anxiety and possibly pain because of the need to remove the wire in the clinic. Several alternatives have been developed. In resection arthroplasty, half of the joint is removed to allow postoperative motion; in arthrodesis, both ends of the joint are removed to achieve fusion.[7-10,13,15,17,20] (**Figure 5**). These techniques use pins, wires, screws, bone dowels, bioabsorbable pins, intramedullary devices, or digital implants.

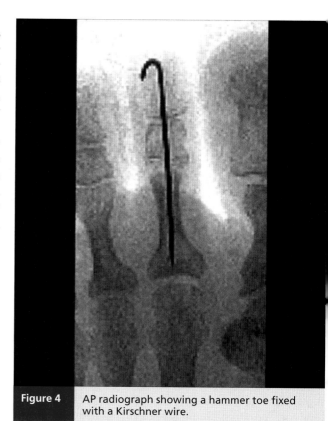

Figure 4 AP radiograph showing a hammer toe fixed with a Kirschner wire.

Claw Toe

By definition, claw toes have pathoanatomy at the MTP joint. Correction of the PIP and/or DIP joint is done as previously described for mallet toes and hammer toes. To fully correct a claw toe, however, the MTP joint also must be corrected. For this purpose, a soft-tissue procedure (MTP joint release of the dorsal capsule, collateral ligaments, and plantar plate, as needed), plantar plate repair, or metatarsal osteotomy is used. A longitudinal incision is made over the MTP joint. The extensor tendons are protected, or they are cut or lengthened, as needed. For a crossover deformity, the extensor digitorum brevis can be cut proximally, rerouted deep to the transverse intermetatarsal ligament, and transferred as a static stabilizer onto the side with laxity (**Figure 6**).

A deformity at the MTP joint after soft-tissue release is corrected with a horizontal oblique metatarsal osteotomy (**Figure 7**). Regardless of attention to detail, the lesser toes frequently drift upward at the MTP joint. The MTP joint can be pinned in slight plantar flexion, or a splint can be used after surgery (**Figure 8**).

Plantar plate instability recently has received increased attention, and a classification system has been described for use in treatment plannning.[21,22] The plantar plate is important to consider in diagnosing and treating claw toe deformity. Novel techniques and devices have been

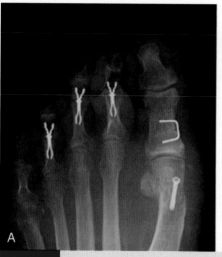 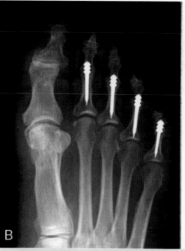 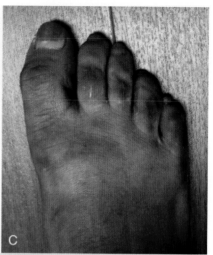

Figure 5 Hammer toe fixation with an intramedullary proximal interphalangeal implant. **A,** AP radiograph showing the Hammerlock device (BioMedical Enterprises). **B,** AP radiograph] showing the Protoe device (Wright Medical). **C,** Postoperative clinical photograph of the foot shown in **B**.

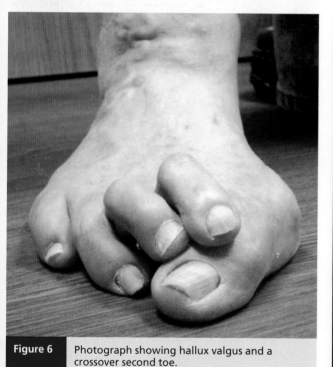

Figure 6 Photograph showing hallux valgus and a crossover second toe.

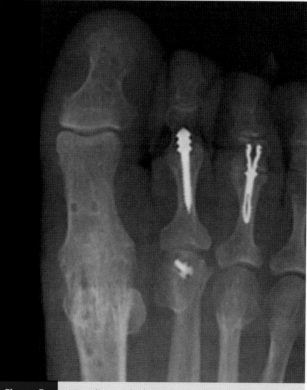

Figure 7 AP radiograph showing a Weil osteotomy.

developed for use in direct anatomic repair of the plantar plate in which the plantar plate is grasped and secured to the base of the proximal phalanx through drill holes (Figure 9).

Bunionette

A bunionette, also called a tailor's bunion, is caused by widening of the fourth-fifth intermetatarsal angle, causing varus deviation of the fifth toe at the MTP joint. As the deformity progresses, the lateral structures are stretched. Sometimes a dorsal contracture of the MTP joint develops, leading to pain under the fifth metatarsal head. Often the patient is asymptomatic because of the mobility of the affected joint, but the condition is exacerbated by shoe wear. A painful callus may develop over the lateral MTP joint.

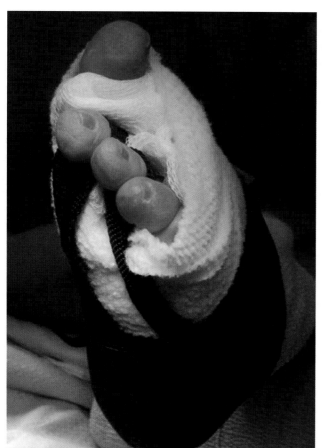

Figure 8   Photograph showing the use of a commercial splint to position the toes immediately after surgery for correction of claw toe.

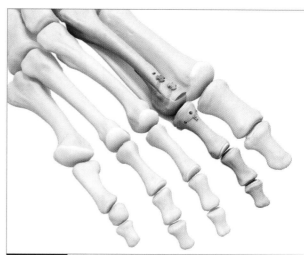

Figure 9   Three-dimensional drawing showing a repair of the plantar plate.

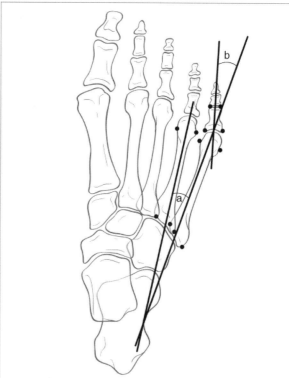

Figure 10   Schematic showing the use of the fourth-fifth intermetatarsal angle (a) and the fifth metatarsophalangeal joint angle (b) to measure bunionette deformity.

Standard weight-bearing radiographs are required to evaluate a bunionette deformity. The fourth-fifth intermetatarsal angle and fifth MTP joint angle are used to measure the deformity (**Figure 10**). The average normal fourth-fifth intermetatarsal angle is 9.1°, but is 10.7° in patients with a bunionette.[23] The average normal MTP joint angle is 10.2°, but it is 16.6° in patients with a bunionette.

A bunionette is classified as type I, enlargement of the metatarsal head; type II, widening of the fourth-fifth intermetatarsal angle; type III, lateral bowing of the fifth metatarsal; or type IV, a combination of types I, II, and III. Type IV is most common in patients with rheumatoid arthritis.

The nonsurgical treatment of a bunionette deformity is directed toward pain relief and includes shoe wear modification, silicone sleeves, and pads over the painful areas.[24] The condition most often is surgically treated as part of another procedure. Many patients have hallux valgus, and concomitant correction greatly decreases the forefoot width. Resection of the fifth metatarsal head is not recommended; at long-term follow-up, recurrence, pain, fourth transfer metatarsalgia, cock-up deformity, and substantial shortening were found.[25] Simple resection of the prominent lateral eminence of the fifth metatarsal head does not correct the underlying deformity, and aggressive resection can destabilize the fifth MTP joint.

Fifth metatarsal osteotomy is the preferred technique for correcting bunionette deformity. Many procedures have been described. A distal chevron or Weil osteotomy is commonly used for a mild to moderate deformity (**Figure 11**). Fixation is completed with a small screw or Kirschner wire. Fifth metatarsal osteotomy can reduce the fourth-fifth intermetatarsal angle by 2.6°, the MTP angle by 7.9°, and forefoot width by 3 mm.[26] Minimally invasive osteotomy, popularized as the SERI osteotomy (simple, effective, rapid, inexpensive), has had good success.[27] A diaphyseal or proximal osteotomy can be used for a large deformity or after an unsuccessful distal osteotomy. These osteotomies are technically demanding and have significant nonunion rates, however.

Summary

Understanding the cause of a lesser toe deformity is important to the success of nonsurgical or surgical treatment. The patient must be thoroughly evaluated, and treatment should be tailored to the patient's deformity, comorbidities, and expectations as well as the surgeon's experience. The goals of treatment are to decrease pain, improve toe alignment and function, and increase the patient's shoe wear options.

Annotated References

1. Menz HB, Gilheany MF, Landorf KB: Foot and ankle surgery in Australia: A descriptive analysis of the Medicare Benefits Schedule database, 1997–2006. *J Foot Ankle Res* 2008;1(1):10.

   Foot and ankle surgery accounted for a considerable healthcare expenditure in Australia, and the number of procedures in patients older than 55 years was found to be increasing.

2. Saro C, Bengtsson AS, Lindgren U, Adami J, Blomqvist P, Felländer-Tsai L: Surgical treatment of hallux valgus and forefoot deformities in Sweden: A population-based study. *Foot Ankle Int* 2008;29(3):298-304.

   Forefoot and hallux valgus surgery was more common in urban than rural regions of Sweden.

3. Coughlin MJ, Dorris J, Polk E: Operative repair of the fixed hammertoe deformity. *Foot Ankle Int* 2000;21(2):94-104.

4. Ellington JK: Hammertoes and clawtoes: Proximal interphalangeal joint correction. *Foot Ankle Clin* 2011;16(4):547-558.

   Understanding the cause of a lesser toe deformity is important to its treatment, which should be tailored to the patient's deformity, comorbidities, and expectations as well as the surgeon's experience.

5. Sarrafian SK, Topouzian LK: Anatomy and physiology of the extensor apparatus of the toes. *J Bone Joint Surg Am* 1969;51(4):669-679.

6. Femino JE, Mueller K: Complications of lesser toe surgery. *Clin Orthop Relat Res* 2001;391:72-88.

7. Caterini R, Farsetti P, Tarantino U, Potenza V, Ippolito E: Arthrodesis of the toe joints with an intramedullary cannulated screw for correction of hammertoe deformity. *Foot Ankle Int* 2004;25(4):256-261.

8. Ellington JK, Anderson RB, Davis WH, Cohen BE, Jones CP: Radiographic analysis of proximal interphalangeal joint arthrodesis with an intramedullary fusion device for lesser toe deformities. *Foot Ankle Int* 2010;31(5):372-376.

   An intramedullary fusion device was efficacious for maintaining PIP alignment in the treatment of lesser toe deformities. The reoperation rate was relatively low at midterm follow-up. Union occurred in 23 of 38 patients (60.5%).

9. Konkel KF, Menger AG, Retzlaff SA: Hammer toe correction using an absorbable intramedullary pin. *Foot Ankle Int* 2007;28(8):916-920.

10. Alvine FG, Garvin KL: Peg and dowel fusion of the proximal interphalangeal joint. *Foot Ankle* 1980;1(2):90-94.

11. Coughlin MJ: Lesser toe deformities. *Orthopedics* 1987;10(1):63-75.

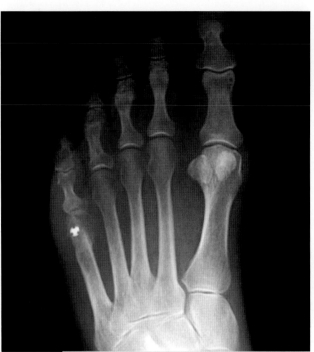

Figure 11 AP radiograph showing correction of a bunionette deformity using a snap-off screw osteotomy.

12. Chadwick C, Saxby TS: Hammertoes/Clawtoes: Metatarsophalangeal joint correction. *Foot Ankle Clin* 2011;16(4):559-571.

The etiology and pathophysiology of hammer toe and claw toe deformities were reviewed, with a well-illustrated description of nonsurgical and surgical treatments.

13. Fernández CS, Wagner E, Ortiz C: Lesser toes proximal interphalangeal joint fusion in rigid claw toes. *Foot Ankle Clin* 2012;17(3):473-480.

The reliability of arthrodesis and arthroplasty of the PIP joint was assessed for the treatment of claw toes. Some of the 95 patients had pain from the tip of the 2.4-mm screw.

14. Lehman DE, Smith RW: Treatment of symptomatic hammertoe with a proximal interphalangeal joint arthrodesis. *Foot Ankle Int* 1995;16(9):535-541.

15. Holinka J, Schuh R, Hofstaetter JG, Wanivenhaus AH: Temporary Kirschner wire transfixation versus strapping dressing after second MTP joint realignment surgery: A comparative study with ten-year follow-up. *Foot Ankle Int* 2013;34(7):984-989.

Fifty-four patients were treated for a claw toe deformity using condylectomy of the proximal phalanx and dorsal capsulotomy of the MTP joint with incision of the extensor hood. The postoperative fixation was with a soft dressing or Kirschner wire. There was a significantly lower recurrence of second MTP joint subluxation if Kirschner wire fixation was used rather than a soft dressing. Level of evidence: III.

16. Atinga M, Dodd L, Foote J, Palmer S: Prospective review of medium term outcomes following interpositional arthroplasty for hammer toe deformity correction. *Foot Ankle Surg* 2011;17(4):256-258.

In a prospective study of 24 patients who underwent interpositional arthroplasty to correct hammer toe deformity, the excisional arthroplasty was modified to include the divided extensor tendon as interpositional by suturing it to the flexor tendon. Follow-up of 16 patients (19 hammer toes) found improved scores, with no infections or nerve injury.

17. Klammer G, Baumann G, Moor BK, Farshad M, Espinosa N: Early complications and recurrence rates after Kirschner wire transfixion in lesser toe surgery: A prospective randomized study. *Foot Ankle Int* 2012;33(2):105-112.

A prospective, randomized study of the use of Kirschner wires for fixation of hammer and claw toes found that 6 weeks of fixation was more beneficial than 3 weeks and was not associated with more complications.

18. Taylor RG: The treatment of claw toes by multiple transfers of flexor into extensor tendons. *J Bone Joint Surg Br* 1951;33(4):539-542.

19. Kwon JY, De Asla RJ: The use of flexor to extensor transfers for the correction of the flexible hammer toe deformity. *Foot Ankle Clin* 2011;16(4):573-582.

An excellent review of techniques and outcomes found that flexor-to-extensor transfer is useful for correcting a flexible hammer toe deformity.

20. Edwards WH, Beischer AD: Interphalangeal joint arthrodesis of the lesser toes. *Foot Ankle Clin* 2002;7(1):43-48.

21. Coughlin MJ, Baumfeld DS, Nery C: Second MTP joint instability: Grading of the deformity and description of surgical repair of capsular insufficiency. *Phys Sportsmed* 2011;39(3):132-141.

A clinical staging and anatomic grading classification combined clinical findings and anatomic aspects of plantar plate tears. The described surgical treatment reconstructs the anatomic structures that lead to instability of the second MTP joint.

22. Coughlin MJ, Schutt SA, Hirose CB, et al: Metatarsophalangeal joint pathology in crossover second toe deformity: A cadaveric study. *Foot Ankle Int* 2012;33(2):133-140.

Sixteen below-knee cadaver specimens with a second crossover toe deformity were examined and dissected by removing the metatarsal head, and the pathologic findings were recorded. The types and extent of plantar plate tears associated with increasing deformity of the second ray were described. An anatomic grading system described the progressive anatomic changes in the plantar plate.

23. Nestor BJ, Kitaoka HB, Ilstrup DM, Berquist TH, Bergmann AD: Radiologic anatomy of the painful bunionette. *Foot Ankle* 1990;11(1):6-11.

24. Coughlin MJ: Treatment of bunionette deformity with longitudinal diaphyseal osteotomy with distal soft tissue repair. *Foot Ankle* 1991;11(4):195-203.

25. Kitaoka HB, Holiday AD Jr: Metatarsal head resection for bunionette: Long-term follow-up. *Foot Ankle* 1991;11(6):345-349.

26. Moran MM, Claridge RJ: Chevron osteotomy for bunionette. *Foot Ankle Int* 1994;15(12):684-688.

27. Magnan B, Samaila E, Merlini M, Bondi M, Mezzari S, Bartolozzi P: Percutaneous distal osteotomy of the fifth metatarsal for correction of bunionette. *J Bone Joint Surg Am* 2011;93(22):2116-2122.

Thirty consecutive percutaneous distal osteotomies of the fifth metatarsal in 21 patients were done to treat a painful prominence of the head of the fifth metatarsal. In 73% of feet there was complete resolution of pain at the fifth MTP joint without any functional limitation. The clinical results were similar to those reported after traditional open techniques, with the advantages of a minimally invasive surgical procedure.

Chapter 16

Metatarsalgia

Anish Raj Kadakia, MD

Introduction

Although the term metatarsalgia generally is used to describe pain in the forefoot, it is better suited to describe the location of pain rather than the diagnosis. The etiologies of forefoot pain include Freiberg disease, intractable plantar keratosis (IPK), lesser metatarsophalangeal (MTP) synovitis, stress fracture, Morton (interdigital) neuroma, sesamoid pathology, transfer metatarsalgia (insufficient loading through the first ray), and equinus contracture. These diagnoses are not mutually exclusive, and the physician must carefully consider the entire foot and ankle to appropriately diagnose and treat the patient's disease process.

Pathoanatomy and Etiology

Freiberg Disease

Freiberg disease (also called Freiberg infraction) is an osteochondrosis of a lesser metatarsal head. The second metatarsal is affected in 68% of patients, and the third metatarsal is affected in 27%.[1] The disease most commonly affects girls and women and is most prevalent during adolescence. Repetitive minor trauma is commonly but not universally associated with the condition. Recurrent microtrauma or overloading of the metatarsal can lead to interruption of the blood supply to the metatarsal head, with resulting ischemia, bone resorption, and collapse. The entire foot must be examined to determine the factors contributing to lesser metatarsal overload in a patient with Freiberg disease. These factors can include a gastrocnemius contracture, an unstable first ray, and relatively long lesser metatarsals.

Dr. Kadakia or an immediate family member is a member of a speakers' bureau or has made paid presentations on behalf of Acumed, serves as a paid consultant to or is an employee of Sythes Acumed, and has received research or institutional support from Acumed.

Intractable Plantar Keratosis

An IPK is a painful callus on the plantar aspect of the foot secondary to excess pressure from the metatarsal head or sesamoid (**Figure 1**). There are two forms, which are treated differently. The discrete form of IPK affects a single metatarsal, has a keratotic core, and may occur secondary to the prominence of a fibular condyle or the tibial sesamoid (**Figure 2**). The diffuse form of IPK appears as a thickening of the skin under an entire metatarsal head or multiple metatarsal heads, and it does not have a discrete keratotic core. In IPK primarily involving the second metatarsal, the overloading is caused by an incompetent first metatarsal and may involve first tarsometatarsal instability, hallux valgus, or an iatrogenically short first metatarsal.[2] An equinus contracture may be the sole underlying etiology if the callus is present over multiple metatarsals including the first ray. An equinus contracture can occur with both the discrete and diffuse forms and must be assessed in every patient. Alternate diagnoses include plantar warts, a foreign body reaction, and epidermal inclusion cysts.

Morton Neuroma

A Morton (interdigital) neuroma is believed to develop as an entrapment neuropathy of the digital nerve. Chronic pressure on the digital nerve as it courses beneath the transverse intermetatarsal ligament leads to perineural and endoneural fibrosis. Degeneration of the myelinated fibers is common and must be histologically verified. The anatomy of the digital nerves formerly was believed to create a predisposition to a Morton neuroma in the third web space. Branches from the lateral and medial plantar nerves enter the web spaces as common digital nerves; it was believed that both the lateral and medial plantar nerves have branches extending to the third web space, thus creating a relatively thick nerve predisposed to microtrauma. The medial communicating branch to the third web space is present in only 27% of the population, however, and if present, the common interdigital nerve is no thicker than other interdigital nerves.[3]

Wearing narrow-toed shoes may contribute to neuroma formation. Dorsiflexion of the MTP joints causes plantar flexion of the metatarsal heads, making the nerve

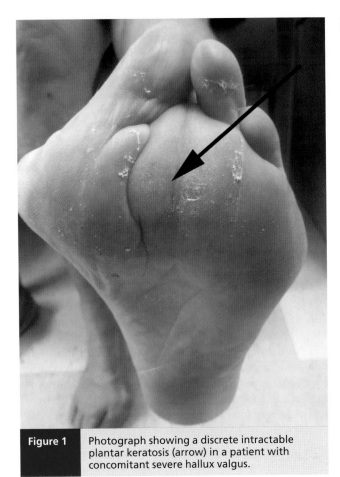

Figure 1   Photograph showing a discrete intractable plantar keratosis (arrow) in a patient with concomitant severe hallux valgus.

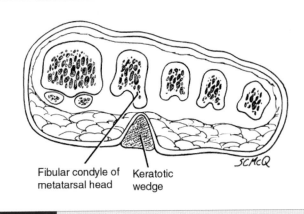

Figure 2   Schematic cross-section showing a prominent plantar condyle that has resulted in an intractable plantar keratosis. (Reproduced with permission from Murphy GA: Lesser toe abnormalities, in Canale ST, ed: *Campbell's Operative Orthopaedics,* ed 9. St. Louis, MO, Mosby, 1998, pp 1746-1783.)

subject to repetitive trauma through increased compression of the metatarsal heads and stretching over the intermetatarsal ligament. Extrinsic factors also can influence neuroma formation. Ganglions or synovial cysts arising from the MTP joint may cause direct pressure on the digital nerve. Degeneration of the MTP joint capsule in a patient with an inflammatory condition such as rheumatoid arthritis often causes subluxation of the joint and stretches the nerve. Distortion of the MTP joint also can compress the bursae surrounding the ligament, increasing pressure on the surrounding tissues.

Sesamoiditis

The sesamoids are primary load-bearing structures of the forefoot, in addition to their function in decreasing friction and increasing the mechanical advantage of the flexor hallucis brevis. The importance of these structures is underscored by their absorption of as much as 32% of the energy generated during the stance phase of sprinting. Sesamoiditis is inflammation and pain affecting the sesamoids resulting from arthrosis, osteonecrosis, acute fracture, stress fracture, or mechanical overloading. The medial (tibial) sesamoid is most commonly involved

because of the increased load on the medial aspect of the foot during gait. Bipartite sesamoids occur in 10% to 30% of the population and should not be confused with acute fracture. Only 85% of these individuals have bipartite sesamoids in both feet; therefore, a normal contralateral radiograph is not sufficient to determine the presence of an acute fracture. These injuries commonly occur in athletes and must be aggressively treated to prevent long-term disability. Unlike lesser metatarsal pain, which can be secondary to an unstable first ray, sesamoid pain may be associated with a plantarflexed rigid first ray (as in a cavus foot).

Transfer Metatarsalgia

Incompetence of the medial column during the load-bearing phases of gait increases stress on the lesser metatarsals.[4] This phenomenon may be a factor in Freiberg disease, IPK, and Morton neuroma as well as stress fracture, synovitis, and joint subluxation, and it must be considered in all patients with lesser metatarsalgia. Hallux valgus with associated first tarsometatarsal instability is a common cause of stress transfer. Iatrogenic shortening or elevation of the first ray also must be considered. The weight-bearing function of the medial column must be restored during an isolated lesser metatarsal correction to avoid increasing the risk of recurrent pain and deformity.

Clinical and Radiographic Evaluation

Clinical Evaluation

The inciting factors and the location of a patient's forefoot pain are critical for determining the underlying cause.

Weight-bearing activities, in particular those associated with running, are a common inciting factor in all forefoot pathologies. Symptoms that worsen with constrictive shoe wear are associated with Freiberg disease or a Morton neuroma. Wearing shoes with very high heels (4 inches or higher) universally exacerbates forefoot pain; patients having an underlying gastrocnemius contracture will have relief from pain in shoes with a 1- to 2-inch heel. Ambulation without shoes typically reduces pain in patients with neuroma but worsens the discomfort in patients with another etiology. The use of a cushioned insole is common but offers little relief to patients with Freiberg disease or a Morton neuroma.

In Freiberg disease, the pain is limited to one lesser MTP joint but never is associated with the first or fifth metatarsal. The primary location is the dorsal aspect of the affected joint. Plantar pain directly over a callus is associated with an IPK. A callus over both the first and fifth metatarsal heads suggests a cavus foot deformity. Pain in multiple lesser metatarsals may be secondary to a Morton neuroma, transfer metatarsalgia, or gastrocnemius contracture. A history of a burning sensation, tingling, or numbness ideally should be elicited before a Morton neuroma is diagnosed. Isolated pain over the plantar aspect of the first metatarsal without an associated callus probably is secondary to sesamoid pathology. Lesser metatarsal symptoms that arise after hallux valgus correction suggest transfer metatarsalgia rather than an isolated lesser metatarsal condition.

The physical examination should begin with a standing examination of the alignment of the foot, with a focus on the medial column. A forefoot-driven cavovarus deformity (a plantarflexed first ray), will contribute to sesamoid pain and possibly to isolated discrete IPK, whereas a midfoot cavus deformity leads to a diffuse IPK. Medial column instability, as may occur in hallux valgus deformity, contributes to lesser metatarsal symptoms. Iatrogenic dorsal elevation of the medial column may be noted clinically if the condition is severe but is more easily identified radiographically. Compression during shoe wear can exacerbate neuroma symptoms in a splay foot with hallux valgus or a bunionette deformity (**Figure 3**). These associated deformities must be treated if nonsurgical or surgical treatment is to be successful.

Inspection of the soft tissues will reveal gastrocnemius contracture, transfer metatarsalgia, calluses in IPK, or swelling in Freiberg disease. The Silfverskiöld test should be used to assess for isolated contracture of the gastrocnemius in all patients. In this test, ankle dorsiflexion is assessed with the knee in full extension and in 90° of flexion (**Figure 4**). The foot must be locked in subtalar neutral position. Lack of dorsiflexion past neutral is consistent with an equinus contracture. An increase in

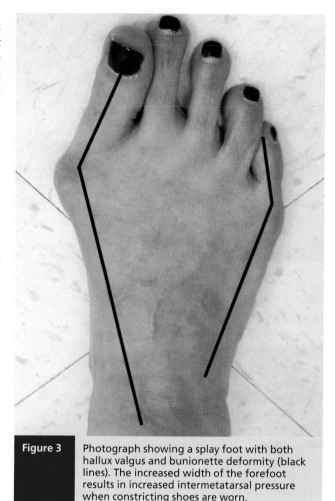

Figure 3 Photograph showing a splay foot with both hallux valgus and bunionette deformity (black lines). The increased width of the forefoot results in increased intermetatarsal pressure when constricting shoes are worn.

dorsiflexion with the knee in flexion is indicative of an isolated gastrocnemius contracture.

Palpation for tenderness is useful for determining the source of the pain and narrowing the differential diagnosis. In Freiberg disease, there is tenderness to palpation at the affected joint when a plantar-directed force is applied from the dorsal surface. Isolated dorsal-directed pressure from the plantar surface typically is painless unless the patient has an IPK. Compression of the joint elicits pain in patients with MTP synovitis or Freiberg disease. To mitigate confounding pain from an IPK, care must be taken to avoid placing pressure on any callus during this test while compressing the joint. The presence of a palpable dorsal osteophyte allows Freiberg disease to be easily differentiated from MTP synovitis. Provocative testing for a neuroma is done by compressing the forefoot while alternating plantar and dorsal pressure at the affected web space. This test may elicit a palpable click (the Mulder click) when the nerve and bursal tissue snap between the metatarsal heads. The Mulder click without pain also may be present in patients without

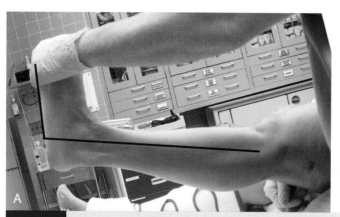
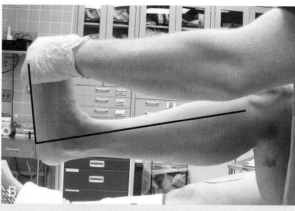

Figure 4 Photographs showing the Silfverskiöld test. **A,** An equinus contracture with the knee in extension denoted by the angle formed by the tibia and the plantar aspect of the foot (black lines). **B,** Dorsiflexion past neutral with 90° flexion of the knee, denoting an isolated gastrocnemius contracture.

foot pathology, however. A positive Mulder sign requires the click to be accompanied by pain radiating into the affected toes, and it is diagnostic for interdigital neuritis. The compression should be applied proximal to the metatarsal head to avoid irritating the joint, possibly leading to a false-positive test in the setting of MTP synovitis or Freiberg disease. The range of motion of the toe typically is normal unless the patient has Freiberg disease, in which the range of motion gradually becomes limited, with progressive articular collapse and osteophyte formation. Absolute dorsiflexion varies, and a comparison with the contralateral foot or the unaffected lesser toes provides a reliable reference. Deformity of the phalanx, as seen with hammer toes, claw toes, or a crossover toe, requires a different treatment algorithm. The vertical drawer test is 99.8% specific and should be performed to rule out the presence of a plantar plate injury.[5] Dorsally directed pressure placed directly along the sesamoids will reproduce pain in patients with sesamoid pathology. Identification of the affected sesamoid is critical because resection of only a single sesamoid can be done without creating a cock-up toe deformity. Metatarsosesamoid pain may be relieved with plantar flexion of the first MTP joint but is exacerbated with dorsiflexion of the joint, which engages the sesamoids onto the plantar aspect of the metatarsal head.

Radiologic Evaluation

Three weight-bearing radiographic views of the foot are necessary to identify a pathologic process of the MTP joint, an elevation of the first metatarsal, or an abnormal relative length of the lesser metatarsals.

Common radiographic findings in Freiberg disease include resorption of the central metatarsal bone adjacent to the articular surface, flattening of the metatarsal head, and osteochondral loose bodies (**Figure 5**). In

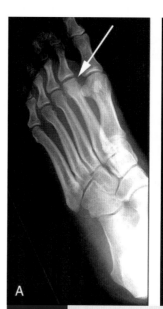
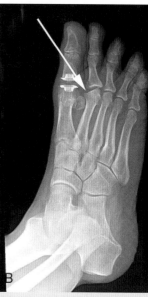

Figure 5 Oblique radiographs of the foot showing resorption of the central metatarsal head with resultant flattening of the articular surface (arrows). The condition is worse in **A** than in **B**. These findings are consistent with Freiberg disease.

late-stage disease, joint space narrowing with osteophyte formation and collapse of the articular surface can be seen (**Figure 6**). An axial view of the forefoot with dorsiflexion of the MTP joints may reveal relative prominence of the fibular condyle in patients with a discrete IPK. A non-weight–bearing medial oblique view and an axial sesamoid view are recommended for patients with suspected sesamoid pathology (**Figure 7**). Radiographs typically are normal in patients with Morton neuroma, but a malunited metatarsal fracture with narrowing of the intermetatarsal space is seen in rare instances. The

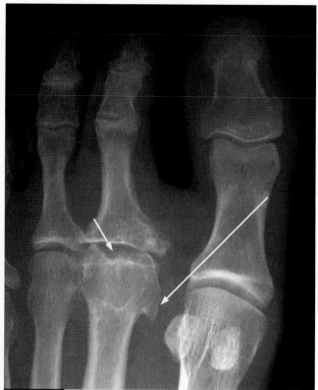

Figure 6 Coned-down AP radiograph of the forefoot showing the natural history and long-term sequelae of untreated Freiberg disease. The significant subchondral cysts (arrowhead) and osteophyte formation (arrow) indicate osteoarthritis.

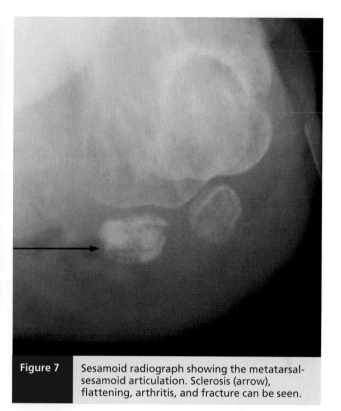

Figure 7 Sesamoid radiograph showing the metatarsal-sesamoid articulation. Sclerosis (arrow), flattening, arthritis, and fracture can be seen.

possibility of a shortened or elevated first metatarsal should be evaluated in all patients and specifically in patients who have had surgery. This deformity may result in transfer metatarsalgia or may be associated with Freiberg disease, and it may require correction in addition to treatment of osteonecrosis of the lesser metatarsal (Figure 8).

Additional imaging is not routinely required for a patient with metatarsalgia. On MRI of a patient with Freiberg disease, the subchondral bone of the metatarsal head has low fat saturation with T1 weighting and variable fat saturation with T2 weighting, and flattening of the metatarsal head is seen. With eventual fragmentation of the bone, intra-articular loose bodies are formed. Arthritis in late-stage disease is indicated by subchondral bone marrow edema involving both the metatarsal and the phalanx (seen as high signal on T2-weighted MRI). The use of MRI in Morton neuroma is controversial. Before the development of high-resolution scanners, the predictive value of MRI was low. Currently, MRI can detect aberrant pathology such as a cyst or ganglion, but its usefulness for detecting and diagnosing an interdigital neuroma remains open to debate.

Ultrasonography has high sensitivity and variable specificity in the diagnosis of a neuroma. One study found that ultrasonography accurately predicted the size and location of the neuroma in 98% of 55 neuromas, with no false-positive readings, but other studies found 95% sensitivity and only 65% specificity.[6] Routine use of ultrasonography is not required because neuroma is a clinical diagnosis.

Nonsurgical Treatment

The term metatarsalgia is relevant when considering treatment to relieve a patient's pain, despite the many underlying pathologies. The patient is instructed to cease any activities that increase the load on the forefoot, such as running, jumping, ballroom dancing, or impact sports. Nonimpact activities such as biking, elliptical equipment exercise, and swimming are encouraged. NSAIDs are useful for minimizing pain and inflammation but require consideration of the gastrointestinal, renal, and liver system complications related to long-term use. The use of narcotic pain medication is not encouraged.

Shoe wear modification and the use of orthotic devices are the mainstay treatments of the underlying conditions and the primary means of achieving long-term pain relief without medication. A stiff-soled shoe, such as a walking shoe, minimizes the force placed on the forefoot and prevents the MTP dorsiflexion that increases the stress

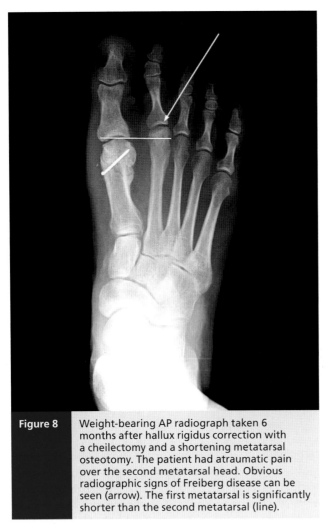

Figure 8 Weight-bearing AP radiograph taken 6 months after hallux rigidus correction with a cheilectomy and a shortening metatarsal osteotomy. The patient had atraumatic pain over the second metatarsal head. Obvious radiographic signs of Freiberg disease can be seen (arrow). The first metatarsal is significantly shorter than the second metatarsal (line).

and increases pain within the forefoot. For patients with lesser metatarsalgia, the use of a Morton extension can provide relief by effectively creating a stiff-soled shoe without placing extra pressure on the metatarsal heads. A Morton extension is a good alternative if the patient wants to avoid modifying shoe wear. Wearing shoes with a wide forefoot is especially helpful in patients with a neuroma to minimize compressive force on the nerve in the coronal plane. Metatarsal pads placed immediately proximal to the metatarsal heads elevate the metatarsal head and thereby stabilize the MTP joint. Silicone pads placed directly along the painful callus may decrease the pain in patients with IPK. In patients with sesamoid pain, a so-called dancer's pad is an effective orthotic device. This C-shaped pad has a recess for the sesamoid that is effective at reducing the pressure and pain of sesamoid pathology. Patients with an equinus contracture may achieve pain relief by using a half-inch heel lift in shoes with a 1- to 2-inch heel. This heel height is contrary to conventional beliefs on forefoot pain but is appropriate

for treating an equinus contracture. The low heel positions the ankle to allow a more functional range of motion and minimize forefoot pressure during the stance phase of gait.

Custom orthotic devices are most appropriate for patients who have had relief while using a simple over-the-counter device and want to achieve long-term nonsurgical relief. Given the cost of a custom orthotic device, it is important to determine that the patient has a reasonable chance of achieving pain relief from a mechanical alteration in foot pressure. A full-length orthotic device with recesses for the affected metatarsal heads is effective (**Figure 9**). Pain relief can be aided by the use of a removable carbon fiber plate with the orthotic device. Although this orthotic device is bulky, it can provide significant relief if the patient is willing to wear athletic or walking shoes. For patients with sesamoid pain, a full-length orthotic device with a built-in dancer's pad and a reverse Morton extension is effective.

Intra-articular injections can be effective but should be used with caution because they can cause further articular damage in Freiberg disease, weaken the surrounding capsular restraints, and lead to an iatrogenic crossover toe. A cortisone injection can be used as both a diagnostic and a therapeutic tool for Morton neuroma. The reported success rates of cortisone injection vary. A prospective study using ultrasound-guided injections found that 28% of patients had complete relief and 44% had significant relief with minor residual pain at 9-month follow-up.[7] No complications were reported. A single cortisone injection is appropriate during the diagnostic workup and management of a neuroma, and it has the potential to provide long-term pain relief with a low risk of complications. However, multiple injections can lead to fat-pad atrophy and soft-tissue disruption, and they should be used with caution. Multiple ethanol injections also have been used as a surgical alternative. The basis for intralesional alcohol injection is the ability of 20% dehydrated alcohol to inhibit neuron cell function in vitro. A 22% success rate was reported after an average of 4.1 injections.[8] In contrast, earlier studies reported an 82% rate of complete pain relief after 1 year.[9] Additionally, the results of alcohol sclerosing therapy were noted to deteriorate over time with 84% pain relief noted at 10 months after injection compared to 29% at 5 years in the same cohort of patients.[10] No major complications have been reported, but extreme pain was reported during some injections, precluding completion of the injection.[8] Given the variability in reported relief and the discomfort associated with multiple ethanol injections, these injections cannot be recommended.

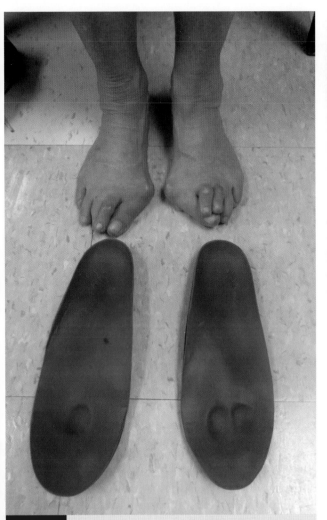

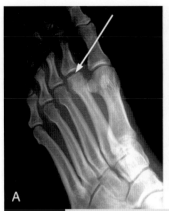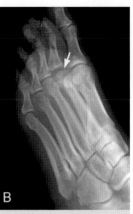

| Figure 10 | Oblique radiographs showing the characteristic flattening of the metatarsal head (arrow) in Freiberg disease before (**A**) and after (**B**) treatment with a dorsal closing-wedge osteotomy. The contour of the metatarsal head has been re-created (arrowhead). |

conjunction with a thorough débridement of synovitis, abnormal cartilage, osteophytes, and necrotic bone (**Figure 10**). The osteotomy serves to rotate the plantar aspect of the articular surface, which typically is well preserved, to a more superior position where it articulates with the phalanx. The metatarsal is shortened by several millimeters to help offloading. Additional joint distraction with a miniexternal fixator used for 6 weeks has been promoted as a means of improving articular self-repair and preventing joint contracture.[11] At a mean 18-month follow-up after joint distraction with a miniexternal fixator was performed, 12 patients had mean improvement from 8.2 to 2.2 on the visual analog scale, with a mean 37° increase in MTP range of motion. Additional studies are required to understand the efficacy of this technique and to compare it with isolated débridement and osteotomy.

The use of an extra-articular osteotomy has been described, with recent results showing a mean improvement from 7.5 to 1 on the visual analog scale and a 6.2° improvement in motion in 12 patients.[12] The benefit of the osteotomy was believed to derive from simple fixation with crossed Kirschner wires that were removed 4 to 8 weeks after surgery. A concomitant débridement was performed without excision of the lesion itself. The amount of the excision was calculated before surgery based on MRI findings. The plantar cartilage was successfully rotated to the center of the joint.

Excisional arthroplasty has been used, but the results have been poorer than those of osteotomy. The results were better after interpositional arthroplasty using the extensor digitorum brevis tendon.[13] Small case studies found osteochondral autografting to be promising.[14,15] All three patients in one study returned to sport (badminton, soccer, or baseball) within 3 months of surgery,

| Figure 9 | Photographs showing multiple foot deformities including hallux valgus and claw toes. Intractable plantar keratoses were diagnosed bilaterally under the second metatarsal head and on the left foot under the third metatarsal. The patient had unrelieved pain for 5 years before evaluation. The use of orthotic devices with metatarsal pads and recesses for the affected metatarsals provided significant relief and mitigated the need for surgical intervention. |

Surgical Treatment

Freiberg Disease

Joint débridement, in which all synovitis, osteophytes, and loose bodies are débrided through a dorsal incision, should be considered for patients with early-stage Freiberg disease after unsuccessful nonsurgical management. The patient should have relatively good articular surface congruity and minimal metatarsal deformity. Many studies have reported good results after a dorsal closing-wedge metaphyseal osteotomy of the affected metatarsal in

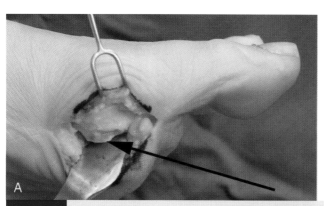
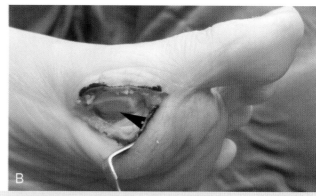

Figure 11 Intraoperative photographs showing a prominent tibial sesamoid (arrow) that caused a discrete intractable plantar keratosis before (A) and after (B) excision of its plantar 50%. The resultant smooth plantar surface (arrowhead) decreased plantar pressure and maintained the integrity of the flexor hallucis brevis.

as reported at a minimum 24-month follow-up.[14] Two patients had an American Orthopaedic Foot and Ankle Society (AOFAS) score of 100, and the third patient had a score of 95. The second study found healing of the plug at 12-month follow-up, based on MRI and arthroscopic findings; two of the four patients had normal cartilage, and the other two had near-normal cartilage.[15] The mean AOFAS score had improved from 70.8 to 97.5 points. Replacement arthroplasty with a silicone prosthesis should be avoided because of the risk of complications. The use of metallic and ceramic implants is being investigated, but adequate evidence is not yet available to recommend their use. Currently, the best evidence is for the use of débridement and dorsal closing-wedge osteotomy.

Intractable Plantar Keratosis
Discrete IPK resulting from a prominent metatarsal head fibular condyle is treated with a plantar condylectomy in which 20% to 30% of the plantar metatarsal head is removed (Figure 9). Care must be taken to avoid notching the plantar cortex by making the cut parallel to the metatarsal shaft.[16] For a discrete IPK inferior to a sesamoid, excision of the plantar 50% of the sesamoid can be performed to decrease the focal pressure (Figure 11).

The focus of treatment of diffuse IPKs should be on the overall deformity rather than narrowly on the metatarsal head. A gastrocnemius contracture may be treated with a gastrocnemius recession. A gastrocnemius recession is a less invasive treatment than multiple metatarsal osteotomies. Any associated deformities, such as a midfoot cavus or an unstable or elevated first ray, should be treated concomitantly. A retrospective study of patients with foot pain found that the use of a gastrocnemius recession to treat isolated metatarsalgia with no other underlying deformity was successful.[17] Six of the 34 feet in this study were treated for metatarsalgia; the patients had improvement on the visual analog scale from 7.5 to

2.2 at a mean 28-week follow-up. This improvement is encouraging but should be interpreted in the setting of the small number of patients, short follow-up time, and lack of a control group.

Morton Neuroma
Surgical excision of a Morton neuroma should be considered if nonsurgical treatment is unsuccessful (Figure 12). Isolated release of the intermetatarsal ligament should not be done secondary to the histopathologic changes known to occur with a Morton neuroma because release of the ligament does not correct the pathologic process and therefore may not lead to pain relief. Metatarsal-shortening osteotomy with release of the intermetatarsal ligament may be considered as an alternative to resection, however. A retrospective review of 86 procedures compared the results of isolated intermetatarsal ligament release with those of release with concomitant metatarsal shortening osteotomy of the longer metatarsal adjacent to the neuroma.[18] Patients treated with the concomitant osteotomy had a 95% rate of good to excellent results, compared with 50% of patients treated with an isolated ligament release. In patients with adjacent neuromas, excision of one neuroma and transection of the intermetatarsal ligament of a web space with a macroscopically normal-appearing nerve can prevent anesthesia of the middle digit. If both nerves appear thickened and abnormal, resection should be performed.

Both the dorsal and plantar approaches have been successful. Results in 125 patients were retrospectively reviewed 2 years after neuroma resection using a dorsal or plantar approach.[19] The intermetatarsal ligament was transected when the dorsal approach was used and was left intact with the plantar approach. Neuroma resection was histologically confirmed in all patients. No significant between-group difference in overall satisfaction was identified, but the patients who underwent surgery with

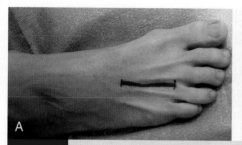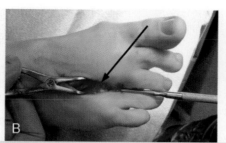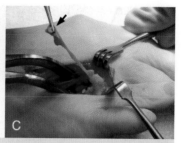

Figure 12 Photographs showing resection of an interdigital neuroma. **A,** The marking for a dorsal approach, showing the proximal extent of the incision required to obtain adequate exposure. **B,** Exposure of the intermetatarsal ligament (arrow) is facilitated by placing a lamina spreader between the metatarsals. **C,** The neuroma is excised from proximal (arrowhead) to distal to ensure that both branches of the nerve are excised distally.

a plantar approach had a substantially lower complication rate, less sensory loss, and a shorter recovery time. There was a 5% rate of missed neuromas with a dorsal approach and a 5% rate of hypertrophic painful scar formation with a plantar approach. Given the similar rates of patient satisfaction, the choice of a dorsal or plantar approach to treating a primary neuroma should be based on the surgeon's comfort level.

A plantar approach is preferable for revision surgery because it allows superior visualization and a more proximal resection. Advanced imaging studies can be obtained before surgical intervention if the patient has undergone unsuccessful nonsurgical management or has an atypical Morton neuroma.

Sesamoiditis

A patient with sesamoiditis who has undergone unsuccessful nonsurgical management, generally for at least 6 months, may be a candidate for surgical treatment. The surgical options include tibial or fibular sesamoidectomy as well as sesamoid shaving. Removal of both tibial and fibular sesamoids is rarely indicated because it predictably leads to development of a cock-up and intrinsic-minus deformity of the hallux. After 26 tibial or fibular sesamoidectomies, all 20 patients returned to sporting activity at a mean of 12 weeks, as reported at a mean 86-month follow-up.[20] The complication rate was 19%, however, with two incidences of hallux valgus, one of hallux varus, and two of postoperative scarring with neuroma-type symptoms. After isolated tibial sesamoidectomy for recalcitrant sesamoid pain, 29 of the 32 patients (90%) were able to return to preoperative levels of activity and said they would choose to have the same surgery again.[21] The mean Foot Function Index score was 18.4. Ten patients (30%) had extreme difficulty standing on their toes, and seven patients (21%) had transfer metatarsalgia or plantar cutaneous neuritis. It is important to be careful during the exposure to avoid damage to the plantar digital nerve and to ensure repair of the flexor hallucis brevis, so as to

decrease the risk of hallux varus or hallux valgus after resection of the fibular or tibial sesamoid, respectively.

Transfer Metatarsalgia

Correction of the deformity of the first metatarsal is the focus of treatment for patients with transfer metatarsalgia. A first metatarsal elevation should be treated with a plantar flexion osteotomy to restore the normal weight-bearing forces (**Figure 13**). Hallux valgus and associated first ray instability are associated with weight transfer to the central metatarsals.[22] Correction of the hallux valgus deformity with a proximal osteotomy led to resolution of plantar pain and callosity in 32 of 40 patients (80%), with no secondary surgery.[2] A Lapidus procedure with plantar flexion of the first metatarsal also is effective if the patient is known to have first tarsometatarsal instability and lesser metatarsalgia. However, the surgery will produce shortening of the medial column that may exacerbate the metatarsalgia. Treating the excessive relative length of the lesser metatarsals was found to relieve the metatarsalgia and to correct the associated hallux deformity. In a retrospective review of propulsive metatarsalgia treated with lesser metatarsal osteotomies, 71 of the 82 patients (86%) were found to require additional surgery.[23] Most of the additional procedures were Scarf osteotomies for correction of hallux valgus, and therefore it was difficult to isolate the effect of the lesser metatarsal osteotomy. The patient satisfaction rate was 80% in patients treated with the Weil or triple Weil osteotomy technique, but the complication rate was relatively high. Recurrence occurred in 4.3% of patients, stiffness in 60.2%, floating toes in 4.3%, and delayed union in 7.5%. The use of a metatarsal shaft osteotomy may mitigate the complications associated with intra-articular osteotomy but requires significant soft-tissue dissection and, because of the diaphyseal nature of the osteotomy, is associated with a higher nonunion rate than distal metatarsal osteotomy.

To correct a rarely occurring severe iatrogenic shortening of the first metatarsal, lengthening can be done with

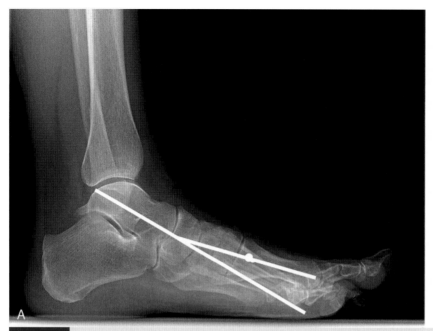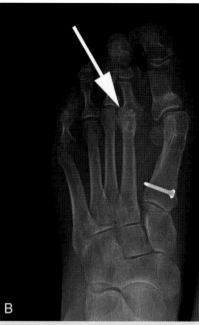

Figure 13	**A,** Lateral standing radiograph showing the lateral talar–first metatarsal angle used to measure a dorsiflexion malunion of the first metatarsal. There is no evidence of collapse of the medial longitudinal arch; the negative angle is caused by iatrogenic elevation of the first ray, leading to increased pressure on the second metatarsal. **B,** AP weightbearing radiograph showing the resulting transfer metatarsalgia with degenerative joint disease (arrow).

a one-stage bone block or gradually with a miniexternal fixator. Long-term longitudinal studies are lacking to determine the efficacy of lengthening, but it can be considered if significant shortening of the lesser metatarsals is necessary to recreate a neutral arc of the forefoot.

Summary

Metatarsalgia is a general term for pain in the forefoot and does not indicate any single diagnosis. Appropriate evaluation of the foot and ankle allows the multiple possible etiologies to be narrowed to the correct diagnosis. Although the nonsurgical management of different conditions can be similar, the surgical interventions are disparate and require an accurate diagnosis to maximize the possibility of pain relief. No single surgical procedure can treat metatarsalgia, and often multiple different procedures are required.

Annotated References

1. Carmont MR, Rees RJ, Blundell CM: Current concepts review: Freiberg's disease. *Foot Ankle Int* 2009;30(2):167-176.

   An overview of the literature on Freiberg disease included a review of recent studies.

2. Lee KB, Park JK, Park YH, Seo HY, Kim MS: Prognosis of painful plantar callosity after hallux valgus correction without lesser metatarsal osteotomy. *Foot Ankle Int* 2009;30(11):1048-1052.

   In a retrospective review of chevron osteotomy for hallux valgus, 32 of 40 feet (80%) had resolution of callosities and pain, with residual symptoms in 7.5%. Level of evidence: IV.

3. Levitsky KA, Alman BA, Jevsevar DS, Morehead J: Digital nerves of the foot: Anatomic variations and implications regarding the pathogenesis of interdigital neuroma. *Foot Ankle* 1993;14(4):208-214.

4. Dietze A, Bahlke U, Martin H, Mittlmeier T: First ray instability in hallux valgus deformity: A radiokinematic and pedobarographic analysis. *Foot Ankle Int* 2013;34(1):124-130.

   An enlarged intermetatarsal angle was associated with an increase in maximal dorsiflexion during gait. The mean maximal dorsiflexion was 2.6° (range, 1.0° to 4.0°). Level of evidence: IV.

5. Klein EE, Weil L Jr, Weil LS Sr, Coughlin MJ, Knight J: Clinical examination of plantar plate abnormality: A diagnostic perspective. *Foot Ankle Int* 2013;34(6):800-804.

   The medical records of 90 patients (109 feet) were reviewed after a plantar plate repair. Clinical examination findings were compared with intraoperative findings, and diagnostic statistics were calculated. Ninety-five percent of patients had a gradual onset of forefoot pain, edema, and a positive drawer sign. Level of evidence: IV.

6. Read JW, Noakes JB, Kerr D, Crichton KJ, Slater HK, Bonar F: Morton's metatarsalgia: Sonographic findings and correlated histopathology. *Foot Ankle Int* 1999;20(3):153-161.

7. Markovic M, Crichton K, Read JW, Lam P, Slater HK: Effectiveness of ultrasound-guided corticosteroid injection in the treatment of Morton's neuroma. *Foot Ankle Int* 2008;29(5):483-487.

   Thirty-five consecutive patients (7 men, 28 women; mean age, 54 years; age range, 29 to 77 years) underwent a single ultrasound-guided corticosteroid injection. Twenty-six of the 39 neuromas (66%) had a positive outcome 9 months later. Level of evidence: IV.

8. Espinosa N, Seybold JD, Jankauskas L, Erschbamer M: Alcohol sclerosing therapy is not an effective treatment for interdigital neuroma. *Foot Ankle Int* 2011;32(6):576-580.

   A retrospective review of 32 consecutive patients who received a series of sclerosing ethanol injections to treat a painful interdigital neuroma found that relief of symptoms was achieved only in 7 patients; 25 had no significant reduction of symptoms and considered or underwent a surgical excision. Level of evidence: IV.

9. Dockery GL: The treatment of intermetatarsal neuromas with 4% alcohol sclerosing injections. *J Foot Ankle Surg* 1999;38(6):403-408.

10. Gurdezi S, White T, Ramesh P: Alcohol injection for Morton's neuroma: A five-year follow-up. *Foot Ankle Int* 2013;34(8):1064-1067.

11. Xie X, Shi Z, Gu W: Late-stage Freiberg's disease treated with dorsal wedge osteotomy and joint distraction arthroplasty: Technique tip. *Foot Ankle Int* 2012;33(11):1015-1017.

    A technique for additional joint distraction to treat Freiberg disease was described.

12. Lee HJ, Kim JW, Min WK: Operative treatment of Freiberg disease using extra-articular dorsal closing-wedge osteotomy: Technical tip and clinical outcomes in 13 patients. *Foot Ankle Int* 2013;34(1):111-116.

    A retrospective review of 13 patients (mean age, 29.1 years) who underwent an extra-articular dorsal closing-wedge osteotomy after débridement of the joint found significant improvement in pain with no nonunions. Level of evidence: IV.

13. Özkan Y, Oztürk A, Ozdemir R, Aykut S, Yalçin N: Interpositional arthroplasty with extensor digitorum brevis tendon in Freiberg's disease: A new surgical technique. *Foot Ankle Int* 2008;29(5):488-492.

    In 10 patients, interpositional arthroplasty for Freiberg disease led to an excellent result in 4 patients, a good result in 5, and a poor result in 1. Level of evidence: IV.

14. Tsuda E, Ishibashi Y, Yamamoto Y, Maeda S, Kimura Y, Sato H: Osteochondral autograft transplantation for advanced stage Freiberg disease in adolescent athletes: A report of 3 cases and surgical procedures. *Am J Sports Med* 2011;39(11):2470-2475.

    A retrospective review of osteochondral autograft transplantation in three young patients with Freiberg disease found that all returned to sports within 12 weeks of surgery. Level of evidence: IV.

15. Miyamoto W, Takao M, Uchio Y, Kono T, Ochi M: Late-stage Freiberg disease treated by osteochondral plug transplantation: A case series. *Foot Ankle Int* 2008;29(9):950-955.

    A retrospective review of osteochondral plug transplantation in four patients with Freiberg disease (mean age, 12 years) found satisfactory results at 12-month follow-up. Two patients had normal cartilage on arthroscopy.

16. Man RA, Mann JA: Keratotic disorders of the plantar skin, in Coughlin MJ, Mann RA, Saltzman CL, eds: *Surgery of the Foot and Ankle,* ed 8. Philadelphia, PA, Mosby Elsevier, 2007, pp 465-490.

17. Maskill JD, Bohay DR, Anderson JG: Gastrocnemius recession to treat isolated foot pain. *Foot Ankle Int* 2010;31(1):19-23.

    A gastrocnemius recession was done in 29 patients (34 feet) for chronic pain without structural abnormality other than an isolated gastrocnemius contracture. At an average 19.5-month follow-up, 27 patients (93%) said they were satisfied with the results of the procedure. Level of evidence: IV.

18. Park EH, Kim YS, Lee HJ, Koh YG: Metatarsal shortening osteotomy for decompression of Morton's neuroma. *Foot Ankle Int* 2013; published online ahead of print July 26.

    Surgical outcomes were retrospectively reviewed in 84 consecutive patients with a total of 86 Morton neuromas. Approximately half were treated with release of the deep transverse metatarsal ligament alone, and the other half were treated with metatarsal shortening osteotomy and deep transverse metatarsal ligament release. The metatarsal shortening osteotomy with deep transverse metatarsal ligament release led to better outcomes. Level of evidence: III.

19. Åkermark C, Crone H, Saartok T, Zuber Z: Plantar versus dorsal incision in the treatment of primary intermetatarsal Morton's neuroma. *Foot Ankle Int* 2008;29(2):136-141.

    Surgical outcomes were retrospectively reviewed after 132 procedures for Morton neuroma. One experienced surgeon used a longitudinal plantar incisions, and another used a dorsal incision. The plantar incision led to significantly better results in terms of long-term sensory loss, postoperative sick leave from work, and complications. Level of evidence: III.

20. Saxena A, Krisdakumtorn T: Return to activity after sesamoidectomy in athletically active individuals. *Foot Ankle Int* 2003;24(5):415-419.

21. Lee S, James WC, Cohen BE, Davis WH, Anderson RB: Evaluation of hallux alignment and functional outcome after isolated tibial sesamoidectomy. *Foot Ankle Int* 2005;26(10):803-809.

22. Greisberg J, Prince D, Sperber L: First ray mobility increase in patients with metatarsalgia. *Foot Ankle Int* 2010;31(11):954-958.

Dynamic metatarsal elevation was prospectively measured in 352 patients. The 64 patients with transfer metatarsalgia had significantly greater first ray mobility (9 mm versus 7 mm; $P < 0.0002$) and metatarsal elevation (5 mm versus 3 mm; $P < 0.0002$) than the 288 patients without symptoms. Level of evidence: II.

23. Pérez-Muñoz I, Escobar-Antón D, Sanz-Gómez TA: The role of Weil and triple Weil osteotomies in the treatment of propulsive metatarsalgia. *Foot Ankle Int* 2012;33(6):501-506.

After Weil or triple Weil osteotomy for the treatment of third rocker metatarsalgia, the median AOFAS score was 90 (range, 34 to 100). The results were satisfactory in 80% of patients.

Special Problems of the Foot and Ankle

SECTION EDITOR:

SHELDON S. LIN, MD

Chapter 17

Nondiabetic Foot Infections

Adolph Samuel Flemister Jr, MD

Introduction

Although most foot and ankle infections occur in patients with diabetic neuropathy, sometimes these infections develop in patients who do not have diabetes.[1,2] Foot or ankle infection can result from penetrating trauma, repetitive microtrauma, a compromised postoperative wound, or hematogenous spread. Foot or ankle infection can be devastating, regardless of whether the patient has diabetes, and potentially can lead to limb loss and permanent dysfunction. Prompt diagnosis and treatment are essential to prevent needless morbidity and prolonged disability.

Diagnosis

History and Physical Examination

Patients with a foot or ankle infection have some combination of pain, swelling, and erythema, with or without an obvious wound. It is important to determine the duration of symptoms, the severity of pain, and the presence of constitutional symptoms such as fevers, chills, and malaise. Chronic renal insufficiency, diabetes mellitus, HIV disease, organ transplantation, or inflammatory arthropathy has the potential to compromise the patient's immune system and ability to fight infection. Current tobacco use affects soft-tissue healing and may affect blood flow.[3] It is important to determine whether the patient has a history of gout because the signs and symptoms of gout can mimic those of infection.

The physical examination begins with the patient's vital signs, including temperature, heart rate, and blood pressure. The patient's overall mental status must be assessed. Tachycardia, hypotension, fever, and altered mental status should alert the provider to the possibility of early sepsis. The affected limb should be inspected for overall alignment, deformity, swelling, and erythema.

Erythema that is not resolved with limb elevation suggests the presence of cellulitis. The skin and interdigital areas of the foot must be closely inspected for calluses, blisters, fissures, and open wounds. The size and depth of a wound should be assessed as well as the presence, amount, and consistency of drainage. The risk of developing osteomyelitis is increased in a wound that can be probed to bone.[4] Exposed tendons or ligaments should be identified. Fluctuant areas should be identified by palpation, with specific attention to gaslike crepitus, regardless of the presence of a wound. Careful inspection and palpation of the surrounding joints are essential to assessing joint range of motion and stability. Diminished range of motion or instability that compromises normal foot mechanics leads to overloading of other areas of the foot, and this repetitive microtrauma increases the risk of skin breakdown. Swollen and painful joints with suspected effusion suggest septic arthritis and may require aspiration.

It is important to perform a thorough neurovascular examination. Although diabetes mellitus is the most common known cause of peripheral neuropathy in the United States, neuropathy can develop in patients without diabetes as a result of idiopathic factors or a known cause such as alcohol abuse, chemotherapy, a viral infection, or a vitamin deficiency. It is essential to determine the patient's gross sensation to light touch and the ability to feel a Semmes-Weinstein 5.07 monofilament.[5] Motor function should be carefully evaluated. If pulses are not palpable, the ankle-brachial index and toe pressure should be measured. An ankle-brachial index of less than 0.45 and an absolute toe pressure of 40 mm Hg or less means that the patient is at risk for poor wound healing and therefore requires a more extensive vascular workup.[6]

Imaging Studies

Plain radiography of the foot and ankle is the primary screening tool for infection. If possible, weight-bearing studies should be obtained to best evaluate bone and joint alignment. Radiographs may show soft-tissue gas or densities representing localized edema, gas gangrene,

Dr. Flemister or an immediate family member serves as an unpaid consultant to Biomimetic and serves as a board member, owner, officer, or committee member of the American Orthopaedic Foot and Ankle Society and the New York State Orthopaedic Society.

or abscess. Bony changes such as erosion, periosteal re-action, and frank destruction indicate osteomyelitis. It is important to realize that negative plain radiographs do not eliminate the possibility of osteomyelitis.[4] Bony change may not appear radiographically during the first 2 to 4 weeks of the acute stage of osteomyelitis. (Figure 1).

CT is more sensitive than plain radiography for de-tecting early-stage bony erosion or destruction. CT also shows air in the soft tissues and is used to locate abscess-es. CT is most commonly used if MRI is contraindicat-ed. Ultrasound also is useful for detecting soft-tissue abscesses and can be used for image-guided aspiration.

MRI is the most effective imaging study for evaluation of soft tissues, and it is the study of choice for detection of a fluid pocket such as an abscess. MRI also readily de-tects bone edema. However, bone marrow edema, shown by increased signal with T2 weighting and decreased signal with T1 weighting, is a nonspecific finding that also is seen in fracture, tumor, Charcot arthropathy, or bony overload related to poor mechanics. The sensitivity and specificity of MRI for detecting osteomyelitis varies among studies.[4,7-9]

Nuclear imaging can provide valuable information about the presence or absence of osteomyelitis.[7,9,10] Triple-phase technetium Tc-99m bone scanning de-tects even subtle bony destruction but can provide a false-positive finding of infection in the presence of fracture, Charcot arthropathy, or stress-related bony changes. The sensitivity and specificity of nuclear testing for chronic osteomyelitis can be improved by combining the triple-phase scan with an indium-111–labeled white blood cell (WBC) scan.[10]

Laboratory Studies

Laboratory studies are an important adjuvant in the diag-nosis and treatment of infection. A complete WBC count with differential, erythrocyte sedimentation rate (ESR), and C-reactive protein (CRP) level should be obtained.[11] In an acute infection, the WBC count normally is elevated; an increase in neutrophils with left shift is noted. Patients who are older than 65 years or who are immunocom-promised may have little or no elevation of the WBC count. The ESR and CRP level are general inflammatory markers that typically are elevated with infection but can be elevated with any inflammatory process or for several weeks after surgery. The ESR and CRP level are useful for monitoring the patient's response to treatment because typically they return to normal with effective treatment of the infection.[11] The CRP level declines rapidly, but the ESR tends to remain somewhat elevated for several weeks, even with effective treatment.[11]

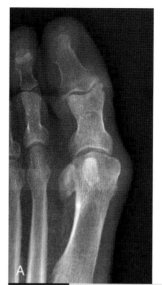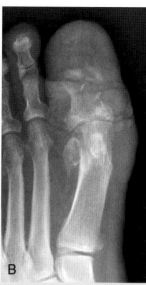

Figure 1 AP radiographs of the great toe showing a dorsal proximal interphalangeal ulcer in a 60-year-old patient (**A**) and destructive osteomyelitis 3 weeks later (**B**).

The patient's nutritional status can have a substan-tial effect on the response to treatment. Albumin, pre-albumin, and transferrin levels all are measures of the patient's nutritional status and should be obtained as part of the infection workup. A total lymphocyte count higher than 1,500 is a useful indicator of general health. A patient found to be nutritionally depleted should take nutritional supplements.[12]

The preferred tissue for culturing contains débrided soft tissue or fluid rather than tissue from a simple swab.[13] Depending on the clinical indications, tissue aspirated from a septic joint should be sent for Gram staining and cultured for aerobic and anaerobic bacteria as well as fungi and acid-fast bacilli. The fluid itself should be sent for WBC count and the presence of crystals. A WBC count higher than 50,000 mL generally indicates an in-fection. The presence or absence of crystals is used to rule out a gouty process.[3,14]

Nail Disorders

Infection surrounding the toenail bed is classified as an infected ingrown nail (paronychia), felon, or onychomy-cosis. An ingrown toenail is caused by a deformity of the nail bed or improper trimming. The irritated surrounding soft tissues become colonized with bacteria. Numerous bacteria have been implicated in such infections, including *Staphylococcus aureus, Streptococcus,* and *Pseudomo-nas.*[15] Patients have a red, swollen, and draining area ad-jacent to the medial or lateral nail fold. Initial radiographs are taken to evaluate for osteomyelitis. In most patients, an early infection responds to local nail débridement. The use of oral antibiotics is not helpful. A resistant or recurrent infection may require partial or complete nail removal for permanent ablation.[15,16]

Felon is a deeper infection occurring in the tissue septi of the distal pulp of the toe. *S aureus* is the most common organism. Patients have a red, swollen, fluctuant area at the distal aspect of the toe. Surgical drainage is essential, followed by culture-specific antibiotic therapy. The wound should be left open and packed as needed, depending on its size. Most such infections respond to an antibiotic that covers gram-positive organisms.

Onychomycosis is a fungal infection that is one of the most common diseases of the nails. The nails become thickened, discolored, and often brittle. The pathogens most often responsible for onychomycosis are dermatophytes, including *Trichophyton rubrum* and *Trichophyton mentagrophytes*.[17] *Candida* and molds are less common causal agents. Onychomycosis can be difficult to treat. Often several months of treatment are required. The systemic antifungal agents carry a risk of liver toxicity, but the use of topical medications may lead to a recurrence after discontinuance. In a healthy patient, onychomycosis rarely is more than a cosmetic concern.[17] The thickened nails may catch on clothing and occasionally cause an ingrown toenail, but frequent débridement usually is sufficient for controlling such issues.

Soft-Tissue Infections

Cellulitis is an infection of skin and subcutaneous tissues. The most common cause is contamination of an obviously open wound or small nondetectable wounds secondary to microtrauma. The incidence of cellulitis increases with patient age, and it is most common in patients with compromised skin from lymphedema, chronic venous stasis, chronic steroid use, or chronic edema.[18] The foot and ankle are inherently predisposed to cellulitis because of their weight-bearing position, multiple bony prominences, and shoe wear requirements, all of which increase the risk of microtrauma to the surrounding soft tissues. Cellulitis appears as erythema, swelling, increasing pain, and induration. Patients may have fever or other constitutional symptoms. Lymphadenopathy may occur proximally at the knee or groin. Initial outlining of the involved area can be helpful in guiding the treatment response.

Methicillin-susceptible *S aureus* and streptococci are the most common organisms responsible for cellulitis. These organisms often reside in the interdigital toe spaces.[19] Usually cellulitis will respond to oral or intravenous antibiotic therapy within the first 1 to 2 days, depending on the severity of the condition. Most such infections can be treated with antibiotics effective against methicillin-susceptible *S aureus* and streptococci. The patient should be closely followed as the symptoms resolve because fluctuant areas or painful joints may become evident, indicating the presence of an abscess or septic arthritis.[20]

Necrotizing fasciitis is an aggressive, rapidly spreading soft-tissue infection that travels along fascial planes. Necrotizing fasciitis is most common in the lower extremities and often starts with a traumatic wound. The foot is particularly at risk for this type of infection. The infection often is polymicrobial, involving both gram-negative and gram-positive species as well as aerobic and anaerobic organisms.[21,22] The commonly found organisms include group A and α-hemolytic streptococci, *S aureus*, *Escherichia coli*, and *Pseudomonas*. Many of these organisms secrete toxins that cause septic shock followed by multiple organ failure.[21-23] Patients who are immunocompromised, such as those with diabetes mellitus, are particularly at risk.

In the early stages of necrotizing fasciitis, the patient has vague muscle joint aches and pains. The symptoms can rapidly deteriorate, however, and the patient may have signs of systemic toxicity such as hypotension.[21] The affected limb rapidly becomes swollen and erythematous. Fluid-filled bullae may be present, signs of necrosis may ensue, and sepsis may progress rapidly.[21,22] A delayed diagnosis resulting from the insidious onset of symptoms can further compromise the outcome.

Emergency surgical débridement of all necrotic tissue including subcutaneous tissues, fascia, and skin is essential to eradicate the infection.[21-23] Multiple repeat débridement is required in a temporally staged manner. Amputation of the limb may be required to avoid mortality. Reconstructive procedures including skin grafting often are necessary after the infection has been eradicated.[21,22]

Deep Infections

Its weight-bearing nature predisposes the foot to multiple forms of trauma, such as penetrating trauma and repetitive microtrauma. A deep infection of the foot may be manifested as a plantar space abscess, osteomyelitis, or septic arthritis. Penetrating trauma most commonly is caused by a puncture injury. *S aureus*, group A streptococci, and *Pseudomonas aeruginosa* are the organisms most commonly identified after such a direct inoculation.[24,25] Most wounds initially can be managed with local irrigation and débridement as well as an oral antibiotic (usually a cephalosporin). A deeper infection may appear days or weeks after the initial injury and will require a thorough surgical débridement. Care should be taken to identify and remove all foreign material.[26]

Patients with peripheral neuropathy are especially prone to wounds secondary to repetitive microtrauma. Superficial ulceration is treated with local débridement and total-contact casting, as for a patient with diabetes. A deeper ulcer with exposed tendon, bone, or joint tissue requires more extensive débridement, followed by the total-contact cast protocol.

A plantar space abscess appears as a red, warm, and swollen foot with tenderness along the plantar surface. An obvious wound or fluctuant area may not be present. In the absence of an obvious abscess location, MRI is helpful for locating the infection and outlining the extent of the process. Surgical drainage, débridement of devitalized tissue, and culture-specific antibiotic therapy are required to eradicate the infection.

Osteomyelitis can result from direct inoculation of tissues in a traumatic or surgical wound or as a result of hematogenous spread. Hematogenous osteomyelitis is most common in children and adults who are immunocompromised.[27] The patient has acute pain, redness, warmth, and tenderness over the affected area. In children, metaphyseal bone is particularly prone to hematogenous spread of infection because of its highly vascularized nature.[27] MRI is helpful in determining the extent of the disease and the presence of an intramedullary abscess. Many infections in children can be adequately treated with intravenous antibiotics. A bone abscess must be drained, however, and an infection that does not respond to intravenous antibiotic therapy in a timely fashion requires surgical débridement.

Osteomyelitis that appears within the first few weeks of surgery or trauma is classified as acute. Acute osteomyelitis has the classic signs of infection: erythema, warmth, tenderness, and usually systemic signs such as fevers, chills, and malaise. In contrast, chronic osteomyelitis commonly has an indolent course characterized by persistent or intermittent drainage from a wound or sinus tract. The consistency of the drainage can be serous, serosanguineous, cloudy, or purulent, depending on the extent of the infection. To eradicate chronic osteomyelitis, removal of infected and necrotic bone is required, followed by culture-specific antibiotic therapy.[28,29]

After early identification, acute osteomyelitis can be treated with culture-specific intravenous antibiotics.[28] Obtaining an accurate culture requires a biopsy of the bone. Biopsy of the bone through an open wound can lead to contamination of the specimen.[30] It is preferable to make a biopsy incision in an area that is outside the wound but allows access to the suspected bony infection. Multiple small bones of the foot often are involved, and obtaining an accurate biopsy specimen can be difficult. The best biopsy specimens are likely to be obtained during débridement to remove necrotic bone and compromised soft tissue.

Septic arthritis appears as an acute onset of pain, swelling, warmth, and erythema as well as a diminished range of motion in the affected joint. Hematogenous spread is most likely to occur in children and adults who are immunocompromised. If hematogenous spread is suspected, care should be taken to closely examine the patient to identify any other source of infection or area of spread. Septic arthritis from direct inoculation of the joint most commonly occurs with a puncture wound or foot ulcer around the metatarsophalangeal joints. The signs and symptoms of septic arthritis are similar to those of a crystalline arthropathy, such as gout, or another inflammatory arthropathy. Joint aspiration is essential for an accurate diagnosis.[14] The analysis of aspirates should include WBC count, Gram staining, culturing, and the presence of crystals. A WBC count of more than 50,000 per mL is suspicious but not diagnostic for infection.[3,14] If the cell count is less than 50,000 per mL, the results of the Gram stain should be used to determine whether there is an early infection.[3] When a diagnosis of septic arthritis is confirmed, surgical drainage should be done on an urgent basis. A delay in treating septic arthritis can lead to early proteoglycan loss, cartilage damage, and severe joint destruction with spread of osteomyelitis to adjacent bones.[31] Open débridement including an aggressive synovectomy is required for most joints of the foot. A larger joint, such as the ankle or subtalar joint, can be treated with arthroscopic débridement, depending on the surgeon's level of comfort and possibly on the extent of the infection.

Surgical Débridement of the Foot and Ankle

The biomechanics and weight-bearing characteristics of the foot and ankle should be considered during surgical débridement. Because the plantar surface of the foot is designed for durability, plantar incisions that compromise the plantar skin and fat should be avoided, if possible. Fortunately, most anatomic structures of the foot can be exposed through a medial, lateral, dorsal, or combined incision.

Osteomyelitis of the Hallux and Lesser Toes

Osteomyelitis of the great and lesser toes is best treated with removal of all involved bone. Toe amputation sometimes is necessary. The best débridement of a lesser toe removes all infected bone and soft tissue and leaves a stable remnant. Leaving a stable residual portion of a lesser toe after débridement or amputation may prevent migration of the adjacent toes. However, leaving a floppy residual toe after bone resection can lead to the formation of new wounds on the toe as well as shoe wear difficulty.

In the great toe, maintaining as much length as possible allows better function than amputation through the metatarsophalangeal joint. The balance of the sesamoid mechanism and relatively normal weight bearing are best preserved when at least 1 cm of the base of the proximal phalanx is maintained.[32] If an amputation through the metatarsophalangeal joint is necessary, it is best to resect the remaining sesamoid bones, which will have no significant function and can be a source of recurrent ulceration or discomfort.

Ray resection (amputation of the toe with all or part of the metatarsal) is required if an infection involves both the metatarsal and phalanx of the toe. Ray resection is preferred even in the absence of infection in the toe itself, if it is necessary to avoid an excessively floppy residual toe after resection of the metatarsal. The foot remains functional and weight bearing after resection of the lateral two rays. Resection of the first ray is more likely to lead to ineffective weight transfer and a less-than-functional foot. The loss of weight-bearing function can be overcome with offloading and an appropriately molded insole, which are preferable to transmetatarsal amputation. Resection of three or more central rays or the first and second medial rays invariably creates an unstable, poorly functioning foot, and transmetatarsal amputation may be the preferable treatment.[32]

Infection of the Midfoot, Hindfoot, or Ankle

Infection about the midfoot, hindfoot, or ankle often involves multiple bones and joints. Multiple aggressive débridement usually is required to eradicate such an infection. Cavitary defects typically remain, which can be temporarily filled with antibiotic-impregnated cement beads, antibiotic biodegradable carrier, or spacers.[33,34] It is critical to determine the extent of bone loss and the relative stability of the bone. External fixation often is used when eradication of the infection leads to bony instability. The use of thin wires with a circular or semicircular frame has the advantage of minimizing soft-tissue trauma. A thin-wire external fixator maintains multiplanar stability and allows earlier weight bearing than a traditional large-pin external fixator.[35-37] Salvage surgery for many infections requires arthrodesis, often followed by thin-wire external fixation, but internal fixation sometimes is indicated. Careful preoperative evaluation before internal fixation is used to be certain the infection is eradicated. Autogenous bone graft is used in preference to allograft.[38] The soft-tissue envelope is relatively sparse around the foot and ankle, and surgical débridement often leaves soft-tissue defects that require a local flap or soft-tissue transfer for coverage.[38] Early consultation with a plastic surgeon is recommended.

Calcaneal osteomyelitis occurs as a consequence of a posttraumatic wound, heel pressure ulcer, or postsurgical infection.[39-41] Many calcaneal infections occur with delayed wound healing. Most postoperative infections follow open reduction and internal fixation of an intra-articular calcaneal fracture.[39] Irrigation and débridement with an attempt at retaining the hardware is initially indicated. If the infection cannot be controlled or an osteomyelitis has been detected, thorough débridement of bone and removal of all infected hardware is indicated. Cavitary defects typically remain and can be filled with antibiotic-impregnated cement. Débridement often creates soft-tissue defects that require flap coverage. The use of a vacuum-assisted device can be helpful for minimizing soft-tissue defects, but early consultation with a plastic surgeon again is recommended.[42] In patients whose calcaneal infection originated in a heel pressure ulcer, the osteomyelitis initially is restricted to the tuberosity. The use of partial or total calcanectomy as a limb-salvage procedure has not been well studied in patients who do not have diabetes, but early results in patients with diabetes were promising. Recent studies found poor functional results and a high reamputation rate after calcanectomy in patients with diabetes.[43-45]

Infection about the ankle most commonly occurs as a complication after treatment of a severe talus or pilon fracture with soft-tissue compromise.[37,38] Total ankle arthroplasty has been done with increasing frequency in recent years, but the incidence of infection after unsuccessful procedures also has increased.[46] Hematogenous spread of infection can occur, leading to septic ankle arthritis and subsequent osteomyelitis, especially in patients who are immunocompromised. Initial management of infection about the ankle involves multiple débridement until all compromised bone and soft tissue have been removed. If the infection occurs during the first weeks after fracture surgery, attempts can be made to retain the hardware. However, infected bone should not be left in place in an effort to retain hardware. Cavitary defects can be filled with antibiotic cement or biodegradable carrier placed as a spacer to maintain height.[33,34] External fixation usually is also required to maintain stability. After the infection has been controlled, arthrodesis is indicated to treat postseptic arthrosis or bone loss. The method of fusion varies with the amount of bone loss, the bone involved, and the surgeon's preference. For osteomyelitis after pilon fracture, a portion of the distal tibia along the joint line usually is left intact to maintain bone length. The defects resulting from tibial bone loss most often are filled with autogenous bone graft.[38] After surgery, the patient is treated with internal or external fixation, depending on the surgeon's preference and confidence that the infection has been eradicated. After talar fracture,

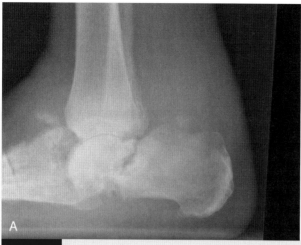
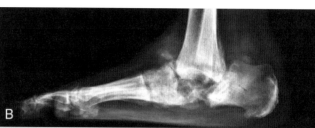

Figure 2 Lateral radiographs of the ankle showing osteomyelitis of the talus in a patient who had neuropathy but did not have diabetes, before (**A**) and 5 months after talectomy and arthrodesis with a circular external fixator (**B**). The patient had a stable plantigrade foot.

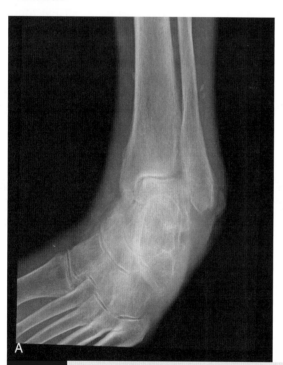
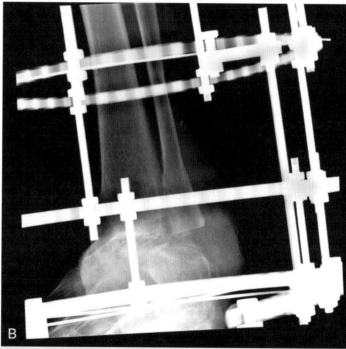

Figure 3 AP radiographs showing a fixed varus deformity in a 75-year-old patient with Charcot-Marie-Tooth disease, osteomyelitis of the fibula, and a 10-cm lateral ulcer before (**A**) and after resection of the involved fibula, partial talus resection, and arthrodesis (**B**). The patient was placed in a static frame circular external fixator.

resection of the entire talar body usually is required, leading to substantial shortening. The surgeon must decide whether to perform a tibiocalcaneal arthrodesis or to place a large-bulk femoral head allograft into the defect in an attempt to maintain height (**Figure 2**). Tibiocalcaneal arthrodesis has variable results but almost always leads to some functional deficits and gait abnormality.[37,47] Internal or external fixation can be used.

Osteomyelitis of the fibula most commonly occurs in patients with a deformity of the foot, many of whom have neuropathy. Abnormal weight bearing on the fibula causes wound breakdown with subsequent infection. Excision of the infected fibula is required. If resection leads to tibiotalar instability, ankle arthrodesis can be done. Because resection of the involved fibula usually completely eradicates the osteomyelitis, a variety of internal or external fixation techniques can be used for arthrodesis (**Figure 3**).

Multidisciplinary Management

The management of foot infection in patients who do not have diabetes can be complex. Often the infection involves significant trauma or severe postoperative infection. Many patients have multiple medical comorbidities or are immunocompromised. The foot or ankle infection is likely to involve soft-tissue compromise and to be polymicrobial. A team approach may be required, involving medical specialists, infectious disease specialists, plastic surgeons, and vascular surgeons.[28,48] The orthopaedic surgeon should not hesitate to involve the necessary subspecialists.

Summary

The goal of managing a nondiabetic foot or ankle infection is to achieve a stable, plantigrade limb devoid of infection. Prompt diagnosis and treatment are required for a successful outcome. Although many superficial infections can be treated nonsurgically, a deep or complicated infection requires repeated aggressive surgical débridement, stabilization, and ultimately reconstruction.

Annotated References

1. Wukich DK, McMillen RL, Lowery NJ, Frykberg RG: Surgical site infections after foot and ankle surgery: A comparison of patients with and without diabetes. *Diabetes Care* 2011;34(10):2211-2213.

   A prospective study of 1,465 consecutive patients treated by a single surgeon found a surgical site infection in 9.5% of patients with diabetes and 2.4% of patients who did not have diabetes. The presence of peripheral neuropathy strongly determined the development of postoperative infection. Level of evidence: II.

2. Wukich DK, Lowery NJ, McMillen RL, Frykberg RG: Postoperative infection rates in foot and ankle surgery: A comparison of patients with and without diabetes mellitus. *J Bone Joint Surg Am* 2010;92(2):287-295.

   A retrospective study of 1,000 patients after orthopaedic foot or ankle surgery found a 2.8% infection rate in those who did not have diabetes. Peripheral neuropathy was a more significant factor than diabetes for the development of postoperative infection. Level of evidence: III.

3. Lee JJ, Patel R, Biermann JS, Dougherty PJ: The musculoskeletal effects of cigarette smoking. *J Bone Joint Surg Am* 2013;95(9):850-859.

   Cigarette smoking was a significant risk factor for perioperative complications including nonunion, delayed union, inadequate wound healing, and infection.

4. Butalia S, Palda VA, Sargeant RJ, Detsky AS, Mourad O: Does this patient with diabetes have osteomyelitis of the lower extremity? *JAMA* 2008;299(7):806-813.

   A systematic review found that the factors most indicative of osteomyelitis of the lower extremity were an ulcer larger than 2 cm², a positive probe-to-bone test, and a positive MRI.

5. Kanji JN, Anglin RE, Hunt DL, Panju A: Does this patient with diabetes have large-fiber peripheral neuropathy? *JAMA* 2010;303(15):1526-1532.

   A systematic literature review found that abnormal results on Semmes-Weinstein 5.07 monofilament and vibratory perception tests were the most helpful signs for detecting large-fiber peripheral neuropathy.

6. Apelqvist J, Castenfors J, Larsson J, Stenström A, Agardh CD: Prognostic value of systolic ankle and toe blood pressure levels in outcome of diabetic foot ulcer. *Diabetes Care* 1989;12(6):373-378.

7. Dinh MT, Abad CL, Safdar N: Diagnostic accuracy of the physical examination and imaging tests for osteomyelitis underlying diabetic foot ulcers: Meta-analysis. *Clin Infect Dis* 2008;47(4):519-527.

   The accuracy of diagnostic tests for osteomyelitis in patients with a foot ulcer was analyzed. MRI was more accurate at diagnosing osteomyelitis than leukocyte scanning. Probe-to-bone testing of a large ulcer was moderately predictive.

8. Kapoor A, Page S, Lavalley M, Gale DR, Felson DT: Magnetic resonance imaging for diagnosing foot osteomyelitis: A meta-analysis. *Arch Intern Med* 2007;167(2):125-132.

9. Termaat MF, Raijmakers PG, Scholten HJ, Bakker FC, Patka P, Haarman HJ: The accuracy of diagnostic imaging for the assessment of chronic osteomyelitis: A systematic review and meta-analysis. *J Bone Joint Surg Am* 2005;87(11):2464-2471.

10. Johnson JE, Kennedy EJ, Shereff MJ, Patel NC, Collier BD: Prospective study of bone, indium-111-labeled white blood cell, and gallium-67 scanning for the evaluation of osteomyelitis in the diabetic foot. *Foot Ankle Int* 1996;17(1):10-16.

11. Michail M, Jude E, Liaskos C, et al: The performance of serum inflammatory markers for the diagnosis and follow-up of patients with osteomyelitis. *Int J Low Extrem Wounds* 2013;12(2):94-99.

   A prospective study found that WBC count, CRP level, and procalcitonin serum level returned to near-normal values at day 7 after initiation of treatment with antibiotics in patients with foot osteomyelitis. The ESR remained high for 3 months. Level of evidence: II.

5: Special Problems of the Foot and Ankle

12. Kavalukas SL, Barbul A: Nutrition and wound healing: An update. *Plast Reconstr Surg* 2011;127(Suppl 1):38S-43S.

Advances in the understanding of nutrition in wound healing were reviewed, with emphasis on the effect of nutritional history and nutritional intervention.

13. Aggarwal VK, Higuera C, Deirmengian G, Parvizi J, Austin MS: Swab cultures are not as effective as tissue cultures for diagnosis of periprosthetic joint infection. *Clin Orthop Relat Res* 2013;471(10):3196-3203.

A prospective study found that tissue cultures had greater sensitivity and specificity for infection than swab cultures. Swab cultures had more false-negative and false-positive results than tissue cultures. Level of evidence: II.

14. Mathews CJ, Kingsley G, Field M, et al: Management of septic arthritis: A systematic review. *Ann Rheum Dis* 2007;66(4):440-445.

15. Heidelbaugh JJ, Lee H: Management of the ingrown toenail. *Am Fam Physician* 2009;79(4):303-308.

Outcomes were not improved by the use of oral antibiotics before or after débridement of an ingrown toenail, with or without phenolization.

16. Eekhof JA, Van Wijk B, Knuistingh Neven A, van der Wouden JC: Interventions for ingrowing toenails. *Cochrane Database Syst Rev* 2012;4:CD001541.

A Cochrane database review of interventions for ingrown toenails cited 24 studies. Surgical interventions were more effective than nonsurgical interventions in preventing the recurrence of ingrown toenails. Surgery in which phenol was used appeared to be least likely to lead to recurrence.

17. de Berker D: Fungal nail disease. *N Engl J Med* 2009;360(20):2108-2116.

A complete review of fungal nail disease emphasized the need for an accurate diagnosis as well as the multiple available medical treatment options. The likelihood of a complete cure was low.

18. McNamara DR, Tleyjeh IM, Berbari EF, et al: Incidence of lower-extremity cellulitis: A population-based study in Olmsted county, Minnesota. *Mayo Clin Proc* 2007;82(7):817-821.

In this population-based survey, the incidence of lower extremity cellulitis was correlated with increasing age but was not influenced by sex. Level of evidence: III.

19. Hirschmann JV, Raugi GJ: Lower limb cellulitis and its mimics: Part I. Lower limb cellulitis. *J Am Acad Dermatol* 2012;67(2):163.

An extensive review pointed to an aging population and obesity as contributors to the incidence of lower extremity cellulitis. The involved organisms were identified. The interdigital toe spaces were identified as the area of colonization.

20. Picard D, Klein A, Grigioni S, Joly P: Risk factors for abscess formation in patients with superficial cellulitis (erysipelas) of the leg. *Br J Dermatol* 2013;168(4):859-863.

A retrospective review of 164 patients with cellulitis of the lower extremity found that abscess formation was correlated with a history of alcohol abuse and delayed initiation of antibiotic treatment. Level of evidence: III.

21. Endorf FW, Cancio LC, Klein MB: Necrotizing soft-tissue infections: Clinical guidelines. *J Burn Care Res* 2009;30(5):769-775.

Clinical guidelines for the management of necrotizing fasciitis were reviewed. Prompt and aggressive surgical débridement with immediate initiation of broad-spectrum antibiotics were found to be essential. The postoperative use of hyperbaric oxygen was noted to be controversial.

22. Wong CH, Chang HC, Pasupathy S, Khin LW, Tan JL, Low CO: Necrotizing fasciitis: Clinical presentation, microbiology, and determinants of mortality. *J Bone Joint Surg Am* 2003;85(8):1454-1460.

23. Tsai YH, Hsu RW, Huang KC, Huang TJ: Laboratory indicators for early detection and surgical treatment of Vibrio necrotizing fasciitis. *Clin Orthop Relat Res* 2010;468(8):2230-2237.

A retrospective review of the laboratory indicators in *Vibrio* necrotizing fasciitis found that initial systolic blood pressure lower than 90 mm Hg, segmented leukocyte counts, hypoalbuminemia, and severe thrombocytopenia were associated with increased mortality. Level of evidence: III.

24. Eidelman M, Bialik V, Miller Y, Kassis I: Plantar puncture wounds in children: Analysis of 80 hospitalized patients and late sequelae. *Isr Med Assoc J* 2003;5(4):268-271.

25. Gale DW, Scott R: Puncture wound of the foot? Persistent pain? Think of Pseudomonas aeroginosa osteomyelitis. *Injury* 1991;22(5):427-428.

26. Chang HC, Verhoeven W, Chay WM: Rubber foreign bodies in puncture wounds of the foot in patients wearing rubber-soled shoes. *Foot Ankle Int* 2001;22(5):409-414.

27. Bouchoucha S, Gafsi K, Trifa M, et al: Intravenous antibiotic therapy for acute hematogenous osteomyelitis in children: Short versus long course. *Arch Pediatr* 2013;20(5):464-469.

A randomized prospective study found that acute hematogenous osteomyelitis in children could be treated with intravenous antibiotics for a period as short as 7 days. Level of evidence: I.

28. Rao N, Ziran BH, Lipsky BA: Treating osteomyelitis: Antibiotics and surgery. *Plast Reconstr Surg* 2011;127(Suppl 1):177S-187S.

A nonsystematic literature review of the treatment of acute and chronic osteomyelitis emphasized the need for a multidisciplinary team approach, surgical débridement, and culture-specific antibiotics to eradicate the infection.

29. Conterno LO, Turchi MD: Antibiotics for treating chronic osteomyelitis in adults. *Cochrane Database Syst Rev* 2013;9:CD004439.

A Cochrane database systematic review of the treatment of chronic osteomyelitis in adults found limited, low-quality evidence to suggest that the route of antibiotic administration affected the rate of disease remission. All patients had surgical débridement in addition to antibiotic treatment.

30. Malone M, Bowling FL, Gannass A, Jude EB, Boulton AJ: Deep wound cultures correlate well with bone biopsy culture in diabetic foot osteomyelitis. *Diabetes Metab Res Rev* 2013;29(7):546-550.

Deep wound cultures were found to be well correlated with osseous cultures. These cultures were believed to be adequate if a bone biopsy was not possible.

31. Montgomery CO, Siegel E, Blasier RD, Suva LJ: Concurrent septic arthritis and osteomyelitis in children. *J Pediatr Orthop* 2013;33(4):464-467.

A retrospective review of 200 children with septic arthritis found that septic elbow, hip, knee, and ankle joints were less likely than shoulder joints to have concurrent osteomyelitis. Advanced imaging was necessary for an early diagnosis of concurrent osteomyelitis.

32. Ng VY, Berlet GC: Evolving techniques in foot and ankle amputation. *J Am Acad Orthop Surg* 2010;18(4):223-235.

Successful amputation planning and techniques for the foot and ankle were extensively reviewed with postoperative prosthetic and orthotic management.

33. Melamed EA, Peled E: Antibiotic impregnated cement spacer for salvage of diabetic osteomyelitis. *Foot Ankle Int* 2012;33(3):213-219.

A retrospective review of 20 patients with diabetic foot osteomyelitis found that extensive débridement and the use of antibiotic-impregnated cement spacers helped surgeons avoid amputation. Level of evidence: IV.

34. Ferrao P, Myerson MS, Schuberth JM, McCourt MJ: Cement spacer as definitive management for postoperative ankle infection. *Foot Ankle Int* 2012;33(3):173-178.

The use of an antibiotic-impregnated cement spacer as definitive treatment to eradicate deep ankle infection was reviewed. The spacer was well tolerated in seven of nine patients. Two of the patients underwent below-knee amputation. Level of evidence: IV.

35. Kugan R, Aslam N, Bose D, McNally MA: Outcome of arthrodesis of the hindfoot as a salvage procedure for complex ankle pathology using the Ilizarov technique. *Bone Joint J* 2013;95-B(3):371-377.

Arthrodesis using a circular external fixator for complex ankle pathology including infection was retrospectively reviewed. Infection was eradicated in all 30 patients with infection, and successful arthrodesis was achieved in 40 of 46 patients. Level of evidence: IV.

36. Pinzur MS, Gil J, Belmares J: Treatment of osteomyelitis in Charcot foot with single-stage resection of infection, correction of deformity, and maintenance with ring fixation. *Foot Ankle Int* 2012;33(12):1069-1074.

In a study of 178 patients with Charcot arthropathy and osteomyelitis of the midfoot who were treated with débridement and realignment using a circular external fixator, limb salvage was achieved in 68 of 71 patients using a single-stage procedure. Level of evidence: IV.

37. Rochman R, Jackson Hutson J, Alade O: Tibiocalcaneal arthrodesis using the Ilizarov technique in the presence of bone loss and infection of the talus. *Foot Ankle Int* 2008;29(10):1001-1008.

In a retrospective review of tibiocalcaneal arthrodesis using an Ilizarov technique, 9 of 11 patients had successful fusion after infected talar nonunion or extrusion. All patients had débridement of all nonviable talus. Level of evidence: IV.

38. Zalavras CG, Patzakis MJ, Thordarson DB, Shah S, Sherman R, Holtom P: Infected fractures of the distal tibial metaphysis and plafond: Achievement of limb salvage with free muscle flaps, bone grafting, and ankle fusion. *Clin Orthop Relat Res* 2004;427:57-62.

39. Kline AJ, Anderson RB, Davis WH, Jones CP, Cohen BE: Minimally invasive technique versus an extensile lateral approach for intra-articular calcaneal fractures. *Foot Ankle Int* 2013;34(6):773-780.

A retrospective comparative review of 112 fractures found a higher rate of patient satisfaction and a significantly lower incidence of wound complications with the use of a minimally invasive approach. Level of evidence: III.

40. Dickens JF, Kilcoyne KG, Kluk MW, Gordon WT, Shawen SB, Potter BK: Risk factors for infection and amputation following open, combat-related calcaneal fractures. *J Bone Joint Surg Am* 2013;95(5):e24.

Lower extremity amputation after an open calcaneal fracture was predicted by the injury mechanism, wound size and location, and severity of the open fracture.

41. Wiersema B, Brokaw D, Weber T, et al: Complications associated with open calcaneus fractures. *Foot Ankle Int* 2011;32(11):1052-1057.

In a retrospective review of 127 open fractures treated with initial débridement and delayed fixation, the superficial wound infection rate was 9.6% and the deep infection rate was 12.2%. Culture-positive osteomyelitis was found in 5.2% of patients. Level of evidence: IV.

42. Mendonca DA, Cosker T, Makwana NK: Vacuum-assisted closure to aid wound healing in foot and ankle surgery. *Foot Ankle Int* 2005;26(9):761-766.

43. Faglia E, Clerici G, Caminiti M, Curci V, Somalvico F: Influence of osteomyelitis location in the foot of diabetic patients with transtibial amputation. *Foot Ankle Int* 2013;34(2):222-227.

    Osteomyelitis of the heel was associated with a higher rate of transtibial amputation than osteomyelitis of the midfoot or forefoot in patients with diabetes. Level of evidence: III.

44. Brown ML, Tang W, Patel A, Baumhauer JF: Partial foot amputation in patients with diabetic foot ulcers. *Foot Ankle Int* 2012;33(9):707-716.

    A retrospective review of partial or total calcanectomy in 33 patients found a higher rate of below-knee amputation and 5-year mortality in patients with diabetic foot ulcers. Level of evidence: III.

45. Bollinger M, Thordarson DB: Partial calcanectomy: An alternative to below knee amputation. *Foot Ankle Int* 2002;23(10):927-932.

46. Jeng CL, Campbell JT, Tang EY, Cerrato RA, Myerson MS: Tibiotalocalcaneal arthrodesis with bulk femoral head allograft for salvage of large defects in the ankle. *Foot Ankle Int* 2013;34(9):1256-1266.

    Thirty-two patients underwent tibiotalar calcaneal arthrodesis using femoral head allograft for large segmental bony defects. The indications included osteomyelitis. Nonunion rates were high, and 19% of patients later required a below-knee amputation.

47. DeVries JG, Berlet GC, Hyer CF: Predictive risk assessment for major amputation after tibiotalocalcaneal arthrodesis. *Foot Ankle Int* 2013;34(6):846-850.

    Tibiotalocalcaneal arthrodesis with a retrograde intramedullary nail was studied in 179 limbs. The likelihood of amputation after this procedure was three times greater if the patient had a preoperative ulcer and six times greater if the patient had undergone revision surgery.

48. Copley LA, Kinsler MA, Gheen T, Shar A, Sun D, Browne R: The impact of evidence-based clinical practice guidelines applied by a multidisciplinary team for the care of children with osteomyelitis. *J Bone Joint Surg Am* 2013;95(8):686-693.

    The use of a multidisciplinary approach in treating children with osteomyelitis was retrospectively studied. Children treated by a multidisciplinary team were believed to have a more efficient diagnostic workup, better adherence to their antibiotic plan, and a shorter hospital stay.

Chapter 18

Plantar Heel Pain

John S. Gould, MD

Introduction

Pain on the plantar aspect of the heel is common and has multiple etiologies. Plantar heel pain is distinguished from pain in the posterior heel, as occurs at the Achilles tendon insertion or in the retrocalcaneal space. Plantar fasciitis is the most commonly diagnosed condition, but a host of other disorders also can be responsible for a patient's symptoms.[1] A careful history and physical examination are essential to accurate diagnosis and treatment.

The Diagnosis

It is important to determine the history and circumstances of the onset of symptoms as well as the details of current symptoms. The physical examination requires precise knowledge of the surface anatomy of the foot. Ancillary testing is helpful for documentation and elimination of some of the possible diagnoses but can be misleading in the absence of a careful history and examination.[2]

The history is useful for determining whether the etiology is mechanical, neurogenic, oncologic, infection based, or traumatic. The possible etiologies are listed in Table 1. The patient may report a remote or recent acute traumatic event. An injury can affect the skin, fat pad, fascia, nerve, vascular system, or bone, or it can introduce a foreign body that causes an infection. The traumatic event is not always related to the disorder, however. An increasingly intense program of walking, running, or weight-bearing activity may strain the plantar tissues and lead to the spontaneous development of pain.

The nature of the patient's current symptoms is useful for determining the responsible anatomic system. It is particularly difficult to sort out a truly mechanical etiology or one that is brought on by activity and appears mechanical but really is not (quasimechanical). Nerve pain can be increased with changes in the patient's

Table 1

Etiologies of Plantar Heel Pain

Nerve syndromes (entrapments and neuromas)

Tarsal tunnel syndrome

Tarsal tunnel syndrome with chronic plantar fasciitis

Lateral plantar nerve entrapment

First branch of the lateral plantar nerve involvement (central heel pad syndrome)

Medial plantar nerve entrapment

Calcaneal nerve lesion

Sural nerve lesion

Osteomyelitis of the calcaneus

Plantar fasciitis

Ruptured plantar fascia

Skin lesion or foreign body of the heel pad

Stress fracture of the calcaneus

Tumor of the heel

positioning or level of activity. The patient should be asked whether the pain begins with the first step in the morning, disappears with further walking, and reappears when arising after sitting; or is the pain made worse by standing or walking? Does the pain occur at night and wake the patient from sleep? It is also helpful to ask the patient to describe the exact location of the pain: Is it in the medial, central, or lateral heel? Does the pain radiate, and, if so, where? Such information should allow the physician to determine the anatomic system or systems involved in the patient's pain.

During the physical examination, the physician locates the precise area of tenderness and often can determine the site of the lesion. The pain may be over the central heel pad, or at the medial soft spot where the neurovascular bundle enters the foot or over the medial tubercle of the calcaneus at the origin of the plantar fascia. Palpation may reveal a subcutaneous foreign body or a lack of prominence of the medial border of the plantar fascia. Dorsiflexion of the ankle and the great toe (the provocative test for a competent plantar fascia) may reveal a structural defect.

The history and physical examination should provide the physician with the information necessary to determine the type of pain, the anatomy involved, and the best means of proceeding to a final diagnosis.[3] The basic ancillary test is the plain radiograph. Any additional imaging is based on the history and physical examination findings. MRI is widely used and quite sensitive, but it is expensive and not particularly specific. Soft-tissue lesions of the heel, such as tumors, foreign bodies, and plantar fascia defects, can be seen with the use of less expensive ultrasonography as well as with MRI. However, the area that can be examined with ultrasonography is more limited, and interpretation of the test results is much difficult than with MRI.

On MRI, a change in signal in the calcaneus is nonspecific and can indicate a stress fracture, osteomyelitis, a bone bruise, or simply plantar fasciitis at the bony origin. If the history suggests infection, blood tests for infection markers should be considered; these should include white blood cell count and differential, erythrocyte sedimentation rate, C-reactive protein level, and labeled white blood cell scan. If a stress fracture is suspected, CT is indicated.

Plantar Heel Disorders and Their Treatment

Plantar Fasciitis

Acute plantar fasciitis is a specific entity that involves the origin of the plantar fascia on the medial tubercle of the calcaneus. This esthesopathy is caused by repeated minor trauma to the fascial origin, which lies plantar and superficial to the origin of the flexor digitorum brevis. A broad ledge of bone may extend into this muscle origin, but the bone itself does not cause heel pain, despite the reputation of the so-called heel spur syndrome. This structure is incorrectly interpreted as a spur on lateral radiographs of the calcaneus.

Plantar fasciitis typically develops with an increase in activity related to weight bearing or a change in running shoes or other type of shoe. Sometimes the symptoms arise spontaneously, however.[4] The classic symptoms are pain in the heel during the first step in the morning that disappears after a few steps but may reoccur with standing or walking after sitting. The pain does not occur at night or before arising in the morning. It does not become worse with activity. A variation on this history of the symptoms suggests a different diagnosis, which may involve a progression of plantar fasciitis into another entity.

The physical examination reveals specific tenderness limited to the origin of the plantar fascia, and provocative

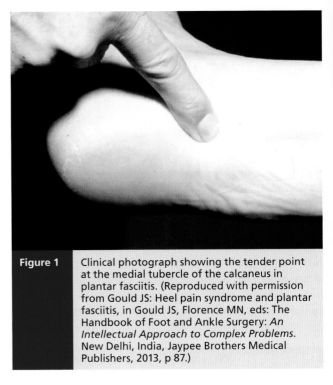

Figure 1 Clinical photograph showing the tender point at the medial tubercle of the calcaneus in plantar fasciitis. (Reproduced with permission from Gould JS: Heel pain syndrome and plantar fasciitis, in Gould JS, Florence MN, eds: The Handbook of Foot and Ankle Surgery: *An Intellectual Approach to Complex Problems.* New Delhi, India, Jaypee Brothers Medical Publishers, 2013, p 87.)

testing determines that the plantar fascia is intact (Figure 1). The plain radiograph is unremarkable, although the so-called spur may be present. Although MRI is not indicated, it shows reaction in the plantar fascial origin and often in the adjacent bone.

Myriad treatments have been suggested. Some are used indiscriminately for both the acute condition and recalcitrant symptoms that are presumed to represent persistent plantar fasciitis.[5] Many such treatments appear to be successful because of spontaneous remission, which is common in plantar fasciitis, or because the treatment was administered in combination with tissue-specific plantar fascial stretching, which is the fundamental effective treatment.[6] The use of a simple heel cup or an over-the-counter orthotic device can provide symptomatic relief by splinting the plantar fascia and gathering the heel pad fat, thereby decreasing the contact of the irritated plantar fascia with the weight-bearing surface.[7] Oral NSAIDs also are helpful for symptom relief.

Open surgical release of the plantar fascia historically has been used to treat persistent symptoms, with or without removal of the so-called heel spur. The extremely variable outcomes have included persistent and worsening pain, pain on the lateral border and dorsum of the foot, and classic neurogenic symptoms.[8] Denervation of the heel, including division of the calcaneal nerves, also has been attempted. Division of only the medial plantar fascia has had variable outcomes. With the advent of endoscopy, partial release of the plantar fascia was recommended but led to complications including laceration of the tibial nerve or vascular structures.[9]

A recent comparison of patients whose symptoms were of less than or more than 6 months' duration found no risk factors related to the development of chronic plantar fasciitis.[10] Patients in the two groups had equivalent pain intensity and functional limitations. MRI confirmation of changes in the origin of the plantar fascia was found on MRI in 15 of the 21 patients (71%) who had atypical plantar heel pain at night, and in 38 of the 50 patients (76%) who had undergone appropriate but unsuccessful nonsurgical management.[11] Five patients with atypical symptoms had an arteriovenous malformation or plantar fascial tearing.

The addition of acupuncture was found to add some benefit to a standard protocol using ice, NSAIDs, and stretching.[12] Physical therapists compared the use of low-dye taping with the use of medial arch supports.[13] Patients in both groups were treated with ultrasonography and stretching. No between-group difference was found, except that the arch support was found to be more convenient. A 57% incidence of isolated gastrocnemius contracture was found in patients with plantar fasciitis.[14] Patients with chronic foot pain, including pain from plantar fasciitis, had a 93% success rate after gastrocnemius recession for an isolated contracture.[15] Proximal medial gastrocnemius release for patients with recalcitrant plantar fasciitis and a gastrocnemius contracture led to pain relief in 81% of patients.[16] The use of a full-length silicone insole was compared with an ultrasonography-guided steroid injection to the origin of the plantar fascia in 42 randomly chosen patients.[17] One month after surgery, the results were equivalent with respect to heel tenderness and pain relief. Patients who received an injection had less thickness of the fascia. The researchers recommended the use of insoles as primary management. In a randomized controlled study of radial extracorporeal shock wave therapy in 245 patients with chronic plantar fasciitis, the success rate was 61%, compared with 42% in those treated with a placebo.[18]

A nonsurgical protocol is recommended for management of acute plantar fasciitis. Tissue-specific stretching, NSAIDs, and a simple full-length orthotic device are used. Parenteral or local steroid injections are not used.

Ruptured Plantar Fascia

Sudden tearing of the plantar fascia during an acute dorsiflexion stretch can occur regardless of whether the patient has a history of plantar fasciitis. Often the tear is associated with a history of steroid injections. The patient reports acute pain in the heel and arch, aching on the lateral border of the foot and in the dorsal arch, and sometimes neurogenic symptoms in the tibial nerve distribution. A sensation of popping or suddenly giving way is classic. The physical findings are acute tenderness in the proximal fascia, midfoot ecchymosis, and a fascial defect. A subtle tear can be confirmed using ultrasonography or MRI.

The usual treatment is immobilization in a cast or walking boot for 7 to 10 days as well as NSAIDs and oral analgesics. A custom-molded orthotic device with posting of the longitudinal arch can be used for an extended period of time. Hypertrophic scarring of the plantar fascia may be palpable at the site of the rupture. Many patients continue to be symptomatic indefinitely after the rupture.[19] Typically, the medial border of the plantar fascia is ruptured, but the central and lateral portions may be left intact. Complete release of the remaining fascia often is recommended and can relieve the mechanical symptoms. If neurogenic symptoms ensue, the recommended treatment is a complete release of the remaining plantar fascia with a detailed tarsal tunnel release.

Nerve Syndromes
Tarsal Tunnel Syndrome
Tarsal tunnel syndrome classically is described as compression of the tibial nerve under the flexor retinaculum (laciniate ligament).[20,21] The compression has variously been attributed to a ganglion, a lipoma, a neurilemoma, a fibroma, a varicose vein, an accessory muscle belly, or a displaced bone after fracture. The results of simple decompression of the flexor retinaculum are quite variable.

The patient has a subtle, spontaneous onset of pain in the heel and medial border of the ankle. The symptoms typically are made worse with activity and slowly relieved by rest, but they may occur at night or at rest. The pain often is described as a boring or aching sensation and occasionally as a burning sensation. There is tenderness over the medial retinaculum of the ankle and/or over the abductor hallucis. Nerve conduction velocity studies only occasionally are positive. The inciting lesion may be seen on MRI or ultrasonography.[22]

If there is a discrete lesion, excision with release of the retinaculum is successful (**Figure 2**). The outcome is less predictable if an accessory muscle or varicose vein is the source of compression.[23]

So-called distal tarsal tunnel syndrome is now recognized as a traction neuropathy of the tibial nerve and its branches[24,25] (**Figure 3**). This condition may be associated with chronic plantar fasciitis, attenuation of the plantar fascia, or unilateral flatfoot secondary to collapse of the medial structures and attenuation of the posterior tibial tendon.[26,27] The patient has a history of heel and medial ankle neurogenic pain made worse with activity and slowly relieved by rest. The pain may occur at rest and at night, however. The onset is gradual and often

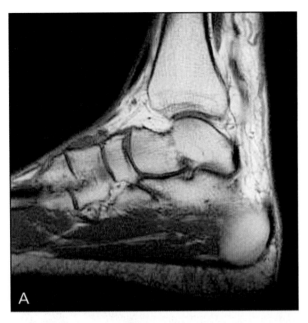
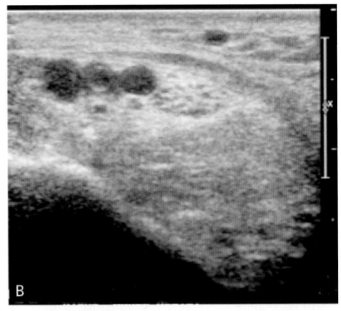
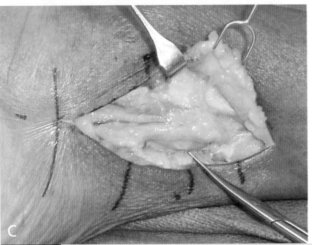
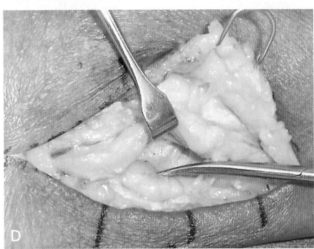

Figure 2 Lipoma in the tarsal tunnel. **A,** MRI showing a lipoma lying under the tibial nerve in the tarsal tunnel. **B,** Ultrasonograph showing a lipoma under the nerve. **C** and **D,** Intraoperative photographs in which the lipoma can be seen at the scissors tip. **C,** The flexor retinaculum has been released and the lipoma is dissected from under the nerve. **D,** The lipoma is dissected free from the nerve. (Panels B, C, and D reproduced with permission from Gould JS: Tarsal tunnel syndrome. *Foot Ankle Clin* 2011;16[2]:275-286.)

progressive. There is tenderness over the distal edge of the abductor hallucis at the soft spot where the neurovascular bundle enters the foot (**Figure 4**). Objective testing may not be helpful. Typical electromyographic testing does not show a conduction delay, but there may be signal abnormalities in the abductor hallucis and the abductor digiti quinti.[28] The condition is treated using a specially constructed total-contact orthotic shoe insert with a posted longitudinal arch and a nerve relief channel filled with a viscoelastic polymer that follows the posteromedial and plantar course of the tibial and lateral plantar nerves[23,29] (**Figure 5**). After treatment, the

neurogenic symptoms often are relieved without the need for a nerve release.

Tarsal Tunnel Syndrome With Chronic Plantar Fasciitis

Plantar fasciitis usually is resolved in 6 weeks to 3 months and often more rapidly with appropriate nonsurgical treatment. In some patients the condition persists, however, and the symptoms change. The pain begins to resolve less quickly after taking the first step in the morning or arising during the day. There seems to be a more prolonged afterburn sensation, and pain characterized as sharp, aching, burning, or intensely itching develops after prolonged

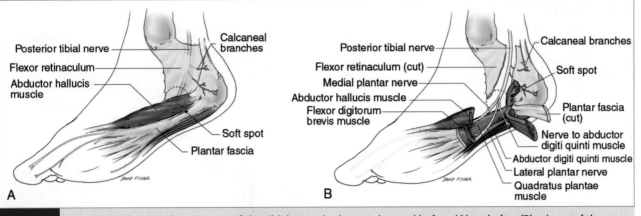

Figure 3 Schematics showing the anatomy of the tibial nerve in the tarsal tunnel before (**A**) and after (**B**) release of the flexor retinaculum (the laciniate ligament), plantar fascia, abductor hallucis.and flexor digitorum brevis.

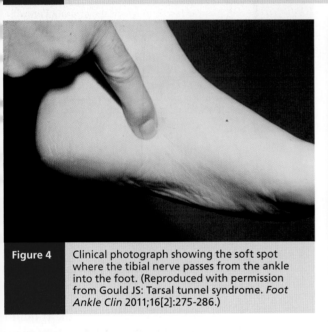

Figure 4 Clinical photograph showing the soft spot where the tibial nerve passes from the ankle into the foot. (Reproduced with permission from Gould JS: Tarsal tunnel syndrome. *Foot Ankle Clin* 2011;16[2]:275-286.)

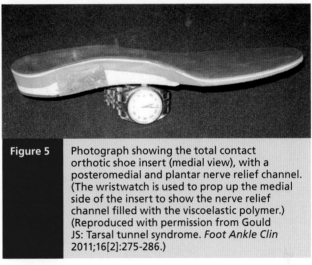

Figure 5 Photograph showing the total contact orthotic shoe insert (medial view), with a posteromedial and plantar nerve relief channel. (The wristwatch is used to prop up the medial side of the insert to show the nerve relief channel filled with the viscoelastic polymer.) (Reproduced with permission from Gould JS: Tarsal tunnel syndrome. *Foot Ankle Clin* 2011;16[2]:275-286.)

standing or walking. Pain may occur while sitting or at night. Some but not necessarily all of the elements of neurogenic pain may be present, such as the prolonged afterburn and first-step pain characteristic of plantar fasciitis. There is tenderness over the nerve at the plantar edge of the abductor hallucis and the medial edge of the plantar fascia (the so-called soft spot), perhaps along the course of the nerve, and at the origin of the plantar fascia on the medial tubercle. During the ankle and great toe provocative dorsiflexion test, loss of definition of the medial border of the plantar fascia is common, indicating attenuation or rupture of the structure.[23] Electromyographic changes in the intrinsic musculature are more likely than with normally resolving plantar fasciitis.[28]

The nonsurgical treatment includes fascia-stretching exercises and use of an orthotic device with a posteromedial nerve channel. If there is no improvement after 6 weeks, surgery may be advisable. If there is some improvement, the orthotic device should be used until the patient reaches a satisfactory resolution of symptoms, completely recovers, or decides to undergo surgical intervention after inadequate improvement.

The preferred surgical procedure is a complete release of the plantar fascia with decompression of the entire tarsal tunnel (**Figure 6**). A posteromedial incision is begun midway between the posterior edge of the medial malleolus and the medial edge of the Achilles tendon. The incision follows the course of the nerve, distally curving forward to cross the soft spot and continuing across the plantar surface just distal to the heel pad until it extends approximately three quarters of the way across the sole of the foot. The flexor retinaculum (laciniate ligament) is divided, as is the superficial fascia of the abductor hallucis. The entire plantar fascia is divided from the abductor hallucis to the abductor digiti quinti. By working under the abductor hallucis muscle, the deep fascia of the muscle is fully divided. On the anterior side of the

5: Special Problems of the Foot and Ankle

interval between the distal edge of the abductor hallucis and the medial edge of the flexor digitorum brevis muscle, the lateral plantar nerve is located and inspected to ensure that a septum is not isolating and constricting the nerve. The nerve is retracted, and the tendinous fibers of the quadratus plantae muscle lying under the nerve are divided.[30-32] At the confluence of the plantar edge of the superficial fascia of the abductor hallucis as it joins its deep fascia, with the medial edge of the plantar fascia lying over the nerve and the quadratus fibers lying under it, the nerve takes a sharp turn from the medial to the plantar foot. Presumably this is the point at which traction on the nerve produces irritation with weight bearing and pronation of the foot. The histologic evidence of nerve injury at this point is not conclusive, although some evidence of change at this location can be seen on ultrasonography and MRI.

If a septum is isolating the nerve, the entire abductor hallucis is released by unipolar cautery to improve visualization, and the septum is fully divided. To explore a so-called failed release, the abductor is similarly divided. The procedure ends with closure of the subcutaneous tissue and skin in the ankle portion of the wound and closure of the skin only in the glabrous plantar portion of the wound.

The patient must avoid weight bearing for 4 weeks to allow the plantar fascia to reconstitute itself in a lengthened position and thereby prevent the development of lateral border and dorsal arch pain. The orthotic device is used for an additional 9 to 12 months. High-heeled shoes can be worn after 3 months. At a mean 19.6-month follow-up (range, 3 to 24 months), 93% of 92 patients (104 feet) had complete or significantly improved outcomes with pain relief after complete release of the plantar fascia and tarsal tunnel, as described.[32]

Lateral Plantar Nerve Involvement

The lateral and medial plantar nerves diverge from the tibial nerve at the upper edge of the abductor hallucis or more proximally. The lateral plantar nerve continues distally and crosses the soft spot entering the foot. The medial plantar nerve runs under the muscle of the abductor, with the medial plantar artery and accompanying vein, and does not cross under the potentially restrictive area of the distal edge of the abductor hallucis fascia and proximal edge of the plantar fascia. The lateral plantar nerve typically is the more affected branch of the tibial nerve in distal tarsal tunnel syndrome. Involvement is managed with the total-contact orthotic shoe insert, and surgical release, if necessary, is the same as for chronic plantar fasciitis. Partial release of the plantar fascia and the tarsal tunnel is not reliably successful.

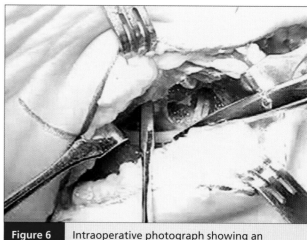

Figure 6   Intraoperative photograph showing an extended surgical release of the tarsal tunnel and plantar fascia, in which the lateral plantar nerve is exposed in the interval between the abductor hallucis and flexor digitorum brevis after release of the laciniate ligament, the superficial and deep fascia of the abductor hallucis, the entire plantar fascia, and the tendinous fibers and fascia of the quadratus plantae. (Reproduced with permission from Gould JS: Tarsal tunnel syndrome. *Foot Ankle Clin* 2011;16[2]:275-286.)

First Branch of the Lateral Plantar Nerve Involvement (Central Heel Pad Syndrome)

The first branch of the lateral plantar nerve typically emerges from the nerve just distal to the branching of the lateral from the tibial nerve, but occasionally it emerges from the tibial nerve itself. The branch runs posteriorly under the abductor hallucis, over the quadratus plantae to innervate it, and over the periosteum and the flexor digitorum brevis; it sends a sensory branch to the central heel pad and continues into the abductor digiti quinti as a motor branch. The first branch of the lateral plantar nerve has been described as the cause of central heel pad syndrome in runners, for which release of the deep fascia of the abductor hallucis and the medial third of the plantar fascia is the surgical treatment of choice.[33,34] The recommended nonsurgical treatment is to use the total-contact orthotic shoe insert, with widening of the nerve relief channel posteriorly on the medial and plantar surfaces, and to modify the patient's running regimen.[29] If surgery is necessary, a relatively complete release is used. This procedure has been successful in football, soccer, baseball, and distance-running athletes.

It is important to differentiate the first branch of the lateral plantar nerve from the calcaneal branches of the tibial nerve, which usually emerge more proximally and end in the subcutaneous tissue and skin of the medial and posteromedial heel. The first branch of the lateral plantar nerve passes under the abductor hallucis, but he calcaneal nerve remains superficial. The distinction between these two nerves is important because they are of similar diameter, and both emerge from the nerve posteriorly and often close together.

A contusion of the central heel with a neuroma of the nerve can be treated by surgical exposure of the first branch through the tarsal tunnel incision, with excision of the branch, insertion into a conduit, and placement of the conduit into the retrocalcaneal space. Resolution of the symptoms can be expected (**Figure 7**).

Medial Plantar Nerve Involvement

The medial plantar nerve can be involved in tarsal tunnel distal or proximal conditions; it also can be involved individually as it leaves the course of the lateral plantar nerve and passes under the abductor hallucis muscle with the medial plantar artery and veins. Slightly more distally, it meets the flexor digitorum longus and flexor hallucis longus at the master knot of Henry. Here, in the proximal longitudinal arch, it may be affected by tenosynovitis of these tendons.[35] The pain typically is in the arch and occurs with active or passive movement of the involved tendons, but the nerve may be tender under the abductor hallucis posteromedially, with referred pain into the tarsal tunnel and the heel. An understanding of the surface anatomy of this entity makes the diagnosis relatively easy. The total-contact orthotic shoe insert is modified by extending the nerve relief channel anteriorly. A shoe with a stiff rocker sole is used, or the insert is stiffened with an extended steel shank or a Morton extension and is used with a rocker sole. Oral NSAIDs also are used.

If the symptoms primarily are in the medial plantar distribution, with pain into the great and second toes and the plantar heel, the same incision is used as in the release just described for the combined tarsal tunnel and plantar fascia release. In the course of the surgery, the abductor hallucis is fully incised to allow the medial plantar nerve to be seen. Crossing small arterial and venous branches are cauterized using bipolar cautery, or small Ligaclips (Ethicon) are used to maintain meticulous hemostasis. After the exact course of the medial plantar nerve is observed, a curvilinear incision is extended from the original incision to follow the medial plantar nerve through the abductor muscle. Uneventful wound healing is likely if the incision is made directly down to the nerve without undermining the subcutaneous tissue. Postoperative treatment is the same as for an extended tarsal tunnel release. The most important consideration with this release is to decide how far it should extend. If the patient has had both heel pain and tenderness proximally along the nerve, the release is carried beyond the bifurcation under the muscle longitudinally until no

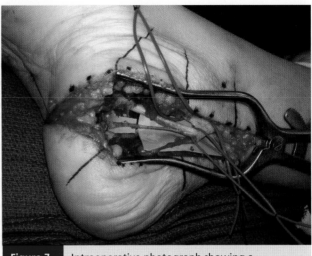

Figure 7 Intraoperative photograph showing a neuroma of the first branch of the lateral plantar nerve. (Reproduced from Gould JS, Florence MN: Neuromas of the foot and ankle. *Orthopaedic Knowledge Online Journal.* 2014;12. http://orthoportal.aaos.org/oko/article.aspx?article=OKO_FOO058#article. Accessed September 9, 2014.)

constricting bands appear and the nerve appears unscarred and normal under loupe magnification.

If the patient has tenosynovitis of the flexor digitorum longus and flexor hallucis longus without significant tarsal tunnel or heel pain, the release is made along the nerve in the longitudinal arch and a synovectomy is done simultaneously. The tarsal tunnel is not opened and the plantar fascia not released.

Calcaneal Branch Involvement

The medial plantar heel is innervated by the calcaneal branch(es) of the tibial nerve, which can cause medial plantar heel pain after contusion or surgery in the area.[36] Palpation should allow relatively straightforward identification of the site of the lesion. The history of injury or a surgical incision over the area should be compatible. The treatment can be difficult, with a variable response to nonsurgical desensitization and cushioning. The use of a backless shoe or sandal is recommended while manual desensitization is attempted, and topical anti-inflammatory and neuritis medications should be used. The calcaneal nerves can be excised by placing them in a vein or collagen conduit and, if possible, directing the conduit into the retrocalcaneal space, which is a more protected area where the nerve conduit is surrounded by retrocalcaneal fat. Although patients have had substantial to complete pain relief, the data on this technique are too limited to be conclusive.

Sural Nerve Involvement

Branches of the sural nerve innervate the lateral plantar heel, the lateral border of the foot, the plantar aspect of the fifth toe, and the dorsal aspects of the fourth and fifth toes. Lesions of the first branch of the lateral plantar nerve can cause both pain in the central heel pad and lateral heel pad aching through the continuation of the branch to the abductor digiti quinti. A history of trauma to the sural nerve, including a surgical procedure that put the nerve at risk, may account for injury to the nerve and resulting pain in the lateral heel.[37,38] The pain may be accompanied by loss of sensibility in the area and tenderness or a positive Tinel sign with palpation over the nerve. Sensory electrical testing may be helpful. A sural nerve block can be a useful adjunctive tool for diagnosis. A backless shoe and manual desensitization with topical medications, are the initial treatments of choice. The use of neurolysis is unpredictable, but excision of the nerve can be curative. If the neuroma from the excision develops, a more proximal excision of the entire nerve just below the popliteal space may be needed.

Stress Fractures of the Calcaneus

Stress fracture of the heel can occur in runners. Young women who are amenorrheic, people who have osteoporosis, and otherwise healthy people who have had an increase in stress to the bone are particularly susceptible.[39] The patient often becomes aware of the pain at the moment the injury occurs or shortly after the inciting activity. The pain initially is constant but becomes worse with activity. Eventually, the pain is present with activity but is relieved by rest, and typically the pain disappears after the requisite 6 weeks of healing. Examination reveals point tenderness with palpation. The examination may be unremarkable aside from some soft-tissue swelling and bruising. Swelling may be seen on radiographs with good soft-tissue definition, but the fracture may not be apparent until 10 to 14 days after the injury, when resorption is seen at the fracture site, followed by new bone formation. MRI shows a change in signal at the site that is not specific for fracture. CT can be used to confirm the diagnosis. Ultrasonography also can confirm the diagnosis in a patient who is thin. The typical fracture in a patient with pain in the plantar heel is a break in the plantar cortex without displacement. The treatment is rest and immobilization in a boot or cast as needed.

Osteomyelitis of the Calcaneus

Direct inoculation of the calcaneus from a penetrating foreign body is the most common cause of osteomyelitis of the calcaneus.[40] The patient's history, physical examination, and radiographs should easily confirm the diagnosis. Constant pain, night pain, and pain unaffected by activity or rest are the diagnostic features of pain with an infectious or oncologic etiology. A subtle penetration by a foreign body may be responsible, especially if the lesion is radiolucent. Such a foreign body can often be more easily seen on MRI or ultrasonography if the foreign body is not radiopaque. Diagnosing osteomyelitis adds another dimension of difficulty, and overreading of an MRI often leads to a spurious diagnosis. Clearly seen bone destruction on radiographs or CT makes the diagnosis more obvious. The definitive diagnosis requires Gram staining and culturing of material obtained through aspiration guided by ultrasonography (the preferred method) or fluoroscopy. The treatment is with immobilization, the use of intravenous antibiotics, and débridement, as indicated.

Foreign Body or Skin Lesion in the Heel Pad

The presence of a foreign body in the heel pad may require MRI or ultrasonography for diagnosis.[41] The history and point tenderness are keys to the diagnosis. A radiopaque object can be removed under sterile conditions with the help of fluoroscopy. Ultrasonographic guidance may be helpful for locating a radiolucent object.

A plantar verrucous lesion (a wart) on the heel pad can be excruciatingly painful. The presence of pain when the lesion is squeezed can distinguish such a wart from a callus, as in a cavus foot with a tripod stance, in which pain occurs with direct pressure. Paring of the lesion and producing pinpoint bleeding can be definitive. A patient with such a dermal lesion ideally is referred to a dermatologist for treatment. A ring curet can be used for curative curettage, with the patient under sedation and local anesthetic injected around the lesion. The treatment of choice often is cryotherapy (liquid nitrogen) with the use of salicylic acid preparations, offloading of the lesion, and frequent débridement. Electrofulguration, including laser surgery, is not recommended because of the risk that the lesion will not heal and will require a difficult plastic reconstruction of the heel pad.

Heel Pad Tumors

Tumors of the heel pad are rare. Such a diagnosis is suggested by constant pain, unaffected by activity or rest and including night pain, as in an infectious etiology. An oncologic diagnosis is possible in the absence of a skin lesion or a history of a penetrating wound. MRI or ultrasonography is definitive. In a case report of heel pain occurring at night and with weight bearing, a palpable vascular leiomyoma (angioleiomyoma) had been present for 3 years; excision was curative.[42]

Summary

Plantar heel pain has multiple etiologies, although plantar fasciitis is the most common. In chronic plantar fasciitis, the neurogenic findings may evolve and require modification of the diagnosis and treatment. Management begins with a proper diagnosis based on a careful history and physical examination followed by the use of inductive reasoning. Adjunctive testing may be indicated to clarify and document the diagnosis. An algorithmic treatment plan is developed and followed to the level indicated. Despite recent studies on plantar heel pain, the fundamentals of diagnosis and management remain unchanged.

Acknowledgment

The author thanks Mason N. Florence, MD, orthopaedic foot and ankle fellow, for assistance with the literature search.

Annotated References

1. Riddle DL, Schappert SM: Volume of ambulatory care visits and patterns of care for patients diagnosed with plantar fasciitis: A national study of medical doctors. *Foot Ankle Int* 2004;25(5):303-310.

2. Gould JS: General workup of the foot and ankle patient, in Gould JS, ed: *The Handbook of Foot and Ankle Surgery: An Intellectual Approach to Complex Problems.* Jaypee Brothers Medical Publishers, New Delhi, India, 2013, pp 3-4.

   The author describes the details of history taking, physical examination, and indicated ancillary examinations required in a proper workup of the foot and ankle patient.

3. Gould JS: Making the diagnosis and the discussion of management with the patient, in Gould JS, ed: *The Handbook of Foot and Ankle Surgery: An Intellectual Approach to Complex Problems.* Jaypee Brothers Medical Publishers, New Delhi, India, 2013, pp 5-7.

   After the diagnosis is made, the patient is apprised of recommended treatment options.

4. Riddle DL, Pulisic M, Pidcoe P, Johnson RE: Risk factors for plantar fasciitis: A matched case-control study. *J Bone Joint Surg Am* 2003;85(5):872-877.

5. Wolgin M, Cook C, Graham C, Mauldin D: Conservative treatment of plantar heel pain: Long-term follow-up. *Foot Ankle Int* 1994;15(3):97-102.

6. DiGiovanni BF, Nawoczenski DA, Lintal ME, et al: Tissue-specific plantar fascia-stretching exercise enhances outcomes in patients with chronic heel pain: A prospective, randomized study. *J Bone Joint Surg Am* 2003;85(7):1270-1277.

7. Pfeffer G, Bacchetti P, Deland J, et al: Comparison of custom and prefabricated orthoses in the initial treatment of proximal plantar fasciitis. *Foot Ankle Int* 1999;20(4):214-221.

8. Sammarco GJ, Helfrey RB: Surgical treatment of recalcitrant plantar fasciitis. *Foot Ankle Int* 1996;17(9):520-526.

9. Hogan KA, Webb D, Shereff M: Endoscopic plantar fascia release. *Foot Ankle Int* 2004;25(12):875-881.

10. Klein SE, Dale AM, Hayes MH, Johnson JE, McCormick JJ, Racette BA: Clinical presentation and self-reported patterns of pain and function in patients with plantar heel pain. *Foot Ankle Int* 2012;33(9):693-698.

    No risk factors were found to determine which patients would have chronic pain. Patients with chronic pain had no increase in pain or functional limitation.

11. Chimutengwende-Gordon M, O'Donnell P, Singh D: Magnetic resonance imaging in plantar heel pain. *Foot Ankle Int* 2010;31(10):865-870.

    MRI of patients with plantar heel pain or atypical symptoms including night pain revealed that 76% had changes in the origin of the plantar fascia. Patients with atypical pain had arteriovenous malformation and plantar fascial tears.

12. Karagounis P, Tsironi M, Prionas G, Tsiganos G, Baltopoulos P: Treatment of plantar fasciitis in recreational athletes: Two different therapeutic protocols. *Foot Ankle Spec* 2011;4(4):226-234.

    A protocol of ice, NSAIDs, and stretching was compared with a protocol that added acupuncture. The addition of acupuncture led to better results.

13. Abd El Salam MS, Abd Elhafz YN: Low-dye taping versus medial arch support in managing pain and pain-related disability in patients with plantar fasciitis. *Foot Ankle Spec* 2011;4(2):86-91.

    A comparison of the use of a taping technique and an orthotic device also used ultrasound treatments and stretching. No difference was found other than a patient preference for the orthotic device.

14. Patel A, DiGiovanni BF: Association between plantar fasciitis and isolated contracture of the gastrocnemius. *Foot Ankle Int* 2011;32(1):5-8.

    An isolated gastrocnemius contracture was found in 57% of patients with a diagnosis of plantar fasciitis.

15. Maskill JD, Bohay DR, Anderson JG: Gastrocnemius recession to treat isolated foot pain. *Foot Ankle Int* 2010;31(1):19-23.

5: Special Problems of the Foot and Ankle

A 93.1% success rate was achieved in patients with an isolated gastrocnemius contracture associated with chronic foot pain, including patients with plantar fasciitis, after a gastrocnemius recession.

16. Abbassian A, Kohls-Gatzoulis J, Solan MC: Proximal medial gastrocnemius release in the treatment of recalcitrant plantar fasciitis. *Foot Ankle Int* 2012;33(1):14-19.

   A proximal medial gastrocnemius release for patients with an isolated gastrocnemius contracture and plantar fasciitis led to pain relief in 81% of patients.

17. Yucel U, Kucuksen S, Cingoz HT, et al: Full-length silicone insoles versus ultrasound-guided corticosteroid injection in the management of plantar fasciitis: A randomized clinical trial. *Prosthet Orthot Int* 2013;37(6):471-476.

   The use of a full-length silicone insole was compared with an ultrasonically guided steroid injection in 42 randomly selected patients. The results related to heel tenderness and pain relief were equivalent at 1-month follow-up, but there was less thickness of the fascia in the patients who received the injection.

18. Gerdesmeyer L, Frey C, Vester J, et al: Radial extracorporeal shock wave therapy is safe and effective in the treatment of chronic recalcitrant plantar fasciitis: Results of a confirmatory randomized placebo-controlled multicenter study. *Am J Sports Med* 2008;36(11):2100-2109.

   In a randomized controlled study, radial extracorporeal shock wave therapy in 245 patients with chronic plantar fasciitis had a 61% success rate.

19. Acevedo JI, Beskin JL: Complications of plantar fascia rupture associated with corticosteroid injection. *Foot Ankle Int* 1998;19(2):91-97.

20. Keck C: The tarsal-tunnel syndrome. *J Bone Joint Surg Am* 1962;44(1):180-182.

21. Lam SJ: A tarsal-tunnel syndrome. *Lancet* 1962;2(7270):1354-1355.

22. Lopez-Ben R: Imaging of nerve entrapment in the foot and ankle. *Foot Ankle Clin* 2011;16(2):213-224.

   MRI and ultrasonography findings are described for nerve entrapment syndrome of the foot and ankle.

23. Gould JS: Tarsal tunnel syndrome. *Foot Ankle Clin* 2011;16(2):275-286.

   Proximal and distal tarsal tunnel syndromes are described, with nonsurgical management and the author's surgical technique.

24. Heimkes B, Posel P, Stotz S, Wolf K: The proximal and distal tarsal tunnel syndromes: An anatomical study. *Int Orthop* 1987;11(3):193-196.

25. Lau JT, Daniels TR: Effects of tarsal tunnel release and stabilization procedures on tibial nerve tension in a surgically created pes planus foot. *Foot Ankle Int* 1998;19(11):770-777.

26. DiGiovanni BF, Gould JS: Tarsal tunnel syndrome and related entities. *Foot Ankle Clin* 1998;3:405-426.

27. Labib SA, Gould JS, Rodriguez-del-Rio FA, Lyman S: Heel pain triad (HPT): The combination of plantar fasciitis, posterior tibial tendon dysfunction and tarsal tunnel syndrome. *Foot Ankle Int* 2002;23(3):212-220.

28. Roy PC: Electrodiagnostic evaluation of lower extremity neurogenic problems. *Foot Ankle Clin* 2011;16(2):225-241.

   The fine points of electrodiagnostic evaluation of nerve entrapment syndromes of the lower extremity are described.

29. Gould JS, Ford D: Orthoses and insert management of common foot and ankle problems, in Schon LC, Porter DA, eds: *Baxter's The Foot and Ankle in Sports*. Philadelphia, PA, Mosby Elsevier, 2008, pp 595-593.

   The orthotic devices and shoe modifications used for foot and ankle diagnoses are described, including tarsal tunnel syndrome.

30. DiGiovanni BF, Abuzzahab FS, Gould JS: Plantar fascia release with proximal and distal tarsal tunnel release: Surgical approach to chronic disabling plantar fasciitis with associated nerve pain. *Tech Foot Ankle Surg* 2003;2:254-261.

31. Gould JS, DiGiovanni BF: Plantar fascia release in combination with proximal and distal tarsal tunnel release, in Weisel SW, ed: *Operative Techniques in Orthopaedic Surgery, vol. 4*. Philadelphia, PA, Wolters Kluwer/Lippincott Williams & Wilkins, 2011, pp 3911-3919.

   A detailed description was provided of the author's technique of combined plantar fascia and tarsal tunnel release.

32. Gould JS: Entrapment syndromes, in Gould JS, ed: *The Handbook of Foot and Ankle Surgery: An Intellectual Approach to Complex Problems*. New Delhi, India, Jaypee Brothers Medical Publishers, 2013, pp 247-269.

   Nerve entrapment syndromes of the foot and ankle are described.

33. Baxter DE, Thigpen CM: Heel pain: Operative results. *Foot Ankle* 1984;5(1):16-25.

34. Rondhuis JJ, Huson A: The first branch of the lateral plantar nerve and heel pain. *Acta Morphol Neerl Scand* 1986;24(4):269-279.

35. Rask MR: Medial plantar neurapraxia (jogger's foot): Report of 3 cases. *Clin Orthop Relat Res* 1978;134:193-195.

36. Govsa F, Bilge O, Ozer MA: Variations in the origin of the medial and inferior calcaneal nerves. *Arch Orthop Trauma Surg* 2006;126(1):6-14.

37. Pringle RM, Protheroe K, Mukherjee SK: Entrapment neuropathy of the sural nerve. *J Bone Joint Surg Br* 1974;56(3):465-468.

38. Flanigan RM, DiGiovanni BF: Peripheral nerve entrapments of the lower leg, ankle, and foot. *Foot Ankle Clin* 2011;16(2):255-274.

   The anatomy, clinical evaluation, diagnostic studies, and treatment of entrapment syndromes including the sural nerve are described.

39. Leabhart JW: Stress fractures of the calcaneus. *J Bone Joint Surg Am* 1959;41:1285-1290.

40. Fukuda T, Reddy V, Ptaszek AJ: The infected calcaneus. *Foot Ankle Clin* 2010;15(3):477-486.

   The etiologies of calcaneal infection, the effect of comorbidities on healing, and treatment options are described in terms of a multidisciplinary approach.

41. Seminario-Vidal L, Cantrell W, Elewski BE: Dermatologic conditions of the foot. *Orthopaedic Knowledge Online Journal* 12(8). http://orthoportal.aaos.org/oko/article.aspx?article=OKO_FOO060. Accessed August 1, 2014.

   This illustrated survey of dermatologic conditions that may be encountered by the orthopaedic surgeon is organized into infectious, neoplastic, and systemic conditions.

42. Cheung MH, Lui TH: Plantar heel pain due to vascular leiomyoma (angioleiomyoma). *Foot Ankle Spec* 2012;5(5):321-323.

   A tumor causing heel pain was cured with excision of the lesion.

5: Special Problems of the Foot and Ankle

Chapter 19

Foot and Ankle Tumors

J.C. Neilson, MD   Joseph Benevenia, MD

Introduction

The evaluation, diagnosis, treatment, and referral of patients with a tumor of the foot or ankle are important in
clinical practice. Orthopaedic surgeons should be vigilant
to detect these tumors. A foot or ankle tumor is classified
as benign or, less often, malignant; and may occur within
the soft tissue or bone. A mass can develop in the foot as
a result of a posttraumatic or neuropathic condition, or
because of bone or soft-tissue infection.

Incidence

Tumors of the foot or ankle are rare, and their incidence
has not been well studied. In a retrospective review of
2,660 musculoskeletal tumors at any anatomic site that
were surgically treated at a tertiary center over 20 years,
153 tumors were in the bone or soft tissue of the foot
or ankle (5.75%; mean patient age, 33.2 years).[1] Sixty
of the foot and ankle tumors (39.2%) were considered
to be malignant, and the remaining 93 were considered
to be benign. Eighty patients (52.3%) had a soft-tissue
tumor, of which giant cell tumor of the tendon sheath and
pigmented villonodular synovitis were the most common.
The remaining 73 patients had a bone tumor (47.7%);
giant cell tumor was the most common type.

Dr. Neilson or an immediate family member has received
nonincome support (such as equipment or services), commercially derived honoraria, or other non–research-related
funding (such as paid travel) from the Musculoskeletal
Transplant Foundation. Dr. Benevenia or an immediate
family member is a member of a speakers' bureau or has
made paid presentations on behalf of the Musculoskeletal
Transplant Foundation; serves as an unpaid consultant to
Merete NJOS; has received research or institutional support
from Biomet, the Musculoskeletal Transplant Foundation,
and Synthes; and serves as a board member, owner, officer, or committee member of the American Academy of
Orthopaedic Surgeons, the Musculoskeletal Transplant
Foundation, and the Musculoskeletal Tumor Society.

Patient Evaluation

History

A thorough patient history is key to the differential diagnosis of a mass or lesion of the foot or ankle. The most
common initial symptom of a bony lesion is pain, and
identifying the onset, duration, location, and character of
the pain can be useful in determining the etiology. Any
aggravating or alleviating activities may be especially important. In general, an aggressive malignant bone lesion is
painful. Many benign bone lesions are found incidentally.
NSAIDs can provide significant pain relief in a patient
with aggressive tumor or some specific types of tumors,
such as osteoid osteoma. A soft-tissue mass, whether
malignant or benign, usually is not painful, although
discomfort may result from displacement or destruction
of adjacent structures or a change in gait pattern. When
a mass has been identified, the duration, onset, as well as
changes in the size, location, and number of masses can
be helpful in determining the best management. Most
masses that have been present for years without increasing
in size are benign, but some benign masses are at risk for
malignant dedifferentiation. A stable tumor that begins to
grow may represent malignant progression to a sarcoma
and should be evaluated and treated by a musculoskeletal
oncologist. Some tumors, such as vascular anomalies,
have a distinct pattern of enlarging and shrinking, especially with activity. Some foot masses, such as Morton
neuroma and plantar fibroma, have a distinct location.

In addition to the history of the tumor itself, the patient history should include a complete discussion of any
earlier tumors, whether benign or malignant, as well
as any risk factors such as tobacco smoking, chemical
exposure, recent or past trauma or infection, or a family
history of tumors.

Physical Examination

In addition to the involved foot and ankle, a complete
examination should include the contralateral extremity,
proximal draining lymph node beds, any masses discovered while taking the history, and any skin lesions. This
evaluation may lead to identification of primary or metastatic tumor sites or a syndrome such as neurofibromatosis

or plantar fascial fibromatosis (Ledderhose disease). The size and depth of the mass should be measured because these are the two factors most useful for determining the likelihood of malignancy. A large subfascial tumor is most likely to be malignant. Direct palpation of the mass may elicit pain. The mass may be firm or fluctuant, although a mass that usually is fluctuant, such as a ganglion, can appear to be firm because of the tension exerted by the many structures in the foot. The mobility of the mass can help in identifying both its depth and its origin; for example, a schwannoma usually is only mobile perpendicular to the plane of the nerve. Provocative testing with percussion for a Tinel sign can be useful in evaluating neural tumors. Transillumination can help characterize solid, rather than fluid-filled, masses. Auscultation and palpation for bruits can be useful in identifying arteriovascular malformations. Evaluation for other common generators of pain in the foot should be undertaken as suggested by the patient's history.

Imaging

Radiographic analysis is important in the evaluation of both soft-tissue and bone tumors. Radiographs can indicate the aggressiveness of an osseocentric tumor. A permeative pattern suggests an aggressive, often malignant process. A geographic pattern often is characterized by a thin, eggshell-like margin of bone around the tumor and connotes a less aggressive process. This observed difference is explained by the response of the bone to the tumor. The bone is able to respond to and even contain a relatively slow-growing, unaggressive tumor. Some types of tumors are most likely to occur in a diaphyseal, metaphyseal, or epiphyseal area, but because the foot bones are small and irregular, the specific origin of a tumor can be difficult to identify. Periosteal elevation may be the result of a mass effect, and subperiosteum elevated off the bone usually indicates a relatively aggressive tumor or infection. The pattern of periosteal elevation is described as a sunburst, onion skinning, or a Codman triangle.

The matrix of any lesion can give important clues to its origin. Cartilage tumors often have a lucent appearance and over time become mineralized in a punctate pattern. Fibrous dysplasia typically has a ground glass radiographic appearance. In comparison with normal bone, other tumors are more or less lucent or have mixed lucency; this characteristic often is helpful in the differential diagnosis of primary and metastatic tumors of bone. Cortical destruction also can indicate a relatively aggressive tumor. Extraosseous mineralization may appear adjacent to a bone lesion or in some soft-tissue masses. The most commonly seen forms of extraskeletal bone are phleboliths in an arteriovascular malformation or synovial sarcoma, mineralization of the necrotic center of a soft-tissue sarcoma, peripheral mineralization of myositis ossificans, or cloudlike mineralization of an extraskeletal osteosarcoma. Radiographs can differentiate soft-tissue masses within different tissue planes by the density of air, fat, water (muscle), and bone.

CT is helpful for evaluating the character of mineralized structures, which have many characteristics in common with those of bone, as seen on plain radiographs. CT of the chest, abdomen, and pelvis is an important part of the workup for a patient with suspected metastatic carcinoma to bone.[2] Although CT angiography is an effective tool for a patient who cannot undergo MRI, usually MRI is superior for precise evaluation of tumors and important surrounding structures in the foot and ankle. Obtaining high-quality MRI results for small structures in areas such as the forefoot requires the use of small coils and a high-Tesla machine. MRI with gadolinium contrast is recommended for all soft-tissue and most bone lesions because this technique shows the amount of blood flow to a mass. By enhancing the rim of a cystic structure such as a ganglion, as well as some arteriovascular malformations and bone cysts, MRI can differentiate between a fluid-filled and a solid mass. Diffusion-weighted MRI sequences are most commonly used to assess the tumor response to radiation, chemotherapy, or ablative treatment. Magnetic resonance angiography has supplanted traditional angiography for most tumor indications, and it is useful for evaluating the blood supply to the foot before resection or reconstruction. The soft-tissue detail provided by a high-quality MRI is critical to the surgical resection of soft-tissue and bone tumors of the foot and ankle.[3]

Technetium Tc-99 bone scanning is useful for evaluating a stress fracture or a stress reaction that can masquerade as an osseous lesion of the foot. Whole body scanning is commonly used to identify malignant metastasis to bone, but it must be interpreted with caution because some tumors, such as multiple myeloma, eosinophilic granulomas, and large renal cell cancers, may not show significant uptake.

The use of ultrasonography in the diagnosis and management of soft-tissue tumors is constantly evolving. Ultrasonography is used to differentiate solid and fluid-filled masses, and it is an excellent tool for measuring flow in vascular anomalies. The usefulness of ultrasonography increases with the surgeon's experience with this modality. In the treatment of tumors, ultrasonography most commonly is used for guidance during soft-tissue biopsy or the treatment of a vascular anomaly.

Positron emission tomography (PET) is useful in the evaluation of many but not all types of malignancies. Inclusion of the lower extremities is not standard during PET staging of many cancerous conditions, and whole body PET should be specified if PET evaluation is appropriate for the patient's lesion. PET is rarely ordered by a physician other than an oncologist. PET can be useful for evaluation of the lymphatic spread of hidradenocarcinoma, melanoma, or epithelioid sarcoma, usually in conjunction with lymphangioscintigraphy and sentinel node resection.[4] Although PET-MRI is a promising tool for identifying tumor metastasis at diagnosis and during subsequent staging, its use has not yet been completely validated.[5]

Laboratory Evaluation

Laboratory testing is not necessary for most tumors of the foot and ankle. However, inflammatory markers, white blood cell analysis, and cultures are appropriate if an infectious origin is suspected. Complete blood cell counts are useful for identifying leukemia or lymphoma and may reveal anemia in a patient with multiple myeloma or a widely metastatic cancer. Protein electrophoresis and light chain evaluations can be diagnostic for multiple myeloma. Some other primary cancers have blood markers, such as prostate-specific antigen. Metabolic analysis can reveal kidney or liver damage, malnutrition, or electrolyte abnormalities.[2] Calcium levels should be checked in all patients with metastatic disease to the bone because increased bone turnover can lead to increased serum calcium or to cardiac conditions including fatal arrhythmias.

Biopsy

Pathologic analysis should be performed for all masses. An excision, incision, or needle technique can be used, depending on the size, location, and imaging characteristics of the lesion as well as the experience of the surgeon. Excisional biopsy is appropriate if a cuff of normal tissue can be obtained around the lesion to ensure negative margins. This saves the patient from a wider re-excision if the lesion is determined to be malignant by pathology. Incisional biopsy should be considered for a relatively large mass, which should be presumed to be malignant until histologic analysis proves otherwise. In general, biopsies should be performed or guided by a surgeon trained in treating primary malignant tumors of the extremity. Frozen section should be obtained during an open biopsy to determine whether lesional tissue is obtained and thereby increase the likelihood of a correct diagnosis. A needle biopsy can be done with or without imaging guidance. Ultrasonography or CT can be used to increase the likelihood of obtaining tissue from the lesion by targeting solid, nonnecrotic areas and correlating these findings with those of contrast-enhanced MRI. A thoughtful approach to needle biopsy is essential because bleeding from deep or subcutaneous vessels could allow tumor tissue to spread along uninvolved tissue planes and thereby increase the

resection area.[6] Fine-needle aspiration biopsy can be used in many masses, but this technique is operator dependent. Core biopsy allows more tissue to be obtained, but its use is limited to tumors large enough to accommodate the throw of the needle.

The small amount of subcutaneous tissue in the foot and ankle often allows relatively early identification of a mass. Usually a mass smaller than 3 cm is benign. A mass larger than 3 cm is more likely to be malignant. However, a recent study found that malignant bone tumors in the foot are 5 to 30 times smaller than those in other skeletal areas.[7] All biopsies should be done with great care; a inexpert biopsy can increase the likelihood that a secondary surgical procedure, tissue transfer, or amputation will be required.[8]

Benign Soft-Tissue Tumors

Synovial Tumors
Ganglion
A synovial ganglion is the most common mass of the foot and ankle. An MRI study found that 5.6% and 0.4% of patients had a ganglion around the ankle or the foot, respectively.[9] Synovial ganglia result from a weakness in the wall of a synovial structure. On MRI, a ganglion most commonly is seen in the tarsal canal and on the dorsum of the foot.[10] These structures often are painless but can create pain when they compress adjacent structures, and they can become irritating with shoe wear. Ganglia can be diagnosed clinically if they increase and decrease in size, are over a joint and superficial tendon, are subcutaneous, or can be transilluminated (if sufficiently large). In addition, fluid can be aspirated using a large-bore needle. If all of these factors are present, resection without advanced imaging may be appropriate. However, if these factors are not present, high-quality gadolinium-enhanced MRI is needed to consolidate the diagnosis. The mass should be characterized by a homogeneous low signal with T1 weighting, a high signal with T2 weighting, and rim enhancement with gadolinium[3] (Figure 1). The use of hand/foot MRI coils decreases the field of view and improves the quality of the image for a small mass. The treatments include observation, corticosteroid injection, and surgical resection. Marginal resection can be undertaken with an attempt to remove the stalk and entire cyst capsule.

Pigmented Villonodular Synovitis
Pigmented villonodular synovitis is an intra-articular process characterized by hemorrhage, hemosiderin deposition, giant cells, histiocytes, and fibrous stroma. The incidence is two per one million people.[9] Although the knee is the most commonly affected joint, pigmented

5: Special Problems of the Foot and Ankle

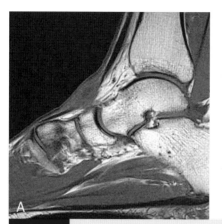
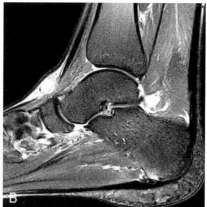
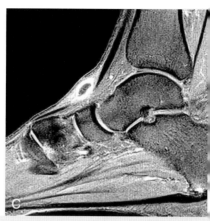

Figure 1 | MRI studies showing the characteristics typical of a synovial ganglion on the dorsum of the ankle. **A,** A homogeneous low signal with T1 weighting. **B,** A high signal with T2 weighting. **C,** Rim enhancement with gadolinium-enhanced T1 weighting.

villonodular synovitis sometimes occurs in the ankle. In the earlier stages, patients may have a painful or painless effusion. Patients with long-standing disease may have large masses, poor joint motion, and arthritis. MRI classically shows a low signal with T1 and T2 weighting, with peripheral contrast enhancement. A blooming pattern can be seen in larger masses. In the foot or ankle the tumor may involve more than one adjacent joint as a result of direct extension.

Pigmented villonodular synovitis is categorized as localized or diffuse. The localized form is treated with open or arthroscopic resection of the nodule, and recurrence rates are low. The diffuse form is treated with open and/or arthroscopic surgery but is associated with high recurrence rates because of the difficulty of obtaining a complete resection. Low-dosage radiation, alone or in conjunction with surgery, has been used for patients with degenerative disease.[11] Some patients with degenerative disease can benefit from fusion or arthroplasty.

Giant Cell Tumor of Tendon Sheath

Giant cell tumor of tendon sheath is histologically identical to pigmented villonodular synovitis but is extra-articular and associated with synovial structures such as tendon sheaths. The mass itself is painless, but it may impinge upon or irritate adjacent structures. The MRI signal characteristics are similar to those of pigmented villonodular synovitis. Marginal resection is the appropriate treatment. Needle or incisional biopsy should be considered for a relatively large and fast-growing tumor because it is possible for such a tumor to degenerate into a malignant giant cell tumor of tendon sheath that, like a sarcoma, should undergo wide resection.

Synovial Chondromatosis

Synovial chondromatosis is much less common than pigmented villonodular synovitis, but it can be no less debilitating. This abnormality is believed to be a cartilaginous metaplasia of the synovium that breaks off to form loose bodies. This tumor has been associated with an abnormality in chromosome 6. Open or arthroscopic treatment is appropriate. Synovial chondromatosis of the foot or ankle recurred locally in as many as 38.5% of patients in a small study, and two thirds of the recurrent tumors degenerated into low-grade chondrosarcoma.[12] Degeneration to chondrosarcoma is difficult to diagnose correctly, and a questionable diagnosis should be reviewed by an experienced musculoskeletal pathologist.

Lipoma Arborescens

Lipoma arborescens is an extremely rare synovial disorder that most likely represents a reactive process made up of intra-articular lipomalike masses of hypertrophic synovial villi distended by fat. Open or arthroscopic treatment usually is curative.[13]

Other Synovial Proliferations

Significant synovial proliferations similar to those of pigmented villonodular synovitis can be caused by medical conditions including acute or chronic infection, gout, calcium pyrophosphate disease, amyloidosis, rheumatologic disease, and foreign material in the joint.

Vascular Anomalies

Vascular anomalies are a broad group of tumors that stem from an abnormality in the arteries, veins, capillaries, or lymph tissues. These tumors can occur in any tissue in the body. A superficial vascular anomaly often is seen as a change in skin color and character. Deeper intramuscular growths often change in size with activity. Often the growth infiltrates areas between the muscle fibers, and as a result complete resection is difficult. A deep tumor can become painful or cause cramping as it grows. Well-circumscribed soft-tissue calcifications often are seen on radiographs. Ultrasound and some MRI sequences can differentiate between high-flow and low-flow lesions. The appearance of the lesion on MRI often is serpiginous and has been described as an axial slice through a bowl of worms. Although surgical resection is an option, many vascular anomalies can be effectively treated with serial percutaneous sclerosing therapy, usually under ultrasound guidance. Very few vascular anomalies of the foot require systemic treatment.[14,15]

Nodular Fasciitis

Nodular fasciitis is a rapidly growing, very cellular tumor with a high mitotic rate. It is sometimes misdiagnosed as a sarcoma, and only an experienced pathologist may be able to arrive at the correct diagnosis. Patients age 20 to 40 years are most often affected. Unclear borders can be seen on MRI as the tumor infiltrates the surrounding soft tissue; T1- and T2-weighted signal intensities are mixed, and there is a mixed pattern with gadolinium enhancement. Pain can come from local irritation as the tumor grows to a significant size within weeks. The tumor is self-limiting and often regresses with biopsy.

Fibroma

Benign fibromas primarily occur in the subcutaneous tissues and can be found in any area of the body. Histologically dense, mature fibrocytes are present. T1- and T2-weighted MRI shows low signal intensity, and there is no enhancement with gadolinium. Marginal resection usually is curative, and recurrence is rare.

Plantar Fibroma/Fibromatosis

Plantar fibroma appears as one or more lesions, usually along the medial border of the plantar fascia, most often in adolescents or young adults. The tissue is histologically similar to that of Dupuytren or Peyronie contracture, which is found in older adults. The lesions rarely grow larger than 2 cm and remain static in size. Bilateral masses occur in as many as half of patients. On MRI, there is low T1 signal and low-to-intermediate T2 signal, with variable enhancement.

Most patients are asymptomatic. A patient with pain should be evaluated for the presence of another pain generator and should undergo extensive nonsurgical treatment including physical therapy and the use of night splints, shoe modification, and over-the-counter pain medications. Resection is rarely recommended. The recurrence rate is 100% after an isolated surgical resection and 25% after complete plantar stripping.[16] Resection

may leave a hypersensitive area on the plantar aspect of the foot. Novel treatments such as extracorporeal shock wave therapy have been used to treat symptomatic patients, with a resulting decrease in pain scores and subjective softening of masses.[17]

Extra-abdominal Fibromatosis

Extra-abdominal fibromatosis (also known as desmoid tumor) is a locally aggressive, monoclonal proliferative disease that occurs anywhere in the musculoskeletal system. The tumor grows at a variable rate and in some patients is latent for long periods of time. The peak incidence is in patients approximately 30 years old. These tumors are firm and may adhere to underlying structures. MRI classically shows low T1 and T2 signal, but some tumors have a mixed T2 signal; enhancement with gadolinium is low or mixed. Unlike a sarcoma, fibromatosis often infiltrates the surrounding tissues, and planning a wide resection is difficult. As many as 28% of these tumors are associated with previous trauma, including a surgical scar. The treatment is evolving. Medical therapies have included the use of NSAIDs, antiestrogen therapies, and other chemotherapies. Radiation has been used alone and in conjunction with surgical resection for tumor control. Local control rates after surgical resection range from 50% to 80%.[18,19]

Epidermoid Inclusion Cyst

An epidermoid inclusion cyst usually is subungual and occurs as the result of traumatic disruption of the nail matrix beneath the skin, with subsequent collection of keratin in a cystlike structure that can erode into the distal phalanx. The treatment is with biopsy and intralesional excision and grafting, if necessary. Secondary infection can complicate the treatment.

Glomus Tumor

The vascular glomus tumor appears as a small, painful red to blue discoloration beneath the nail bed. Pain usually is associated with cold exposure or pressure. Other subungual tumors, especially malignant melanoma, should be considered in the differential diagnosis. A glomus tumor usually is smaller than 1 cm. Imaging is difficult, but MRI signal is low with T1 weighting and high with T2 weighting; a low-intensity central nidus is seen with gadolinium enhancement. Tumor pressure on the bone can cause erosion of the phalanx. This tumor usually occurs in early adulthood and is treated with marginal excision.[20]

Morton Interdigital Neuroma

Morton neuroma is a fibrosing process of the plantar digital nerve that causes pain in the plantar aspect of the foot.

5: Special Problems of the Foot and Ankle

This disorder most commonly occurs between the heads of the third and forth metatarsals and less often between the second and third metatarsals. Pain radiates proximally along the innervations and into the toes. A mass may be palpable on physical examination; squeezing the forefoot or palpating the mass aggravates the symptoms. On MRI, a large Morton neuroma has a characteristic low-intensity signal with T1 weighting, a intermediate-intensity signal with T2 weighting, and mild uptake with gadolinium enhancement (**Figure 2**). Nonsurgical treatment including shoe wear modification and the use of an in-shoe orthotic device may alleviate the symptoms. Corticosteroid injections may decrease the symptoms and tumor size. If these measures are unsuccessful, marginal surgical resection leads to pain relief in most patients.

Neurilemmoma or Schwannoma

Neurilemmoma or schwannoma is a benign proliferation of Schwann cells in the nerve sheath. This tumor is most common in patients age 20 to 50 years. Tumors usually occur on the flexor surfaces of the extremities, and 90% are isolated. The tumor often is identifiable on physical examination because of a positive Tinel sign and restriction of the movement of the mass to one plane as a result of nerve tethering. MRI characteristically shows a mass along the tract of a nerve with a central low signal known as a target sign. When left untreated for a long period of time, a tumor can develop atypia; such a tumor is called an ancient schwannoma. This transformation does not necessarily have malignant potential. Most patients have an isolated tumor, but schwannomatosis syndromes do exist. The tumor can be resected by marginal excision, leaving the nerve intact.

Neurofibroma

Neurofibroma is a benign spindle cell tumor of a peripheral nerve that usually is superficial. Like schwannoma, neurofibroma is isolated in 90% of patients. The tumor occurs in patients age 20 to 30 years. Multiple lesions are seen in patients with neurofibromatosis.[1] These patients have a 10% risk of dedifferentiation of one of their many tumors into a neurosarcoma. Resection of these tumors from major nerves is not recommended because no plane exists between the neurofibroma and the nerve.

Lipoma

Lipomas are fatty tumors that can occur in any part of the body. Most lipomas appear in patients age 40 to 60 years. The lipoma itself is painless, but it can compress other structures or painfully herniate out of the fascial covering. A small superficial tumor has a soft, doughy consistency, rarely grows larger than 10 cm, and can be monitored with simple observation. A large subfascial

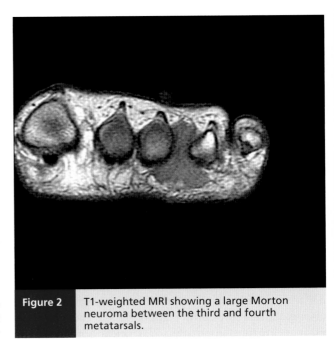

| Figure 2 | T1-weighted MRI showing a large Morton neuroma between the third and fourth metatarsals. |

tumor often is excised because of the difficulty of monitoring and the risk of malignant dedifferentiation. MRI can be used to diagnose lipoma without a biopsy. The key is to examine every MRI sequence to ensure that the tumor has the signal characteristics of subcutaneous fat. Further evaluation by an orthopaedic oncologist is advised if any of the sequences differ in even a portion of the tumor because this signal change might represent progression of the tumor to a well-differentiated or dedifferentiated liposarcoma. The many subtypes of lipomas, including angiolipoma, spindle cell lipoma, lipoblastoma, hibernoma, myolipoma, chondroid lipoma, and myelolipoma, also may have signal characteristics different from those of subcutaneous fat. For a true lipoma, a marginal excision of less than 5 cm is sufficient, and no follow-up is necessary.

Malignant Soft-Tissue Tumors

Soft-Tissue Sarcomas

Most types of soft-tissue sarcomas can occur in the foot or ankle. A low-grade tumor may be slow growing and exist in the foot for a long time, but a high-grade tumor can progress in a short period of time to a large and fungating mass within the thin soft-tissue covering of the ankle (**Figure 3**). Benign or low-grade tumors that have been present for many years can dedifferentiate into a higher grade sarcoma and suddenly begin to grow. Sarcomas often have an indeterminate profile on MRI, and the diagnosis must be confirmed by biopsy. In general, sarcomas have a low T1 signal intensity and a mixed or high T2 intensity, with significant gadolinium enhancement. A patient with a suspected soft-tissue sarcoma should be referred to a sarcoma center for a wide surgical excision with adjuvant or neoadjuvant radiotherapy and/or chemotherapy.

Synovial Sarcoma

Synovial sarcoma is the most common sarcoma of the foot. More than 25% of synovial sarcomas occur below the knee, with 13% in the foot alone.[9] Like other sarcomas, synovial sarcoma often is smaller in the distal extremities than in the rest of the body. Mineralization occurs in many synovial sarcomas.[21] Synovial sarcoma can appear as a cystic mass similar in appearance to a synovial ganglion on MRI.[22]

Acryl Myxoinflammatory Fibroblastic Sarcoma

Acryl myxoinflammatory fibroblastic sarcoma is a poorly defined, slow-growing, painless mass that involves the underlying tendon sheath. Most patients are age 30 to 50 years. Thirty percent of these rare tumors occur in the foot or ankle.[9] On MRI, the tumor is seen as less well encapsulated than most sarcomas. Metastasis is uncommon, but the tumor can be locally recurrent.[23]

Epithelioid Sarcoma

Nine percent of epithelioid sarcomas occur in the foot or ankle.[9] Most patients are age 10 to 35 years, and two-thirds of these tumors occur in boys or men. Metastasis occurs through lymphatic chains. PET and sentinel node evaluation should be considered. The use of isolated limb infusion, a relatively new technique for treating regional metastasis, may preclude the need for amputation.

Clear Cell Sarcoma

Clear cell sarcoma is rare. Most patients are age 20 to 40 years, and the foot or ankle is the primary tumor site in 38% of patients.[35] This tumor usually is found deep to the fascia and produces melanin. Sometimes clear cell sarcoma is believed to be a deep-tissue variant of malignant melanoma. Because the tumor often is spread throughout the lymphatic system, the sentinel nodes should be evaluated. Isolated limb infusion may be an option for a patient with clear cell sarcoma. The prognosis is poor because of a high incidence of pulmonary metastasis.

Malignant Melanoma

Acral lentiginous melanoma is the most common malignancy of the foot. Most patients are in the fourth decade of life, and more women than men are affected. A patient with a pigmented or otherwise concerning skin lesion should be referred to a melanoma specialist. The acral variant of melanoma has a worse prognosis than all other types of melanoma.[24] Sentinel lymph node biopsy

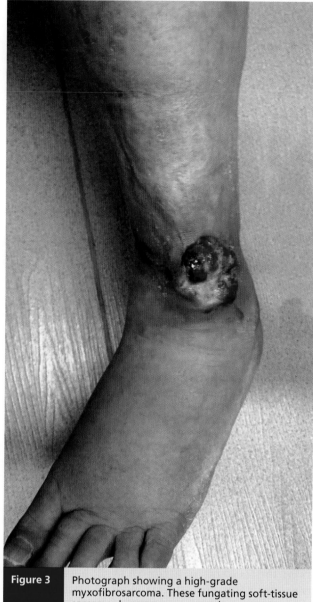

Figure 3 Photograph showing a high-grade myxofibrosarcoma. These fungating soft-tissue sarcomas have a poor prognosis.

is commonly done for these tumors, and involvement of the node is the dominant factor predicting recurrence or survival with acral disease.[25] Isolated limb infusion commonly is used to treat patients with in-transit melanoma.

Benign Osseous Tumors

Osteochondroma

Osteochondroma is the most common tumor of bone, and it can occur anywhere in the body. The tumors can be isolated or multiple. Osteochondroma develops during childhood or adolescence, and the tumors grow until the patient reaches skeletal maturity. Although many masses go unnoticed, the thin covering of the foot and ankle often allows detection. The growths are pedunculated (growing from a single stalk) or sessile (having a broad base similar in size to the tumor). Resection of the tumor, with or without subsequent protected weight bearing, may be appropriate for tumors that are unsightly or are irritating surrounding structures. Observation is recommended for asymptomatic tumors. The diagnosis requires the identification of a continuum between the marrow space of the bone and the marrow space of the osteochondroma. Plain radiographs often are sufficient for diagnosis, but advanced imaging sometimes is necessary. Biopsies are not necessary for tumors with cartilage caps smaller than 3 cm that have not changed in size. Chondrosarcomatous differentiation should be considered if a tumor enlarges substantially after adolescence. Patients with multiple hereditary exostosis have a loss of function related to one of three known exostosin (*EXT*) tumor suppressor genes. Patients with multiple hereditary exostosis have an increased risk of malignant differentiation of the tumor in up to 25% of patients.[26]

Subungual Exostosis

Subungual exostosis is a benign osteochondral lesion that does not arise from a physis but rather from the tip of the distal phalanx. This tumor often is painful and causes nail deformity. The treatment involves removing the nail to gain access to the bone below, and usually it is curative.

Enchondroma/Chondroma

Enchondroma is a benign proliferation of hyaline cartilage that occurs when dysplastic embryonal cartilage becomes trapped in a bone. Eight percent of these tumors occur in the bones of the foot, most commonly in the forefoot.[27] The lesions usually are centrally located in the bone along the trajectory of a growth plate. Enchondromas most commonly are incidentally found after they have begun normal mineralization in a specified pattern. MRI shows a low T1 and a high T2 signal with a well-defined popcorn-type margin. Observation is the treatment of choice for lesions with a benign appearance.

There is a very low risk of malignant transformation. Malignant presentations are more common in the midfoot and hindfoot.[28] Radiographic features causing concern include cortical thinning, soft-tissue masses, and growth. The most common symptom of malignant degeneration is pain from weakening of the bone. Biopsy is appropriate for suspicious lesions; for small foot and ankle lesions, simple curettage may be an appropriate excisional biopsy. The risk of local recurrence for lesions excised with simple curettage is very low. Patients with Ollier disease or Maffucci syndrome are at increased risk

for malignant transformation and should be observed closely.

Periosteal Chondroma

Periosteal chondroma is a rare benign eccentric tumor of bone that is more common in the long bones of the body than in the foot or ankle. Usually this tumor is found incidentally, and excision biopsy or curettage is the usual treatment.[29]

Chondroblastoma

Chondroblastoma is a rare benign lesion that accounts for fewer than 1% of primary bone tumors and is one of very few epiphyseal or apophyseal tumors. More than 80% of patients are younger than 25 years, and often they have open growth plates.[27] In the foot, chondroblastoma usually occurs in the talus or calcaneus. Despite its benign nature, chondroblastoma carries a small (less than 1%) risk of pulmonary metastasis, and plain radiography of the chest should be part of the initial workup. Radiographs and CT show dystrophic calcification in the epiphysis, with possible enlargement of the bone. MRI often shows low signal with T1 weighting and high signal with T2 weighting. Many lesions are cystic or have secondary aneurysmal bone cysts; this characteristic can make diagnosis difficult because of the small epiphysis of the small bones. Microscopically, these tumors have a characteristic chicken wire appearance between the chondroid cells. Lesions are treated with curettage and high-speed burring. Often adjuvant peroxide, phenol, cryotherapy, or argon beam laser treatment is useful for extending the margin and decreasing the risk of local recurrence.

Giant Cell Tumor of Bone

Giant cell tumor of bone is a locally aggressive epiphyseal neoplasm that accounts for 5% of primary bone tumors. Only 6% of these tumors occur in the foot or ankle.[27] This disease is most common in patients age 20 to 40 years. In contrast to patients with chondroblastoma, patients with giant cell tumor of bone usually have closed growth plates, and there is no significant mineralization within the lesion. The risk of benign metastasis to the lung is approximately 1%, but in patients with metastasis the risk of mortality is 15% to 20%. Malignant giant cell tumors are found in 1% of patients with giant cell tumor of bone.[30] This high-grade sarcoma often represents a recurrence of a tumor treated with radiation. Radiographically, these lesions are purely lytic, and they may enlarge to destroy the metaphysis. MRI shows low signal with T1 weighting and high signal with T2 weighting, often with fluid levels that may represent secondary aneurysmal bone cysts. The pathologic findings classically are described as the nuclei

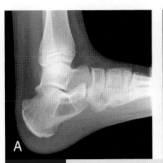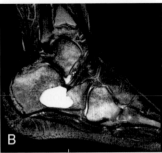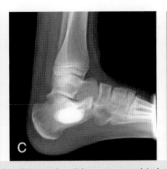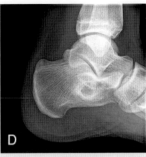

Figure 4 A painful unicameral cyst in the calcaneus. **A,** Lateral radiograph with a geographic lesion of the calcaneus. **B,** T2 sagittal MRI demonstrating fluid signal within the calcaneous lesion. **C,** Postoperative radiograph after irrigation and percutaneous injection of calcium sulfate-calcium phosphate. **D,** Radiograph showing near-complete resolution 1 year after surgery.

of the giant cells having an appearance similar to that of the nuclei of the surrounding stromal cells. The treatment usually entails biopsy followed by wide curettage, mechanical burring, adjuvant treatment, and cementing and/or bone grafting of the lesion. Completely destructive lesions may require bone replacement with allograft or endoprosthesis. In a recent review of 31 patients with a distal tibial giant cell tumor of bone who underwent an extended curettage, the recurrence rate was 29%. This rate was higher than that reported in other studies.[31] The use of alternative treatments including embolization, bisphosphonates, and denosumab is becoming more common in the treatment of giant cell tumors, especially those in difficult locations such as the spine and pelvis.

Unicameral Bone Cyst

Unicameral bone cyst is a destructive tumor that most commonly occurs in the calcaneus of teenagers. The tumor may or may not be symptomatic and often is discovered incidentally. The lesions usually are lateral on the calcaneus and adjacent to the middle facet. MRI shows a fluid-filled lesion with few or no fluid-fluid levels; peripheral rim enhancement is seen with gadolinium enhancement. The risk of fracture is low in patients with these lesions. Observation is appropriate for an asymptomatic patient. A painful cyst usually is treated with percutaneous techniques including the injection of steroids, bone marrow, a sclerosing agent, and/or a bone graft substitute (**Figure 4**). Open surgery may be indicated for a displaced fracture.

Aneurysmal Bone Cyst

Approximately 10% of aneurysmal bone cysts are found in the distal tibia or foot.[27] Patients with this lesion commonly report pain during weight bearing or activity. Most patients are in the first or second decades of life. In the long bones, radiographs classically show aggressive, eccentric, expansile lucent lesions with a surrounding thin sclerotic layer of reactive bone. MRI shows multiple

fluid-fluid levels throughout the lesion. These lesions classically are treated with extended curettage, with or without adjuvant treatments or bone grafting. Some patients currently are treated with sclerosing agents, however. This technique often involves multiple fluoroscopic injections of sodium tetradecyl sulfate or a similar agent into the lesions, causing involution of the tumor and mineralization of the bone. A sclerosing agent often is used to treat lesions, including some foot and ankle tumors, that are difficult to reach surgically, are small and carry a low risk of fracture, or have caused too much bone destruction to allow allograft reconstruction. Aneurysmal bone cysts can arise secondary to another type of bone lesion, including but not limited to nonossifying fibroma, chondromyxoid fibroma, chondroblastoma, or giant cell tumor. Caution is necessary in diagnosing aneurysmal bone cyst because the differential diagnosis includes telangiectatic osteosarcoma, which can have an identical appearance on imaging studies. Biopsy is recommended before treatment is initiated.

Chondromyxoid Fibroma

Chondromyxoid fibroma is a tumor of adolescence that occurs in the foot or ankle in as many as 25% of patients.[27] In the long bones chondromyxoid fibroma commonly is an eccentric metaphyseal lesion and has a sclerotic margin with cortical scalloping or expansion. There is little matrix calcification. On MRI, lesions often have a high signal with T2 weighting. The preferred treatment is aggressive curettage with optional adjuvant treatment and grafting. A 20% recurrence rate recently has been documented in the foot and ankle.[32]

Nonossifying Fibroma

Approximately 25% of nonossifying fibromas (also called fibroxanthomas) occur in the distal tibia or fibula,[27] but this tumor is rare in the bones of the foot. Patients often are adolescents with an ankle sprain; the tumor is an incidental geographic lesion separate from the area of pain. Observation is the most common treatment. Surgical curettage and grafting are reserved for lesions that are painful or at a high risk for fracture.

Osteoid Osteoma

Osteoid osteoma is a small, cortically based tumor that occurs in the foot or ankle in approximately 10% of patients.[27] Patients classically describe night pain that is relieved by the use of NSAIDs. Sometimes the pain is referred from or perceived as coming from an adjacent joint. Tumors near a joint may cause early arthritis. The lesion is smaller than 2 cm on radiography and has a sclerotic rim around a lucent area with a central, small, dense sclerotic nidus resembling a target. Significant local sclerosis may be present. CT is preferable to MRI for imaging these lesions. If adequate relief cannot be obtained with NSAID therapy, the treatment of choice is radiofrequency ablation, which has excellent results. En bloc excision also is an option.

Osteoblastoma

Osteoblastoma in the foot or ankle is rare. The symptoms are similar to those of osteoid osteoma, but pain is not usually relieved with NSAIDs. Osteoblastomas have a varied appearance, and many have aggressive radiographic characteristics.[27] The tumor is treated with curettage and grafting.

Intraosseous Lipoma

Intraosseous lipoma in the calcaneus is common and often is found incidentally in a patient with plantar fasciitis or Achilles tendinitis. Radiographically, this benign-appearing lesion has well-defined borders and central lucency with occasional areas of mineralized septa. MRI or CT can confirm the presence of adipose tissue. Asymptomatic patients do not require treatment. Patients with corresponding bone edema or fracture are best treated with simple curettage and grafting.

Malignant Osseous Tumors

Primary malignant bone tumors of the foot or ankle classically have been treated with amputation. Patients can achieve an excellent functional outcome after below-knee amputation. Limb salvage is now offered to most patients as a primary treatment. A patient with a suspicious lesion should be referred to a musculoskeletal oncologist before biopsy to decrease the risk of morbidity.

Chondrosarcoma

Chondrosarcoma occurs in the foot or ankle in only 3% of patients.[27] Sixty percent of high-grade tumors are partially calcified, with cortical destruction.[27] Relatively large lesions may have associated soft-tissue masses. The treatment is primarily based on tumor grade. Grade 1 chondrosarcomas in the lower extremity can be treated with extended curettage using a high-speed burr, with adjuvant treatment using cryotherapy, argon beam, phenol, or cementation grafting. Resection of the lesion may be necessary with allograft or autograft reconstruction. Grade 2 and 3 lesions are treated with wide resection and reconstruction or amputation. For grade 4 (dedifferentiated) lesions, primary amputation should be considered because of the high risk of local recurrence and metastasis.

Osteosarcoma

Approximately 3% of osteosarcomas occur in the foot or ankle.[27] Most patients are adolescents. The tumor usually is painful, and patients often report night pain. Aggressive lucent or mixed lesions often have periosteal new bone formation and mineralized soft-tissue masses. Pathologic analysis shows malignant osteoid. The treatment routinely includes neoadjuvant and adjuvant chemotherapy, with surgery for removal of the primary tumor and any metastases.

Ewing Sarcoma

Approximately 8% of Ewing sarcomas occur in the distal tibia, fibula, or foot.[27] Patients report pain with activity and at night. These tumors often have fast-growing soft-tissue masses that expand from the bone. Radiographs show lucency within the bone and often impressive periosteal reactions. The histopathologic finding is of a small round blue cell tumor, with little surrounding stroma. The course of treatment is similar to that of osteosarcoma. Radiation can be substituted for surgical excision, but because of slightly inferior outcomes radiation usually is reserved for tumors in areas that are extremely difficult to resect, such as the spine.

Metastatic Carcinoma

The incidence of metastatic bone tumors greatly increases with advancing patient age. Metastatic carcinoma is the most common destructive bone lesion in patients older than 40 years, many of whom have no known history of cancer. The initial symptom is pain. Because of their metastatic nature, these tumors are stage IV. With advances in the treatment of carcinomas, many patients live with the disease for years or decades. As patient survival rates improve, so does the need for durable reconstruction of the destroyed bone. If possible, an intervention to stabilize a foot or ankle metastatic site must create a strong construct that will bear the patient's weight soon and for many years to come.

Patients older than 40 years are more likely to have a destructive metastatic carcinoma than a primary bone sarcoma. The primary tumor site and sites of metastasis must be identified. For a patient with newly diagnosed lesions, a thorough history and physical examination are important for identifying risk-increasing behaviors, a family history of cancer, or other relevant factors. A laboratory evaluation should be considered, including a complete blood cell count to identify any blood disorder or anemia, a metabolic panel to identify renal dysfunction in multiple myeloma, and disease-specific markers such as prostate-specific antigen, thyroid-specific hormone, and electrophoresis in multiple myeloma. The most useful means of identifying a primary tumor is contrast CT of the chest, abdomen, and pelvis. A bone scan is recommended for a patient believed to have metastatic carcinoma to identify sites at risk for fracture and possibly to identify a biopsy site that will not increase the risk of fracture.

The most common primary sites of metastatic carcinoma are the breast, kidney, thyroid gland, lung, and prostate gland. Because of its acral metastases, lung cancer most often leads to destructive carcinoma of the foot and ankle. Many lung cancers are radioresponsive, and excellent pain relief usually is achieved early in the course of radiation. With a large, painful lesion that is at risk for pathologic fracture, the patient may be able to bear weight soon after biopsy, curettage, adjuvant treatment, and stabilization with plates, screws, and cementation of the defect. In treating characteristically vascular tumors, as in kidney or thyroid cancers, embolization should be considered to limit blood loss during surgical stabilization (**Figure 5**). Amputation rarely is necessary.

Multiple Myeloma
Multiple myeloma is the most common primary bone tumor in patients older than 40 years. Many patients have multiple purely radiolucent lesions. Patients who have a lesion, anemia, and renal dysfunction rarely require biopsy; the diagnosis usually can be made with serum protein electrophoresis, urine protein electrophoresis, and serum light chains. Lesions with a low risk of fracture usually can be treated with chemotherapy and/or radiation. Painful lesions with significant structural loss may be quite vascular, and the treatment should be similar to that of metastatic carcinoma.

Reconstructive Treatments

Amputation and Prosthetic Replacement
Some patients choose amputation to treat their malignant tumor. Excellent functional outcomes can be achieved after amputation. Prosthesis design continues to progress and to lead to increases in normal patient function. A German group has pioneered the use of transcutaneous

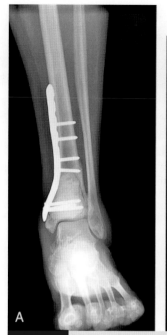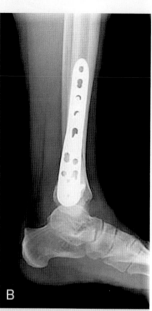

Figure 5 AP (**A**) and lateral (**B**) radiographs showing a treated metastatic lesion to the distal tibia. The patient was able to bear weight as tolerated immediately after surgery.

prostheses that are biologically anchored to bone, thus allowing the patient to attach the prosthesis with a mechanical latch and completely eliminating the need for a socket. Prostheses with this design primarily are used after transfemoral amputation. However, some patients with transtibial amputations with fit issues and short residual bone may be candidates for an endo-exo prosthesis. This technique creates a permanent bone prosthesis interface with an endoprosthesis that extends outside of the bone through a chronic fistula. This endo-exo metal shaft connects mechanically to a prosthetic leg, negating the need for a socket.[33]

Osseous Grafting
Masquelet Technique
The Masquelet technique of bone formation, also called the induced membrane technique, most commonly is used in long bones. This technique also is useful for smaller bone defects of the foot and ankle caused by tumor, trauma, or infection. The two-step surgical process is designed to create structural bone from cancellous graft. A block of polymethyl methacrylate is placed to conform to the shape of the bone defect. The wound is closed, the skin is allowed to heal, and a granulation membrane is induced and matures before the polymethyl methacrylate block is removed. In vitro studies have demonstrated improved alkaline phosphatase activity and calcium deposition if the autograft is placed 1 month after the spacer.[34]

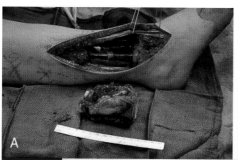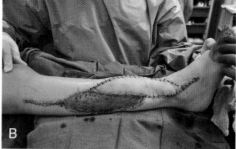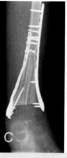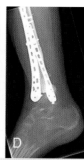

Figure 6 Intraoperative photographs and postoperative radiographs showing the surgical treatment of periosteal osteosarcoma of the distal tibia and fibula. The allograft-autograft reconstruction used tissue from the patient's ipsilateral vascularized fibula. **A,** Intraoperative image after resection of the periosteal osteosarcoma. **B,** Intraoperative image after reconstruction of the distal tibia including free fibula osseocutaneous transfer and skin grafting of host site. Six month postoperative AP (**C**) and lateral (**D**) radiographs with evidence of osseous healing.

Vascularized Autograft

The most common source of vascularized free-osseous transfers is the fibula, but other bones also are used. Because of its native shape, a vascularized portion of the iliac crest can be used to recreate the medial arch of the foot after resection of portions of the midfoot and forefoot. A vascularized portion of the medial femoral condyle has been used to treat osteonecrosis, nonunion, and small bone defects.[35]

Allograft

The use of osteoarticular allograft in a large joint is fraught with complications, but it can be successful in a small segment (less than 3 to 5 cm). Frozen or freeze-dried morcellized allograft is commonly used to fill defects after curettage of a benign tumor.

Synthetic Bone Fillers

The broad group of synthetic bone fillers includes products with a range of material properties that the treating surgeon may consider desirable. Some products can be percutaneously injected into cystic structures and allowed to harden. Others products can be mixed with an antibiotic to create beads that are absorbed into the body and act as a scaffolding for bone formation.

Allograft-Autograft Composite

The treatment of some tumors of the distal tibia creates massive bone loss. Although some patients choose transtibial amputation as a reliable and functionally satisfactory treatment, others prefer to avoid amputation if at all possible. Intercalary bulk allografting has a high failure rate in massive tibial defects as a result of allograft fracture and junctional nonunion. A technique for structural allografting coupled with intramedullary fibular autografting has led to improved rates of union and allograft vascularization, thereby decreasing fracture rates and improving healing after fracture.[36] This use of

this technique allows patients to retain the native ankle joint after cryogenic treatment or radiation of autograft (**Figure 6**).

Allograft Prosthetic Reconstruction

The availability of modular tibial components with long stems for ankle arthroplasty has increased the feasibility of allograft prosthetic reconstruction of the ankle. Outcomes research is needed to determine whether this technique is superior to allograft fusion or transtibial amputation.

Bone Transport

Ring fixators and rails for bone transport, with or without a rod, can be used for reconstruction of distal tibial bone. The lengthening process can be prolonged depending on the defect size. Patient compliance varies.

Bracing and Shoe Inserts

Orthotic devices can be used after tumor resection in the foot and ankle. Simple inserts are used for offloading if anatomic changes have led to pain in a portion of the foot after tumor resection. Some orthotic devices are contoured to compensate for the loss of a major portion of the foot.

Isolated Limb Infusion

In isolated limb infusion, high-dosage chemotherapy is circulated through the extremity in a closed loop after tourniquet inflation proximally to the catheters. Isolation of the leg allows for administration of much higher dosages than is possible systemically without damaging solid organs. Isolated limb infusion is a well-established treatment of in-transit metastatic melanoma of the extremities, and it is now being used for other lymphatically spread diseases, such as Merkel cell carcinoma and epithelioid sarcoma. Recently this technique was found to be useful in shrinking unresectable extremity tumors to allow limb salvage.[37] Isolated limb infusion has great potential for treating foot and ankle tumors, but it should be used with caution because of the risk of severe toxicity to the skin.[38]

Nononcologically Excised Malignant Tumors

Nononcologic excision of malignant tumors continues to be a major concern for orthopaedic oncologists. Patients are referred to oncologists not only by orthopaedic surgeons but also by podiatrists and general surgeons after removal of a small mass that was believed to be benign. Most such masses are soft-tissue sarcomas, and routine reexcision is recommended if negative margins were not obtained during the original surgery. This protocol decreases the risk of recurrence to the same level as in a wide primary excision. Unfortunately, reexcision requires greater flap coverage, and in some patients amputation may be necessary to control the disease.

Summary

A thorough understanding of the common benign and malignant tumors of the foot and ankle are essential to the evaluation, diagnosis, and treatment of masses in the foot. Despite the small size of tumors on presentation, the possibility of malignancy should be considered before any surgical intervention is undertaken.

Annotated References

1. Chou LB, Ho YY, Malawer MM: Tumors of the foot and ankle: Experience with 153 cases. *Foot Ankle Int* 2009;30(9):836-841.

   A retrospective single-surgeon study cataloged tumors treated at a referral center. Of all studied tumors, 5.75% were in the foot or ankle. Level of evidence: IV.

2. Rougraff BT: Evaluation of the patient with carcinoma of unknown origin metastatic to bone. *Clin Orthop Relat Res* 2003;(415, suppl):S105-S109.

3. Woertler K: Soft tissue masses in the foot and ankle: Characteristics on MR imaging. *Semin Musculoskelet Radiol* 2005;9(3):227-242.

4. Gauerke S, Driscoll JJ: Hidradenocarcinomas: A brief review and future directions. *Arch Pathol Lab Med* 2010;134(5):781-785.

   The literature on hidradenocarcinoma was reviewed. Diagnosis, staging with sentinel node biopsy, and surgical resection of this uncommon tumor were discussed.

5. Buchbender C, Heusner TA, Lauenstein TC, Bockisch A, Antoch G: Oncologic PET/MRI: Part 2. Bone tumors, soft-tissue tumors, melanoma, and lymphoma. *J Nucl Med* 2012;53(8):1244-1252.

   PET-MRI of bone tumors, soft-tissue sarcoma, melanoma, and lymphoma was reviewed. PET-MRI appears to be of benefit in T-staging of primary bone tumors and soft-tissue sarcomas. For whole-body N-staging, PET-MRI has accuracy similar to that of PET-CT.

6. Binitie O, Tejiram S, Conway S, Cheong D, Temple HT, Letson GD: Adult soft tissue sarcoma local recurrence after adjuvant treatment without resection of core needle biopsy tract. *Clin Orthop Relat Res* 2013;471(3):891-898.

   A retrospective review of 59 patients with deep, large soft-tissue sarcomas resected without removal of the needle biopsy tract found no increase in local recurrence or metastatic disease. Level of evidence: IV.

7. Brotzmann M, Hefti F, Baumhoer D, Krieg AH: Do malignant bone tumors of the foot have a different biological behavior than sarcomas at other skeletal sites? *Sarcoma* 2013;2013:767960.

   A retrospective review of 32 patients with malignant tumors of the foot found delays in diagnosis, relatively small tumor volumes, and outcomes similar to those of tumors at other locations. Level of evidence: IV.

8. Mankin HJ, Mankin CJ, Simon MA; Members of the Musculoskeletal Tumor Society: The hazards of the biopsy, revisited. *J Bone Joint Surg Am* 1996;78(5):656-663.

9. Weiss SW, Goldblum JR: *Enzinger and Weiss's Soft Tissue Tumors,* ed 5. Philadelphia, PA, Mosby, 2008.

10. Weishaupt D, Schweitzer ME, Morrison WB, Haims AH, Wapner K, Kahn M: MRI of the foot and ankle: Prevalence and distribution of occult and palpable ganglia. *J Magn Reson Imaging* 2001;14(4):464-471.

11. Ma X, Shi G, Xia C, Liu H, He J, Jin W: Pigmented villonodular synovitis: A retrospective study of seventy five cases (eighty one joints). *Int Orthop* 2013;37(6):1165-1170.

    Pigmented villonodular synovitis in the ankle was found in 4 of 75 patients. All patients were treated with open débridement, and one patient had arthroplasty. There were no recurrences. Level of evidence: IV.

12. Galat DD, Ackerman DB, Spoon D, Turner NS, Shives TC: Synovial chondromatosis of the foot and ankle. *Foot Ankle Int* 2008;29(3):312-317.

    Eight patients were identified as having synovial chondromatosis of the foot and/or ankle during a 36-year period. Four patients were pain free after synovectomy, and two patients underwent amputation for malignant degeneration. Level of evidence: IV.

13. Babar SA, Sandison A, Mitchell AW: Synovial and tenosynovial lipoma arborescens of the ankle in an adult: A case report. *Skeletal Radiol* 2008;37(1):75-77.

5: Special Problems of the Foot and Ankle

Lipoma arborescens of the ankle joint was found in an adult, with involvement of the intra-articular synovium as well as the synovial sheath of the tendons around the ankle.

14. Behr GG, Johnson C: Vascular anomalies: Hemangiomas and beyond. Part 1: Fast-flow lesions. *AJR Am J Roentgenol* 2013;200(2):414-422.

   A two-part review of the medical literature and the classification of vascular anomalies clarified common misconceptions and provided guidance for imaging and treatment. Part 1 focused on the fast-flow vascular anomalies.

15. Behr GG, Johnson CM: Vascular anomalies: Hemangiomas and beyond. Part 2: Slow-flow lesions. *AJR Am J Roentgenol* 2013;200(2):423-436.

   Part 2 focused on the slow-flow vascular anomalies.

16. Veith NT, Tschernig T, Histing T, Madry H: Plantar fibromatosis: Topical review. *Foot Ankle Int* 2013;34(12):1742-1746.

   Established procedures and experimental strategies were reviewed for the treatment of Ledderhose disease.

17. Knobloch K, Vogt PM: High-energy focussed extracorporeal shockwave therapy reduces pain in plantar fibromatosis (Ledderhose's disease). *BMC Res Notes* 2012;5(1):542.

   All six patients with painful plantar fibromatosis had excellent pain relief 3 months after treatment. Level of evidence: IV.

18. Pritchard DJ, Nascimento AG, Petersen IA: Local control of extra-abdominal desmoid tumors. *J Bone Joint Surg Am* 1996;78(6):848-854.

19. Bonvalot S, Desai A, Coppola S, et al: The treatment of desmoid tumors: A stepwise clinical approach. *Ann Oncol* 2012;23(Suppl 10):x158-x166.

   Medical, surgical, and minimally invasive treatment of desmoid tumors was comprehensively reviewed.

20. Netscher DT, Aburto J, Koepplinger M: Subungual glomus tumor. *J Hand Surg Am* 2012;37(4):821-824.

   The literature on the diagnosis and treatment of subungual glomus tumor was reviewed.

21. Wilkerson BW, Crim JR, Hung M, Layfield LJ: Characterization of synovial sarcoma calcification. *AJR Am J Roentgenol* 2012;199(6):W730-W734.

   Fine stippled calcifications in a soft-tissue mass should raise suspicion for synovial sarcoma, based on a review of imaging studies in 29 patients. Level of evidence: IV.

22. Bixby SD, Hettmer S, Taylor GA, Voss SD: Synovial sarcoma in children: Imaging features and common benign mimics. *AJR Am J Roentgenol* 2010;195(4):1026-1032.

   Imaging studies of synovial sarcoma were reviewed, with a description of common mimicking conditions.

23. Montgomery EA, Devaney KO, Giordano TJ, Weiss SW: Inflammatory myxohyaline tumor of distal extremities with virocyte or Reed–Sternberg-like cells: A distinctive lesion with features simulating inflammatory conditions, Hodgkin's disease, and various sarcomas. *Mod Pathol* 1998;11(4):384-391.

24. Durbec F, Martin L, Derancourt C, Grange F: Melanoma of the hand and foot: Epidemiological, prognostic and genetic features. A systematic review. *Br J Dermatol* 2012;166(4):727-739.

   A global review of the literature found that hand and foot melanomas represent a subgroup of rare, potentially severe melanomas that require specific management.

25. Egger ME, McMasters KM, Callender GG, et al: Unique prognostic factors in acral lentiginous melanoma. *Am J Surg* 2012;204(6):874-879, discussion 879-880.

   A retrospective study of 85 patients found that sentinel node biopsy was the dominant factor predicting recurrence and survival in acral lentiginous melanoma. Level of evidence: III.

26. Peterson HA: Multiple hereditary osteochondromata. *Clin Orthop Relat Res* 1989;239:222-230.

27. Wold LE, Unni KK, Sim FH, Sundaram M: *Atlas of Orthopaedic Pathology*, ed 3. Philadelphia, PA, Saunders, 2008.

28. Gajewski DA, Burnette JB, Murphey MD, Temple HT: Differentiating clinical and radiographic features of enchondroma and secondary chondrosarcoma in the foot. *Foot Ankle Int* 2006;27(4):240-244.

29. Parodi KK, Farrett W, Paden MH, Stone PA: A report of a rare phalangeal periosteal chondroma of the foot. *J Foot Ankle Surg* 2011;50(1):122-125.

30. Siebenrock KA, Unni KK, Rock MG: Giant-cell tumour of bone metastasising to the lungs. A long-term follow-up. *J Bone Joint Surg Br* 1998;80(1):43-47.

31. AlSulaimani SA, Turcotte RE; Canadian Orthopaedic Oncology Society (CANOOS) collaborators: Iterative curettage is associated with local control in giant cell tumors involving the distal tibia. *Clin Orthop Relat Res* 2013;471(8):2668-2674.

   This case series of 31 patients demonstrated a higher local recurrence rate than other giant cell tumor sites. Level of evidence: IV.

32. Roberts EJ, Meier MJ, Hild G, Masadeh S, Hardy M, Bakotic BW: Chondromyxoid fibroma of the calcaneus: Two case reports and literature review. *J Foot Ankle Surg* 2013;52(5):643-649.

33. Frölke JP, van de Meent H: The endo-exo prosthesis for patients with a problematic amputation stump. *Ned Tijdschr Geneeskd* 2010;154:A2010.

    This case series of two patients describes the early use of endo-exo prosthesis for selected patients with prosthetic fitting issues.

34. Aho OM, Lehenkari P, Ristiniemi J, Lehtonen S, Risteli J, Leskelä HV: The mechanism of action of induced membranes in bone repair. *J Bone Joint Surg Am* 2013;95(7):597-604.

    Retrospective study of 14 patients who underwent biopsy of their induced membranes at the time of bone grafting. Biopsies demonstrated in vitro evidence of improved alkaline phosphate activity and calcium deposition at 1 month over 2 months after spacer placement. Level of evidence: IV.

35. Haddock NT, Alosh H, Easley ME, Levin LS, Wapner KL: Applications of the medial femoral condyle free flap for foot and ankle reconstruction. *Foot Ankle Int* 2013;34(10):1395-1402.

    This article is a retrospective case series of five medial femoral condyle flaps used for reconstruction of bone defects in the foot and ankle. There were no flap failures, and all patients went on to union with an average follow-up of 20 months. Level of evidence: IV.

36. Bakri K, Stans AA, Mardini S, Moran SL: Combined massive allograft and intramedullary vascularized fibula transfer: The capanna technique for lower-limb reconstruction. *Semin Plast Surg* 2008;22(3):234-241.

37. Vohra NA, Turaga KK, Gonzalez RJ, et al: The use of isolated limb infusion in limb-threatening extremity sarcomas. *Int J Hyperthermia* 2013;29(1):1-7.

    Twenty-two patients underwent isolated limb infusion to treat soft-tissue sarcomas. At a median 11-month follow-up, nine (41%) had a response. Two patients underwent surgical resection of previously unresectable disease. Level of evidence: IV.

38. Kroon HM, Thompson JF: Isolated limb infusion: A review. *J Surg Oncol* 2009;100(2):169-177.

    Isolated limb infusion is the preferred treatment option for locally advanced melanoma and sarcoma confined to a limb. The indications, techniques, and risks were discussed.

Chapter 20

Nail and Skin Disorders of the Foot and Ankle

Edward Lansang, MD, FRCSC   Perla Lansang, MD, FRCPC   Andrea Veljkovic, MD, BComm, FRCSC

Johnny Lau, MD, MSc, FRCSC

Introduction

Nail and skin diseases of the foot and ankle represent a heterogeneous group of disorders, ranging from tumors to inflammatory conditions to infections. They may have a significant effect on the quality of life of patients; some tumors, such as melanoma, may even be life-threatening. This chapter reviews important diseases of the skin and nails of the foot.

Nail Disorders

Nail Anatomy

The five distinct anatomic regions of the nail apparatus are the nail plate, the proximal nail fold, the nail matrix, the nail bed, and the hyponychium. The nail plate is a fully cornified structure composed of tightly layered keratinized cells generated by the nail matrix. The proximal third of the nail plate is covered by the proximal nail fold, the tip of which forms the cuticle. The nail matrix

Dr. Perla Lansang or an immediate family member is a member of a speakers' bureau or has made paid presentations on behalf of Abbott, Amgen, and Johnson & Johnson. Dr. Lau or an immediate family member has received royalties from Zimmer; has made paid presentations on behalf of Zimmer; serves as a paid consultant to or is an employee of Olumpus Biotech Corporation and Zimmer; has received nonincome support (such as equipment or services), commercially derived honoraria, or other non-research–related funding (such as paid travel) from Stryker; and serves as a board member, owner, officer, or committee member of the American Academy of Orthopaedic Surgeons. Neither of the following authors nor any immediate family member has received anything of value from or has stock or stock options held in a commercial company or institution related directly or indirectly to the subject of this chapter: Dr. Edward Lansang and Dr. Veljkovic.

Table 1

Morphologic Terms Related to Nail Disorders

Term	Description
Onycholysis	Detachment of the nail plate from the nail bed, leading to a yellow-white nail appearance
Onychomadesis	Detachment of the nail plate from the proximal nail fold
Onychorrhexis	Longitudinal ridging and fissuring of the nail plate
Onychoschizia	Splitting of the nail plate into layers, especially at the distal edge
Pitting	Punctate depressions on the nail plate resulting from proximal nail matrix damage
Subungual hyperkeratosis	Accumulation of keratin underneath the nail plate

also is part of the proximal nail fold. The visible white half-moon–shaped area of the nail, called the lunula, corresponds to the distal portion of the nail matrix. The nail bed begins where the lunula ends, and it underlies the entire nail plate. The hyponychium connects the nail bed to the epithelium of the fingertip.[1] Morphologic terms related to nail disorders are outlined in Table 1.

Traumatic Subungual Hematoma

Subungual hematoma occurs when a traumatic injury leads to accumulation of blood between the nail plate and the nail bed. Compression of the nail matrix may cause secondary nail dystrophy. The color of a subungual hematoma can range from purple red to black. The possibility of a subungual melanoma should be considered in

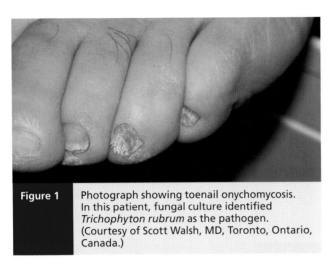

Figure 1 Photograph showing toenail onychomycosis. In this patient, fungal culture identified *Trichophyton rubrum* as the pathogen. (Courtesy of Scott Walsh, MD, Toronto, Ontario, Canada.)

Table 2

Oral Drugs for Treating Toenail Onychomycosis

Drug	Dosage	Duration
Terbinafine	250 mg once daily	12–16 weeks
Itraconazole	200 mg twice daily for 1 week; three 1-week pulses, each followed by a 3-week interval	12 weeks (three pulses)

the diagnosis. Because nail bed lacerations and fractures of the distal phalanx are associated with subungual hematomas, a radiograph should be obtained. It may be necessary to evacuate a large hematoma by creating a hole through the nail plate. A nail bed laceration with a distal phalangeal fracture should be treated with irrigation, débridement, and antibiotics.[2]

The nail bed can be repaired after thorough cleansing and assessment using loupe magnification. The nail plate is removed to allow adequate visualization and repair, and the repair is done using simple interrupted sutures with an absorbable monofilament (size 5 to 7).[3] Replacing the nail plate after traumatic injury was found to delay healing and increase the risk of infection.[4] A fractured distal phalanx can be reduced or stabilized using a fine Kirschner wire or hypodermic needle.[3]

Infectious Conditions
Onychomycosis
The term onychomycosis encompasses both dermatophytic and nondermatophytic infections of the nail. Dermatophytic nail infection is more specifically called tinea unguium and often is associated with tinea pedis. *Trichophyton rubrum* is the most common pathogen, but *Trichophyton mentagrophytes* and *Epidermophyton floccosum* also are common. The infection appears as subungual hyperkeratosis, thickening of the nail plate, and onycholysis (**Figure 1**).

The diagnosis of onychomycosis involves potassium hydroxide preparation and examination of nail scrapings and fungal cultures to identify the pathogen. Specimens are best taken by clipping part of the affected nail for laboratory microscopic examination and culture.

Topical treatment of onychomycosis usually is ineffective, and systemic treatment is required. The use of an antifungal agent such as itraconazole, fluconazole, or terbinafine provides a cure rate as high as 80%, but

recurrent disease is common. Liver toxicity and drug interaction, especially with the azoles, must be considered when a systemic antifungal agent is used.[5] The treatment of choice for onychomycosis is oral terbinafine. In clinical studies, terbinafine was found to be more effective for treatment than azoles such as itraconazole and fluconazole.[6-9] Oral therapeutic options for toenail onychomycosis are listed in **Table 2**. Surgical avulsion with topical therapy can be considered, especially for single nail involvement, but a low response rate and a high recurrence rate were reported when this treatment modality was used.[10]

Recent studies show promising results using novel topical antifungal therapy for onychomycosis. Efinaconazole has been shown to be superior to placebo in randomized controlled trials.[11]

Paronychia
Acute paronychia appears as redness, swelling, and pain of the periungual area. The most common cause of acute paronychia is *Staphylococcus aureus*. The infection may be secondary to trauma or toenail ingrowth. Recurrence of acute paronychia should raise suspicion of a herpes simplex infection. The treatment of acute paronychia depends on the causative agent, and culturing is necessary to identify the agent. Incision and drainage can relieve pain if there is a local collection of pus.

Chronic paronychia is characterized by redness and swelling of the proximal nail fold. There is much less pain than in acute paronychia, and the absence of the cuticle is a hallmark finding. *Candida* is a common pathogen. Chronic paronychia is common in workers whose feet are exposed to water and irritants. The treatment consists of avoidance of water and irritants. There is evidence that the use of topical steroids and topical azole antifungal agents is effective.[1]

Inflammatory Conditions
Psoriasis
Nail involvement is extremely common in psoriasis and may be the only manifestation of the disease. Pitting is the most common finding in nail psoriasis. Onycholysis and the appearance of an oil drop under the nail (the oil drop sign) also are common. Other findings include subungual hyperkeratosis, thickening of the nail plate, and splinter hemorrhages. A diagnosis of nail psoriasis should alert the clinician to search for psoriatic arthritis because there is an association between the two conditions.

Nail psoriasis is difficult to treat. The first-line treatment is with topical steroids and/or calcipotriol. Systemic therapy with methotrexate, cyclosporine, or biologic agents is effective but reserved for patients with moderate to severe skin involvement.[12-14]

Lichen Planus
Lichen planus of the nail appears as nail thinning, ridging, and fissuring. Severe lichen planus can progress to pterygium formation. Because lichen planus can lead to permanent scarring of the nail matrix and total loss of the nail unit, prompt treatment is essential. The diagnosis is based on the clinical appearance and involvement of skin, scalp, and mucosa. The treatment involves the use of topical, intralesional, or systemic steroids, depending on the severity of the condition and the response to treatment.[15]

Tumors
Subungual Exostosis
Subungual exostosis is the most common benign bony proliferation associated with nail abnormalities, and it is histologically similar to an osteochondroma. Type I, which typically occurs in women age 20 to 40 years, appears as an outgrowth on the dorsomedial phalanx and causes pain and shoe wear difficulty. Type II appears in older women on the distal aspect of the hallux as an elevation of the tip of the nail. The patient has pain with palpation of the distal nail plate. The diagnosis is confirmed with radiographs. The surgical treatment is resection of the exostosis, approached through the nail bed or the tip of the toe. Recurrence of the exostosis is associated with inadequate resection or perforation of the nail bed.[16]

Glomus Tumor
A glomus tumor arises from the neuromyoarterial glomus cells of the nail bed. It appears as a red-blue macule and characteristically is severely painful. The pain is exacerbated by pressure and cold. Although glomus tumors are benign, the symptoms often require them to be surgically excised.[1]

Melanoma
Nail melanoma is rare, accounting for 0.7% to 3.5% of all melanomas. In 25% of patients the tumor is amelanotic, and as a result the diagnosis is delayed. A pigmented nail melanoma most commonly is characterized by longitudinal melanonychia. Pigment encroaching on the proximal nail fold (the Hutchinson sign) should raise suspicion of a nail melanoma but is not pathognomonic for the disease. The diagnosis is based on histologic examination of the involved area. The treatment is surgical, but there is controversy regarding the margins of resection. Patients should be referred to a melanoma specialist for staging and therapy.[1]

Ingrown Toenail
An ingrown toenail, also called onychocryptosis, occurs when the nail plate grows into the lateral nail folds, causing pain as well as secondary infection and possibly the development of hypergranulation tissue. The hallux is the most commonly affected toe, and congenital malalignment of the hallux may play a role. Ingrown toenail is most common in young adults. The precipitating factors include improper or aggressive nail cutting, ill-fitting shoes, and trauma. The preferred treatment of an ingrown toenail is removal of the embedded spicule and maintenance of proper nail length. Partial or total nail avulsion may be required for a severely ingrown toenail, accompanied by partial or total matricectomy. Matricectomy can be done by chemical or surgical means. Oral antibiotics should be administered to treat a secondary bacterial infection.[17,18]

Skin Disorders

Infectious Conditions
Tinea Pedis
The foot is the most common site of fungal infections. The most important factors in the development of tinea pedis are the lack of sebaceous glands in the foot and the wearing of occlusive shoes[19] (**Figure 2**). Tinea pedis has four clinical types: moccasin, interdigital, inflammatory, and ulcerative. Bacterial superinfection, cellulitis, and osteomyelitis are possible complications of untreated tinea pedis.

A patient with tinea pedis should be examined for concurrent onychomycosis because untreated onychomycosis can serve as a nidus for recurrent tinea pedis infection. The most common dermatophytes are *T rubrum* and *T mentagrophytes*. The diagnosis is based on the presence of fungal elements on potassium hydroxide examination of skin scrapings. Ideally, fungal cultures should guide the choice of therapeutic options. Topical therapy with antifungal agents may be sufficient for most

5: Special Problems of the Foot and Ankle

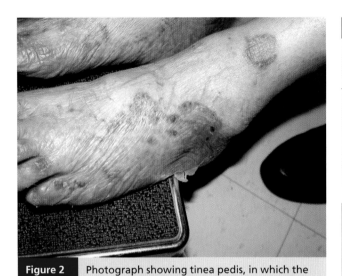

| Figure 2 | Photograph showing tinea pedis, in which the active border and annular configuration of the plaques can be seen. (Courtesy of Scott Walsh, MD, Toronto, Ontario, Canada.) |

infections. Options include topical azoles, terbinafine cream, ciclopirox gel, and newer agents such as naftifine gel.[20] Systemic therapy should be considered in patients who have diabetes, are immunocompromised, or have moccasin-type tinea pedis. The oral therapeutic options for tinea pedis are listed in Table 3.

Plantar Warts

Plantar warts are caused by the human papilloma virus. Warts appear as hyperkeratotic papules, often with the punctate black dots representing thrombosed capillaries and pinpoint bleeding. Multiple warts sometimes coalesce to form a large plaque called a mosaic wart.

Plantar warts are extremely resistant to therapy. There is no specific antiviral treatment for the human papilloma virus. The goal of treatment is to destroy and remove infected skin cells. The warts are benign and often self-limiting, and aggressive treatment, especially treatment that causes scarring and severe pain, is unnecessary. Several options are available for destroying infected tissue, including the use of salicylic acid, cryotherapy, surgical curettage, laser surgery, and electrosurgery. Salicylic acid was found to be a safe and effective treatment; other modalities including cryotherapy and surgical therapies were not found to be superior.[21] The nonsurgical treatment options for recalcitrant warts include topical imiquimod, intralesional bleomycin, and immunotherapy.

Inflammatory Conditions

Psoriasis

Psoriasis of the foot can be nonpustular or pustular. Nonpustular psoriasis often appears as red, sharply demarcated, scaly plaques that can lead to significant keratoderma.

Table 3

Oral Drugs for Treating Tinea Pedis

Drug	Dosage	Duration
Terbinafine	250 mg once daily	2 weeks
Itraconazole	200 mg twice daily	1 week
	100 mg once daily	2–4 weeks
Fluconazole	150 mg once weekly	2–4 weeks

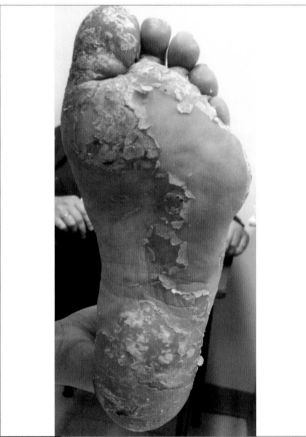

| Figure 3 | Photograph showing pustular psoriasis on the plantar surface of the foot. |

In pustular psoriasis, multiple small, superficial pustules may coalesce to form lakes of pus (Figure 3). Psoriasis must be differentiated from tinea pedis and dermatitis. Culturing can be done to rule out fungal infection. Examining the scalp, elbows, knees, umbilicus, or nails for psoriasis can be helpful in the diagnosis.

Psoriasis of the foot is debilitating and greatly diminishes the patient's quality of life. The treatment depends on the severity of the disease, and referral to a dermatologist is recommended.

Contact Dermatitis

Contact dermatitis appears as chronic scaly and pruritic plaques. The condition often is allergic in nature, and the distribution of the plaques corresponds to the sites of exposure to the allergen. The common allergens include preservatives in topical pharmaceuticals and materials used in shoes such as leather, rubber, and adhesives.[22] Occupational exposure to allergens also should be investigated. If contact dermatitis is suspected, the patient should be referred for patch testing. The mainstay of treatment is allergen avoidance, but topical steroids are helpful for resolving the inflammatory process.

Traumatic Conditions

Corns and Calluses

Corns and calluses are hyperkeratotic papules that develop as the skin's natural protective response to repeated mechanical injury at bony prominences and areas of constant friction. Although the resulting hyperkeratosis is completely benign and often physiologic, it can cause pressure and subsequent pain.

The treatment of corns and calluses consists of relief of symptoms and correction of the underlying predisposing condition. Pain relief can be achieved with the use of padding, an orthotic device, and chemical or mechanical callus paring. Surgical treatment of the underlying condition may involve correcting the mechanical alignment and excising the exostoses.[23]

Tache Noir

Tache noir (black heel) results from intraepidermal hemorrhage and appears as a black macule on a weight-bearing surface of the foot. The process is self-healing but can be disconcerting because of the color. The acuteness of the lesion and a history of trauma lead to the diagnosis. Melanoma is the most important differential diagnosis. Tache noir is common in athletes and probably occurs when the shearing forces produced by sudden stopping cause dermal blood vessels to rupture and leak blood into the epidermis.[24]

Melanoma of the Foot

Melanomas of the foot are rare and comprise only about 3% of all melanomas. Although rare, melanomas often present late and are very challenging to treat. In a recent review, acral lentiginous melanomas represented approximately one-half of all foot melanomas.[25,26] Perhaps because foot melanomas present later and other genetic or intrinsic factors play a role in the pathogenesis, the prognosis of foot melanomas is worse than melanomas in other cutaneous sites. Thicker melanomas, male sex, and amelanosis are associated with poorer survival rates.[27]

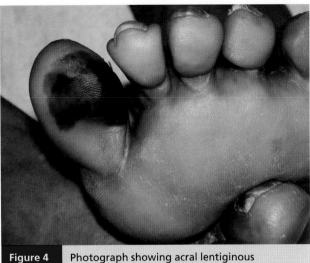

Figure 4 Photograph showing acral lentiginous melanoma. The variegated color and indistinct borders can be seen. (Courtesy of Scott Walsh, MD, Toronto, Ontario, Canada.)

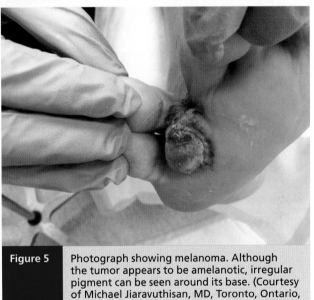

Figure 5 Photograph showing melanoma. Although the tumor appears to be amelanotic, irregular pigment can be seen around its base. (Courtesy of Michael Jiaravuthisan, MD, Toronto, Ontario, Canada.)

Melanomas on the foot can present as pigmented lesions but, as already mentioned, amelanosis is not uncommon. Any changing pigmented lesion on the foot or any tumor that is bleeding, ulcerated, or rapidly changing should be biopsied for histopathological diagnosis. Because the treatment of melanomas is dependent on the thickness of the lesion, it is best to excise a lesion to ensure adequate depth. If this is not feasible, an incisional biopsy may be acceptable, again ensuring that it is taken at an adequate depth (**Figures 4** and **5**).

Summary

Diseases of the nails and skin of the foot can be traumatic, infectious, or inflammatory in origin. These conditions can cause significant morbidity and can affect the patient's quality of life. Melanoma is one such disease that can be fatal. Prompt diagnosis and treatment are essential, and appropriate referral is helpful.

Annotated References

1. Bolognia JL, Rapini RP, Jorizzo JL: *Dermatology.* Philadelphia, PA, Mosby, 2003.

2. Kensinger DR, Guille JT, Horn BD, Herman MJ: The stubbed great toe: Importance of early recognition and treatment of open fractures of the distal phalanx. *J Pediatr Orthop* 2001;21(1):31-34.

3. Inglefield CJ, D'Arcangelo M, Kolhe PS: Injuries to the nail bed in childhood. *J Hand Surg Br* 1995;20(2):258-261.

4. Miranda BH, Vokshi I, Milroy CJ: Pediatric nailbed repair study: Nail replacement increases morbidity. *Plast Reconstr Surg* 2012;129(2):394e-396e.

   This retrospective study reviews 111 patients with traumatic nail bed injuries, assessing rates of complication in patients where the nail plate is replaced versus those where the nail plate is discarded. Overall complications occurred more frequently in the nail replacement group. Complications included delayed wound healing, infection, persistent pain, and overgranulation.

5. Elewski BE, Hazen PG: The superficial mycoses and the dermatophytes. *J Am Acad Dermatol* 1989;21(4 Pt 1):655-673.

6. Evans EG, Sigurgeirsson B; The LION Study Group: Double blind, randomised study of continuous terbinafine compared with intermittent itraconazole in treatment of toenail onychomycosis. *BMJ* 1999;318(7190):1031-1035.

7. Havu V, Heikkilä H, Kuokkanen K, et al: A double-blind, randomized study to compare the efficacy and safety of terbinafine (Lamisil) with fluconazole (Diflucan) in the treatment of onychomycosis. *Br J Dermatol* 2000;142(1):97-102.

8. Warshaw EM, Fett DD, Bloomfield HE, et al: Pulse versus continuous terbinafine for onychomycosis: A randomized, double-blind, controlled trial. *J Am Acad Dermatol* 2005;53(4):578-584.

9. Sigurgeirsson B, Elewski BE, Rich PA, et al: Intermittent versus continuous terbinafine in the treatment of toenail onychomycosis: A randomized, double-blind comparison. *J Dermatolog Treat* 2006;17(1):38-44.

10. Grover C, Bansal S, Nanda S, Reddy BS, Kumar V: Combination of surgical avulsion and topical therapy for single nail onychomycosis: A randomized controlled trial. *Br J Dermatol* 2007;157(2):364-368.

11. Elewski BE, Rich P, Pollak R, et al: Efinaconazole 10% solution in the treatment of toenail onychomycosis: Two phase III multicenter, randomized, double-blind studies. *J Am Acad Dermatol* 2013;68(4):600-608.

    This placebo-controlled randomized trial shows higher mycologic cure rates for efinaconazole 10% solution compared to placebo in the treatment of distal lateral subungual onychomycosis. Treatment success with efinaconazole ranged from 17% to 45% versus 5% to 17% for placebo.

12. de Berker D: Management of nail psoriasis. *Clin Exp Dermatol* 2000;25(5):357-362.

13. Jiaravuthisan MM, Sasseville D, Vender RB, Murphy F, Muhn CY: Psoriasis of the nail: Anatomy, pathology, clinical presentation, and a review of the literature on therapy. *J Am Acad Dermatol* 2007;57(1):1-27.

14. Paul C, Reich K, Gottlieb AB, et al; the CAIN457A2211 study group: Secukinumab improves hand, foot and nail lesions in moderate-to-severe plaque psoriasis: Subanalysis of a randomized, double-blind, placebo-controlled, regimen-finding phase 2 trial. *J Eur Acad Dermatol Venereol* 2014; Jan 7 [Epub ahead of print].

    This subgroup analysis of a randomized controlled trial in moderate to severe psoriasis shows substantial improvement in nail psoriasis as compared to placebo. These results are congruent with efficacy for psoriasis of the hands and feet as well.

15. Tosti A, Peluso AM, Fanti PA, Piraccini BM: Nail lichen planus: Clinical and pathologic study of twenty-four patients. *J Am Acad Dermatol* 1993;28(5 Pt 1):724-730.

16. Lemont H, Christman RA: Subungual exostosis and nail disease and radiologic aspects, in Sher RK, Daniel CR, eds: *Nails: Therapy, Diagnosis, Surgery,* ed 2. Philadelphia, PA, WB Saunders, 1997.

17. de Berker DA: Phenolic ablation of the nail matrix. *Australas J Dermatol* 2001;42(1):59-61.

18. Ikard RW: Onychocryptosis. *J Am Coll Surg* 1998;187(1):96-102.

19. Leyden JJ, Aly R: Tinea pedis. *Semin Dermatol* 1993;12(4):280-284.

20. Stein Gold LF, Parish LC, Vlahovic T, et al: Efficacy and safety of naftifine HCl Gel 2% in the treatment of interdigital and moccasin type tinea pedis: Pooled results from two multicenter, randomized, double-blind, vehicle-controlled trials. *J Drugs Dermatol* 2013;12(8):911-918.

This study shows that nafitifine gel 2% once daily for 2 weeks provides mycologic and clinical cure for interdigital and moccasin-type tinea pedis. Results are evident as early as 2 weeks, but highest response rates were observed 4 weeks after treatment.

21. Gibbs S, Harvey I, Sterling JC, Stark R: Local treatments for cutaneous warts. *Cochrane Database Syst Rev* 2003;3:CD001781.

22. Landeck L, Uter W, John SM: Patch test characteristics of patients referred for suspected contact allergy of the feet—retrospective 10-year cross-sectional study of the IVDK data. *Contact Dermatitis* 2012;66(5):271-278.

   This cross-sectional study of 2,671 patients who underwent patch testing for suspected contact dermatitis of the feet showed that potassium dichromate, colophony and p-tert-butylphenol-formaldehyde resin were the most common allergens.

23. Singh D, Bentley G, Trevino SG: Callosities, corns, and calluses. *BMJ* 1996;312(7043):1403-1406.

24. Wilkinson DS: Black heel: A minor hazard of sport. *Cutis* 1977;20(3):393-396.

25. Rashid OM, Schaum JC, Wolfe LG, Brinster NK, Neifeld JP: Prognostic variables and surgical management of foot melanoma: Review of a 25-year institutional experience. *ISRN Dermatol* 2011;2011:384729.

   This is a retrospective review of 46 patients with foot melanomas treated from 1985-2010. The age of diagnosis was 16 to 99 years, with a median of 62 years. This study describes subtypes, pathologic variants, site of origin, and treatment for these patients.

26. Durbec F, Martin L, Derancourt C, Grange F: Melanoma of the hand and foot: Epidemiological, prognostic and genetic features. A systematic review. *Br J Dermatol* 2012;166(4):727-739.

   This systematic review includes 37 articles on melanomas of the hand and foot. The review states that acral lentiginous melanomas represent half of all melanomas. The review also suggests that previous trauma and nevi may be risk factors. The prognosis of hand and foot melanoma is thought to be poorer than melanomas on other sites.

27. Phan A, Touzet S, Dalle S, Ronger-Savlé S, Balme B, Thomas L: Acral lentiginous melanoma: A clinicoprognostic study of 126 cases. *Br J Dermatol* 2006;155(3):561-569.

5: Special Problems of the Foot and Ankle

Chapter 21

Amputations of the Foot and Ankle

G. Alexander Simpson, DO   Terrence M. Philbin, DO

Introduction

Amputations of the foot and ankle have been described for many centuries. In the United States, the most common reasons for foot and ankle amputation include complications of diabetes and vascular disease; more than 60% of nontraumatic lower limb amputations are in patients with diabetes. More than 6% of patients older than 60 years have symptoms of peripheral artery disease. Furthermore, the incidence of lower limb amputation is five to ten times greater than those patients without diabetes.[1,2] Other reasons for amputation of the foot and ankle include severe trauma, chronic pain, infection, congenital abnormality, and malignancy.

The purpose of amputation can be defined in terms of restoring the function of a nonfunctioning or nonviable limb. Amputation should be considered the first step in a patient's rehabilitation, rather than a failure of treatment.[3,4] The goals of every amputation are to obtain wound healing, avoid infection, and return a patient to his or her preamputation ambulatory level. Additional goals include adequate balancing of the

Table 1

Tests Predicting Wound Healing After Lower Extremity Amputation

Test	Positive Predictor
Serum albumin level	> 2.5 g/dL
Total lymphocyte count	> 1,500/μL
Transcutaneous oxygen pressure	20–30 mm Hg
Ultrasound Doppler ankle-brachial index	> 0.5

remaining muscles to avoid contracture formation and retain residual limb control.[5] Amputations of the foot and ankle range from simple phalangeal amputation to midfoot or hindfoot amputation, ankle disarticulation, and transtibial amputation. Amputation of the midfoot and hindfoot can preserve ambulation and thereby decrease patient morbidity.[6]

Preoperative Management

Many patients in need of an amputation have multiple medical comorbidities, such as diabetes and vascular disease. The preoperative evaluation is extremely important to a good outcome. The extremity should be evaluated for color, temperature, pulses, sensation, and tissue quality. Any contributing factor such as malunion or equinus contracture should be detected preoperatively, if possible. Radiographs and advanced imaging studies should be ordered to evaluate the bony structure and determine the extent of any underlying osteomyelitis. The evaluation should include the patient's functional ability, social environment, nutritional and immune status, and mental state. A thorough preoperative evaluation including laboratory and vascular studies helps determine the patient's potential for wound healing. The predictors of wound healing include serum albumin level, total lymphocyte count, transcutaneous oxygen pressure, and ankle-brachial index[7,8] (Table 1).

A well-organized multidisciplinary team must care for a patient undergoing an amputation. The medical specialists include an orthopaedic surgeon, a vascular surgeon, a medical doctor, physical therapists, a social worker, a physiatrist, and a mental health professional. The patient should feel a rapport with the medical specialists. A psychiatric evaluation is important before surgery because an amputation is a life-changing event.[9] The surgeon must be well versed in surgical technique, postoperative treatment, prosthetics, and footwear modification.

Indications for Amputation

Vascular Disease and Diabetes

The indications for an amputation may be multiple and multifactorial. The combination of peripheral vascular disease and diabetes results in dysvascularity, and severe infection of the foot and ankle with sepsis may ensue. Patients at high risk of dysvascularity represent an important target group for systematic efforts to reduce the number of foot and ankle amputations.[10] The most prominent subgroup is composed of patients who are African American, have diabetes, and live in a region with inadequate vascular care. In the population age 45 years or older, the incidence of vascular lower extremity amputation at or proximal to the transmetatarsal level is eight times higher in people who have diabetes than in those who do not have diabetes. One in four patients who undergo amputation may require a contralateral amputation and/or reamputation at a higher level.[11] During the past decade, the use of lower extremity amputation declined markedly in the Medicare population, and there was an increase in the nonsurgical care of diabetic ulcers.[12-14] However, patients with diabetes in the Medicare population had an increasing incidence of amputation at a distal, limb-conserving location.[14] Patients with poorly controlled diabetes were more likely than other patients with diabetes to undergo amputation rather than limb-salvage techniques.[15,16] Limb salvage was found to represent a greater cost burden than amputation in patients with diabetes who were diagnosed with severe Charcot foot deformity.[17]

Trauma

Approximately 16% of amputations in the United States are necessitated by a traumatic etiology. Traditional injury severity scores do not predict the need for amputation after trauma.[18] Despite the relatively low proportion of amputations performed after trauma, individuals with a traumatic amputation account for almost 45% of the estimated 1.6 million living people with an amputation.[5] Patients who undergo a traumatic amputation frequently have complications as well as chronic pain and a relatively low likelihood of returning to work.[19,20] Wartime blast injuries have resulted in a focus on amputation-related care

after military trauma. US service personnel increasingly have sustained complex blast injuries that affect limb tissue availability and limit reconstruction efforts.[21,22] Patients undergoing amputation after combat trauma were found to have better function and fewer psychologic symptoms than those undergoing limb salvage surgery.[23,24] Regardless of treatment, however, high levels of morbidity are associated with the effects of combat warfare.[25]

Malignancy

Amputation once was the treatment of choice for a malignant bone tumor, but reconstruction is used increasingly as a result of advances in radiography, pharmacology, and surgery.[26] If amputation is needed, the primary consideration is to fully excise the malignancy while diminishing the risk of local recurrence and increasing the likelihood of patient survival.[26]

Level of Amputation

The functional goal of an amputation is to maintain the greatest possible residual limb length for the purpose of allowing maximal function to be restored.[27] The patient's mobility and functional independence should be maintained to the greatest extent possible. Because the level of amputation will affect the amount of energy the patient must expend, maintaining maximal limb length is important.[27,28] The overall length of the residual limb is affected by the preoperative condition of the limb, the associated pathology, and general intraoperative findings. Coverage of residual osseous structures is important to prevent tissue breakdown; therefore, it is important to maintain thick myocutaneous flap coverage. After blast trauma, the level of amputation is greatly affected by the amount of residual tissue available for wound closure.[29]

An amputation can be performed through a joint (a disarticulation) or through bone (a transosseus amputation). A disarticulation is end bearing; loads are directly transmitted through the joint surface and metaphyseal bone. Compared with a disarticulation, a transosseous amputation has a smaller residual cross-sectional area, through which the weight is transferred indirectly. After a transosseous amputation, load transfer is through the entire limb from a total-contact prosthesis.[30]

Depending on the level of amputation, the energy required for ambulation differs dramatically. Children who have undergone a Syme, transtibial, or bilateral transtibial amputation do not have an increased energy cost of walking, however, and are able to walk at speeds similar to those of their peers.[31]

Types of Amputations

Toe Amputation
Great Toe Amputation
Great toe amputation may be indicated for pathology of the distal aspect of the hallux or a chronic condition of the nail plate. The benefits of this amputation over a disarticulation of the metatarsophalangeal joint include maintenance of the plantar flexion mechanism of the first ray and some preservation of the weight-bearing function of the hallux, which decreases the transfer stress of the adjacent rays. It is important to preserve at least 1 cm of the proximal phalangeal base during a great toe amputation.[32]

Metatarsophalangeal Disarticulation
If the entire great toe is affected by poor vascularity or infection, metatarsophalangeal disarticulation may be indicated to resect the entire phalanx. Several technical aspects of metatarsophalangeal joint disarticulation are important. Adequate viable soft-tissue flaps must be maintained and be capable of being closed without tension. The patient must be monitored for wound complications after surgery. When the wound has healed, the patient should be fitted with an orthotic device that prevents undue pressure on the residual first ray.[32]

Lesser Toe Amputation
Amputation of a lesser toe may be necessary because of ischemia or an infection such as osteomyelitis (**Figure 1**). A disarticulation from the metatarsophalangeal joint or a proximal phalanx resection can be performed. Maintenance of adequate flaps is important to decrease the risk of wound complications. After amputation, the patient may have adjacent toe drift or dorsal drift of the remaining phalangeal stump.

Ray Resection
Ray resection is an amputation of a toe with its corresponding metatarsal. Indications for ray amputation are osteomyelitis of a toe/metatarsal, as occurs in many patients with a plantar foot ulcer. The resection can affect one or more border or central rays. A border ray resection is the easiest to perform, with the use of a direct medial or lateral incision for the first or fifth ray, respectively (**Figure 2**). Care must be taken during a border ray amputation to allow for adequate flap closure, which decreases the risk of wound complications.[32] Ray resections maintain foot length, and patients have good function with the aid of a shoe filler or custom insert.

A central ray resection, affecting the second, third, or fourth ray, is less often indicated than a border ray amputation. Closing the initial central ray incision is

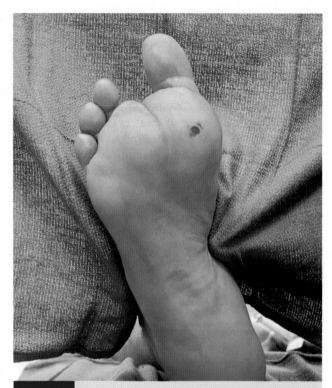

Figure 1   Photograph showing a lesser toe amputation.

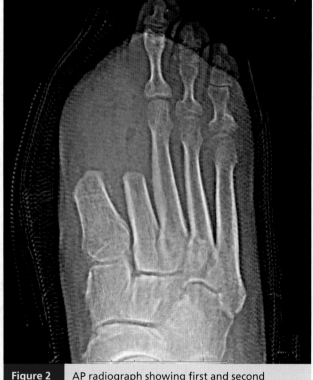

Figure 2   AP radiograph showing first and second (border and central) ray resections.

challenging and should be performed by using as much of the original skin flap as possible.

Multiple ray amputation may be necessary in patients who have a traumatic injury, diabetes, or vascular disease. A transmetatarsal amputation may be indicated if three rays are nonviable.[32] A medial-side amputation can result in the development of transfer lesions and loss of balance. To promote wound healing, as much of the flap length as possible should be maintained. Postoperative shoe wear modification is important for proper balance and foot propulsion.

Transmetatarsal Amputation

Transmetatarsal amputation is indicated if the patient has a severe infection, traumatic injury, deformity, or vascular disease in the forefoot (**Figure 3**). A transmetatarsal amputation may be of any length, but shoe wear is better accommodated with a relatively long residual limb. A short residual limb may heal more successfully, however. The advantages of a transmetatarsal amputation are that it is less technically demanding than other hindfoot amputations, and it preserves ambulation.[33] A transmetatarsal amputation preserves the attachment of the ankle dorsiflexors and plantar flexors. Most patients can wear regular shoes with the addition of a custom insert to fill the shoe. Wound complications and ulcerations can occur after a transmetatarsal amputation because of recurrent equinus contractures, which can be corrected by a gastrocnemius or Achilles tendon release.

Midfoot Amputation

Lisfranc Amputation

The Lisfranc amputation, named after a surgeon in the French army of Napoleon, is a disarticulation of the tarsometatarsal joint. After a Lisfranc amputation, the pull of the gastrocnemius-soleus complex and the tibialis posterior may result in an equinus contracture. Therefore, it is important to restore muscle balance by maintaining the attachment of the tibialis anterior and the peroneus brevis.

Chopart Amputation

The Chopart amputation, named after a French surgeon of the late 1700s, involves a disarticulation of the talonavicular and calcaneocuboid joints.[34] In comparison with other hindfoot and transtibial amputations, the Chopart amputation has several benefits, the most important of which is that it retains the heel pad tissues to allow weight bearing through the amputated residual limb. The patient can be fitted for an ankle-foot orthosis rather than a below-knee prosthesis. In addition, the technique is less technically demanding than that of other amputations. The limitations of the Chopart amputation include the risk of equinus contractures and residual limb ulceration.

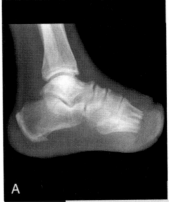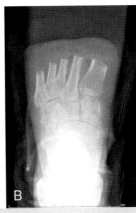

Figure 3 Lateral (**A**) and AP (**B**) radiographs showing a transmetatarsal amputation.

It is important that the ankle dorsiflexors and plantar flexors be repositioned and that the Achilles tendon be released.

Hindfoot Amputation

Pirogoff Amputation

In the Pirogoff amputation, as originally described in Russia, the forefoot, midfoot, talus, distal part of the calcaneus, and distal tibial articular cartilage are removed. The plantar skin flap is left attached to the calcaneus, which is rotated 90° dorsally to create a sensate weight-bearing surface with minimal loss of leg length (usually less than 5 cm).[35] Because of the risk of wound failure, infection, or nonunion of the tibiocalcaneal arthrodesis, the Pirogoff amputation is rarely used for limb salvage. The use of the Ilizarov external frame has resulted in a better rate of fusion while allowing immediate weight bearing.[36]

Boyd Amputation

In a Boyd amputation, the forefoot, midfoot, and a portion of the hindfoot are removed, with maintenance of the calcaneus. The talus is removed, and the calcaneus is shaped to articulate with the ankle mortise. The articular surfaces of the tibial plafond, malleoli, and calcaneus are débrided to achieve a fusion of the calcaneus to the tibial plafond. Achieving a successful fusion is the most difficult challenge of this amputation.[37]

Syme Amputation

The Syme amputation is a disarticulation of the ankle joint, in which the calcaneus and talus are removed. The Syme amputation allows weight bearing by the distal tibia through the preserved heel pad and heel skin. The residual limb is longer than in a transtibial amputation, and as a result, ambulation requires a lower expenditure of energy. The complications include wound-healing difficulty,

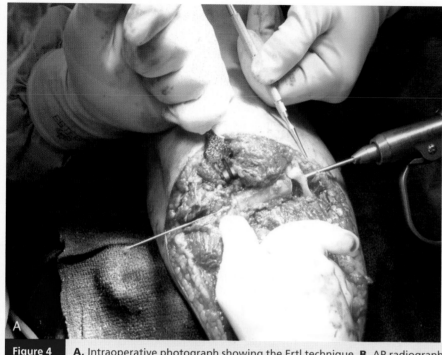
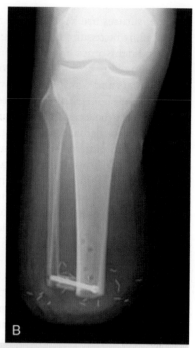

Figure 4   **A,** Intraoperative photograph showing the Ertl technique. **B,** AP radiograph showing an Ertl amputation.

especially in a dysvascular heel pad, and pressure ulcerations from the residual malleoli of the distal tibia.

Transtibial Amputation

Transtibial (below-knee) amputation is commonly performed if the foot and ankle cannot be preserved. Often this amputation is necessary in patients with diabetes who have an infected, dysvascular lower extremity. Although partial foot amputation is more durable than transtibial amputation, it may not be an option in a patient with diabetes because of osteomyelitis of the hindfoot.[6,38] A crush or penetrating injury also can result in the need for a transtibial amputation.

As with any amputation, the surgeon must maintain the longest possible residual limb. The traditional residual limb length is 12.5 to 17.5 cm below the knee joint. In a complex injury, such as a blast injury as sustained during military combat, it may not be possible to achieve the desired residual limb length. The Ertl technique, described in 1949, is a modification of the traditional transtibial amputation designed to decrease pain and difficulty with ambulation after transtibial amputation, as caused by movement of the remaining distal tibia and fibula during direct load bearing[39] (**Figure 4**). By increasing direct end bearing, the Ertl technique results in an improved functional outcome in young, active patients.[30,40] The original bone-bridging Ertl amputation required a corticoperiosteal flap. Most subsequent modifications use a fibular strut graft with preserved muscle attachments to create the synostosis. These methods collectively are known as modified Ertl amputations or simply bone-bridging or bridging-synostosis amputations.[41]

Patients who underwent a modified transtibial amputation were found to have a substantially higher rate of return to work, a lower rate of revision, and substantially higher physical and psychosocial outcome scores than patients who underwent a traditional transtibial amputation.[42] Noninfectious complications were found to result in a higher rate of reoperation after the Ertl amputation than after the modified Burgess amputation, in which the posterior myocutaneous flap is transferred anteriorly, covering the residual bony limb.[25] In patients with a combat injury, no evidence was found to support the belief that bone bridging contributes to a more efficient platform in the total surface-bearing socket.[43]

The common complications of transtibial amputation include wound infection and neuroma formation. Heterotopic ossification, nonunion, or hardware failure also can occur after bone-bridging synostosis.[44]

Postoperative Care

The postoperative treatment goals of amputation are to promote wound healing, decrease pain, decrease contracture, control edema and swelling, and obtain a well-fitting prosthesis. The residual limb often is wrapped in a compression dressing to decrease swelling. The incision is kept dry, and the dressing is frequently changed. On average, sutures are kept for 2 to 3 weeks, but a longer period many be required if swelling has increased the risk of wound dehiscence.

An immediate postoperative prosthesis can be used in some patients and was found to have psychologic benefits and to lower the overall cost of treatment, the reoperation rate, and the length of hospital stay.[45] Despite these advantages, immediate postoperative prostheses are not widely used in patients with a traumatic injury because of expense and time requirements, the need for adequate wound healing and early detection of infection, and the presence of associated injuries that can preclude early mobilization.[5] Weight bearing often is delayed until the incision is healed. After bone-bridging synostosis, full weight bearing is delayed until the bone has healed, typically at 10 to 12 weeks.

Rehabilitation begins when the wound is healed and the patient is able to bear weight. A team approach is used. The overall goal is achieve maximal function, and the specific goals commonly include functional, pain-free ambulation; a return to work; a decrease in psychosocial stress, and the elimination of pain.[46,47] After combat trauma, patients with amputation were found to have a better rehabilitation outcome than those who underwent limb salvage surgery.[46]

The patient's pain may be difficult to control after amputation and can cause long-term dysfunction. The patient may have residual limb pain, back or hip pain, or phantom pain. Reduction in the intensity of acute residual limb pain appears to allow the central nervous system to lessen the memory of the pain and the likelihood of phantom pain.[48] An increased level of activity also can decrease phantom pain. The tools for pain management include medications and implantable pain control devices. Pain control after a traumatic amputation is achieved through a multimodal approach.[48,49]

Summary

Amputation of the foot and ankle often is required to treat infection caused by ischemia in patients with diabetes and peripheral vascular disease. The treatment of patients with traumatic injury, especially combat-related injury, is particularly challenging. Patients must undergo a thorough multidisciplinary evaluation before amputation and be optimally prepared for the procedure. The surgeon must be diligent in deciding how maximal function can be obtained. The different levels of amputation require different surgical techniques, which continue to advance. After the amputation, a team approach is used to help the patient reach functional and pain control goals.

Annotated References

1. Norgren L, Hiatt WR, Dormandy JA, et al; TASC II Working Group: Inter-society consensus for the management of peripheral arterial disease (TASC II). *Eur J Vasc Endovasc Surg* 2007;33(Suppl 1):S1-S75.

2. Centers for Disease Control and Prevention: *National Diabetes Fact Sheet: National Estimates and General Information on Diabetes and Pre-Diabetes in the United States, 2011.* Atlanta, GA, US Department of Health and Human Services, Centers for Disease Control and Prevention, 2011.

   Information on diabetes in the United States was summarized.

3. Pinzur MS, Beck J, Himes R, Callaci J: Distal tibiofibular bone-bridging in transtibial amputation. *J Bone Joint Surg Am* 2008;90(12):2682-2687.

   Patients treated with distal tibiofibular bone bridging did not appear to have better outcomes than patients treated with standard transtibial amputation. More information is needed before the bone-bridging technique can be recommended for standard transtibial amputation surgery. Level of evidence: III.

4. Ng VY, Berlet GC: Evolving techniques in foot and ankle amputation. *J Am Acad Orthop Surg* 2010;18(4):223-235.

   Foot and ankle amputation techniques were reviewed. Level of evidence: V.

5. Tintle SM, Keeling JJ, Forsberg JA, Shawen SB, Andersen RC, Potter BK: Operative complications of combat-related transtibial amputations: A comparison of the modified Burgess and modified Ertl tibiofibular synostosis techniques. *J Bone Joint Surg Am* 2011;93(11):1016-1021.

   A retrospective review of combat-related amputations found that reoperation was needed at a significantly higher rate overall and to treat noninfectious complications after modified Ertl bone-bridging synostosis compared with modified Burgess transtibial amputation. Level of evidence: III.

6. Brown ML, Tang W, Patel A, Baumhauer JF: Partial foot amputation in patients with diabetic foot ulcers. *Foot Ankle Int* 2012;33(9):707-716.

   Longevity, outcome, and mortality after partial foot amputation were examined. The high ambulatory levels and the long durability of transmetatarsal and Chopart amputations suggest these amputations provide an ambulatory advantage over transtibial amputation. Level of evidence: III.

7. Pinzur MS, Pinto MA, Schon LC, Smith DG: Controversies in amputation surgery. *Instr Course Lect* 2003;52:445-451.

8. Bunt TJ, Holloway GA: TcPO2 as an accurate predictor of therapy in limb salvage. *Ann Vasc Surg* 1996;10(3):224-227.

9. Boutoille D, Féraille A, Maulaz D, Krempf M: Quality of life with diabetes-associated foot complications: Comparison between lower-limb amputation and chronic foot ulceration. *Foot Ankle Int* 2008;29(11):1074-1078.

    An improved understanding of the consequences of diabetic foot complications would benefit the general population and general practitioners in particular. Psychologic evaluation and support are important before and after amputation. Level of evidence: III.

10. Goodney PP, Holman K, Henke PK, et al: Regional intensity of vascular care and lower extremity amputation rates. *J Vasc Surg* 2013;57(6):1471-1479.

    The intensity of vascular care provided to patients at risk for amputation varies. Regions with the most intensive vascular care have the lowest amputation rates. Level of evidence: IV.

11. Johannesson A, Larsson GU, Ramstrand N, Turkiewicz A, Wiréhn AB, Atroshi I: Incidence of lower-limb amputation in the diabetic and nondiabetic general population: A 10-year population-based cohort study of initial unilateral and contralateral amputations and reamputations. *Diabetes Care* 2009;32(2):275-280.

    Comparison of the incidence of vascular lower limb amputation in patients with or without diabetes found an eightfold greater incidence at or proximal to the transmetatarsal level in patients with diabetes age 45 years or older. Level of evidence: IV.

12. Shojaiefard A, Khorgami Z, Mohajeri-Tehrani MR, Larijani B: Large and deep diabetic heel ulcers need not lead to amputation. *Foot Ankle Int* 2013;34(2):215-221.

    A study of large, deep heel ulcers in 37 patients with diabetes found that 33 ulcers healed in 4 to 7 months. Transtibial amputation was performed on 4 feet. Patients with heel ulcers can be treated using a multidisciplinary approach to prevent amputation. Level of evidence: IV.

13. Kim BS, Choi WJ, Baek MK, Kim YS, Lee JW: Limb salvage in severe diabetic foot infection. *Foot Ankle Int* 2011;32(1):31-37.

    Forty-five septic feet in patients with diabetes were treated using negative pressure wound therapy between 2006 and 2008. With immediate evacuation of abscess, early vascular intervention, and appropriate débridement, this therapy is a useful adjunct to the management of limb-threatening diabetic foot infections. Level of evidence: IV.

14. Belatti DA, Phisitkul P: Declines in lower extremity amputation in the US Medicare population, 2000-2010. *Foot Ankle Int* 2013;34(7):923-931.

    A cost analysis found a marked decline over 10 years in the use of amputation in the Medicare population. Lower extremity amputation was more likely to be performed at distal, limb-conserving locations. Over the same period, orthopaedic treatment of ulcers increased in frequency.

15. Wukich DK, Hobizal KB, Brooks MM: Severity of diabetic foot infection and rate of limb salvage. *Foot Ankle Int* 2013;34(3):351-358.

    Patients with a severe diabetic infection had a median hospital stay 60% longer than patients with a moderate infection, and 55% of the patients with a severe infection required an amputation compared with 42% of patients with a moderate infection. Level of evidence: IV.

16. Younger AS, Awwad MA, Kalla TP, de Vries G: Risk factors for failure of transmetatarsal amputation in diabetic patients: A cohort study. *Foot Ankle Int* 2009;30(12):1177-1182.

    Glucose control was the primary factor determining the success of a transmetatarsal amputation. The glycohemoglobin value should be less than 8 as a prerequisite for surgery. Level of evidence: III.

17. Gil J, Schiff AP, Pinzur MS: Cost comparison: Limb salvage versus amputation in diabetic patients with Charcot foot. *Foot Ankle Int* 2013;34(8):1097-1099.

    Preliminary data on the relative cost of transtibial amputation and prosthetic limb fitting compared with limb salvage in 76 patients found that amputation was less costly than limb salvage. Level of evidence: IV.

18. Brown KV, Ramasamy A, McLeod J, Stapley S, Clasper JC: Predicting the need for early amputation in ballistic mangled extremity injuries. *J Trauma* 2009;66(suppl 4):S93-S97.

    Patients who had undergone amputation or limb salvage were retrospectively evaluated with the Mangled Extremity Severity Score for lower extremity trauma. This system was not helpful for deciding whether amputation was appropriate.

19. Ferreira RC, Sakata MA, Costa MT, Frizzo GG, Santin RA: Long-term results of salvage surgery in severely injured feet. *Foot Ankle Int* 2010;31(2):113-123.

    Five years after severe foot injury, most patients had painful stiffness and only 40% had returned to work. The long-term clinical and functional outcomes after treatment of a severely injured foot may be disappointing. Level of evidence: IV.

20. Harris AM, Althausen PL, Kellam J, Bosse MJ, Castillo R; Lower Extremity Assessment Project (LEAP) Study Group: Complications following limb-threatening lower extremity trauma. *J Orthop Trauma* 2009;23(1):1-6.

    A review of 545 patients with lower extremity trauma found that patients with severe injury had a higher rate of complications, most notably infection, nonunion, wound necrosis, and osteomyelitis.

5: Special Problems of the Foot and Ankle

21. Ramasamy A, Hill AM, Masouros S, et al: Outcomes of IED foot and ankle blast injuries. *J Bone Joint Surg Am* 2013;95(5):e25.

    Of 63 soldiers with a blast injury to a total of 89 limbs, 32 (51%) had multisegmental injuries to the foot and ankle. Amputation of 26 legs (29%) was required. Improvised explosive devices were associated with a high amputation rate and a poor clinical outcome. Level of evidence: IV.

22. Fleming ME, Watson JT, Gaines RJ, O'Toole RV; Extremity War Injuries VII Reconstruction Panel: Evolution of orthopedic reconstructive care. *J Am Acad Orthop Surg* 2012;20(Suppl 1):S74-S79.

    Limb salvage after war-related injury is complex and challenging. Innovations have been developed for complex limb reconstruction and salvage.

23. Rispoli DM, Mackenzie EJ; Extremity War Injuries VII Outcomes Panel: Orthopaedic outcomes: Combat and civilian trauma care. *J Am Acad Orthop Surg* 2012;20(Suppl 1):S84-S87.

    Analysis of two studies determined that a multidisciplinary approach and treatment environment greatly influences patient function.

24. Doukas WC, Hayda RA, Frisch HM, et al: The Military Extremity Trauma Amputation/Limb Salvage (METALS) study: Outcomes of amputation versus limb salvage following major lower-extremity trauma. *J Bone Joint Surg Am* 2013;95(2):138-145.

    A retrospective review of 324 soldiers with lower extremity trauma found that those who underwent amputation had a better functional outcome than those who underwent limb salvage. Level of evidence: III.

25. MacKenzie EJ, Bosse MJ: Factors influencing outcome following limb-threatening lower limb trauma: Lessons learned from the Lower Extremity Assessment Project (LEAP). *J Am Acad Orthop Surg* 2006;14(10 Spec No.):S205-S210.

26. DiCaprio MR, Friedlaender GE: Malignant bone tumors: Limb sparing versus amputation. *J Am Acad Orthop Surg* 2003;11(1):25-37.

27. Pinzur MS, Gold J, Schwartz D, Gross N: Energy demands for walking in dysvascular amputees as related to the level of amputation. *Orthopedics* 1992;15(9):1033-1036, discussion 1036-1037.

28. Waters RL, Perry J, Antonelli D, Hislop H: Energy cost of walking of amputees: The influence of level of amputation. *J Bone Joint Surg Am* 1976;58(1):42-46.

29. Andersen RC, Swiontkowski MF: Perceived performance differences: Limb salvage versus amputation in the lower extremity. *J Am Acad Orthop Surg* 2011;19(Suppl 1):S20-S22.

Functional limitations resulting from loss of muscle needed to cover bone and provide limb function are a major factor in the decision to amputate a salvaged limb.

30. Pinzur MS, Gottschalk FA, Pinto MA, Smith DG; American Academy of Orthopaedic Surgeons: Controversies in lower-extremity amputation. *J Bone Joint Surg Am* 2007;89(5):1118-1127.

31. Jeans KA, Browne RH, Karol LA: Effect of amputation level on energy expenditure during overground walking by children with an amputation. *J Bone Joint Surg Am* 2011;93(1):49-56.

    Oxygen consumption was measured during overground walking in 73 children with an amputation at a variety of levels. Children with an amputation through the knee or distal to the knee were able to maintain a normal walking speed without substantially increasing their energy cost. Level of evidence: IV.

32. Brodsky J: Amputations of the foot and ankle, in Coughlin M, Mann R, Saltzman C, eds: *Surgery of the Foot and Ankle*, ed 8. Philadelphia, PA, Mosby Elsevier, 2007, pp 1369-1398.

33. Landry GJ, Silverman DA, Liem TK, Mitchell EL, Moneta GL: Predictors of healing and functional outcome following transmetatarsal amputations. *Arch Surg* 2011;146(9):1005-1009.

    Factors that predict healing, functional outcome, and survival were evaluated in 62 patients with a transmetatarsal amputation. Healing was found to significantly predict subsequent ambulatory status. Level of evidence: III.

34. Philbin TM, Berlet GC, Lee TH: Lower-extremity amputations in association with diabetes mellitus. *Foot Ankle Clin* 2006;11(4):791-804.

35. Taniguchi A, Tanaka Y, Kadono K, Inada Y, Takakura Y: Pirogoff ankle disarticulation as an option for ankle disarticulation. *Clin Orthop Relat Res* 2003;414:322-328.

36. Gessmann J, Citak M, Fehmer T, Schildhauer TA, Seybold D: Ilizarov external frame technique for Pirogoff amputations with ankle disarticulation and tibiocalcaneal fusion. *Foot Ankle Int* 2013;34(6):856-864.

    After 24 patients with infection and Charcot arthropathy underwent Pirogoff amputation with an Ilizarov external frame, 21 patients healed well, and 16 (67%) had a good or excellent functional result. The frame allowed immediate weight bearing and soft-tissue control. Level of evidence: IV.

37. Tosun B, Buluc L, Gok U, Unal C: Boyd amputation in adults. *Foot Ankle Int* 2011;32(11):1063-1068.

    Complete wound healing was documented in 7 of 15 feet in 14 patients after Boyd amputation. Revision to a more proximal amputation level was required in 7 feet. Boyd amputation is an option for preserving limb length. Level of evidence: IV.

38. Faglia E, Clerici G, Caminiti M, Curci V, Somalvico F: Influence of osteomyelitis location in the foot of diabetic patients with transtibial amputation. *Foot Ankle Int* 2013;34(2):222-227.

    The rate of transtibial amputation was higher if osteomyelitis involved the heel rather than the midfoot or forefoot in patients with diabetes. Level of evidence: III.

39. Taylor BC, Poka A: Osteomyoplastic transtibial amputation: Technique and tips. *J Orthop Surg Res* 2011;6:13.

    Distal bone-bridge creation and osteomyoplasty add time and potential morbidity to a transtibial amputation procedure but are intended to lead to a more functional and physiologic residual extremity.

40. Pinzur MS, Stuck RM, Sage R, Hunt N, Rabinovich Z: Syme ankle disarticulation in patients with diabetes. *J Bone Joint Surg Am* 2003;85(9):1667-1672.

41. Berlet GC, Pokabla C, Serynek P: An alternative technique for the Ertl osteomyoplasty. *Foot Ankle Int* 2009;30(5):443-446.

    In a modified Ertl technique, tightrope fixation can decrease time to union through compressive forces. Level of evidence: V.

42. Taylor BC, French B, Poka A, Blint A, Mehta S: Osteomyoplastic and traditional transtibial amputations in the trauma patient: Perioperative comparisons and outcomes. *Orthopedics* 2010;33(6):390.

    A retrospective comparison of 26 patients with transtibial amputation osteomyoplasty and 10 patients with traditional amputation after severe lower-extremity trauma found that amputation osteomyoplasty appeared to be safe and possibly was more beneficial than traditional amputation in terms of functional outcome.

43. Tucker CJ, Wilken JM, Stinner PD, Kirk KL: A comparison of limb-socket kinematics of bone-bridging and non-bone-bridging wartime transtibial amputations. *J Bone Joint Surg Am* 2012;94(10):924-930.

    No difference was found between surgical techniques with respect to bone-socket displacement. These data provided no evidence to support statements that bone bridging contributes to a more efficient platform in the total surface-bearing socket. Level of evidence: III.

44. Gwinn DE, Keeling J, Froehner JW, McGuigan FX, Andersen R: Perioperative differences between bone bridging and non-bone bridging transtibial amputations for wartime lower extremity trauma. *Foot Ankle Int* 2008;29(8):787-793.

    Longer surgical and tourniquet times should not be considered a contraindication to using the bone-bridging amputation technique in relatively young and healthy patients. Bone-bridging and non–bone-bridging amputation techniques have comparable rates of short-term wound complications and blood loss. Level of evidence: IV.

45. Schon LC, Short KW, Soupiou O, Noll K, Rheinstein J: Benefits of early prosthetic management of transtibial amputees: A prospective clinical study of a prefabricated prosthesis. *Foot Ankle Int* 2002;23(6):509-514.

46. Gordon WT, Stannard JP, Pasquina PF, Archer KR; Extremity War Injuries VII Rehabilitation Panel: Evolution of orthopaedic rehabilitation care. *J Am Acad Orthop Surg* 2012;20(Suppl 1):S80-S83.

    The goal of rehabilitation of patients with severe injury is to restore limb function in the interest of reintegration into society. The US Department of Defense has developed a network of rehabilitation centers to optimize outcomes.

47. Smith DG, Ehde DM, Legro MW, Reiber GE, del Aguila M, Boone DA: Phantom limb, residual limb, and back pain after lower extremity amputations. *Clin Orthop Relat Res* 1999;361:29-38.

48. Richardson C, Glenn S, Nurmikko T, Horgan M: Incidence of phantom phenomena including phantom limb pain 6 months after major lower limb amputation in patients with peripheral vascular disease. *Clin J Pain* 2006;22(4):353-358.

49. Buckenmaier CC III: The role of pain management in recovery following trauma and orthopaedic surgery. *J Am Acad Orthop Surg* 2012;20(Suppl 1):S35-S38.

    The US Army Pain Management Task Force evaluated pain medicine practices at 28 military and civilian institutions and provided recommendations.

Chapter 22

Osteonecrosis of the Talus

Keun-Bae Lee, MD, PhD   Jae-Wook Byun, MD   Thomas H. Lee, MD

Introduction

Osteonecrosis of the talus is difficult to diagnose and treat because the anatomic location of the talus means that it is hidden and its blood supply is precarious.[1] Osteonecrosis of the talus is not always clinically symptomatic, and patients should be followed until revascularization and consolidation are completed. No consensus exists as to the pathophysiology or natural course of the disease. Many treatments and surgical techniques have been tried, but few long-term outcome reports have been published.

The incidence of talar osteonecrosis is rising with the increasing incidence of high-energy trauma.[1] Injury to the talus requires great force; falls from a substantial height and motor vehicle crashes are the primary causes of the condition.[2] Survivors of a high-speed motor vehicle crash often have injuries to the distal extremities. The use of highly developed imaging techniques has led to an increase in the number of patients diagnosed with an early talar lesion.

Anatomy and Vascular Supply

An understanding of the unique anatomy of the talus and its blood supply is crucial for comprehending talar osteonecrosis. The orientation of the talar neck differs

Dr. Thomas Lee or an immediate family member has received royalties from Wright Medical Technology and Bledsoe; is a member of a speakers' bureau or has made paid presentations on behalf of Wright Medical Technology, Integra, Biomet, Stryker, and SBI; serves as a paid consultant to Wright Medical Technology, Stryker, DJ Orthopaedics, Biomet, and Amniox; has received research or institutional support from Wright Medical Technology, Zimmer, and DJ Orthopaedics; and serves as a board member, owner, officer, or committee member of the American Orthopaedic Foot and Ankle Society. Neither of the following authors nor any immediate family member has received anything of value from or has stock or stock options held in a commercial company or institution related directly or indirectly to the subject of this chapter: Dr. Keun-Bae Lee and Dr. Byun.

from that of the body of the talus in both the horizontal and sagittal planes. In the horizontal plane, the neck shifts medially with deviation. In the sagittal plane, the neck deviates downward. This complicated shape can lead to difficulty in determining the accuracy of reduction on radiographs. The talus has seven articular surfaces, which make up almost 60% of its surface, and screw fixation using the anteromedial approach is complicated[1] (**Figure 1**). The talus is most stable in the mortise at dorsiflexion because it is wider anteriorly than posteriorly. The bone is recessed for dorsiflexion at the neck of the talus, which is the most common site of talar fracture, especially during hyperdorsiflexion with axial loading.

The talus has no tendinous attachments or muscular origins. The entire blood supply comes from several direct vascular insertions, and understanding each contribution is important for avoiding iatrogenic vascular injury. The posterior tibial, dorsalis pedis, and perforating peroneal arteries are the three main extraosseous arteries that supply the talus[3] (**Figure 2**). The posterior tibial artery contributes the principal blood supply of the talar body through the artery of the tarsal canal and the deltoid artery.[4] The artery of the tarsal canal arises from the posterior tibial artery within the deltoid ligament below the medial malleolus, and it passes between the sheath of the flexor digitorum longus and flexor hallucis to enter the tarsal canal. The deltoid artery, which travels between deep and superficial deltoid ligament and arises near the origin of the artery of the tarsal canal, is an important source of extraosseous circulation to the body of the talus. Preservation of the deltoid artery is critical during stabilization or reduction of the talar neck and body. The artery of the tarsal sinus is formed from the anatomic loop between the dorsalis pedis and perforating peroneal arteries, and it merges with the artery of the tarsal canal. Together these arteries feed most of the talar neck and head.[1,3,4]

Etiology and Incidence

Osteonecrosis of the talus has three primary causes. Approximately 75% of patients have a history of trauma including talar neck or body fracture. Fifteen percent of

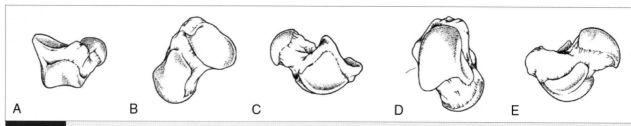

Schematic drawings showing the important anatomic features of the talus. **A,** Posterior view. **B,** Inferior view. **C,** Lateral view. **D,** Superior view. **E,** Medial surface of the talus.

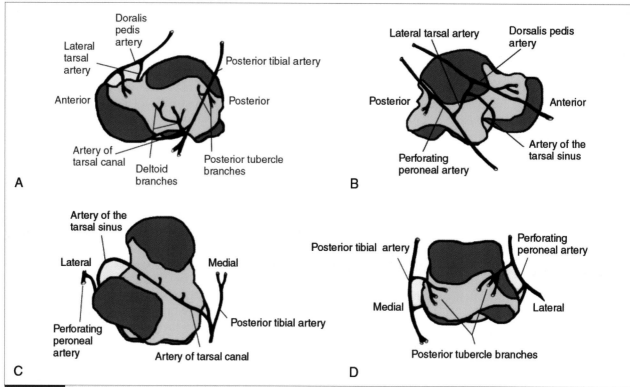

Figure 2 Schematic drawings showing the blood supply of the talus. **A,** The medial talar blood supply. The first branches of the posterior tibial artery are the posterior tubercle branches. More distally, the posterior tibial artery gives off the tarsal canal artery with its deltoid branches. This artery courses through the tarsal canal. **B,** The lateral talar blood supply. The lateral tarsal artery connects the dorsalis pedis artery to the perforating peroneal artery and branches to form the tarsal sinus artery. **C,** The inferior talar blood supply. The tarsal sinus artery and the tarsal canal artery form an anastomotic loop within the tarsal canal. **D,** The posterior talar blood supply. The posterior tubercle branches of the posterior tibial artery and perforating peroneal artery supply the medial and lateral tubercles.

patients have a nontraumatic medical condition as well as a history of steroid usage (regardless of dosage or duration of use).[1] Some of these patients have alcoholism, sickle cell disease, dialysis, hemophilia, hyperuricemia, or lymphoma.[4-8] The remaining 10% of patients have idiopathic talar necrosis without a determined traumatic or medical cause.

The Hawkins classification system for talar neck fractures stratifies the future risk of osteonecrosis based on fracture displacement and joint congruency.[9] The risk after a type I talar fracture is 10%; after a type II fracture,

almost 40%; and after a type III fracture, approximately 90%. Type IV implies the development of talar osteonecrosis to an even greater extent than type III.[4,10] Talar body and talar neck fractures do not differ significantly in terms of the risk of developing osteonecrosis.[11]

The death of hematopoietic cells, capillary endothelial cells, and lipocytes usually can be confirmed microscopically after 1 to 2 weeks of circulatory compromise. Lipocytes release lysosomes that acidify the tissue, osteocytes begin to shrink, and the water content in the bone increases. As a consequence of bone collapse,

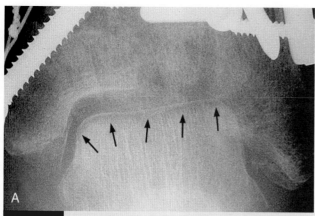 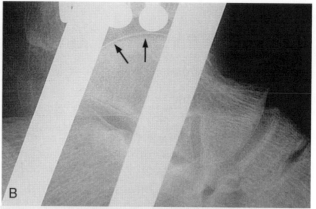

Figure 3 The Hawkins sign in a woman who had undergone external and internal fixation of a complex pilon fracture. Mortise view (**A**) and lateral (**B**) radiographs of the ankle reveal striking subchondral radiolucency (arrows), indicating talar viability.

saponification of fat or creeping substitution occurs, which means gradual replacement of necrotic tissue with new osteogenic tissue followed by bone formation. Without the ability to repair itself, the dysvascular bone eventually collapses, appearing fragmented and sclerotic. This process accelerates with additive microtrauma, which can occur during unprotected weight bearing with ambulation.[4,12]

Symptoms and Diagnosis

Pain is the most common symptom of talar osteonecrosis and is strongly associated with loss of articular integrity.[13] Before the collapse of the articular surface, a patient may be asymptomatic. With osteonecrosis of subchondral bone, subchondral collapse can occur because of the lack of structural support against pressure from body weight on the articular surface. This sequence is regarded as subchondral fracture, and it can cause pain as well as mechanical symptoms.[1]

Although MRI and bone scanning are useful for early detection of talar osteonecrosis, the evaluation should begin with plain radiography of the ankle. Early sclerotic changes, cystic changes, and advanced changes related to subchondral collapse can be seen on plain radiographs. The Hawkins sign may provide evidence of revascularization and is believed to be a reliable early indicator of vascular viability, with few false-negative results[1] (**Figure 3**). The Hawkins sign is a subchondral radiolucent band in the dome of the talus that can be seen on AP radiographs of the ankle 6 to 8 weeks after fracture and on lateral radiographs 10 to 12 weeks after fracture. Subchondral collapse often has no symptoms, and it is rare to detect lesions on plain radiographs during the early stage of talar osteonecrosis. MRI is considered to be a key diagnostic tool at the early stage.[3] MRI is used

to diagnose and quantify the extent of osteonecrosis because of its sensitivity to altered fat cell signals. Bone marrow predominantly is composed of fat components responsible for strong T1-weighted images, and bone marrow necrosis with subsequent edema is an early part of osteonecrosis.[1] The necrotized materials show density of water, which is revealed with high signal intensity on T2-weighted images. MRI also can be used to examine advanced stages of talar osteonecrosis. To minimize the signal interference, titanium screws should be used for fixation of a talar fracture. Titanium implants are preferable to stainless steel implants because of their nonmagnetic properties. Technetium Tc 99m bone scanning also is helpful for diagnosing early-stage talar osteonecrosis; usually it is done 6 to 12 weeks after internal fixation of the talar fracture and shows decreased uptake in the talar body. Radiographic findings are commonly used with the Ficat and Arlet classification system to determine the extent of talar osteonecrosis[13] (**Table 1**).

Nonsurgical Treatment

Many treatments of talar osteonecrosis have been described, but few long-term or critical outcome studies have been published, and there is no consensus as to the best treatment. Nonsurgical treatment is preferred for talar osteonecrosis at Ficat and Arlet stage I, II, or III. Some early studies found benefit to avoiding weight bearing until revascularization is complete.[14-16] A study of 23 patients with posttraumatic osteonecrosis found that patients who were non–weight bearing on crutches for an average of 8 months had a fair to excellent result.[6] Those who were partially weight bearing in a patellar tendon brace or short leg brace with limited ankle motion had a poor to good result. Most of those who received no treatment (defined as not bearing weight for less than 3 months)

Table 1

The Ficat and Arlet Classification of the Radiographic Appearance of Talar Osteonecrosis

Stage	Radiographic Appearance
I	Normal
II	Cystic and sclerotic lesions Normal talar contour
III	Crescent sign Subchondral collapse
IV	Narrowing of the joint space Secondary changes in the tibia

Adapted with permission from Delanois RE, Mont MA, Yoon TR, Mizell M, Hungerford DS: Atraumatic osteonecrosis of the talus. *J Bone Joint Surg Am* 1998;80(4):529-536.

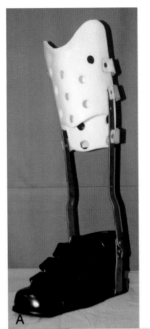
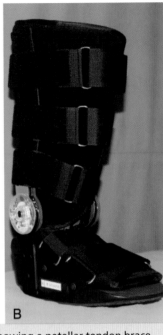

Figure 4 Photographs showing a patellar tendon brace (**A**) and a cam boot walker (**B**).

had a poor result. Other investigators reported that protected weight bearing using a patellar tendon brace had a favorable outcome and that delayed weight bearing had no benefit.[17,18] The amount and duration of weight bearing should be determined for the individual patient based on the location of the lesion and its symptoms. There is no need to restrict weight-bearing ambulation if sufficient bony structures remain to support weight bearing.[18] Regardless of the extent of weight bearing, however, it is important to preserve ankle motion, especially flexion and extension, and to protect the ankle from varus and valgus stress by using a patellar tendon brace or a cam boot walker (Figure 4).

The use of oral or intravenous bisphosphonates can be tried for patients with talar osteonecrosis.[19] Bisphosphonates are antiresorptive agents that inhibit the action of mature osteoclasts on bone, thereby changing the balance between resorption and deposition of bone to allow more deposition. Bisphosphonates appear to transiently stimulate the proliferation of pro-osteoblast cells, increase their differentiation, increase the production of antiresorptive protein osteoprotegerin by osteoblasts, and decrease edema at the site of osteonecrosis.[20] Although bisphosphonates have been used widely for patients with osteonecrosis of the femoral head, their use for talar osteonecrosis is off label and controversial.

Ultrasound bone stimulators also can be used for bone regeneration.[19] Low-intensity pulsed ultrasound was found to enhance the osteogenic differentiation of mesenchymal stem cells, stimulate the differentiation and proliferation of osteoblasts, inhibit activities of osteoclasts, improve local blood perfusion and angiogenesis, and accelerate stress fracture healing.[21] Extracorporal shock wave therapy was found to be an effective treatment for

osteonecrosis of the femoral head but is a controversial off-label use for treating talar osteonecrosis.[22]

Surgical Treatment

Core Decompression

An increase in pressure in the osteonecrotic area is believed to be the result of edema associated with cell death. This reparative process causes additional damage by increasing local compartment pressure and inhibiting revascularization.[23] The purpose of core decompression is to decrease core pressure, using multiple drilling procedures, and thereby enhance revascularization. Decompression also is effective in decreasing pain. In a rabbit model, the effect of core decompression was enhanced by negative pressure in necrotic areas of the femoral head.[24] Histologic analysis revealed better healing in animals treated with additional negative pressure than in those who underwent core decompression only.

Drills with a 1.5- to 4-mm diameter usually are used for decompression of the talar lesion. Two to 10 holes are made into the osteonecrotic lesion using a traditional posterolateral, a lateral, or a medial approach, depending on the location of the lesion.[25] Thirty-two of 37 ankles with stage II talar osteonecrosis remained severely symptomatic after standard nonsurgical treatment and received core decompression.[13] At a mean 7-year follow-up (range, 2 to 15 years), 29 of the ankles had a fair to excellent clinical outcome; the remaining

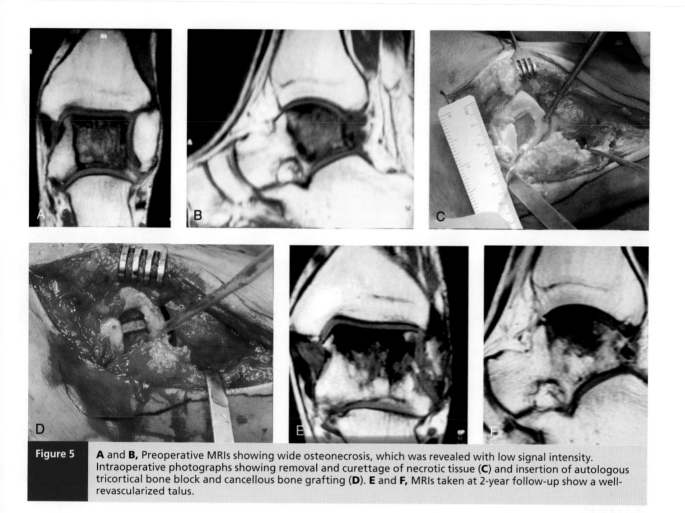

Figure 5 **A** and **B,** Preoperative MRIs showing wide osteonecrosis, which was revealed with low signal intensity. Intraoperative photographs showing removal and curettage of necrotic tissue (**C**) and insertion of autologous tricortical bone block and cancellous bone grafting (**D**). **E** and **F,** MRIs taken at 2-year follow-up show a well-revascularized talus.

3 ankles underwent arthrodesis after unsuccessful core decompression. In a recent case report, a patient with stage I talar osteonecrosis had a satisfactory outcome after percutaneous core decompression using a 3.5-mm cannulated drill through a small stab incision.[26] Core decompression is a relatively simple, short procedure that does not preclude subsequent arthrodesis or arthroplasty. However, core decompression can be used only before the collapse of the talar dome. After the articular surface collapses, core pressure has been decompressed and the necrotic anatomic changes are too far advanced for treatment with decompression.

Bone Grafting

Autograft or allograft bone grafting can be used before a salvage procedure is considered.[25] Nonvascularized autograft from the iliac crest is the most widely used bone graft, followed by allograft. The advantages of autograft over allograft include biocompatibility and rapid union; the disadvantages include donor site pain and limitation in the amount and size of grafting bone. Autologous bone grafting usually is done with resection or curettage of the necrotic area. Tricortical bone block and cancellous bone can be used for filling the defects. Favorable outcomes were reported when autologous bone grafting was used after 6 months of unsuccessful nonsurgical treatment in patients with a wide area of talar osteonecrosis[25] (**Figure 5**). At 2-year follow-up, the patients were almost symptom free with ongoing creeping substitution. Patients treated with iliac bone grafting followed by matrix-associated autologous chondrocyte transplantation returned to their former activities of daily living and recreation without restriction and only a slight deficit in range of motion.[27] Morphologic and biochemical MRI at 12-month follow-up showed excellent bone healing with no intraosseous edema.

If the lesion is large and primarily involves the articular surface, structural talar allograft can be a good choice. Osteochondral allograft can be considered for partial joint resurfacing in a young patient with focal lesions[19] (**Figure 6**). Talar allograft has a narrow range of indications, because of the difficulty of matching talar size, the limited supply of fresh allograft, and the extremely high cost. No long-term outcome data are

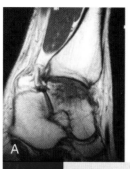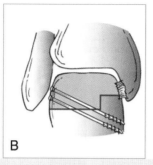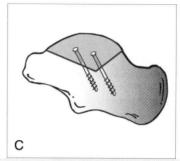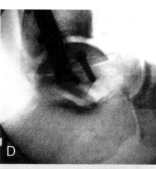

Figure 6 Segmental osteochondral allograft resurfacing for an ankle with focal talar osteonecrosis. **A,** Preoperative MRI showing large segmental involvement. **B** and **C,** Schematics showing preoperative planning for partial joint arthroplasty. **D,** Lateral radiograph showing placement of prepared allograft with screws from a transmalleolar approach.

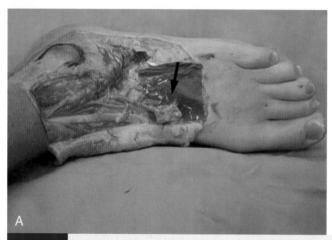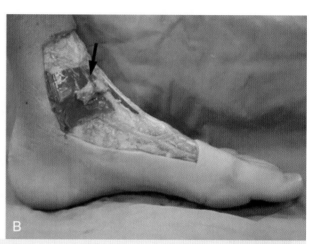

Figure 7 Photographs showing the transverse pedicle branch of the proximal lateral tarsal artery with the cuboid pedicle (arrow) (**A**) and its range (arrow), which can be rotated even to the medial malleolus (**B**).

available to guide decisions about revascularization of talar allograft. Vascularized autologous bone graft has long been used for treating osteonecrosis of the femoral head. Its theoretic advantages are a direct vascular supply to the necrotic area and mechanical support for prevention of further collapse. This procedure often is chosen despite its technical demands; microsurgical techniques and a long surgical time are required. Free vascularized bone graft is more difficult to use in the talus than in the femoral head because the vessels are smaller around the ankle than the hip. A vascularized bone graft from the iliac crest was used for revascularization in a 16-year-old patient with posttraumatic talar osteonecrosis.[28] Vessel-pedicled bone graft also can be used, although the technique is demanding. The sacrifice of small bones around the talus as a donor is required, and multiple joints around donor bone must be destroyed and fused. A cadaver study identified a consistent blood supply to the distal fibula, the cuboid, and the first and second cuneiforms with reliable nutrient arteries.[29] In every cadaver specimen, the transverse pedicle branch of the

proximal lateral tarsal artery reached and supplied the cuboid, which is approximately 4.1 cm long and can be rotated even far to the medial malleolus (**Figure 7**). The transverse segment of the anterolateral malleolar artery to the lateral malleolus is approximately 4 cm long but usually is an extremely small vessel. When 20 patients with talar osteonecrosis were treated with transposition of a vascularized cuneiform bone flap and iliac cancellous bone grafting, clinical symptoms were completely or partially relieved, the necrotic area was filled with newly formed bone, and 18 patients (90%) had a good or excellent result.[30] Vessel-pedicled bone grafts are promising but technically demanding, and additional outcome studies are warranted.

Arthrodesis

Arthrodesis can be considered as one of the last options if other treatments have been unsuccessful or in patients with stage IV talar osteonecrosis. Subtalar arthrodesis was used in an attempt to hasten ingrowth of blood vessels to the talus and thus avoid osteonecrosis and subsequent

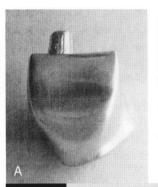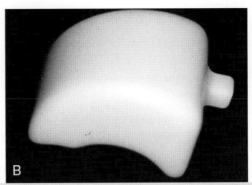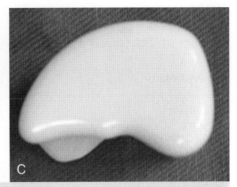

Figure 8 Photographs showing a stainless steel talar prosthesis (**A**), a first-generation ceramic talar prosthesis with a peg for an intact talar neck (**B**), and a second-generation implant without the peg (**C**).

arthrosis, but subsequent researchers reported poor results after this procedure.[1,31,32] Arthrodesis between the tibia and talar neck and head initially was used for patients with fracture and collapse of the talar body.[33] The procedure involves removing the fragments of the talar body and inserting a sliding tibial graft into the talar neck. Modified procedures have had favorable outcomes.[34-36]

Large cannulated screws, blade plates, locking plates, locked intramedullary rods, or multiplane thin–wire external fixators have been extensively studied for ankle fusion in patients with talar osteonecrosis.[19,37] The choice of technique should be based on the status of the patient, the location and range of the lesion, and the surgeon's preference.

If there is little or no malalignment of the ankle joint, it is possible to perform an arthroscopic ankle arthrodesis.[38] The anterolateral, anteromedial, and posterolateral portals are used to denude the entire cartilage while maintaining the contour of the bony surfaces. Internal or external fixation in situ is accomplished using two or three percutaneous, cancellous, cannulated or noncannulated screws placed parallel or converging. The advantages of an arthroscopic procedure include minimal blood loss, a relatively short time to union, and minimal interruption of the surrounding soft tissue. The subsequent blood supply leads to a better union rate than after an open procedure. A multicenter comparative study found that arthroscopic arthrodesis required a shorter hospital stay and led to better outcomes than an open procedure at 1- and 2-year follow-up.[39]

The mini-open technique, which is similar to the arthroscopic technique, uses an extended small incision at the same location as the arthroscopic portal. The advantages and disadvantages are similar to those of the arthroscopic technique, but the mini-open technique allows additional iliac crest grafting.[25] Nine patients treated using the mini-open technique had a satisfactory clinical and radiographic outcome at a mean 55-month follow-up.[40]

Curettage or resection of the necrotic area during ankle arthrodesis can cause shortening. The risk is minimal during the early stages of osteonecrosis if the necrotic area is small and shallow. Most patients who undergo ankle arthrodesis have stage III or IV talar osteonecrosis, however, and shortening from resection is an important consideration. A critical analysis of arthrodesis for the treatment of ankle arthrosis and talar body osteonecrosis found that the osteonecrotic talus was retained, thereby preserving ankle biomechanics and leg length.[41] Fusion was obtained in 16 of the 19 ankles, perhaps disproving the belief that fusion cannot be achieved in an osteonecrotic talus.

Talar Body Prostheses and Total Ankle Arthroplasty
A talar body prosthesis has been used in an attempt to avoid the drawbacks of arthrodesis or total talectomy in a wide area of talar osteonecrosis and to save the function of the talus. The difficulties of using a talar body prosthesis have included shrinkage, loosening, instability attributable to loss of ligamentous attachments, inexact prosthesis shape, and expense. Fourteen of 16 patients had a favorable outcome with respect to pain and function after receiving a talar body prosthesis made of stainless steel[42] (**Figure 8, A**). An alumina-ceramic prosthesis and a second-generation ceramic talar body prosthesis have been designed[43,44] (**Figure 8, B and C**). In the latter prosthesis, the peg for fixation on the neck of the surviving talus was removed to avoid the loosening found with the first-generation prosthesis, which appeared to be the result of concentrated stress.

Total ankle arthroplasty for a patient with talar osteonecrosis was first reported more than 35 years ago.[45] A few published studies are available, all of which reported unsatisfactory outcomes as well as some revisions to arthrodesis[46-49] (**Table 2**). Arthrodesis is the treatment of choice for end-stage talar osteonecrosis. Surgeons rarely use total ankle arthroplasty in patients with talar

Table 2

Studies of Cementless Total Ankle Arthroplasty for Talar Osteonecrosis

Study (Year)	Number of Patients	Follow-Up (Years)	Implant (Manufacturer)	Results
Newton[48] (1982)	3	3	Scandinavian Total Ankle Replacement (Small Bone Innovations)	Collapse in two patients, conversion to fusion in one Persistent pain in one patient
Buechel et al[46] (1988)	2	2	Buechel-Pappas (Endotec)	Complex regional pain syndrome in one patient
Buechel et al[47] (2003)	2	5	Buechel-Pappas	Collapse in one patient Complex regional pain syndrome in one patient
Takakura et al[49] (2004)	2	2	TNK Ankle (Japan Medical Materials)	Collapse in both patients, conversion to fusion

Adapted with permission from Lee KB, Cho SG, Jung ST, Kim MS: Total ankle arthroplasty following revascularization of osteonecrosis of the talar body: Two case reports and literature review. *Foot Ankle Int* 2008;29:852-858.

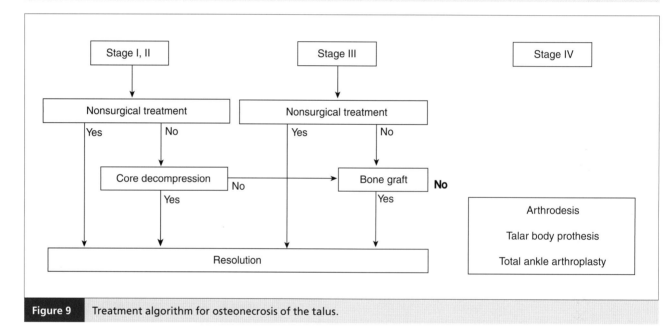

Figure 9   Treatment algorithm for osteonecrosis of the talus.

osteonecrosis because of poor bone ingrowth and the lack of supporting bony structures.

Treatment Algorithm

The treatment of talar osteonecrosis is marked by many controversies and little consensus. The recommended algorithm begins with the use of the Ficat and Arlet classification (**Figure 9**). Treatment success is defined as relief of pain or cessation of articular collapse. A widened necrotic area on MRI or a widened sclerotic margin on plain radiographs does not mean failure of the treatment. If collapse of the articular surface has been halted, even with the progression of necrosis, the surgeon can wait for revascularization and resolution of the lesion. Nonsurgical treatment is absolutely indicated for patients with stage I or II talar osteonecrosis. If there is no effect, core decompression or bone graft can be considered. A patient with stage III talar osteonecrosis with collapse of the articular surface will not benefit from core decompression; bone grafting is the only possible procedure. A salvage procedure such as arthrodesis can be done if there are arthritic changes.

Summary

Osteonecrosis of the talus is not a common disease, but if untreated it can lead to collapse of the talus and progressive pain with arthritic change. After a displaced fracture of the talar neck, as many as 90% of patients may be at risk of talar osteonecrosis, depending on the fracture pattern, because of the vulnerable vascular structure around the talar bone. In particular, osteonecrosis of the talus in a young patient can lead to end-stage arthritis requiring arthrodesis or arthroplasty later in life. Only a few comparative outcome studies on the treatment of osteonecrosis of the talus have been published. Careful evaluation and treatment decision making are of utmost importance. Radiographs should be used in conjunction with CT, bone scanning, or MRI, which is the most useful imaging modality for the disease. Identification of revascularization using bone scanning or MRI is essential to deciding on the best treatment plan. Before the collapse of the articular surface, nonsurgical treatment designed to protect the joint with limited weight bearing should be used until revascularization. For a patient who has undergone unsuccessful nonsurgical treatment or has articular collapse of the talar dome, the treatment options may include core decompression and bone grafting. A salvage procedure should be considered as a last resort or for a patient with end-stage arthritic changes.

Annotated References

1. Adelaar RS, Madrian JR: Avascular necrosis of the talus. *Orthop Clin North Am* 2004;35(3):383-395, xi.

2. Zwipp H: Severe foot trauma in combination with talar injuries, in Tscherne H, Schatzker J, ed: *Major Fractures of the Pilon, the Talus, and the Calcaneus: Current Concepts of Treatment.* Berlin, Germany, Springer-Verlag, 1993, pp 123-135.

3. Pearce DH, Mongiardi CN, Fornasier VL, Daniels TR: Avascular necrosis of the talus: A pictorial essay. *Radiographics* 2005;25(2):399-410.

4. DiGiovanni CW, Patel A, Calfee R, Nickisch F: Osteonecrosis in the foot. *J Am Acad Orthop Surg* 2007;15(4):208-217.

5. Langevitz P, Buskila D, Stewart J, Sherrard DJ, Hercz G: Osteonecrosis in patients receiving dialysis: Report of two cases and review of the literature. *J Rheumatol* 1990;17(3):402-406.

6. Kemnitz S, Moens P, Peerlinck K, Fabry G: Avascular necrosis of the talus in children with haemophilia. *J Pediatr Orthop B* 2002;11(1):73-78.

7. Miskew DB, Goldflies ML: Atraumatic avascular necrosis of the talus associated with hyperuricemia. *Clin Orthop Relat Res* 1980;148:156-159.

8. David RR: Sports injuries of the ankle, in Canale ST, James HB, eds: *Campbell's Operative Orthopaedics,* ed 12. Philadelphia, PA, Mosby, 2013, pp 4234-4249.

9. Hawkins LG: Fractures of the neck of the talus. *J Bone Joint Surg Am* 1970;52(5):991-1002.

10. Canale ST, Kelly FB Jr: Fractures of the neck of the talus: Long-term evaluation of seventy-one cases. *J Bone Joint Surg Am* 1978;60(2):143-156.

11. Lindvall E, Haidukewych G, DiPasquale T, Herscovici D Jr, Sanders R: Open reduction and stable fixation of isolated, displaced talar neck and body fractures. *J Bone Joint Surg Am* 2004;86(10):2229-2234.

12. Day S, Ostrum R, Chao E, Rubin C, Aro H, Einhorn T: Bone injury, regeneration and repair, in Buckwalter J, Einhorn T, Simon S, eds: *Orthopaedic Basic Science,* ed 2. Rosemont, IL, American Academy of Orthopaedic Surgeons, 2000, pp 317-370.

13. Delanois RE, Mont MA, Yoon TR, Mizell M, Hungerford DS: Atraumatic osteonecrosis of the talus. *J Bone Joint Surg Am* 1998;80(4):529-536.

14. Adelaar RS: The treatment of complex fractures of the talus. *Orthop Clin North Am* 1989;20(4):691-707.

15. Canale ST: Fractures of the neck of the talus. *Orthopedics* 1990;13(10):1105-1115.

16. Kenwright J, Taylor RG: Major injuries of the talus. *J Bone Joint Surg Br* 1970;52(1):36-48.

17. Penny JN, Davis LA: Fractures and fracture-dislocations of the neck of the talus. *J Trauma* 1980;20(12):1029-1037.

18. Comfort TH, Behrens F, Gaither DW, Denis F, Sigmond M: Long-term results of displaced talar neck fractures. *Clin Orthop Relat Res* 1985;199:81-87.

19. Saltzmann CL: Talar avascular necrosis, in Coughlin MJ, Mann RA, Saltzmann CL, eds: *Surgery of the Foot and Ankle,* ed 8. Philadelphia, PA, Mosby, 2007, pp 952-960.

20. Agarwala S, Jain D, Joshi VR, Sule A: Efficacy of alendronate, a bisphosphonate, in the treatment of osteonecrosis of the hip: A prospective open-label study. *Rheumatology (Oxford)* 2005;44(3):352-359.

21. Yan SG, Huang LY, Cai XZ: Low-intensity pulsed ultrasound: A potential non-invasive therapy for femoral head osteonecrosis. *Med Hypotheses* 2011;76(1):4-7.

    This study introduces low-intensity pulsed ultrasound for the early stage of osteonecrosis of femoral head. It is indicated to enhance the osteogenic differentiation of mesenchymal stem cells, stimulate the differentiation and the proliferation of osteoblasts, inhibit osteoclasts, and improve the local blood perfusion and angiogenesis.

22. Wang CJ, Wang FS, Yang KD, et al: Treatment of osteonecrosis of the hip: Comparison of extracorporeal shockwave with shockwave and alendronate. *Arch Orthop Trauma Surg* 2008;128(9):901-908.

This prospective study compared the results of ESWT (30 hips) and alendronate with that of ESWT without alendronate (30 hips) in early osteonecrosis of femoral head. They concluded that ESWT is effective with or without the concurrent use of alendronate

23. Urbaniak JR, Harvey EJ: Revascularization of the femoral head in osteonecrosis. *J Am Acad Orthop Surg* 1998;6(1):44-54.

24. Zhang YG, Wang X, Yang Z, et al: The therapeutic effect of negative pressure in treating femoral head necrosis in rabbits. *PLoS One* 2013;8(1):e55745.

The therapeutic effect of negative pressure on femoral head necrosis was found to be superior to that of core decompression.

25. Horst F, Gilbert BJ, Nunley JA: Avascular necrosis of the talus: Current treatment options. *Foot Ankle Clin* 2004;9(4):757-773.

26. Grice J, Cannon L: Percutaneous core decompression: A successful method of treatment of stage I avascular necrosis of the talus. *Foot Ankle Surg* 2011;17(4):317-318.

Stage I osteonecrosis, diagnosed clinically and on MRI, was successfully treated with percutaneous core decompression of the talus.

27. Dickschas J, Welsch G, Strecker W, Schöffl V: Matrix-associated autologous chondrocyte transplantation combined with iliac crest bone graft for reconstruction of talus necrosis due to villonodular synovitis. *J Foot Ankle Surg* 2012;51(1):87-90.

Matrix-associated autologous chondrocyte transplantation led to a good clinical outcome, with 100% defect filling as well as excellent integration and surface and signal intensity of the cartilage repair tissue. The American Orthopaedic Foot and Ankle Society ankle-hindfoot score improved from 47 to 79 points.

28. Hussl H, Sailer R, Daniaux H, Pechlaner S: Revascularization of a partially necrotic talus with a vascularized bone graft from the iliac crest. *Arch Orthop Trauma Surg* 1989;108(1):27-29.

29. Gilbert BJ, Horst F, Nunley JA: Potential donor rotational bone grafts using vascular territories in the foot and ankle. *J Bone Joint Surg Am* 2004;86(9):1857-1873.

30. Yu XG, Zhao DW, Sun Q, et al: Treatment of non-traumatic avascular talar necrosis by transposition of vascularized cuneiform bone flap plus iliac cancellous bone grafting. *Zhonghua Yi Xue Za Zhi* 2010;90(15):1035-1038.

Clinical observation and radiographic examination revealed that function of the ankle joint was completely or almost normal in 16 patients, and the bone repair was excellent after vascularized bone graft. This method may be effective for treating talar osteonecrosis.

31. McKeever FM: Treatment of complications of fractures and dislocations of the talus. *Clin Orthop Relat Res* 1963;30:45-52.

32. Pennal GF: Fractures of the talus. *Clin Orthop Relat Res* 1963;30:53-63.

33. Blair HC: Comminuted fractures and fracture dislocations of the body of the astragalus: Operative treatment. *Am J Surg* 1943;59:37-43.

34. Lionberger DR, Bishop JO, Tullos HS: The modified Blair fusion. *Foot Ankle* 1982;3(1):60-62.

35. Lin SY, Cheng YM, Huang PJ, Tien YC, Yap WK: Modified Blair method for ankle arthrodesis. *Kaohsiung J Med Sci* 1998;14(4):217-220.

36. Hantira H, Al Sayed H, Barghash I: Primary ankle fusion using Blair technique for severely comminuted fracture of the talus. *Med Princ Pract* 2003;12(1):47-50.

37. Devries JG, Philbin TM, Hyer CF: Retrograde intramedullary nail arthrodesis for avascular necrosis of the talus. *Foot Ankle Int* 2010;31(11):965-972.

The authors present their results in 14 patients undergoing tibiotalocalcaneal arthrodesis with a retrograde nail for talar osteonecrosis, and concluded that it is a possible salvage option and has a high likelihood of successful fusion.

38. Myerson MS, Quill G: Ankle arthrodesis: A comparison of an arthroscopic and an open method of treatment. *Clin Orthop Relat Res* 1991;268:84-95.

39. Townshend D, Di Silvestro M, Krause F, et al: Arthroscopic versus open ankle arthrodesis: A multicenter comparative case series. *J Bone Joint Surg Am* 2013;95(2):98-102.

Patients treated with arthroscopic ankle arthrodesis had significantly greater improvement on the Ankle Osteoarthritis Scale than those treated with an open procedure at 1- and 2-year follow-up, as well as a shorter hospital stay. Complication rate, surgical time, and radiographic alignment were similar in the two patient groups.

40. Wrotslavsky P, Giorgini R, Japour C, Emmanuel J: The mini-arthrotomy ankle arthrodesis: A review of nine cases. *J Foot Ankle Surg* 2006;45(6):424-430.

41. Kitaoka HB, Patzer GL: Arthrodesis for the treatment of arthrosis of the ankle and osteonecrosis of the talus. *J Bone Joint Surg Am* 1998;80(3):370-379.

42. Harnroongroj T, Vanadurongwan V: The talar body prosthesis. *J Bone Joint Surg Am* 1997;79(9):1313-1322.

43. Tanaka Y, Takakura Y, Kadono K, et al: Alumina ceramic talar body prosthesis for idiopathic aseptic necrosis of the talus. *Bioceramics* 2002;15:805-808.

44. Taniguchi A, Takakura Y, Sugimoto K, et al: The use of a ceramic talar body prosthesis in patients with aseptic necrosis of the talus. *J Bone Joint Surg Br* 2012;94(11):1529-1533.

  Although the use of a second-generation prosthesis improved results, the talar body prosthesis was not recommended. The total talar implant is preferred.

45. Manes HR, Alvarez E, Llevine LS: Preliminary report of total ankle arthroplasty for osteonecrosis of the talus. *Clin Orthop Relat Res* 1977;127:200-202.

46. Buechel FF, Pappas MJ, Iorio LJ: New Jersey low contact stress total ankle replacement: Biomechanical rationale and review of 23 cementless cases. *Foot Ankle* 1988;8(6):279-290.

47. Buechel FF Sr, Buechel FF Jr, Pappas MJ: Ten-year evaluation of cementless Buechel-Pappas meniscal bearing total ankle replacement. *Foot Ankle Int* 2003;24(6):462-472.

48. Newton SE III: Total ankle arthroplasty: Clinical study of fifty cases. *J Bone Joint Surg Am* 1982;64(1):104-111.

49. Takakura Y, Tanaka Y, Kumai T, Sugimoto K, Ohgushi H: Ankle arthroplasty using three generations of metal and ceramic prostheses. *Clin Orthop Relat Res* 2004;424:130-136.

5: Special Problems of the Foot and Ankle

Foot and Ankle Trauma

SECTION EDITOR:

ANDREW HASKELL, MD

Chapter 23

Ankle and Pilon Fractures

André Spiguel, MD   Mark J. Jo, MD   Michael J. Gardner, MD

Ankle Fractures

Introduction

The ankle is the most frequently injured weight-bearing joint. Ankle fractures are among the most common of all fractures; the annual incidence was found to be 71 to 187 per 100,000 people.[1-3] Fractures about the ankle range from a malleolar avulsion fracture to a comminuted fracture of the articular surface, with a resulting spectrum of stability and congruity of the mortise. Ankle fracture often is considered to be a simple fracture that sometimes is used in introductory surgical training. However, the evaluation, diagnosis, and decision making for an apparently simple ankle fracture can prove to be difficult.

A small incongruity in the ankle leads to dramatic changes in the pressure distribution of the joint surface and subsequently leads to arthritis.[4,5] Even a 1-mm shift of the talus can result in a 40% loss of contact area with the plafond. The goal of treating an ankle fracture should be to restore congruity and stability to the ankle and to maintain them through the healing process. Whether this goal is best achieved by surgical or nonsurgical means is best decided by weighing the risks and benefits of the treatment options while taking patient-specific factors into account.

Evaluation

Patient History

A thorough patient history should give particular attention to any medical comorbidities. The presence of

Dr. Gardner or an immediate family member serves as a paid consultant to or is an employee of DGIMed, RTI Biologics, Stryker, and Synthes; has received research or institutional support from Smith & Nephew and Synthes; and serves as a board member, owner, officer, or committee member of the Orthopaedic Trauma Association. Neither of the following authors nor any immediate family member has received anything of value from or has stock or stock options held in a commercial company or institution related directly or indirectly to the subject of this chapter: Dr. Spiguel and Dr. Jo.

diabetes, peripheral neuropathy, or peripheral vascular disease is important for risk stratification and decision making.[6,7] The patient's age, preinjury activity level, occupation, and recreational activities also can be important in decision making. Patients should be asked if osteoporosis has been diagnosed or if they have had a fragility fracture, such as a compression fracture of the spine, a hip fracture, or a distal radius fracture.[8] The presence of a medical comorbidity can increase the risk of infection, nonunion, malunion, or soft-tissue complications.[7,9] A patient who is obese is at increased risk for soft-tissue complications.[10] A patient who uses tobacco or abuses alcohol should be counseled about the associated fracture- and wound-healing risks as well as the potential benefits of cessation.[7,11]

The details of the injury should be noted because an understanding of the mechanism and energy of the injury can be helpful for evaluation, initial reduction, and treatment planning.

Physical Examination

A thorough 360° examination of the ankle should be performed to evaluate the soft tissue of the entire ankle region, including the posterior aspect. Evaluation of the soft-tissue envelope around an ankle fracture is paramount because its condition can be the determining factor during treatment decision making. The ankle has little soft-tissue coverage, and substantial edema, fracture blisters, and soft-tissue compromise can occur even with a low-energy ankle fracture. An ankle fracture-dislocation may require urgent reduction to minimize the comorbidity associated with inside-out pressure on the soft tissue. An open fracture can cause a transverse medial wound over the medial malleolus. Findings such as venous stasis skin changes, chronic skin discoloration, and ulceration may be signs of diabetes or peripheral vascular disease.

Tenderness in the medial and lateral malleoli and the collateral ligaments should be noted, regardless of the presence of a fracture. Tenderness to palpation in the absence of a fracture may indicate ligamentous injury, although the accuracy of this finding has been challenged.[12,13] Evaluation of a syndesmotic injury can be difficult. Tenderness over the anterior tibiofibular joint or a positive squeeze test (performed 5 cm above the distal tibiofibular joint) may indicate the presence of a syndesmotic injury. The entire tibia and fibula should be palpated up to the knee joint. Tenderness to palpation about the proximal fibula may indicate a Maisonneuve fracture variant with injury to the syndesmosis.

A thorough neurovascular examination and contralateral-side comparison should be done. Decreased sensation in a stocking distribution indicates advanced peripheral neuropathy. A size 5.07 Semmes-Weinstein monofilament should be used to test sensation if there is a question about peripheral neuropathy.[9] The ankle-brachial index can be measured to detect a vascular injury or peripheral vascular disease, and a vascular consultation may be warranted.

Radiographic Studies

Urgent intervention may be required for an ankle dislocation, open fracture, or acutely evolving neurovascular injury. An ankle dislocation with skin tenting or neurovascular compromise may need immediate reduction after only the most pertinent history and physical examination are obtained. Imaging studies done with the ankle in a roughly reduced position may provide more detail about the fracture pattern than studies with the joint in a grossly deformed state.

Imaging of an ankle fracture should begin with AP, lateral, and mortise radiographic views. A full-length tibiofibular series is helpful for diagnosing a proximal fibula fracture. The radiographs should be used to understand the fracture pattern and detect signs of instability. Any incongruity of the talus and the plafond is a sign of instability. Displacement of the medial or lateral malleolus or a talar shift of less than 2 mm historically was associated with a satisfactory result and was used as a criterion for fracture fixation.[14] On the AP radiograph, tibiofibular overlap of less than 10 mm or a clear space of more than 5 mm suggests a syndesmotic injury.[15] On the mortise view radiograph, a medial clear space that is larger than 5 mm or unequal to the superior clear space suggests a medial-side ligament injury. Tibiofibular overlap of less than 10 mm on the mortise view also may indicate a syndesmotic injury. The lateral radiograph may show a posterior malleolus fracture, malpositioning of the fibula relative to the tibia, and/or talar subluxation. The positioning of the ankle during radiographs is important; the medial clear space was found to become wider with increasing plantar flexion of the ankle, possibly leading to an incorrect diagnosis of deep deltoid injury.[16] Comparison views of the contralateral side may be helpful for detecting asymmetry or associated instability.

Stress radiographs may be indicated to assess stability if the talus and syndesmosis appear reduced but the injury mechanism or pattern suggests an unstable ankle. A manual external rotation or gravity stress mortise view radiograph can be used to assess deltoid ligament integrity and talus stability in an isolated lateral malleolus fracture.[12,13,17] With instability, this fracture pattern commonly is called a bimalleolar-equivalent fracture. Similarly, a stress view can be used to assess for syndesmotic injury, as in a proximal fibula fracture with a well-reduced ankle. Widening of the tibiofibular joint with an associated lateral shift of the talus is a positive finding. Evaluation of the syndesmosis may be more sensitive in the sagittal plane than in the coronal plane.[18]

CT is essential for evaluating the fracture pattern and planning treatment of an axial-loading injury or a suspected plafond or pilon-type fracture. CT also is beneficial for a complex fracture or a fracture with posterior malleolus fragments.

MRI is useful for detecting ligamentous injury. Although MRI may not be economically feasible for every ankle fracture, it can be beneficial if the diagnosis is difficult. MRI was found to be useful for distinguishing partial and complete tears of the deltoid ligament.[19,20]

Classification

An ideal classification system is reliable, reproducible, useful for treatment decision making, and able to provide prognostic information. Although no system for classifying ankle fractures meets all of these goals, the Lauge-Hansen, Denis-Weber, and AO Foundation–Orthopaedic Trauma Association (AO/OTA) systems are most commonly used.

The Lauge-Hansen classification uses the position of the foot at the time of injury as well as the direction of the force causing the injury to define four types of injuries: supination–external rotation (SER), supination-adduction (SAD), pronation–external rotation (PER), and pronation-abduction (PAB).[21] Each of these types has four subtypes (I through IV) denoting injury severity. The Lauge-Hansen system is popular but difficult to reproduce. A cadaver study found that a short oblique fracture of the distal fibula can occur with the foot in the pronated position, and a high fibular fracture can occur with abduction of the ankle.[22] A novel study compared online videotape clips showing the mechanism of ankle fractures with postinjury radiographs showing the same injuries.[23] The Lauge-Hansen classification was correctly correlated with SAD-type injuries but had only a 29% correlation with PER-type injuries. The Lauge-Hansen classification system is not useful for making treatment decisions or providing prognostic information. Because this system correlates the mechanism of injury with the fracture pattern, it may be useful for communicating patterns of injury and guiding closed reduction techniques.

Countering the injuring force with a splint, cast, or external fixator may improve the reduction.

The Denis-Weber classification, commonly described as a Weber A, B, or C, is based on the level of a lateral malleolus fracture.[24,25] A type A fracture is below the level of the plafond; a type B fracture, at the level of the plafond; and a type C fracture, above the plafond. A type A fracture without a medial fracture probably is an avulsion-type fracture that does not lead to lateral instability of the talus and can be treated nonsurgically. A type C fracture is inherently unstable and may involve the syndesmosis. The stability of a type B fracture is more difficult to assess because it may combine a syndesmotic injury with a deltoid ligament injury or may be a stable injury.[26] A stress radiograph can be helpful.

The combined AO/OTA system uses alphanumeric labels to systematically classify fractures.[27] This classification system is reproducible and can be used to describe a wide range of injury types as well as specific fracture patterns. Although the AO/OTA system is useful in data collection and research endeavors, it is cumbersome to use clinically and lacks specific diagnostic and prognostic components.

Initial Management

Reduction and splinting of an ankle fracture should be done in a timely manner. The health of the soft tissue is paramount. Reduction of any dislocation or subluxation will help to alleviate pressure on the skin and subcutaneous tissues, and proper reduction can alleviate any pressure, tethering, or kinking of the neurovascular structures. Reduction helps to alleviate atypical joint contact pressure that can contribute to posttraumatic arthritis. A successful reduction typically depends on recognizing the fracture pattern and reversing the deforming force. For example, the commonly used Quigley maneuver for laterally translated or externally rotated ankle fractures applies a varus and internal rotation force through the first toe.[28] An unsuccessful reduction may result from the use of an incorrect technique, inadequate anesthesia, or the interposition of structures such as surrounding tendons or fracture fragments. An open reduction may be needed if reduction with closed methods is unsuccessful.

Timely splinting also is beneficial for soft-tissue preservation. The splint can help hold the reduction while decreasing shear forces as well as the risk of further soft-tissue injury. Incorrect splinting technique can cause serious damage, however. The combination of insufficient padding and the pressures added during molding can create pressure points and lead to ulceration. Excess padding can cause the splint to be too loose, increase the shear forces, and even lead to loss of reduction. A study of plaster splints showed that dipping the plaster in water

hotter than 24°C can lead to thermal injury.[29] The use of multiple plaster layers, as when excess plaster is folded over at its end or layers are added to create a stirrup or strut, also was found to increase the temperature. The recommended method is to cut the plaster to the exact length needed. Placing the curing splint on a pillow or overwrapping it with fiberglass also can increase the temperature to a dangerous level.[29,30]

Routine postsplinting radiographs of a minimally or nondisplaced fracture that was not unnecessarily manipulated exposes patients to radiation, increases clinical waiting times, increases health care costs, and does not provide meaningful information.[31]

Definitive Management

The treatment goal for a rotational ankle fracture is healing with the mortise in an anatomic position. Attaining this goal may or may not require anatomic positioning of the fibular fracture. Nonsurgical treatment is appropriate if there is no medial malleolar fracture, the deep deltoid remains competent, and the mortise is stable, as can be confirmed using an external rotation or gravity stress mortise radiograph. A positive stress test typically is considered to be lateral translation of the talus, in which the medial clear space is larger than the superior clear space. The larger the medial clear space is on a stress radiograph, the greater the likelihood of syndesmotic injury.[32] If the mortise stress radiograph is negative, nonsurgical management typically consists of early functional treatment, with weight bearing as tolerated. A soft orthosis, walking boot, or walking cast initially can provide comfort and protection from further injury. Its use can be discontinued as symptoms allow.

A fracture-dislocation or subluxation requires an immediate closed reduction. The Quigley maneuver consists of rolling the patient onto the affected side and suspending the limb by the great toe to allow the talus to internally rotate and translate medially, thus reversing the most common dislocation vector and reducing the ankle joint. Ankle fracture-dislocations are inherently unstable and typically require open reduction and internal fixation of the malleoli to ensure anatomic healing. A Weber type B ankle fracture with a positive stress radiograph that remains well reduced within the mortise without stress can be considered for nonsurgical treatment. A recent prospective randomized study found that nonsurgically and surgically treated fractures had similar outcomes at 1-year follow-up, although 20% of the patients who were nonsurgically treated had medial clear space widening, and 20% had a delayed union or nonunion.[33]

If surgical treatment is indicated, attention to the fibular fracture is the key to restoring ankle reduction and stability. Care must be taken to accurately re-create fibular length, alignment, and rotation. The most common fracture pattern is a Weber type B with a spiral configuration at the level of the distal tibiofibular joint. Effective fixation methods include the use of multiple lag screws, one or more lag screws with neutralization plating, or antiglide plating. The plating surfaces are directly lateral or posterolateral. Laterally based plates tend to be more prominent because this is a subcutaneous location, and posterolateral plates can cause peroneal irritation if placed too distally.

The medial side of the ankle can fail through the medial malleolus or the ligamentous structures. The medial malleolus consists of the anterior colliculus, to which the superficial deltoid attaches, and the posterior colliculus, to which the deep deltoid attaches. The clinical significance is that when the anterior colliculus is reduced and stabilized, the deep deltoid, and thus the ankle mortise, may remain incompetent.[34] Medial malleolar fixation typically consists of two lag screws directed from the tip of the malleolus into the distal tibia after open reduction. Depending on the size of the fragment, one screw, a screw and pin, or a tension band technique can be used. Biomechanical and clinical data indicate that cortical lag screws engaged in the far lateral cortex of the distal tibia provide better fixation than screws ending in the distal tibial metaphysis.[35] Although most medial malleolus fractures are transverse, a medially directed traumatic force may create a vertical shear fracture, often with marginal impaction of the distal tibia joint surface at the fracture edge. This fracture pattern requires disimpaction and possibly grafting of any joint irregularity, typically followed by spring plate and screw fixation with screws directed from medial to lateral rather than from the tip of the malleolus (**Figure 1**). Outcomes research found no difference in functional result based on whether the medial-side injury was ligamentous or bony.[36]

Treatment of the posterior malleolus component has received increased attention. The decision to fix the posterior malleolus historically was based on the percentage of the articular surface involved, as measured on a lateral radiograph. A fracture involving more than one quarter to one third of the articular surface area or a fracture in which the talus is subluxated posteriorly with the posterior malleolar fragment typically requires reduction and fixation (**Figure 2**). It is now recognized that a posterior malleolus fracture involving the posterolateral corner of the distal tibia represents avulsion of the posterior tibiofibular ligaments, which are a component of the syndesmosis complex. Thus, reduction and fixation of the posterior malleolar component restores the tension and competence of the syndesmosis in this fracture type, and it may provide better stability than a syndesmotic screw.[37] The posterior malleolus contributes to the posterior lip

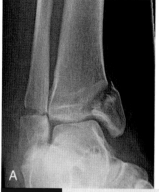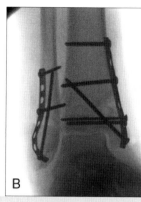

Figure 1 **A,** Preoperative mortise view radiograph showing a typical supination-adduction ankle fracture that demonstrates a transverse fibular fracture pattern at the level of the plafond and a relatively vertical medial malleolus fracture line and is associated with articular impaction of the medial shoulder. **B,** Intraoperative fluoroscopic mortise view showing the use of horizontal screws and a medial antiglide plate to buttress the impaction after reduction. (Courtesy of Michael J. Gardner, MD, St. Louis, MO.)

of the tibial incisura, and reduction and fixation may improve syndesmotic reduction accuracy. The less common transverse-type posterior malleolus fracture typically involves a greater percentage of the articular surface and may extend to the medial malleolus. This fracture typically requires open reduction and internal fixation, either percutaneously or through a direct posterior approach. CT can be used to improve the characterization of the transverse-type posterior malleolus fracture.

Reduction and fixation of the syndesmosis has been a source of controversy (**Figure 3**). Two key points have been established: syndesmosis malreduction is common, and it has a substantial effect on functional outcomes.[38-40] Instability of the syndesmosis can be diagnosed intraoperatively with an external rotation stress test after fixation of the malleolar fracture, although the accuracy of this test has been questioned.[41] Evidence of syndesmosis injury should be sought in all ankle fractures requiring surgical treatment; its incidence is as high as 40% in Weber type B fractures and is even higher in Weber type C fractures.[42] The risk of anterior or posterior translation of the syndesmosis can be minimized by reduction of the posterior malleolus fragment, meticulous clamp placement, direct visualization, and comparing the true talar dome lateral fluoroscopic views of the injured ankle to that of the contralateral ankle.[43-45] Overcompression of the syndesmosis previously was believed to be impossible, regardless of the position of the ankle during reduction.[46] Recent evidence suggests that overcompression is possible, however, and can affect the functional outcome.[43,47]

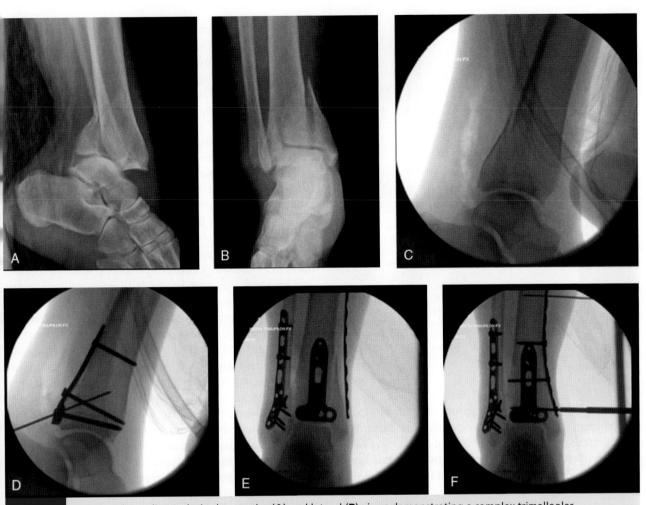

Figure 2 Preoperative radiographs in the mortise (**A**) and lateral (**B**) views demonstrating a complex trimalleolar fracture-dislocation of the ankle. **A,** Note the vertical fracture pattern of the medial malleolus but with no evidence of articular impaction in this case. **B,** The posterior dislocation of the talus is placing pressure on the anterior soft tissues. This will necessitate prompt reduction to protect the articular surfaces and soft tissue. Preoperative planning should include whether the posterior malleolus fracture needs to be addressed surgically as well as consideration of the planned approach (anterior or posterior) and positioning of the patient. **C** and **D,** Intraoperative fluoroscopic images in the lateral view. **C,** After appropriate reduction of the talus, there is concomitant reduction of the posterior malleolus fragment. **D,** The posterior malleolus fragment was initially secured using a Kirschner wire. The plate was then placed using a buttress technique with the initial screw placed through the plate just proximal to the apex of the fracture. The construct was then finalized utilizing lag screws through the fragment. **E** and **F,** Intraoperative fluoroscopic images in the mortise view. **E,** After appropriate reduction of the posterior malleolus and fibula, that medial malleolus has a near-anatomic reduction. A low profile plate was placed in the appropriate position using a percutaneous technique. The plate was undercontoured to achieve the desired buttress affect. **F,** The initial screw was placed at the apex of the fracture and with tightening of the screw, anatomic reduction was achieved with the plate. The construct was then completed using horizontal screws placed with a lag technique. For both the posterior and medial malleolus fragment a lag screw was placed in the subchondral bone to provide compression close to the articular surface.

Fixation of the syndesmosis with quadricortical or tricortical screws does not affect long-term outcomes.[48]

Postoperative Management

A splint is used to keep patients from bearing weight immediately after surgery. Elevation can be used to reduce swelling. The splint and sutures are removed 2 weeks after surgery. If the fracture fixation is believed to be stable, the patient begins to use a removable boot, and physical therapy is initiated to increase range of motion. Weight bearing is initiated at 4 to 6 weeks in patients who do not have diabetes and whose fracture healing is progressing as expected. To minimize the risk of neuroarthropathic (Charcot) collapse, immobilization and protection from weight bearing should be continued for a longer period in patients who have neuropathy from any

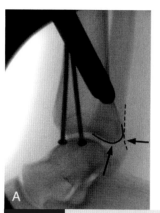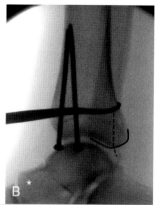

Figure 3 **A,** True talar dome lateral fluoroscopic view showing syndesmotic malreduction after clamp placement, indicated by the relative posterior position of the posterior border of the fibula (dashed line) in relation to the posterior edge of the plafond (solid line). **B,** Fluoroscopic view showing reduction of the fibular anterior translation using a hook after clamp removal. Note the intersection of the posterior border of the fibular at the posterior corner of the plafond. (Courtesy of Michael J. Gardner, MD, St. Louis, MO.)

source or diabetes-related nephropathy or retinopathy. For patients older than 70 years, with unstable surgical ankle fractures, poor bone quality, and difficulty adhering to restrictions on bearing weight, a novel construct using Kirschner wires and cement augmentation was found to permit safe early weight bearing.[49]

Complications

Nonunion is a rare complication usually related to nonsurgical treatment of the medial malleolus. This is often a fibrous nonunion and not painful. Malunion is most common in fractures treated nonsurgically. In surgically treated fractures, care must be taken to obtain anatomic reduction of the mortise and syndesmosis to avoid posttraumatic arthrosis and recurrent instability.[50] Wound-healing complications are uncommon, particularly with 2 weeks of splint immobilization to prevent tissue shearing. Tobacco smoking substantially increases the risk of all complications, including impaired wound healing.[51]

Pilon Fractures

Introduction

Fractures of the distal tibial articular surface, called pilon fractures, are among the most difficult fractures to treat. Usually these fractures are caused by axial loading to the tibial plafond, where the talus is forced cranially into the distal tibia. A high- or low-energy mechanism can be responsible. The fracture pattern and articular

impaction are determined by the direction of the force and position of the foot at the time of injury. There is no consensus on the optimal treatment of these fractures. Surgical treatment is technically demanding and requires careful planning. The outcomes tend to be unpredictable and are often disappointing.

Clinical and Radiographic Evaluation

As in any initial patient evaluation, a history and physical examination are essential. A thorough medical history helps to determine whether the patient is at increased risk for a poor outcome (soft-tissue complications, poor fracture healing, or fixation failure). Patients at increased risk include those who smoke tobacco; abuse alcohol; are long-term users of steroids; or have diabetes, neuropathy, malnutrition, osteoporosis, or peripheral vascular disease.

The mechanism of injury is directly related to the amount of force sustained by the limb, and initially the soft-tissue injury is more important than the fracture itself. Perfusion, swelling, tissue necrosis, and fracture blisters must be carefully assessed and will influence the treatment algorithm. Early intervention, including limb realignment with closed reduction, is imperative to minimize impending skin compromise from fracture fragments and to restore circulation and nerve function.

The radiographic evaluation of the ankle should begin with standard AP, lateral, and mortise radiographic views as well as full-length tibiofibular radiographic views. For a complex pilon fracture, radiographs of the contralateral limb sometimes are needed to understand unique morphologic variations of the distal tibia and provide a preoperative planning template. CT always should be obtained after restoration of limb length and alignment. CT is useful for understanding the fracture pattern and determining the extent of articular involvement for purposes of preoperative planning as well as determination of the appropriate surgical approach and fixation strategies.[52,53]

Classification

Fracture classification systems are tools for describing the fracture pattern and understanding factors related to the prognosis and treatment. The Ruedi and Allgöwer classification, described in 1968, is moderately useful. The three Ruedi and Allgöwer injury types increase in severity from a low-energy to a high-energy injury. Type I fractures are nondisplaced, type II fractures are characterized by articular displacement, and type III fractures have associated articular comminution and impaction.[54]

The AO/OTA system is much more detailed than the Ruedi and Allgöwer classification. All fractures of the distal tibia, including extra-articular metaphyseal fractures, are classified in a manner similar to that of other periarticular fractures, with differentiation between partial and complete articular injuries. Type A is an extra-articular fracture, type B is a partial articular fracture, and type C is a complete articular fracture (**Figure 4**).

Initial Management

The timing of definitive surgery for pilon fractures is critical. Typically a staged protocol is used to minimize the risk of complications and soft-tissue compromise. The initial focus should be on treating the soft-tissue envelope and the swelling, restoring the length and alignment of the tibia, and unloading the joint surface. Premature definitive open reduction and internal fixation can lead to wound complications including skin necrosis, dehiscence, and infection. Clinical studies from the 1980s and 1990s found high complication rates and poor clinical outcomes after definitive fixation was performed in the acute period.[52] In the staged protocol most surgeons currently use, external fixation with or without limited internal fixation is performed in the acute period. Definitive fixation is done when the soft tissues are optimized and swelling has diminished. This treatment plan has led to a substantial reduction in the rate of complications associated with pilon fractures.[55,56] A recent retrospective review of high-energy open pilon fractures treated using a staged treatment protocol with external fixation and serial débridement as needed, followed by definitive open reduction and internal fixation (ORIF), found acceptable outcomes and a low rate of soft-tissue complications.[57] Adequate fracture reduction was achieved and maintained in all patients.

Limited internal fixation with external fixation can be used in a pilon fracture with a long oblique or spiral fracture extending into the diaphysis. The soft tissues along the diaphysis are typically outside the area of greatest injury and can be treated with minimal exposure and reduction using an antiglide-type plate application. This method can help reestablish limb length, rotation, and alignment, and can provide early intimate contact of fracture fragments at the diaphysis to encourage early union and minimize the need for secondary procedures. However, limited internal fixation with external fixation should be used only in specific situations in which the articular block is spanned and the limited internal fixation will assist in obtaining the final reduction.[58]

Despite the known benefits of provisional external fixation, soft-tissue rest, and future definitive management, some surgeons still prefer early surgical fixation. Although some studies found similar complication rates and overall functional scores regardless of whether a staged protocol or single-stage ORIF was used to treat high-energy pilon fractures during the acute period, each

Tibia/fibula, distal, extra-articular (43-A)

1. Metaphyseal simple (43-A1)
2. Metaphyseal wedge (43-A2)
3. Metaphyseal complex (43-A3)

Tibia/fibula, distal, partial articular (43-B)

1. Pure split (43-B1)
2. Split depression (43-B2)
3. Multifragmentary depression (43-B3)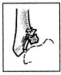

Tibia/fibula, distal, complete articular (43-C)

1. Articular simple, metaphysis simple (43-C1)
2. Articular simple metaphysis multifragmentary (43-C2)
3. Articular multifragmentary (43-C3)

Figure 4 Schematic drawings showing the AO/OTA classification of pilon fractures. (Adapted with permission from Marsh JL, Slongo TF, Agel J, et al: Fracture and dislocation classification compendium, 2007: Orthopaedic Trauma Association classification, database and outcomes committee. *J Orthop Trauma* 2007;21[suppl 10]:S1-133.)

of these studies was limited to a single surgeon, and the results may not be generalizable.[59]

Surgical Treatment
Surgical Approaches

The surgical approach for a pilon fracture must be carefully chosen and is based on the fracture pattern as well as the soft-tissue injuries. Anteromedial, anterolateral, posterolateral, posteromedial, and direct medial incisions have been described (**Figure 5**). The anteromedial approach, traditionally used for ORIF of pilon fractures, is the most extensile approach, providing access to the entire distal tibial articular surface and offering the ability to place a plate medially, laterally, or anteriorly. The anteromedial approach is associated with difficulty in reaching

6: Foot and Ankle Trauma

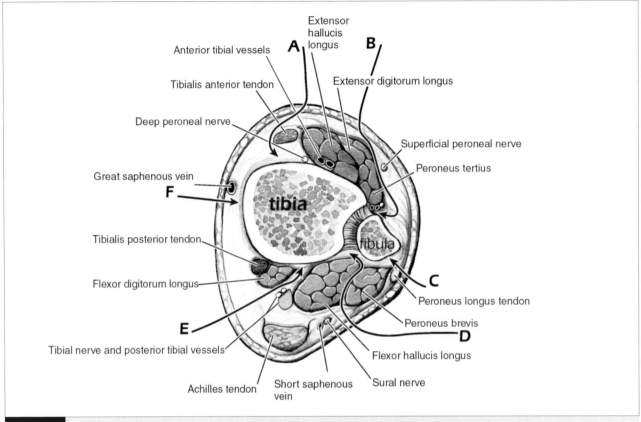

Figure 5 Axial-view schematic showing the anteromedial (**A**), anterolateral (**B**), posterolateral (fibula) (**C**), posterolateral (tibia) (**D**), posteromedial (**E**), and medial (**F**) approaches used to treat tibial plafond and associated fibula fractures. (Adapted with permission from Howard JL, Agel J, Barei DP, et al: A prospective study evaluating incision placement and wound healing for tibial plafond fractures. *J Orthop Trauma* 2008;22[5]:299-305.)

the lateral Chaput fragment. In addition, there may be wound complications over the anteromedial tibia because it is necessary to rely on the survival of full-thickness skin flaps that have undergone significant trauma. When an extensile version of the anteromedial approach was used to treat 21 patients after provisional stabilization with a spanning external fixator, all wounds healed, there were no nonunions, and one superficial infection occurred.[60]

The anterolateral approach is useful for most complete articular fractures. This approach allows good visualization of the medial shoulder of the ankle, avoids dissection over the anteromedial surface of the distal tibia, and may lead to fewer wound complications (**Figure 6**). The muscles of the anterior compartment provide good soft-tissue coverage over an implant, but the anterior tibial artery and vein as well as the superficial and deep peroneal nerves are at risk of injury or impingement. Impaction of the medial articular surface is difficult to reduce when this exposure is used, and the proximal extent of the exposure is limited because of the muscle origins of the anterior compartment on the fibula and the intraosseous membrane distally.[61]

The tibia and fibula also can be reached through the posterolateral or posteromedial approach. The posterolateral approach is useful in primarily posterior and partial articular fractures (AO/OTA type 43B). Articular visualization is almost impossible; the articular reduction usually is done indirectly with cortical reductions of the metaphysis and diaphysis. The posteromedial approach is rarely required for fixation of a pilon fracture. As in the posterolateral approach, it is difficult to see the articular surface, and reduction is done indirectly with an extra-articular cortical reduction. These posterior approaches sometimes are used as an adjunct to an anterior approach for the purpose of treating a complex pilon fracture.[54]

A staged protocol has been described for surgical fixation of a high-energy pilon fracture (AO/OTA type 43C) in which the articular fracture has a displaced posterior component.[62] The researchers believed that it was difficult to obtain an accurate reduction through an anterior approach alone, with an indirect reduction of the posterior fragment, and the result would be less than optimal. Their staged approach involved application of

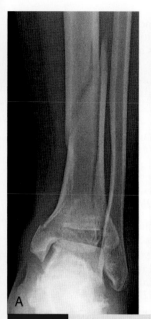 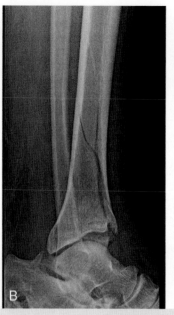 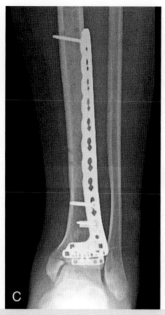 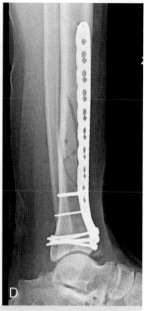

Figure 6 Preoperative radiographs showing AP (**A**) and lateral (**B**) views of a complex pilon fracture with extension into the diaphysis. Postoperative radiographs showing mortise (**C**) and lateral (**D**) views. An anterolateral approach to treat a pilon fracture allows excellent access to the anterior distal tibial articular surface. After the impaction was reduced and stabilized, the metaphysis was fixed with an anterolateral plate. (Courtesy of Michael J. Gardner, MD, St. Louis, MO.)

an initial external fixator followed by a limited ORIF through a posterolateral approach. When the soft tissues were amenable, an anterior approach was used to reduce the anterior and medial fragments to a stable posterior fragment. On the basis of CT, the researchers concluded that the use of this protocol improved their ability to obtain an anatomic articular reduction in comparison with the use of an anterior approach only and an indirect posterior reduction. There was no significant between-group difference in postoperative complications, and the functional outcomes were significantly improved in the patients treated with posterior plating.[62]

Internal Fixation

Pilon fractures in the past typically were treated nonsurgically. A 1979 comparison of nonsurgical treatment with ORIF found better results in surgically treated patients.[63] The researchers recommended four principles to guide the surgical treatment of a pilon fracture: restoration of fibular length, reconstruction of the articular surface and metaphysis, bone grafting, and medial buttressing to stabilize the metaphysis and assist the diaphyseal reduction. The results of this study were difficult to reproduce, however, probably because the patients in the study had a relatively low-energy mechanism of injury (for example, from a skiing accident) in contrast to the high-energy mechanisms (for example, from a motor vehicle crash) that have become increasingly common.

Despite advances in implant technology and surgical approaches, the four principles from 1979 still guide surgeons treating pilon fractures. Precontoured locked distal tibia and fibula plates are available for use in osteoporotic bone and/or fractures with significant metaphyseal comminution. Attention to soft-tissue devitalization has led to minimally invasive plate osteosynthesis using small incisions and indirect or percutaneous reduction techniques. This technique may minimize soft-tissue complications, but the surgeon should not compromise the articular reduction and restoration of the mechanical axis.

External Fixation

Definitive external fixation with hybrid external fixators usually is reserved for a fracture with large articular fragments, a contaminated open fracture, or soft-tissue injury that compromises standard surgical exposures. A limited open reduction of the articular surface sometimes can be done in addition to hybrid external or percutaneous fixation.

A retrospective study evaluated the clinical, radiographic, and functional outcomes of high-energy pilon fractures (AO/OTA type 43C) treated with ORIF or hinged bridging external fixation with limited internal fixation.[64] No between-group difference was found in the clinical or functional outcome or the overall complication and union rates. ORIF and external fixation with limited internal fixation were found to be equivalent for the treatment of high-energy pilon fractures. A retrospective evaluation of union rates and complications in high-energy pilon fractures (AO/OTA type 43C) treated with two-stage ORIF or definitive external fixation using an Ilizarov ring fixator found no statistically significant between-group differences.[65] The two treatment methods led to similar rates of union, times to union, and complications rates.

Summary

The treatment of ankle fractures continues to be challenging. Even seemingly simple ankle fractures can present difficulties. The understanding of the mechanisms that cause ankle fractures and the best means of treating these fractures continues to improve. Soft-tissue preservation is paramount because the ankle is a subcutaneous joint with a very thin soft-tissue envelope. As the prevalence of diabetes and obesity continues to increase, the need to manage fractures with compromised soft tissue will become a common challenge. As patients live longer and continue to lead active lives, the incidence of trauma in patients with poor bone quality also will rise. Although the development of new implants and techniques will continue to provide treatment options, a thorough understanding of ankle anatomy and fracture patterns will continue to provide the foundation for successful treatment of these injuries.

Surgical intervention for pilon fractures historically has led to high complication rates and poor outcomes. To minimize the risk of complications, definitive surgical treatment typically should be delayed until the soft-tissue envelope is optimal. There is still no consensus on the surgical management of these difficult fractures, and it is important that patients understand that pilon fracture is a life-altering injury.

Annotated References

1. Phillips WA, Schwartz HS, Keller CS, et al: A prospective, randomized study of the management of severe ankle fractures. *J Bone Joint Surg Am* 1985;67(1):67-78.

2. Daly PJ, Fitzgerald RH Jr, Melton LJ, Ilstrup DM: Epidemiology of ankle fractures in Rochester, Minnesota. *Acta Orthop Scand* 1987;58(5):539-544.

3. Thur CK, Edgren G, Jansson KA, Wretenberg P: Epidemiology of adult ankle fractures in Sweden between 1987 and 2004: A population-based study of 91,410 Swedish inpatients. *Acta Orthop* 2012;83(3):276-281.

    The Swedish National Patient Register was examined to determine the epidemiology of ankle fractures. Over a 17-year period the annual incidence was approximately 71 ankle fractures per 100,000 persons, and there was a notable increase in fractures among older women.

4. Ramsey PL, Hamilton W: Changes in tibiotalar area of contact caused by lateral talar shift. *J Bone Joint Surg Am* 1976;58(3):356-357.

5. Lloyd J, Elsayed S, Hariharan K, Tanaka H: Revisiting the concept of talar shift in ankle fractures. *Foot Ankle Int* 2006;27(10):793-796.

6. Olsen JR, Hunter J, Baumhauer JF: Osteoporotic ankle fractures. *Orthop Clin North Am* 2013;44(2):225-241.

    A review article examined the unique characteristics of osteoporotic ankle fractures.

7. Miller AG, Margules A, Raikin SM: Risk factors for wound complications after ankle fracture surgery. *J Bone Joint Surg Am* 2012;94(22):2047-2052.

    A review of 478 surgically treated ankle fractures found 20 patients requiring intervention for wound complications. The risk factors included diabetes, peripheral neuropathy, wound-compromising drugs, open fracture, and postoperative noncompliance. Time to surgery did not seem to have an effect. Level of evidence: I.

8. Cummings SR, Melton LJ: Epidemiology and outcomes of osteoporotic fractures. *Lancet* 2002;359(9319):1761-1767.

9. Wukich DK, Kline AJ: The management of ankle fractures in patients with diabetes. *J Bone Joint Surg Am* 2008;90(7):1570-1578.

    This current concepts review discusses the effect of diabetes on the management of ankle fractures. The authors examine the epidemiology of diabetes as it pertains to ankle fractures, characteristics of diabetes that lead to complications in the management of ankle fractures, and evidence regarding the optimal treatment of these patients.

10. Chaudhry S, Egol KA: Ankle injuries and fractures in the obese patient. *Orthop Clin North Am* 2011;42(1):45-53.

    The unique characteristics, diagnosis, and management of ankle fractures in patients who are obese are described.

11. Ovaska MT, Mäkinen TJ, Madanat R, et al: Risk factors for deep surgical site infection following operative treatment of ankle fractures. *J Bone Joint Surg Am* 2013;95(4):348-353.

    This study was performed to identify modifiable risk factors for deep surgical site infection following operative treatment of ankle fractures. The authors found patient-related risk factors for the incidence of deep infection to be diabetes, alcohol abuse, fracture-dislocation, and soft-tissue injury. Surgery-related risk factors included suboptimal timing of prophylactic antibiotics, difficulties during surgery, wound complications, and fracture malreduction. Independent risk factors were identified as tobacco use and duration of surgery more than 90 minutes. Level of evidence: III.

12. Egol KA, Amirtharajah M, Tejwani NC, Capla EL, Koval KJ: Ankle stress test for predicting the need for surgical fixation of isolated fibular fractures. *J Bone Joint Surg Am* 2004;86(11):2393-2398.

13. McConnell T, Creevy W, Tornetta P III: Stress examination of supination external rotation-type fibular fractures. *J Bone Joint Surg Am* 2004;86(10):2171-2178.

14. de Souza LJ, Gustilo RB, Meyer TJ: Results of operative treatment of displaced external rotation-abduction fractures of the ankle. *J Bone Joint Surg Am* 1985;67(7):1066-1074.

15. Joy G, Patzakis MJ, Harvey JP Jr: Precise evaluation of the reduction of severe ankle fractures. *J Bone Joint Surg Am* 1974;56(5):979-993.

16. Saldua NS, Harris JF, LeClere LE, Girard PJ, Carney JR: Plantar flexion influences radiographic measurements of the ankle mortise. *J Bone Joint Surg Am* 2010;92(4):911-915.

   A study of the effect of foot positioning on radiographic appearance of the ankle mortise found that with increasing plantar flexion the medial clear space increased to 0.38 mm at 45°.

17. Michelson JD, Varner KE, Checcone M: Diagnosing deltoid injury in ankle fractures: The gravity stress view. *Clin Orthop Relat Res* 2001;387:178-182.

18. Candal-Couto JJ, Burrow D, Bromage S, Briggs PJ: Instability of the tibio-fibular syndesmosis: Have we been pulling in the wrong direction? *Injury* 2004;35(8):814-818.

19. Koval KJ, Egol KA, Cheung Y, Goodwin DW, Spratt KF: Does a positive ankle stress test indicate the need for operative treatment after lateral malleolus fracture? A preliminary report. *J Orthop Trauma* 2007;21(7):449-455.

20. Cheung Y, Perrich KD, Gui J, Koval KJ, Goodwin DW: MRI of isolated distal fibular fractures with widened medial clear space on stressed radiographs: Which ligaments are interrupted? *AJR Am J Roentgenol* 2009;192(1):W7-12.

   MRI was used to evaluate ligamentous injuries in stress-positive ankle fractures in 19 patients. Partial- to full-thickness tears were seen in all patients, usually of the deltoid or syndesmotic complex. The anteroinferior tibiofibular ligament was disrupted in all patients.

21. Lauge-Hansen N: Fractures of the ankle. II. Combined experimental-surgical and experimental-roentgenologic investigations. *Arch Surg* 1950;60(5):957-985.

22. Haraguchi N, Armiger RS: A new interpretation of the mechanism of ankle fracture. *J Bone Joint Surg Am* 2009;91(4):821-829.

   A cadaver study attempted to recreate the Lauge-Hansen SER ankle fracture. This study generated counterexamples to the Lauge-Hansen classification system showing that pronation and external rotation could cause a short oblique fracture of the distal end of the fibula, and if a lateral abduction force was added, this could result in a high fibular fracture.

23. Kwon JY, Chacko AT, Kadzielski JJ, Appleton PT, Rodriguez EK: A novel methodology for the study of injury mechanism: Ankle fracture analysis using injury videos posted on YouTube.com. *J Orthop Trauma* 2010;24(8):477-482.

   Internet videotaped clips showing incidents of ankle injury were analyzed to identify the mechanism of injury using the Lauge-Hansen classification system, and the result was compared with radiographs of the injured ankle. Injuries of the SAD type had good correlation between the videotape clip and the corresponding radiographs, but videotaped PER-type injuries were found to cause a radiographic PER fracture pattern only in 29% of patients.

24. Danis R: *Theorie et pratique de l' osteosynthese.* Paris, Masson & Cie, 1949.

25. Weber B: *Die verletzungen des oberen sprungge-lenkes. Aktuelle Probleme in der Chirurgie.* Stuttgart, Huber, 1966.

26. Ebraheim NA, Elgafy H, Padanilam T: Syndesmotic disruption in low fibular fractures associated with deltoid ligament injury. *Clin Orthop Relat Res* 2003;409:260-267.

27. Marsh JL, Slongo TF, Agel J, et al: Fracture and dislocation classification compendium, 2007: Orthopaedic Trauma Association classification, database and outcomes committee. *J Orthop Trauma* 2007;21(10, Suppl):S1-S133.

28. Quigley TB: A simple aid to the reduction of abduction-external rotation fractures of the ankle. *Am J Surg* 1959;97(4):488-493.

29. Halanski MA, Halanski AD, Oza A, Vanderby R, Munoz A, Noonan KJ: Thermal injury with contemporary cast-application techniques and methods to circumvent morbidity. *J Bone Joint Surg Am* 2007;89(11):2369-2377.

30. Deignan BJ, Iaquinto JM, Eskildsen SM, et al: Effect of pressure applied during casting on temperatures beneath casts. *J Pediatr Orthop* 2011;31(7):791-797.

   The application of pressure during cast curing was found to increase the cast temperature. In plaster casts overwrapped with fiberglass, the temperature reached 47.9°. Temperatures did not reach the threshold of thermal injury (49° to 50°C). Allowing the plaster cast to cure before applying the fiberglass overwrap substantially reduced the temperature.

6: Foot and Ankle Trauma

31. Chaudhry S, DelSole EM, Egol KA: Post-splinting radiographs of minimally displaced fractures: Good medicine or medicolegal protection? *J Bone Joint Surg Am* 2012;94(17):e128.

The usefulness of postsplinting radiographs was evaluated for fractures that did not require manipulation. None of the 204 analyzed fractures had any displacement after reduction. Requiring postsplinting radiographs only added to patient waiting time, radiation exposure, and health care cost. Level of evidence: II.

32. Tornetta P III, Axelrad TW, Sibai TA, Creevy WR: Treatment of the stress positive ligamentous SE4 ankle fracture: Incidence of syndesmotic injury and clinical decision making. *J Orthop Trauma* 2012;26(11):659-661.

Patients with surgically treated stress-positive supination and external rotation type 4 ankle injuries (SE4) had greater medial clear space widening than those treated nonsurgically. Patients treated nonsurgically healed with no subluxation.

33. Sanders DW, Tieszer C, Corbett B; Canadian Orthopedic Trauma Society: Operative versus nonoperative treatment of unstable lateral malleolar fractures: A randomized multicenter trial. *J Orthop Trauma* 2012;26(3):129-134.

A randomized comparison study of surgical and nonsurgical treatment of stress-positive SE4 ankle fractures found no difference in functional outcomes at 1-year follow-up. Twenty percent of patients treated nonsurgically had at least 5 mm of medial clear space widening at healing.

34. Tornetta P III: Competence of the deltoid ligament in bimalleolar ankle fractures after medial malleolar fixation. *J Bone Joint Surg Am* 2000;82(6):843-848.

35. Ricci WM, Tornetta P, Borrelli J Jr: Lag screw fixation of medial malleolar fractures: A biomechanical, radiographic, and clinical comparison of unicortical partially threaded lag screws and bicortical fully threaded lag screws. *J Orthop Trauma* 2012;26(10):602-606.

Medial malleolar fractures treated with bicortical lag screws had better clinical and radiographic outcomes than those treated with partially threaded cancellous lag screws. Biomechanical strength also was superior.

36. Berkes MB, Little MT, Lazaro LE, et al: Malleolar fractures and their ligamentous injury equivalents have similar outcomes in supination-external rotation type IV fractures of the ankle treated by anatomical internal fixation. *J Bone Joint Surg Br* 2012;94(11):1567-1572.

A prospective cohort study found no difference in functional outcome between SER IV ankle fractures with a medial malleolus fracture and those with a medial ligamentous injury.

37. Gardner MJ, Brodsky A, Briggs SM, Nielson JH, Lorich DG: Fixation of posterior malleolar fractures provides greater syndesmotic stability. *Clin Orthop Relat Res* 2006;447:165-171.

38. Gardner MJ, Demetrakopoulos D, Briggs SM, Helfet DL, Lorich DG: Malreduction of the tibiofibular syndesmosis in ankle fractures. *Foot Ankle Int* 2006;27(10):788-792.

39. Sagi HC, Shah AR, Sanders RW: The functional consequence of syndesmotic joint malreduction at a minimum 2-year follow-up. *J Orthop Trauma* 2012;26(7):439-443.

Patients with syndesmotic injury had bilateral CT at 2-year follow-up. The malreduction rate was 39%. Those with a malreduced syndesmosis had a significantly worse functional outcome.

40. Weening B, Bhandari M: Predictors of functional outcome following transsyndesmotic screw fixation of ankle fractures. *J Orthop Trauma* 2005;19(2):102-108.

41. Pakarinen H, Flinkkilä T, Ohtonen P, et al: Intraoperative assessment of the stability of the distal tibiofibular joint in supination-external rotation injuries of the ankle: Sensitivity, specificity, and reliability of two clinical tests. *J Bone Joint Surg Am* 2011;93(22):2057-2061.

An intraoperative study of 140 ankle fractures found that the hook test and external rotation test had poor sensitivity for detecting syndesmotic injury.

42. Stark E, Tornetta P III, Creevy WR: Syndesmotic instability in Weber B ankle fractures: A clinical evaluation. *J Orthop Trauma* 2007;21(9):643-646.

43. Miller AN, Barei DP, Iaquinto JM, Ledoux WR, Beingessner DM: Iatrogenic syndesmosis malreduction via clamp and screw placement. *J Orthop Trauma* 2013;27(2):100-106.

A cadaver study found that malreduction of the syndesmosis was highly sensitive to clamp position and screw vector.

44. Miller AN, Carroll EA, Parker RJ, Boraiah S, Helfet DL, Lorich DG: Direct visualization for syndesmotic stabilization of ankle fractures. *Foot Ankle Int* 2009;30(5):419-426.

Direct visualization of the syndesmotic reduction led to a significantly lower rate of malpositioning of the fibula within the incisura.

45. Summers HD, Sinclair MK, Stover MD: A reliable method for intraoperative evaluation of syndesmotic reduction. *J Orthop Trauma* 2013;27(4):196-200.

Intraoperative use of mortise and true talar dome lateral fluoroscopic views predictably allowed accurate syndesmotic reduction.

46. Tornetta P III, Spoo JE, Reynolds FA, Lee C: Overtightening of the ankle syndesmosis: Is it really possible? *J Bone Joint Surg Am* 2001;83(4):489-492.

47. Phisitkul P, Ebinger T, Goetz J, Vaseenon T, Marsh JL: Forceps reduction of the syndesmosis in rotational

ankle fractures: A cadaveric study. *J Bone Joint Surg Am* 2012;94(24):2256-2261.

An eccentric clamp vector used for reducing the syndesmosis was found to lead to malreduction. Overcompression of the syndesmosis was common.

48. Wikerøy AK, Høiness PR, Andreassen GS, Hellund JC, Madsen JE: No difference in functional and radiographic results 8.4 years after quadricortical compared with tricortical syndesmosis fixation in ankle fractures. *J Orthop Trauma* 2010;24(1):17-23.

Long-term follow-up of an earlier study of 48 ankle fractures found no difference between tricortical and quadricortical syndesmotic fixation.

49. Assal M, Christofilopoulos P, Lübbeke A, Stern R: Augmented osteosynthesis of OTA 44-B fractures in older patients: A technique allowing early weightbearing. *J Orthop Trauma* 2011;25(12):742-747.

A fibular fixation construct for ankle fractures, consisting of a lateral plate, intramedullary wires, and cement augmentation, was found to avoid nonunion or reduction loss in older patients.

50. Lübbeke A, Salvo D, Stern R, Hoffmeyer P, Holzer N, Assal M: Risk factors for post-traumatic osteoarthritis of the ankle: An eighteen year follow-up study. *Int Orthop* 2012;36(7):1403-1410.

Advanced radiographic osteoarthritis was common 12 to 22 years after ankle fracture open reduction and internal fixation. The risk factors included Weber type C fibular fracture, medial malleolar fracture, fracture-dislocation, high body mass index, and age older than 30 years.

51. Nåsell H, Ottosson C, Törnqvist H, Lindé J, Ponzer S: The impact of smoking on complications after operatively treated ankle fractures: A follow-up study of 906 patients. *J Orthop Trauma* 2011;25(12):748-755.

Cigarette smoking substantially increased the risk of postoperative complications in patients with an unstable ankle fracture requiring surgery.

52. Liporace FA, Yoon RS: Decisions and staging leading to definitive open management of pilon fractures: Where have we come from and where are we now? *J Orthop Trauma* 2012;26(8):488-498.

Current strategies, decision-making processes, and definitive treatment options for pilon fractures were reviewed. Level of evidence: V.

53. Crist BD, Khazzam M, Murtha YM, Della Rocca GJ: Pilon fractures: Advances in surgical management. *J Am Acad Orthop Surg* 2011;19(10):612-622.

The diagnosis, evaluation, and treatment of pilon fractures were reviewed, with particular attention to advances in surgical management.

54. Stannard JP, Schmidt AH, Kregor PJ: *Surgical Treatment of Orthopaedic Trauma*. New York, NY, Thieme, 2007.

55. Sirkin M, Sanders R, DiPasquale T, Herscovici D Jr: A staged protocol for soft tissue management in the treatment of complex pilon fractures. *J Orthop Trauma* 1999;13(2):78-84.

56. Patterson MJ, Cole JD: Two-staged delayed open reduction and internal fixation of severe pilon fractures. *J Orthop Trauma* 1999;13(2):85-91.

57. Boraiah S, Kemp TJ, Erwteman A, Lucas PA, Asprinio DE: Outcome following open reduction and internal fixation of open pilon fractures. *J Bone Joint Surg Am* 2010;92(2):346-352.

A staged protocol was designed to minimize the risk of soft-tissue complications and allow optimal fracture reduction of open pilon fractures. Clinical, radiographic, and functional outcomes were assessed. ORIF of open pilon fractures using the staged treatment protocol was found to have an acceptable outcome and a low rate of soft-tissue complications. Level of evidence: IV.

58. Dunbar RP, Barei DP, Kubiak EN, Nork SE, Henley MB: Early limited internal fixation of diaphyseal extensions in select pilon fractures: Upgrading AO/OTA type C fractures to AO/OTA type B. *J Orthop Trauma* 2008;22(6):426-429.

In pilon fractures with an oblique fracture extension into the diaphysis, the diaphyseal portion of the fracture was reduced during application of the temporary external fixator. Typically a small incision over the fracture spike and application of an antiglide plate were required to help with the reduction and alignment of the fracture fragments and prevent more extensive dissection than may be needed 1 to 3 weeks after injury, when the soft tissues were amenable to definitive fixation and the fracture had begun to heal. The goal was to convert the fracture from an AO/OTA type 43C to a type 43B pattern.

59. White TO, Guy P, Cooke CJ, et al: The results of early primary open reduction and internal fixation for treatment of OTA 43.C-type tibial pilon fractures: A cohort study. *J Orthop Trauma* 2010;24(12):757-763.

The safety and efficacy of early single-stage ORIF to treat pilon fractures was evaluated in 95 patients with an AO/OTA type 43C injury. Wound dehiscence, deep infection requiring surgery, quality of fracture reduction, and functional outcome scores were evaluated. Surgery was performed within 48 hours in 88% of patients, with anatomic reduction in 90%. A deep wound infection or dehiscence requiring surgical débridement developed in six patients.

60. Assal M, Ray A, Stern R: The extensile approach for the operative treatment of high-energy pilon fractures: Surgical technique and soft-tissue healing. *J Orthop Trauma* 2007;21(3):198-206.

6: Foot and Ankle Trauma

61. Mehta S, Gardner MJ, Barei DP, Benirschke SK, Nork SE: Reduction strategies through the anterolateral exposure for fixation of type B and C pilon fractures. *J Orthop Trauma* 2011;25(2):116-122.

    The anterolateral exposure was found to have advantages for pilon fractures. Novel reduction strategies and implant placement could be used through this approach.

62. Ketz J, Sanders R: Staged posterior tibial plating for the treatment of Orthopaedic Trauma Association 43C2 and 43C3 tibial pilon fractures. *J Orthop Trauma* 2012;26(6):341-347.

    A direct approach with posterior malleolar plating was used in combination with staged anterior fixation in high-energy AO/OTA 43C pilon fractures. Nine patients were treated with posterior plating of the tibia followed by staged surgery using a direct anterior approach, and 10 patients were treated using a standard anterior or anteromedial incision. Four of the 10 patients treated with a direct anterior approach and no patients treated with posterior plating had more than 2 mm of joint incongruity at the posterior articular fracture edge.

63. Rüedi TP, Allgöwer M: The operative treatment of intra-articular fractures of the lower end of the tibia. *Clin Orthop Relat Res* 1979;138:105-110.

64. Davidovitch RI, Elkhechen RJ, Romo S, Walsh M, Egol KA: Open reduction with internal fixation versus limited internal fixation and external fixation for high grade pilon fractures (OTA type 43C). *Foot Ankle Int* 2011;32(10):955-961.

    High-energy pilon fractures in 62 patients were treated with ORIF or external fixation with limited internal fixation. Between-group functional outcome scores, complication rates, and union rates were similar. ORIF and external fixation appeared to be comparable with regard to final range of ankle motion, development of arthritis, and hindfoot scores.

65. Bacon S, Smith WR, Morgan SJ, et al: A retrospective analysis of comminuted intra-articular fractures of the tibial plafond: Open reduction and internal fixation versus external Ilizarov fixation. *Injury* 2008;39(2):196-202.

    A retrospective analysis compared a subset of AO/OTA type C pilon fractures in 42 patients after treatment with definitive external Ilizarov fixation or staged external fixation and conversion to ORIF. Patients treated with ORIF required a longer time to healing, but rates of nonunion, malunion, and infection were lower than in patients treated with Ilizarov fixation. No clinical recommendations could be made.

Chapter 24

Talus Fractures

David J. Hak, MD, MBA, FACS

Introduction

The anatomic shape of the talus is unique. Three-fifths of the talar surface is covered by articular cartilage, and the seven separate articular surfaces form complex articulations with the tibia, fibula, calcaneus, and navicular. The calcaneal articular facets form the subtalar joint. Approximately 25% of the subtalar joint is made up of the posterior process of the talus. The anteromedial trochlear surface, central trochlear surface, and lateral process form the talar portion of the ankle joint. The talus is held in position by the bony constraints of the medial and lateral malleolus and by the constraining ligaments of the ankle joint. The smallest cross-sectional area of the talus is in the region of the talar neck, which is covered by a relatively weak cortex and therefore is susceptible to fracture from high-energy trauma.

Talus fractures represent only 3% to 6% of all foot fractures.[1] Talar neck and body fractures commonly result from high-energy trauma and therefore are likely to be associated with other injuries. The high-energy trauma that produces displaced talar neck fractures often damages the limited blood supply to the talus and/or causes articular cartilage damage. Talar process fractures are more likely to be isolated injuries from lower energy trauma.

Talar Neck Fractures

Mechanism of Injury

Great force, as in high-energy trauma, is required to cause a fracture of the thick subchondral bone of the talar neck. The fracture mechanism most commonly is a hyperdorsiflexion force.

Dr. Hak or an immediate family member serves as a paid consultant to RTI Biologics, Baxter, and Invibio; has stock or stock options held in Emerge; has received research or institutional support from Synthes and Stryker; and serves as a board member, owner, officer, or committee member of the Orthopaedic Trauma Association and the International Society for Fracture Repair.

Classification

The most widely accepted classification of talar neck fractures is the Hawkins classification, which is based on displacement and dislocation and therefore is correlated with the presumed extent of disruption to talar blood supply[2] (**Figure 1**). A Hawkins type I fracture is a nondisplaced fracture without subluxation or dislocation, a type II fracture is a displaced vertical talar neck fracture with a subluxation or dislocation of the subtalar joint, and a Hawkins type III fracture is a displaced fracture extending through the talar neck with dislocation at both the subtalar and tibiotalar joints. A type IV fracture, which is a dislocation of the ankle and subtalar joint, along with a dislocation or subluxation of the head of the talus at the talonavicular joint, was added to the classification.[3] The extent of displacement and dislocation at the time of injury is believed to primarily determine damage to the blood supply and therefore the risk of osteonecrosis.

Radiologic Evaluation

Routine radiographs of the ankle (AP, mortise, and lateral views) and/or the foot (AP, oblique, and lateral views) are used to identify talar fractures. The Canale oblique view of the talar neck allows the best evaluation of talar neck angulation and shortening[3] (**Figure 2**). This view is obtained with the ankle in maximum equinus and the foot pronated 15° while the x-ray tube is angled 75° from the horizontal plane. CT should be obtained if plain radiographs do not clearly identify a fracture but talar neck fracture is strongly suspected. Preoperative CT is useful for assessing fracture comminution and displacement and obtaining accurate images of the ankle, subtalar, and transverse tarsal joints.

Emergency Treatment and Timing of Surgical Fixation

Historically, talar neck fracture was considered a surgical emergency requiring immediate reduction and fixation to minimize the risk of osteonecrosis. Recent studies, however, have found no correlation between surgical timing and the development of osteonecrosis. In a retrospective review of 102 talar neck fractures, the mean time to fixation was 3.4 days for patients in whom osteonecrosis later

6: Foot and Ankle Trauma

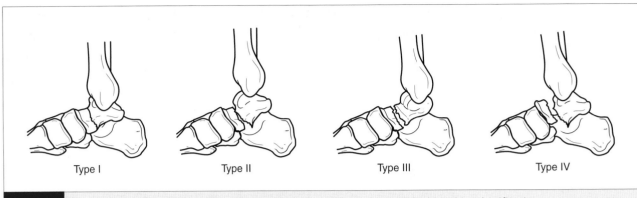

Figure 1 Schematics showing talar neck fracture types I through IV in the modified Hawkins classification.

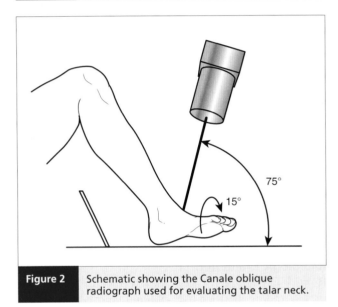

Figure 2 Schematic showing the Canale oblique radiograph used for evaluating the talar neck.

developed, compared with 5 days for patients in whom osteonecrosis did not develop. Instead, osteonecrosis was found to be associated with talar neck comminution (*P* < 0.03) and open fracture (*P* < 0.05).[4]

A retrospective review found evidence of a Hawkins sign, which is considered a prognostic indicator of talar body vascularity, in 59% of active duty soldiers with a combat-related talus fracture, despite an average time to fixation of 12.9 days.[5] No correlation was found between delayed fixation and the development of osteonecrosis or posttraumatic arthritis.

A survey of expert orthopaedic trauma surgeons found that most did not believe that immediate surgical treatment was essential for displaced talar neck fractures.[6] Most of the surgeons believed that the surgery could be delayed more than 8 hours, and a significant number believed that a delay of more than 24 hours was acceptable. Because of the high-energy mechanism and the limited soft-tissue envelope, 21% of talar neck fractures are open, and these fractures require emergency

surgical débridement and irrigation to reduce the risk of infection.[2]

An initial closed reduction is recommended for any dislocation associated with talar neck fracture, with the goal of achieving near-anatomic alignment of the talar neck. Once reduced, the dislocated joint typically stabilizes because of the shape and fit of the articular surfaces and surrounding structures. Both provisional Kirschner wire fixation and spanning external fixation have been used, however.[7] Some researchers recommend the use of an external fixator to provide distraction of the ankle joint and unload the talus, with the hope of reducing the incidence of osteonecrosis.[8,9] Others have found that external fixation has no effect on the prevention of osteonecrosis after talar neck fracture.[10]

Open Reduction and Internal Fixation

Surgical treatment is indicated for Hawkins type II, III, and IV talar neck fractures. Although a completely nondisplaced fracture can be treated nonsurgically, it must be carefully followed with serial radiographs to ensure that the fracture does not become displaced during treatment. To avoid subsequent displacement and deformity, some researchers recommend internal fixation for even nondisplaced talar neck fractures.[7] In addition, internal fixation permits early ankle and subtalar motion.

Anatomic reduction of both the talar neck and subtalar joint is the goal of talar neck fracture treatment. Even a minimal residual displacement can adversely affect subtalar joint mechanics.[11] Rotational alignment can be difficult to judge, but it is important to avoid reducing the fracture in supination, pronation, or axial malalignment. Most surgeons recommend using a two-incision technique (anteromedial and anterolateral) to allow accurate visualization, anatomic reduction, and placement of fixation.[12,13] The anteromedial approach begins at the medial malleolus anterior border and extends toward the navicular tuberosity running between the anterior tibial

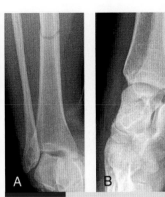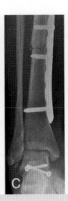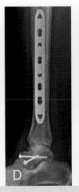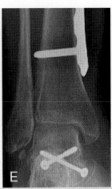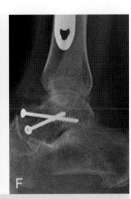

Figure 3 AP (**A**) and lateral (**B**) radiographs show a minimally displaced talar neck fracture with subluxation-dislocation of the ankle and subtalar joints in a 37-year-old woman who sustained multiple injuries in a automobile crash. AP (**C**) and lateral (**D**) radiographs after initial treatment with closed reduction and ankle-spanning external fixation, followed by open reduction and internal fixation using dual surgical approaches on the fifth postinjury day. AP (**E**) and lateral (**F**) radiographs 20 months after surgery show no evidence of osteonecrosis but some narrowing of the joint space.

and posterior tibial tendons. The anterolateral incision begins at the Chaput tubercle on the tibia and extends toward the bases of the third and fourth metatarsals.[14] The Ollier approach, in which an oblique incision is made from the tip of the lateral malleolus to the neck of the talus, also is effective and may permit better control of the lateral process and the anterior part of the posterior subtalar joint.[15] A medial malleolar osteotomy may be desirable if the fracture extends posteriorly into the body of the talus, but it is more likely to be required for a talar body fracture.[16]

Kirschner wires placed in the talar head and body fragments can be used as joysticks to manipulate the reduction and correct the displacement and deformity. At least two screws are required to achieve stable internal fixation and decrease the risk of malunion.

Screw placement from anterior to posterior usually is recommended because the entrance site is routinely exposed during the anterior approach[7] (**Figure 3**). Screw fixation from posterior to anterior was found to be biomechanically stronger, however, in a transverse noncomminuted talar neck fracture model.[17] Another biomechanical study compared fixation in a comminuted talar neck fracture model using three anteroposterior screws, two cannulated posteroanterior screws, or one screw from anterior to posterior with a medially applied blade plate. No significant difference in yield point or stiffness was found among these three fixation methods, all of which exceeded the theoretical stress across the talar neck during active motion.[18] Posterior-to-anterior screw fixation also requires an additional posterior approach with potential injury to the peroneal artery and its branches, and screw head prominence can limit ankle plantar flexion.

Fixation screws typically are placed in lag fashion to compress the talar neck fracture and enable it to withstand early ankle and subtalar motion. Lag screw technique may be contraindicated if there is comminution, especially of the medial column, as it will lead to deformity and malunion. With comminution, transfixion screws can be used to maintain the correct neck length.[13,19] Bone grafting occasionally is needed to replace impaction defects and restore the neck length. Many researchers have recommended plate fixation, with or without neutralization screw fixation, for comminuted talar neck fractures.[7,12,13,20] A plate ranging in size from 2.0 to 2.7 mm can be placed medially, laterally, or bilaterally on the most comminuted column of the talus (**Figure 4**). In addition to providing longitudinal structural support, plate fixation resists supination or pronation of the distal fragment.

Intraoperative fluoroscopy is useful for assessing the accuracy of the reduction and implant positioning. Arthroscopic evaluation can improve visualization of the articular surface to enhance reduction accuracy and allow débridement of any loose intra-articular debris.

Postoperative active motion is begun when the wounds are healed. Joint motion is believed to improve cartilage healing. Full weight bearing generally is restricted for 6 to 12 weeks, until radiographs show sufficient evidence of fracture healing.

Complications
Osteonecrosis
The most feared complication of talar neck fracture is osteonecrosis of the talar body as a consequence of interruption of the precarious blood supply to the talus. The risk of osteonecrosis is almost completely determined by the severity of the injury, but its likelihood may be

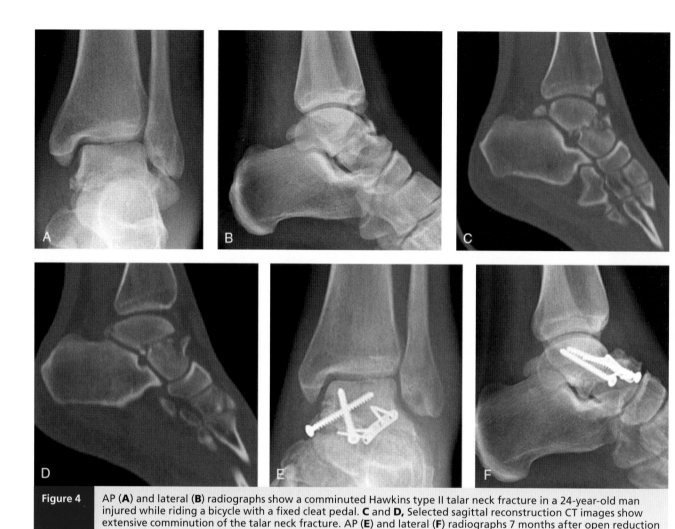

Figure 4 AP (**A**) and lateral (**B**) radiographs show a comminuted Hawkins type II talar neck fracture in a 24-year-old man injured while riding a bicycle with a fixed cleat pedal. **C** and **D,** Selected sagittal reconstruction CT images show extensive comminution of the talar neck fracture. AP (**E**) and lateral (**F**) radiographs 7 months after open reduction and internal fixation show a 2.0-mm plate used laterally and a fully threaded screw used medially to prevent compression and shortening of the talar neck.

decreased by prompt and accurate surgical reduction, with meticulous surgical dissection that avoids further vascular damage. The risk of osteonecrosis in a Hawkins type I fracture is 15% or less because only the blood supply entering through the neck is disrupted. A Hawkins type II fracture, in which both the artery of the tarsal canal and the dorsal blood supply from the neck are disrupted, has a 20% to 50% risk of osteonecrosis. Type III and IV fractures, in which all three main sources of blood supply are damaged, have a 69% to 100% risk of osteonecrosis.[2,3,21] With partial or full collapse of the talar dome, subsequent degenerative changes lead to pain and disability in the ankle and subtalar joints as well as shortening of the affected leg.[2,22,23]

The Hawkins sign can appear 6 to 8 weeks after talar neck fracture and is seen on an ankle AP or mortise view radiograph. In the absence of weight bearing, the preserved blood supply permits resorption of the subchondral bone of the talar dome, which appears as

a radiolucency of the talar dome.[2] In clinical practice, the presence of the Hawkins sign strongly predicts the absence of osteonecrosis. The Hawkins sign is highly sensitive but less specific, and its absence does not universally predict the development of osteonecrosis.[3,21,24]

On plain radiographs osteonecrosis appears as a relative sclerosis of the talar body compared with the surrounding bone. This relative sclerosis may not appear until 4 to 6 months after injury. MRI is the most sensitive test for evaluating the presence and extent of osteonecrosis and can help direct appropriate treatment.[25] For this reason, some surgeons advocate the use of titanium screws to minimize hardware artifact.

The optimal treatment of diagnosed osteonecrosis is unclear. Total or partial avoidance of weight bearing may be recommended to prevent talar collapse. The talus may revascularize through creeping substitution, but this process may require several years, during which the patient would be required to avoid weight bearing.[2] In a study of 71 patients with a talar neck fracture, those who avoided weight bearing for an average of 8 months had a fair to excellent result, but most patients who avoided weight bearing for less than 3 months had a poor result.[3] Patients who were permitted partial weight bearing in a patellar tendon brace or a short leg brace with limited ankle motion had a poor to good result. Some researchers believe that avoidance of weight bearing is of questionable value in preventing collapse after osteonecrosis develops.[2,26] There is no consensus as to the duration or extent of restricted weight bearing or the usefulness of bracing or immobilization for minimizing the sequelae of osteonecrosis.[27]

The surgical treatment of talar osteonecrosis is extremely challenging. Arthrodesis, which can be difficult to achieve in the presence of osteonecrosis, should be a last resort.[28] Core decompression was reported to be successful in selected patients with talar osteonecrosis without collapse.[29,30] Successful revascularization of a partially necrotic talus in a 16-year-old patient was achieved using a vascularized iliac crest bone graft.[31] A stainless steel talar body prosthesis was used in treating osteonecrosis or severe crush injury of the talus.[32] Talectomy has poor outcomes, with frequent pain, a short limb, and significant loss of ankle and subtalar motion.

Malunion and Nonunion
The incidence of malunion after talar neck fracture has been reported to be approximately 30%.[3,23] The typical malunion findings include varus malalignment of the talar neck and medial column deformity. Malalignment of only 2 mm results in significant changes in subtalar contact characteristics that could lead to the progressive development of posttraumatic arthritis.[11] It is difficult to accurately evaluate residual step-offs and alignment on plain radiographs. CT is the most accurate method of measuring malunion and can be helpful in preoperative planning.[33]

Secondary reconstruction of the normal anatomic shape of the talus is recommended for the treatment of malunion, but success depends on the status of the soft tissues and joint cartilage as well as the presence of osteonecrosis.[34] This salvage procedure corrects the foot malposition by an osteotomy through the malunited fracture to restore the medial neck length, using additional bone grafting if necessary. Arthrodesis is the primary salvage procedure for talar neck malunion, but it does not restore normal foot function.[23,35]

Nonunion is rare after talar neck fracture, with an incidence of approximately 2.5%.[4,19] Vascularized bone grafting is one option for the treatment of talar neck nonunion.[36] Delayed union is more common than nonunion.

Posttraumatic Arthritis
Long-term follow-up studies found that posttraumatic arthritis was more common than osteonecrosis after talar neck fractures, with an incidence of 50% to 100%.[23,37] The causes of posttraumatic arthritis are multifactorial and include articular cartilage damage at the time of injury, osteonecrosis, and progressive cartilage degeneration from fracture malunion, leading to malalignment and incongruence. Posttraumatic arthritis primarily involves the subtalar joint but also can affect the ankle and talonavicular joints. Posttraumatic arthritis does not always become symptomatic. Severe posttraumatic arthritis, with chronic pain and function-limiting stiffness, may necessitate arthrodesis if nonsurgical treatment is ineffective.

Talar Body Fractures
Fractures of the talar body are uncommon, accounting for only 7% to 38% of talus fractures.[38] A wide spectrum of fractures can occur in the talar body, ranging from small osteochondral shear injury to severe crush injury involving the entire talar body. These fractures commonly result from a high-energy axial loading injury, such as a fall from height.

Small osteochondral injuries may not be readily apparent but should be strongly suspected in patients with persistent ankle pain 6 to 8 weeks after an apparent simple ankle sprain. Osteochondral injuries commonly are located in the anterolateral and posteromedial talar dome.

A high rate of complications was reported in a study of 38 patients with a talar body fracture. At an average 33-month follow-up, full radiographs of 26 patients revealed evidence of osteonecrosis in 10, posttraumatic tibiotalar arthritis in 17, and posttraumatic subtalar arthritis in 9. In all, 23 of the 26 patients (88%) had evidence of osteonecrosis and/or posttraumatic osteoarthritis. Osteonecrosis and posttraumatic osteoarthritis were most common among the patients who had sustained an open injury and those with an associated talar neck fracture.[38] In 19 patients with a talar body fracture, 7 had osteonecrosis, 1 had a delayed union, and 1 had a malunion at an average 26-month follow-up (range, 18 to 43 months).[39] The clinical outcome, as rated using the American Orthopaedic Foot and Ankle Society ankle-hindfoot score, was excellent in four patients, good in six, fair in four, and poor in five.

Lateral Process Fractures
The lateral process of the talus is a wedge-shaped prominence that has two articular facets. The smaller facet articulates with the distal fibula, and the larger facet forms

6: Foot and Ankle Trauma

the anterolateral portion of the subtalar joint. The high prevalence of lateral process fracture in patients injured while snowboarding has led to its being called snowboarder's fracture. The exact mechanism that produces a fracture of the lateral process is the subject of debate. Some experts believe that this fracture is caused by axial loading, ankle dorsiflexion, and inversion, but others believe an external rotation or eversion force is necessary.[40] In one series of lateral process fractures sustained while snowboarding, the injury mechanisms included axial impact in all 20 patients (100%), dorsiflexion in 19 (95%), external rotation in 16 (80%), and eversion in 9 (45%).[41] Fractures of the lateral process of the talus often are missed on plain radiographs, and ankle sprain usually is the diagnosis. CT best identifies the size and position of a lateral process fracture (**Figure 5**).

Nondisplaced fractures usually are treated with 6 weeks of immobilization followed by partial weight bearing until there is radiographic evidence of healing. Larger noncomminuted displaced fractures require open reduction and internal fixation with 2.0- or 2.7-mm lag screws. The surgical approach is a 5- to 8-cm gently curved incision over the sinus tarsi to expose the subtalar joint. Primary surgical treatment was found to improve outcomes and lower the risk of subtalar arthritis.[41] A displaced comminuted fracture that is not amenable to internal fixation may require excision.

Posterior Process Fractures

The posterior process of the talus usually makes up approximately 25% of the posterior subtalar articulation and consists of a medial and lateral tubercle separated by a groove for the flexor hallucis longus tendon. Posterior process fractures of the talus are uncommon, and most involve an isolated fracture of either the medial or lateral tubercle. An unfused os trigonum may be confused with a fracture of the posterior process.

The cause of a fracture of the entire posterior talar process usually is forceful maximal plantar flexion of the ankle, producing a nutcracker-like compression of the posterior talus process between the posterior malleolus and the calcaneus.[42] Fracture of the medial tubercle of the posterior process can occur when the foot is suddenly forced into combined dorsiflexion and pronation, which places the posterior talotibial portion of the deltoid ligament under tension and causes avulsion of the tubercle.[43] The lateral tubercle of the posterior process may be fractured as a result of repetitive plantar flexion, as in a stress fracture.[42]

Fractures of the entire posterior talar process affect a significant portion of the subtalar joint and usually are treated with open reduction and internal fixation.

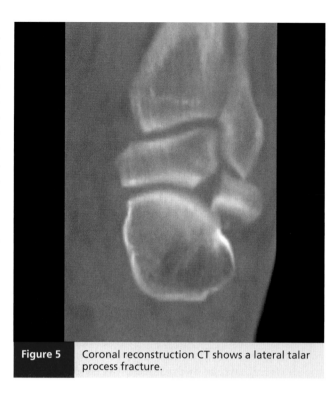

Figure 5 Coronal reconstruction CT shows a lateral talar process fracture.

The surgical approach for fixation is selected based on the direction of major displacement. A posteromedial approach between the flexor digitorum longus tendon and the neurovascular bundle is used if the fragment is displaced posteromedially; a posterolateral approach between the peroneal tendons and the Achilles tendon is used if the fragment is displaced posterolaterally.[42]

Summary

Fractures of the talus are uncommon but often represent serious injury. The high-energy force required to produce a displaced talar neck fracture can cause severe associated soft-tissue damage, including damage to the precarious blood supply. Anatomic reduction and stable internal fixation of a displaced talar neck fracture may minimize the risk of complications, but posttraumatic sequelae may be inevitable. The risk of osteonecrosis is almost completely determined by the severity of injury. Nonetheless, the likelihood of osteonecrosis may be decreased by prompt and accurate surgical reduction as well as meticulous surgical dissection that avoids further vascular damage. Osteonecrosis and posttraumatic arthritis are challenging complications to treat. Talar body fractures are associated with a high rate of complications. Lateral process fractures of the talus can easily be overlooked and may lead to posttraumatic sequelae.

Annotated References

1. Adelaar RS: The treatment of complex fractures of the talus. *Orthop Clin North Am* 1989;20(4):691-707.

2. Hawkins LG: Fractures of the neck of the talus. *J Bone Joint Surg Am* 1970;52(5):991-1002.

3. Canale ST, Kelly FB Jr: Fractures of the neck of the talus: Long-term evaluation of seventy-one cases. *J Bone Joint Surg Am* 1978;60(2):143-156.

4. Vallier HA, Nork SE, Barei DP, Benirschke SK, Sangeorzan BJ: Talar neck fractures: Results and outcomes. *J Bone Joint Surg Am* 2004;86(8):1616-1624.

5. Bellamy JL, Keeling JJ, Wenke J, Hsu JR: Does a longer delay in fixation of talus fractures cause osteonecrosis? *J Surg Orthop Adv* 2011;20(1):34-37.

   A retrospective review of talus fractures in the military Joint Theater Trauma Registry found that the mean time to fixation was 12.9 days. At a mean 16-month follow-up, no correlation was found between osteonecrosis or posttraumatic arthritis and the timing of fixation.

6. Patel R, Van Bergeyk A, Pinney S: Are displaced talar neck fractures surgical emergencies? A survey of orthopaedic trauma experts. *Foot Ankle Int* 2005;26(5):378-381.

7. Rammelt S, Zwipp H: Talar neck and body fractures. *Injury* 2009;40(2):120-135.

   The acute management of talar neck and body fractures and the management of subsequent complications were reviewed.

8. Milenkovic S, Radenkovic M, Mitkovic M: Open subtalar dislocation treated by distractional external fixation. *J Orthop Trauma* 2004;18(9):638-640.

9. Tang H, Han K, Li M, et al: Treatment of Hawkins type II fractures of talar neck by a vascularized cuboid pedicle bone graft and combined internal and external fixation: A preliminary report on nine cases. *J Trauma* 2010;69(4):E1-E5.

   Nine patients with a Hawkins type II fracture were treated with open reduction and internal fixation with screws, external fixation to unload the talus, and a vascularized cuboid pedicle bone graft based on the lateral tarsal artery to improve the talar blood supply. No osteonecrosis was noted in a retrospective review at an average 39-month follow-up.

10. Besch L, Drost J, Egbers HJ: Treatment of rare talus dislocation fractures: An analysis of 23 injuries [in German]. *Unfallchirurg* 2002;105(7):595-601.

11. Sangeorzan BJ, Wagner UA, Harrington RM, Tencer AF: Contact characteristics of the subtalar joint: The effect of talar neck misalignment. *J Orthop Res* 1992;10(4):544-551.

12. Sanders DW, Busam M, Hattwick E, Edwards JR, McAndrew MP, Johnson KD: Functional outcomes following displaced talar neck fractures. *J Orthop Trauma* 2004;18(5):265-270.

13. Herscovici D Jr, Anglen JO, Archdeacon M, Cannada L, Scaduto JM: Avoiding complications in the treatment of pronation-external rotation ankle fractures, syndesmotic injuries, and talar neck fractures. *J Bone Joint Surg Am* 2008;90(4):898-908.

    The potential complications of treatment for three foot and ankle injuries were reviewed, with strategies for preventing common complications.

14. Herscovici D Jr, Sanders RW, Infante A, DiPasquale T: Bohler incision: An extensile anterolateral approach to the foot and ankle. *J Orthop Trauma* 2000;14(6):429-432.

15. Cronier P, Talha A, Massin P: Central talar fractures: Therapeutic considerations. *Injury* 2004;35(suppl 2):SB10-SB22.

16. Gonzalez A, Stern R, Assal M: Reduction of irreducible Hawkins III talar neck fracture by means of a medial malleolar osteotomy: A report of three cases with a 4-year mean follow-up. *J Orthop Trauma* 2011;25(5):e47-e50.

    Clinical case report of three patients with a closed Hawkins type III talar neck fracture in which the posteromedially dislocated talar body was irreducible with combined anteromedial and anterolateral approaches. The talus was successfully reduced using a medial malleolar osteotomy.

17. Swanson TV, Bray TJ, Holmes GB Jr: Fractures of the talar neck: A mechanical study of fixation. *J Bone Joint Surg Am* 1992;74(4):544-551.

18. Attiah M, Sanders DW, Valdivia G, et al: Comminuted talar neck fractures: A mechanical comparison of fixation techniques. *J Orthop Trauma* 2007;21(1):47-51.

19. Fortin PT, Balazsy JE: Talus fractures: Evaluation and treatment. *J Am Acad Orthop Surg* 2001;9(2):114-127.

20. Fleuriau Chateau PB, Brokaw DS, Jelen BA, Scheid DK, Weber TG: Plate fixation of talar neck fractures: Preliminary review of a new technique in twenty-three patients. *J Orthop Trauma* 2002;16(4):213-219.

21. Adelaar RS, Madrian JR: Avascular necrosis of the talus. *Orthop Clin North Am* 2004;35(3):383-395, xi.

22. Berlet GC, Lee TH, Massa EG: Talar neck fractures. *Orthop Clin North Am* 2001;32(1):53-64.

23. Frawley PA, Hart JA, Young DA: Treatment outcome of major fractures of the talus. *Foot Ankle Int* 1995;16(6):339-345.

6: Foot and Ankle Trauma

24. Tezval M, Dumont C, Stürmer KM: Prognostic reliability of the Hawkins sign in fractures of the talus. *J Orthop Trauma* 2007;21(8):538-543.

25. Thordarson DB, Triffon MJ, Terk MR: Magnetic resonance imaging to detect avascular necrosis after open reduction and internal fixation of talar neck fractures. *Foot Ankle Int* 1996;17(12):742-747.

26. Penny JN, Davis LA: Fractures and fracture-dislocations of the neck of the talus. *J Trauma* 1980;20(12):1029-1037.

27. DiGiovanni CW, Patel A, Calfee R, Nickisch F: Osteonecrosis in the foot. *J Am Acad Orthop Surg* 2007;15(4):208-217.

28. Horst F, Gilbert BJ, Nunley JA: Avascular necrosis of the talus: Current treatment options. *Foot Ankle Clin* 2004;9(4):757-773.

29. Mont MA, Schon LC, Hungerford MW, Hungerford DS: Avascular necrosis of the talus treated by core decompression. *J Bone Joint Surg Br* 1996;78(5):827-830.

30. Grice J, Cannon L: Percutaneous core decompression: A successful method of treatment of stage I avascular necrosis of the talus. *Foot Ankle Surg* 2011;17(4):317-318.

   Stage I talar osteonecrosis was successfully treated by percutaneous core decompression in a 41-year-old woman with systemic lupus erythematosus who was on long-term steroid therapy.

31. Hussl H, Sailer R, Daniaux H, Pechlaner S: Revascularization of a partially necrotic talus with a vascularized bone graft from the iliac crest. *Arch Orthop Trauma Surg* 1989;108(1):27-29.

32. Harnroongroj T, Vanadurongwan V: The talar body prosthesis. *J Bone Joint Surg Am* 1997;79(9):1313-1322.

33. Chan G, Sanders DW, Yuan X, Jenkinson RJ, Willits K: Clinical accuracy of imaging techniques for talar neck malunion. *J Orthop Trauma* 2008;22(6):415-418.

   A cadaver study compared the ability of plain radiographs, CT, and radiostereometric analysis to detect changes in talus fracture fragment position and alignment. All methods underestimated talar neck displacement and rotation as measured, but CT was the most accurate imaging technique for measuring displacement in talar neck malunion.

34. Rammelt S, Winkler J, Heineck J, Zwipp H: Anatomical reconstruction of malunited talus fractures: A prospective study of 10 patients followed for 4 years. *Acta Orthop* 2005;76(4):588-596.

35. Easley ME, Trnka HJ, Schon LC, Myerson MS: Isolated subtalar arthrodesis. *J Bone Joint Surg Am* 2000;82(5):613-624.

36. Doi K, Hattori Y: Vascularized bone graft from the supracondylar region of the femur. *Microsurgery* 2009;29(5):379-384.

   Forty-six patients with osteonecrosis of the talus, scaphoid, or lunate were treated with a free vascularized thin corticoperiosteal graft harvested from the supracondylar region of the femur. The graft consisted of periosteum with a thin layer of outer cortical bone, which is elastic and readily conforms to the recipient bed configuration.

37. Lindvall E, Haidukewych G, DiPasquale T, Herscovici D Jr, Sanders R: Open reduction and stable fixation of isolated, displaced talar neck and body fractures. *J Bone Joint Surg Am* 2004;86(10):2229-2234.

38. Vallier HA, Nork SE, Benirschke SK, Sangeorzan BJ: Surgical treatment of talar body fractures. *J Bone Joint Surg Am* 2003;85(9):1716-1724.

39. Ebraheim NA, Patil V, Owens C, Kandimalla Y: Clinical outcome of fractures of the talar body. *Int Orthop* 2008;32(6):773-777.

   Medium-term results were retrospectively reviewed in 19 patients with a displaced talar body fracture treated with internal fixation.

40. Funk JR, Srinivasan SC, Crandall JR: Snowboarder's talus fractures experimentally produced by eversion and dorsiflexion. *Am J Sports Med* 2003;31(6):921-928.

41. Valderrabano V, Perren T, Ryf C, Rillmann P, Hintermann B: Snowboarder's talus fracture: Treatment outcome of 20 cases after 3.5 years. *Am J Sports Med* 2005;33(6):871-880.

42. Berkowitz MJ, Kim DH: Process and tubercle fractures of the hindfoot. *J Am Acad Orthop Surg* 2005;13(8):492-502.

43. Kim DH, Berkowitz MJ, Pressman DN: Avulsion fractures of the medial tubercle of the posterior process of the talus. *Foot Ankle Int* 2003;24(2):172-175.

Chapter 25

Fractures of the Calcaneus

Todd S. Kim, MD

Introduction

Calcaneal fractures are among the most disabling lower extremity injuries. Early complications, long-term pain, posttraumatic arthritis, and reoperation are common. These injuries are challenging to manage, and the best treatment approach remains controversial. Alternative and minimally invasive surgical approaches have gained popularity in recent years and may have potential for minimizing the risk of complications and improving outcomes.

Pathoanatomy and Epidemiology

Most calcaneal fractures are intra-articular injuries from a high-energy mechanism, the most common of which are a fall from a height and a motor vehicle crash. Although the injury can occur at any age, often it affects a relatively young individual in an industrial setting. The socioeconomic effect is great because of this demographic pattern and the disability associated with the injury. Significant impairment has been reported to last 3 to 5 years after injury. The general health outcomes of patients with calcaneal fracture were found to be worse than those of patients with other orthopaedic injuries or patients who had a serious medical event such as an organ transplant or myocardial infarction. Calcaneal fracture is considered to be a serious, life-changing event.[1,2]

The typical calcaneal fracture involves an axial load on the lower limb that drives the talus down into the calcaneus. The exact fracture pattern can depend on the position of the foot at the time of impact, the patient's bone quality, and the amount of energy.[3] The heel is shortened, widened, and displaced into varus. Almost always the patient has significant associated soft-tissue swelling and damage. Severe swelling, fracture, blisters, and even compartment syndrome can occur. Associated

lumbar spine fracture or another lower extremity fracture is common.

The involvement of the posterior facet of the subtalar joint is one of the major challenging factors in achieving successful treatment and outcomes. Articular cartilage injury at the time of the impact and subsequent displacement of the articular fragments can lead to the development of posttraumatic arthritis. The classification of a fracture classification and the treatment algorithm are largely determined by the extent of involvement of the subtalar joint.

Intra-articular Fractures

Classification and Imaging

The initial radiographic assessment of a calcaneal fracture involves plain radiographs and often CT. Plain radiographs should include lateral and AP views of the foot and a Harris axial heel view. On the lateral view, a decreased Böhler angle, an increased angle of Gissane, and an inferior displacement of the posterior facet can be seen (**Figure 1**). If only the lateral portion of the joint is displaced, a double density sign (when two portions of the posterior facet articular surface are visible on the lateral radiograph) can be seen at the posterior facet (**Figure 2**). The AP foot view may show extension of the fracture into the anterior process and calcaneocuboid joint. The axial view may show varus displacement and shortening of the tuberosity. CT is indicated for most intra-articular fractures to evaluate the extent of joint involvement and displacement (**Figure 2 B, C, and D, and Figure 3, A and B**).[4]

A displaced intra-articular calcaneal fracture is identified as a joint depression fracture or a tongue-type fracture, based on the Essex-Lopresti[5] classification. With a relatively posterior-directed force, the fracture line extends into the posterior facet to produce a joint depression fracture. If the force is directed more inferiorly, the fracture line extends inferior to the posterior facet and produces a tongue-type fracture pattern.

The classification of Soeur and Remy[6] was expanded by Sanders[7] to define a system based on the number and location of articular fragments at the posterior facet, as

---

Dr. Kim or an immediate family member serves as a board member, owner, officer, or committee member of the American Orthopaedic Foot and Ankle Society.

6: Foot and Ankle Trauma

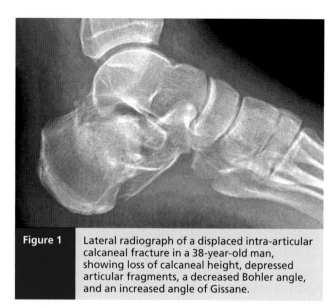

Figure 1 Lateral radiograph of a displaced intra-articular calcaneal fracture in a 38-year-old man, showing loss of calcaneal height, depressed articular fragments, a decreased Bohler angle, and an increased angle of Gissane.

seen on semicoronal CT[6,7] (**Figure 4**). A type I fracture is nondisplaced. A type II fracture is a two-part fracture with a subtype based on the location of the primary fracture line. A type III fracture has three parts, often with a centrally depressed fragment. A type IV fracture has at least four articular fragments and typically is highly comminuted.

Nonsurgical Treatment

A nondisplaced (Sanders type I) fracture usually is treated nonsurgically. A displaced fracture in a patient with significant perioperative risk factors can be treated nonsurgically. Smoking, poorly controlled diabetes, peripheral neuropathy, and a serious medical comorbidity are relative contraindications to surgical treatment. Chronologic age probably should not be considered a contraindication to surgical treatment; a retrospective study found equivalent outcomes after surgical treatment in patients who were older or younger than 50 years.[8]

Surgical Versus Nonsurgical Treatment of a Displaced Fracture

The definitive treatment of patients with displaced intra-articular calcaneal fracture remains controversial. Historically, these fractures were treated nonsurgically. The benefit of surgical treatment was difficult to establish, and the rate of perioperative complications was considered too high to justify surgical treatment. In recent decades, however, surgical treatment has become the standard of care for many of these injuries. Improved understanding and management of the associated soft-tissue injury have led to the development of surgical techniques with relatively low complication rates. At the same time, developments in preoperative and intraoperative imaging

and newer implants have improved the ability to perform open reduction and internal fixation.

Several studies compared the surgical and nonsurgical treatment of intra-articular calcaneal fractures. Many of these studies were limited by a small patient population, a lack of consistency in fracture classification, and variations in surgical technique. A randomized prospective study of 30 patients with a displaced fracture (Sanders type II or III) found that the patients treated surgically had a statistically significant improvement in outcome at 17-month follow-up over those treated nonsurgically.[9]

In a large multicenter randomized study comparing surgical and nonsurgical treatment of displaced intra-articular calcaneal fracture, validated outcomes measures revealed no overall difference between patients in the two treatment groups at 2- to 8-year follow-up.[10] However, among patients who did not have a workers' compensation claim, surgical treatment led to better satisfaction scores than nonsurgical treatment. Women, younger patients, and patients with a greatly displaced fracture also had a better outcome after surgical treatment. Patients treated nonsurgically were much more likely than those treated surgically to require subsequent subtalar arthrodesis for posttraumatic arthritis. Despite the large number of enrolled patients and the sound methodology, this study did not clearly establish the optimal treatment of patients with a displaced intra-articular calcaneal fracture.

Open Reduction and Internal Fixation of a Displaced Fracture

Prospective studies are needed to define the patient groups that will benefit from surgical treatment, but open reduction and internal fixation generally is recommended for patients with a Sanders type II or III intra-articular fracture, as long as there is no clear contraindication.[3] It is clear that outcomes are poor if these injuries are treated nonsurgically.

Although several surgical approaches have been described, most studies have reported open reduction and internal fixation through an extensile lateral approach[3,11-13] (**Figure 5**). This approach remains the most common for surgical treatment of displaced intra-articular calcaneal fractures.

One of the key elements in this surgical treatment approach is the management of the associated soft-tissue injury and swelling. The most common and serious early complications of surgical treatment are delayed wound healing and infection.[14,15] To minimize wound complications, surgical treatment should not be attempted before resolution of the soft-tissue swelling, as indicated by the absence of pitting edema and by the presence of skin wrinkling at the lateral heel[16,17] (**Figure 6**). Some surgeons

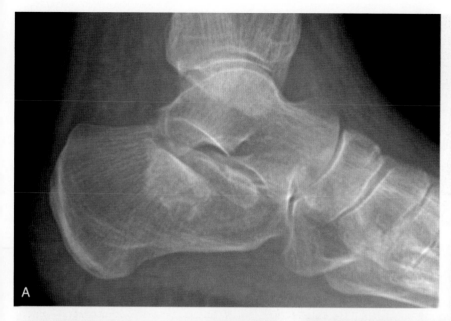
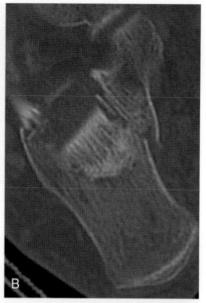
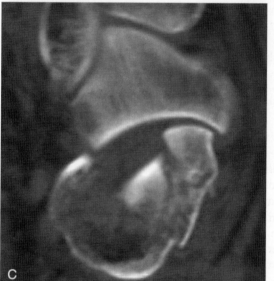
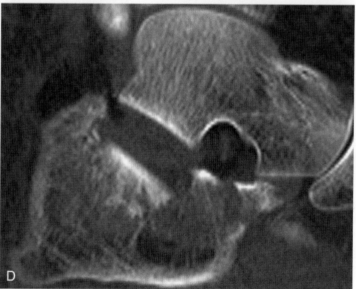

Figure 2 A displaced intra-articular fracture in a 78-year-old woman. **A,** Lateral radiograph showing the double density sign of a depressed articular fragment. Axial (**B**), coronal (**C**), and sagittal (**D**) CT images demonstrating the displaced intra-articular fracture pattern.

recommend the use of an aggressive soft-tissue protocol to decrease the delay to surgery and minimize the risk of complications.[18] Delay of more than 3 weeks after the injury makes fracture reduction extremely difficult because early fracture healing has occurred.

Surgical Treatment of a Tongue-Type Fracture

A displaced tongue-type fracture may require urgent surgical treatment. A severely displaced superior tuberosity fragment places the posterior skin under tension and can lead to soft-tissue injury and even skin necrosis within a few hours (**Figure 7**). A 21% incidence of

posterior soft-tissue compromise was found in a study of 139 tongue-type fractures.[19] Six soft-tissue coverage procedures and one amputation resulted. The patients treated with emergency percutaneous reduction avoided soft-tissue complications.

In general, simple or extra-articular tongue-type fractures (Sanders type IIC) are treated with percutaneous fixation (**Figure 8**). Guidewires are placed percutaneously on either side of the Achilles tendon and into the displaced tuberosity.[20] The guidewires are used to reduce the fracture and subsequently are advanced toward the anterior process. Definitive fixation can be achieved with

6: Foot and Ankle Trauma

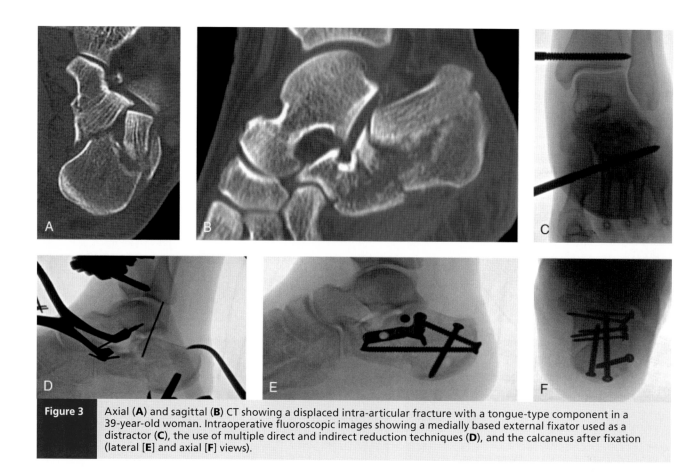

Figure 3 Axial (**A**) and sagittal (**B**) CT showing a displaced intra-articular fracture with a tongue-type component in a 39-year-old woman. Intraoperative fluoroscopic images showing a medially based external fixator used as a distractor (**C**), the use of multiple direct and indirect reduction techniques (**D**), and the calcaneus after fixation (lateral [**E**] and axial [**F**] views).

large cannulated screws placed over the guidewires. Alternatively, multiple small fragment screws can be placed percutaneously to maintain the reduction. Early mobilization is generally encouraged to minimize stiffness.

Complex intra-articular fractures with a tongue-type component (Sanders types IIA, IIB, and III) may not be amenable to reduction using the percutaneous Essex-Lopresti technique. Sagittal fracture lines and comminution at the articular surface cannot be appropriately reduced. These fractures should be treated with open reduction and internal fixation through an extensile lateral approach or with a minimally invasive technique.

Primary Arthrodesis for a Type IV Fracture

Because of multiple joint fragments and comminution, Sanders type IV fractures generally are not amenable to anatomic reduction and stable fixation. Even if anatomic reduction is possible, the articular cartilage damage from the time of impact is significant, and progression to posttraumatic arthritis is inevitable. For these reasons, primary arthrodesis is the surgical treatment of choice. Multiple researchers have reported on open reduction and internal fixation of the calcaneus combined with primary arthrodesis of the subtalar joint, using the extensile lateral approach.[21,22] In this technique, the extra-articular

calcaneal anatomy is restored with open reduction and internal fixation, and iliac crest bone graft is used at the arthrodesis site. High union rates, more rapid return to work, and generally good clinical outcomes have been reported when this method was used to treat these severe injuries.[23] Primary subtalar arthrodesis may be a good treatment option for a type IV fracture even without formal fracture reduction. Good results were obtained in a series of seven fractures treated with primary arthrodesis but not with formal open reduction and internal fixation.[24]

Minimally Invasive Techniques for a Displaced Fracture

In recent years, interest has increased in surgical approaches less invasive than the extensile lateral approach. These alternate approaches may carry less risk of wound complications. In addition, some researchers have suggested that the extensive soft-tissue stripping required for the extensile approach may compromise calcaneal vascularization and may lead to scarring and stiffness of the subtalar joint.[25] It is possible that a minimally invasive technique can lead to better outcomes and an improved subtalar range of motion than surgery through the extensile lateral approach. The described procedures

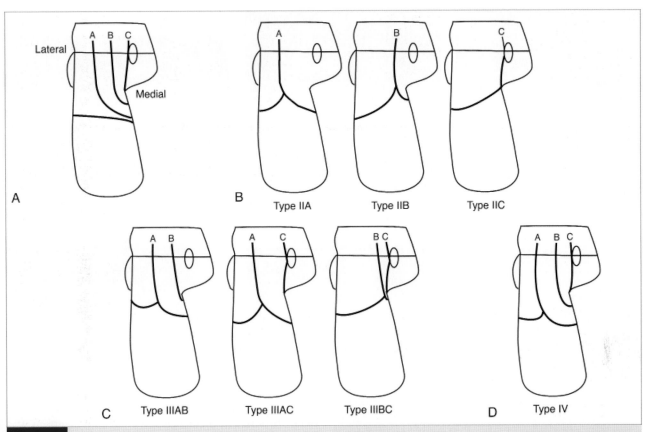

Figure 4 Drawings showing types II, III, and IV in the Sanders classification of intra-articular calcaneal fractures. **A,** Drawing correlates to a coronal CT image. Lateral, central, and medial fracture lines, which are identified as A, B, and C, respectively, are shown for the purpose of classifying the fracture subtype. In **B,C,** and **D,** the image on the left is the representation of fracture pattern on a coronal CT image and the image on the right represents the fracture pattern in the transverse or axial plane. **B,** Patterns of displaced two-part fractures (type II). The black area is the portion of the posterior facet articular surface involved/displaced with the given fracture pattern. **C,** Patterns of displaced three-part fractures (type III). **D,** Comminuted fracture (type IV). (Adapted from Buckley RE, Tough S: Displaced intra-articular calcaneal fractures. *J Am Acad Orthop Surg* 2004;12[3]:172-178.)

have included limited open reduction, closed and percutaneous reduction, percutaneous internal fixation, and external fixation. Regardless of technique, the goals of the minimally invasive approach are similar to those of open reduction and internal fixation through an extensile lateral approach: anatomic reduction of the articular surface, restoration of the height and valgus position of the tuberosity, and stable fixation to allow early mobilization.

With minimally invasive incisions, it is safe to proceed with surgery before the complete resolution of swelling. Because percutaneous and indirect reduction techniques are used, surgery must take place before early consolidation of the fracture. The general recommendation is that surgery be undertaken within 5 days of the injury.

Percutaneous Reduction and Fixation
Of 54 consecutive displaced calcaneal fractures treated with percutaneous reduction and external fixation, 49 (90.7%) had an excellent or good clinical and radiographic result.[26] There were no deep infections and only three superficial pin site infections. These results were comparable to those of conventional open reduction and internal fixation except for the absence of serious wound infections.

In 37 displaced calcaneal fractures treated with closed reduction and percutaneous screw fixation, the patients were positioned prone and the initial closed reduction was done with a temporary external fixator spanning the distal tibia to the calcaneal tuberosity.[27] The joint surface was reduced percutaneously, and internal fixation was obtained with multiple cannulated screws placed percutaneously. Five wound infections occurred. At a mean 66-month follow-up, 2 patients had required subtalar arthrodesis, and 17 (46%) had undergone removal of painful screws. Patient-reported scores revealed good overall results: the mean American Orthopaedic Foot and Ankle Society score was 84 of a possible 100 points, the Medical Outcomes Study Short Form–36 score was 76 points, and the patient satisfaction score was 7.9 of a

6: Foot and Ankle Trauma

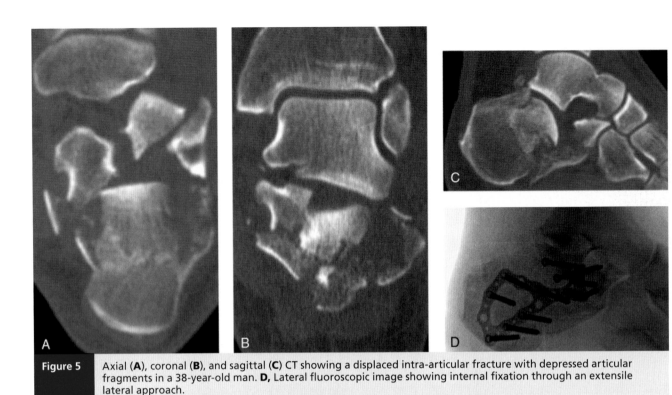

Figure 5 Axial (**A**), coronal (**B**), and sagittal (**C**) CT showing a displaced intra-articular fracture with depressed articular fragments in a 38-year-old man. **D,** Lateral fluoroscopic image showing internal fixation through an extensile lateral approach.

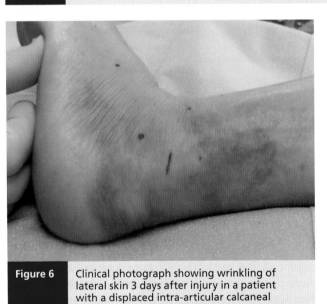

Figure 6 Clinical photograph showing wrinkling of lateral skin 3 days after injury in a patient with a displaced intra-articular calcaneal fracture. The patient had been treated with an aggressive inpatient soft-tissue protocol since the day of injury.

possible 10 points. The study showed that this treatment is viable and relatively safe.

A retrospective study compared 83 fractures treated with percutaneous reduction and fixation with 42 fractures treated with traditional open reduction and internal fixation.[28] The outcomes were similar in terms of the Böhler angle, maintenance of reduction, and rates of late fusion. The incidence of wound complications was significantly decreased in the patients treated percutaneously. No deep infections occurred in the patients treated percutaneously, but six deep infections occurred in those treated with open surgery.

Limited Open Reduction Using the Sinus Tarsi Approach

The sinus tarsi approach to the subtalar joint is commonly used in elective procedures such as subtalar arthrodesis. The use of the sinus tarsi approach for displaced calcaneal fracture allows open reduction and fixation of the articular fragments through a relatively small and safe incision.

Research Findings

A prospective study of displaced fractures treated using a mini-open sinus tarsi approach and percutaneous fixation found a good to excellent clinical result in 16 of 19 patients available for follow-up.[25] Reduction of the posterior facet was graded as good to excellent on CT in 14 of 22 fractures. Three of 21 patients (14%) had a superficial wound complication that resolved within 2 weeks with appropriate treatment.

The limited open approach was used in 24 patients and compared with the extensile lateral approach used in 26 patients.[29] Patients treated using the limited open approach had a shorter surgical time and no wound complications (compared with four wound complications in

6: Foot and Ankle Trauma

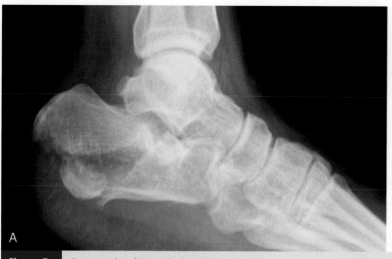
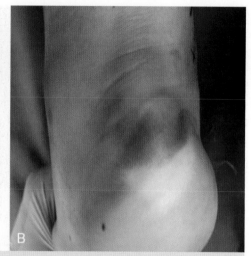

Figure 7 **A,** Lateral radiograph showing a displaced tongue-type calcaneal fracture. **B,** Clinical photograph showing impending skin necrosis in the same patient, caused by tuberosity fragment displacement. (Courtesy of Utku Kandemir, MD, San Francisco, CA.)

those treated using the extensile lateral approach). The functional results were similar, but a minor secondary procedure for screw removal was more common in the patients treated with the limited open approach.

In the largest study to compare the minimally invasive sinus tarsi approach with the extensile lateral approach, no statistically significant differences in patient satisfaction or patient-reported outcomes (using the Medical Outcomes Study Short Form–36, Foot Function Index, and visual analog pain scale) were found between the 33 fractures treated with a minimally invasive approach and the 79 fractures treated with an extensile lateral approach.[30] There was a significant difference in rates of wound complications. Twenty-nine percent of those treated using the extensile lateral approach had a wound complication, compared with only 6% of patients treated using the minimally invasive approach. Despite the inherent limitations of a retrospective study, these results appear to corroborate the finding that effective reduction of a displaced fracture can be achieved through a minimally invasive approach and that the incidence of wound complications is decreased when a minimally invasive technique is used.

The gold standard for surgical treatment of a displaced calcaneal fracture remains the extensile lateral approach. Alternative approaches, especially early in a surgeon's learning curve, should be reserved for relatively simple fracture patterns. Some complex and difficult fractures require the use of the extensile lateral approach for optimal reduction and fixation.

Surgical Technique

The lateral decubitus patient position is used with the sinus tarsi approach. The pelvis is rotated slightly back to allow access to the medial aspect of the foot when the hip is externally rotated and to facilitate positioning of the foot for the axial fluoroscopic view. An external fixator can be used as an intraoperative reduction tool. External fixator pins are placed in the medial distal tibia and the calcaneal tuberosity. Placement of the fixator on the medial side allows reduction of the varus angulation of the tuberosity and the restoration of calcaneal height (**Figure 3, C** and **Figure 9, A**).

A longitudinal incision is made from the distal tip of the fibula toward the base of the fourth metatarsal for a standard sinus tarsi approach to the subtalar joint. Specialized distractors using Kirschner wires inserted into the talus and the distal calcaneus can be helpful for visualization and reduction of the articular fragments (**Figure 3, D** and **Figure 9, B**). The medial fixator sometimes must be loosened temporarily to allow reduction and fixation of the posterior facet from the lateral side. The ability to reduce the tuberosity in relation to the sustentaculum tali at the medial cortex should be confirmed fluoroscopically before final fixation of the posterior facet. Indirect reduction of the tuberosity with the distracting fixator sometimes is not sufficient. Direct reduction maneuvers through the fracture from the lateral side are necessary but are not possible after reduction and fixation of the posterior facet is completed.

Once adequate exposure of the posterior facet of the subtalar joint is established, direct and indirect reduction maneuvers can be employed to achieve reduction of the articular surface (**Figure 9, D**). Initial fixation of the articular reduction typically is done with a 2.7-mm cortical screw placed from the lateral articular fragment toward the sustentaculum tali (**Figure 10, A and B**). Additional fixation can be achieved with screws or with a

6: Foot and Ankle Trauma

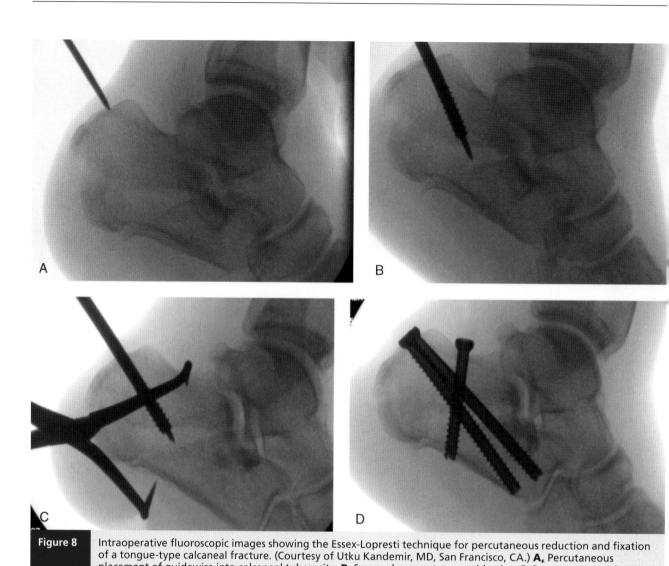

Figure 8 Intraoperative fluoroscopic images showing the Essex-Lopresti technique for percutaneous reduction and fixation of a tongue-type calcaneal fracture. (Courtesy of Utku Kandemir, MD, San Francisco, CA.) **A,** Percutaneous placement of guidewire into calcaneal tuberosity. **B,** Screw placement over guidewire. **C,** Percutaneous reduction technique. **D,** Internal fixation with multiple percutaneous screws.

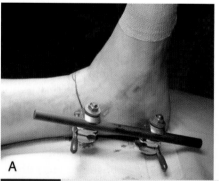 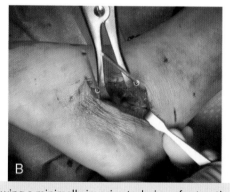 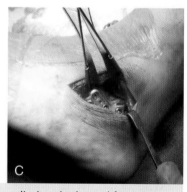

Figure 9 Intraoperative photographs showing a minimally invasive technique for treating a displaced calcaneal fracture. **A,** A distracting external fixator placed on the medial side from the distal tibia to the calcaneal tuberosity. **B,** The sinus tarsi exposure of the subtalar joint, showing articular reduction, and the use of a lateral Kirschner-wire distractor for joint visualization. **C,** Placement of a lateral periarticular plate through the sinus tarsi exposure, after reduction of the articular fragments.

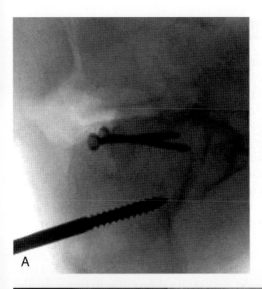
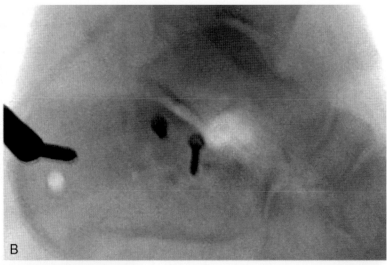
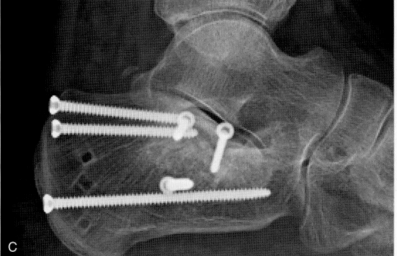
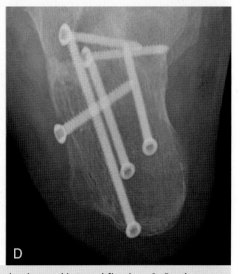

Figure 10 A minimally invasive sinus tarsi approach was used for limited open reduction and internal fixation. **A,** Broden view intraoperative fluoroscopic image showing articular reduction **B,** Lateral view fluoroscopic image showing placement of the external fixator. Lateral (**C**) and axial (**D**) radiographs showing the healed fracture 6 months after surgery.

periarticular plate, depending on the fracture pattern and the surgeon's preference (**Figure 3, E** and **F** and **Figure 8, C**). The approach can be safely extended to allow reduction of additional fracture fragments and percutaneous plate placement.[31] As long as dissection is not carried into the deep portion of the superficial peroneal retinaculum, the blood supply to the lateral skin flap through the lateral calcaneal artery is preserved.

Reduction of the tuberosity and the anterior process is confirmed fluoroscopically. Multiple percutaneous screws can be placed from the tuberosity and from the anterior process, depending on the fracture pattern, to complete fixation (**Figure 3, E** and **F** and **Figure 10, C** and **D**). The distracting fixator usually is removed when percutaneous fixation of the tuberosity is complete. In

an extremely unstable or comminuted fracture, the external fixator can be left in place until early fracture consolidation occurs. To minimize stiffness, patients are kept non–weight bearing until fracture healing at 8 to 12 weeks, but early mobilization is encouraged when the wounds have healed.

Extra-articular Fractures

One third of calcaneal fractures are considered extra-articular because they do not extend into or involve the posterior facet of the subtalar joint. The mechanism of injury is similar to that of an intra-articular fracture, but generally there is less force at impact. An extra-articular fracture is most common in children. The predominance

6: Foot and Ankle Trauma

of boys and men among the patients is less pronounced than with intra-articular fractures. Most of these injuries can be effectively treated nonsurgically, especially if the displacement is minimal.[32]

Calcaneal body fractures (Sanders type I) most commonly are treated nonsurgically. Surgery is indicated to prevent a problematic malunion with severe shortening, which could affect the gastrocnemius-soleus complex, or with widening, which could affect the peroneal tendons. Most authors recommend surgical treatment of displaced body fractures with more than 30° of angulation or more than 1 cm of translation.[3]

Tuberosity fractures result from forced dorsiflexion and can involve a portion of the Achilles tendon insertion. Like a displaced tongue-type fractures, a displaced tuberosity avulsion fracture can place the posterior skin at risk. Without immediate treatment, skin necrosis and wound complications can occur.[33] Urgent surgical treatment with open reduction and internal fixation is indicated. A recent review of calcaneal tuberosity avulsion fractures led to a modified classification scheme.[34] Simple extra-articular avulsion fracture (type I) was found to be the most common type. This fracture generally occurred with a low-energy mechanism in older patients. A true nondisplaced fracture can be treated nonsurgically with immobilization in plantar flexion. Because of the inherent risk to the strength of the gastrocnemius-soleus complex, a displaced fracture should be treated with open reduction and internal fixation. Depending on the size of the fracture fragment and the bone quality, fixation can be achieved with lag screws or a tension-band construct.

Isolated fracture of the sustentaculum tali is rare. CT usually is necessary because the fracture characteristics can be difficult to appreciate on plain radiographs. Fractures that involve the posterior facet or are displaced more than 2 mm require surgical treatment.[35] A study of 15 patients who underwent open reduction and internal fixation through a medial approach to the sustentaculum tali found that all fractures healed with maintained reduction, and there were no complications related to the surgical approach.[36]

Most anterior process fractures can be treated nonsurgically with cast or boot immobilization. Surgical treatment is reserved for fracture fragments that involve more than 25% of the calcaneocuboid joint.[3] If the fracture fragments are too small or comminuted to allow open reduction and internal fixation, primary excision may be necessary. Delayed excision sometimes is necessary to treat painful nonunion of small fragments. Successful endoscopic excision of a symptomatic nonunion recently was reported.[37]

Complications

Wound Complications

The most common and serious early complication of surgical treatment of calcaneal fracture is delayed wound healing and infection, which was reported to occur in as many as 25% of patients after open reduction and internal fixation using a lateral extensile approach.[13-15,17] Despite awareness of soft-tissue swelling, attention to intraoperative handling of the flap, and meticulous two-layer closure, delayed healing and necrosis at the apex of the flap can occur. Treatment using local wound care, antibiotics, and occasionally surgical débridement generally is effective. Fewer than 5% of closed fractures progress to deep infection and osteomyelitis.

A recent study of 490 calcaneal fractures treated with open reduction and internal fixation found a wound complication rate of 17.8%.[15] Patient-related risk factors were identified as tobacco smoking, diabetes, and a Sanders type fracture. Surgery-related risk factors were the presence of residents or fellows in the operating room, duration of surgery, estimated blood loss, and a total of 10 or more people in the operating room at any time during the surgery. Use of a tourniquet was associated with a lower risk of wound complications. An earlier study identified high body mass index, increased time from injury to surgery, and a single-layer closure as risk factors for wound complications.[17]

Open calcaneal fractures have a much higher complication rate than closed calcaneal fractures. A recent study of 115 surgically treated open fractures found superficial wound infection in 9.6%, deep infection in 12.2%, and culture-positive osteomyelitis in 5.2%.[38] Six patients (5.2%) required amputation. The overall complication rate of 23.5% was lower than expected for open fracture. A study of 12 fractures with a plantar medial wound found that this subtype of open fracture was associated with a very high rate of complications.[39] Infection developed in five patients, and three required a soft-tissue coverage procedure. Nonunion developed in three patients, and one patient required a below-knee amputation.

Posttraumatic Arthritis

Posttraumatic arthritis of the subtalar joint is a common complication of calcaneal fracture, whether the fracture was treated surgically or nonsurgically. Displaced intra-articular calcaneal fractures result from a high-energy mechanism; the energy on impact often causes direct and irreversible articular cartilage injury that can be seen at the time of surgery. The mechanisms of chondrocyte injury and death with impact loading have been well described.[40-43] Further joint destruction will occur in a displaced fracture if the articular surface is not anatomically reduced. Fractures treated nonsurgically and fractures treated surgically with a suboptimal articular reduction will progress rapidly to subtalar arthrosis. An analysis of the risk factors reported a 10% rate of late subtalar fusion.[44] The strongest factor for predicting the risk of long-term sequelae was the severity of the initial injury, based on the Böhler angle and Sanders classification. Nonsurgical treatment and the existence of a workers' compensation claim also predicted a poor outcome and the need for late subtalar fusion.

A patient with pain and disability from posttraumatic arthritis often requires surgical treatment with subtalar fusion. Removal of the internal fixation and in situ arthrodesis are recommended.[45] A large study of patients who underwent subtalar fusion to treat a late complication of calcaneal fracture found that the patients who had undergone initial surgical treatment had fewer wound complications and better functional outcomes than those who initially had been treated nonsurgically.[46] The researchers concluded that long-term outcomes were improved because the initial open reduction and internal fixation restored the calcaneal shape, alignment, and height, even if subtalar fusion later was required.

Calcaneal Malunion

Nonsurgical treatment of a displaced calcaneal fracture often leads to a problematic malunion. Loss of calcaneal height results in shortening of the gastrocnemius-soleus complex and can affect ankle dorsiflexion. Varus malalignment of the tuberosity can negatively affect gait and ankle stability. Widening of the calcaneus can lead to subfibular impingement and peroneal tendon dysfunction.

The classification of calcaneal malunion is based on the presence of a lateral wall exostosis, subtalar joint arthrosis, and varus malunion.[47] If subtalar joint arthrosis is present, fusion with an attempt to restore calcaneal height is recommended. A 93% union rate was reported in a study of 40 subtalar arthrodesis procedures to correct malunion.[48] The functional results were good, but there was difficulty in restoring calcaneal height. The researchers recommended initial surgical treatment to prevent calcaneal malunion.

A recent study of 20 patients with calcaneal malunion who underwent corrective osteotomy with preservation of the subtalar joint found a significant improvement in patient functional scores as well as improvement in radiographic parameters.[49] At average 34-month follow-up, only one conversion to a subtalar fusion had been required. Corrective osteotomy with preservation of the subtalar joint may be an alternative to subtalar arthrodesis in some patients with calcaneal malunion.

Summary

Calcaneal fracture can be a devastating injury. Regardless of the initial treatment, chronic pain and disability often ensue. Surgical treatment is technically challenging, even for an experienced surgeon, and serious complications are common. Alternative minimally invasive approaches have shown early promise and carry a decreased risk of wound complications. Future study is needed to determine whether the use of newer techniques improves long-term patient outcomes.

Annotated References

1. van Tetering EA, Buckley RE: Functional outcome (SF-36) of patients with displaced calcaneal fractures compared to SF-36 normative data. *Foot Ankle Int* 2004;25(10):733-738.

2. Potter MQ, Nunley JA: Long-term functional outcomes after operative treatment for intra-articular fractures of the calcaneus. *J Bone Joint Surg Am* 2009;91(8):1854-1860.

   At a mean 12.8-year follow-up, 81 surgically treated calcaneal fractures were retrospectively reviewed with patient-reported functional scores. Level of evidence: III.

3. Sanders R, Clare MP: Fractures of the calcaneus, in Coughlin MJ, Mann RA, Saltzman CL, eds: *Surgery of the Foot and Ankle,* ed 8. Philadelphia, PA, Mosby Elsevier, 2007, pp 2017-2073.

4. Sanders R: Displaced intra-articular fractures of the calcaneus. *J Bone Joint Surg Am* 2000;82(2):225-250.

5. Essex-Lopresti P: The mechanism, reduction technique, and results in fractures of the os calcis. *Br J Surg* 1952;39(157):395-419.

6. Soeur R, Remy R: Fractures of the calcaneus with displacement of the thalamic portion. *J Bone Joint Surg Br* 1975;57(4):413-421.

7. Sanders R: Intra-articular fractures of the calcaneus: Present state of the art. *J Orthop Trauma* 1992;6(2):252-265.

8. Gaskill T, Schweitzer K, Nunley J: Comparison of surgical outcomes of intra-articular calcaneal fractures by age. *J Bone Joint Surg Am* 2010;92(18):2884-2889.

   A retrospective review of 175 patients with patient-reported scores and other clinical outcomes found no significant difference based on age group. Level of evidence: III.

9. Thordarson DB, Krieger LE: Operative vs. nonoperative treatment of intra-articular fractures of the calcaneus: A prospective randomized trial. *Foot Ankle Int* 1996;17(1):2-9.

6: Foot and Ankle Trauma

10. Buckley R, Tough S, McCormack R, et al: Operative compared with nonoperative treatment of displaced intra-articular calcaneal fractures: A prospective, randomized, controlled multicenter trial. *J Bone Joint Surg Am* 2002;84(10):1733-1744.

11. Benirschke SK, Sangeorzan BJ: Extensive intraarticular fractures of the foot: Surgical management of calcaneal fractures. *Clin Orthop Relat Res* 1993;292:128-134.

12. Gould N: Lateral approach to the os calcis. *Foot Ankle* 1984;4(4):218-220.

13. Sanders R, Fortin P, DiPasquale T, Walling A: Operative treatment in 120 displaced intraarticular calcaneal fractures: Results using a prognostic computed tomography scan classification. *Clin Orthop Relat Res* 1993;290:87-95.

14. Folk JW, Starr AJ, Early JS: Early wound complications of operative treatment of calcaneus fractures: Analysis of 190 fractures. *J Orthop Trauma* 1999;13(5):369-372.

15. Ding L, He Z, Xiao H, Chai L, Xue F: Risk factors for postoperative wound complications of calcaneal fractures following plate fixation. *Foot Ankle Int* 2013;34(9):1238-1244.

    A retrospective review of a large group of patients identified risk factors for development of postoperative wound complications. The overall wound complication rate was 17.8%. Level of evidence: III.

16. Shuler FD, Conti SF, Gruen GS, Abidi NA: Wound-healing risk factors after open reduction and internal fixation of calcaneal fractures: Does correction of Bohler's angle alter outcomes? *Orthop Clin North Am* 2001;32(1):187-192, x.

17. Abidi NA, Dhawan S, Gruen GS, Vogt MT, Conti SF: Wound-healing risk factors after open reduction and internal fixation of calcaneal fractures. *Foot Ankle Int* 1998;19(12):856-861.

18. Bergin PF, Psaradellis T, Krosin MT, et al: Inpatient soft tissue protocol and wound complications in calcaneus fractures. *Foot Ankle Int* 2012;33(6):492-497.

    A retrospective study found a decreased time to surgery and a lower complication rate after use of an inpatient soft-tissue protocol. Level of evidence: III.

19. Gardner MJ, Nork SE, Barei DP, Kramer PA, Sangeorzan BJ, Benirschke SK: Secondary soft tissue compromise in tongue-type calcaneus fractures. *J Orthop Trauma* 2008;22(7):439-445.

    A retrospective study of 127 patients found a 21% rate of posterior skin compromise in 139 tongue-type fractures. Level of evidence: III.

20. Tornetta P III: The Essex-Lopresti reduction for calcaneal fractures revisited. *J Orthop Trauma* 1998;12(7):469-473.

21. Buch BD, Myerson MS, Miller SD: Primary subtaler arthrodesis for the treatment of comminuted calcaneal fractures. *Foot Ankle Int* 1996;17(2):61-70.

22. Huefner T, Thermann H, Geerling J, Pape HC, Pohlemann T: Primary subtalar arthrodesis of calcaneal fractures. *Foot Ankle Int* 2001;22(1):9-14.

23. Schepers T: The primary arthrodesis for severely comminuted intra-articular fractures of the calcaneus: A systematic review. *Foot Ankle Surg* 2012;18(2):84-88.

    A systematic review of published studies found high union rates and good outcomes after primary arthrodesis for severely comminuted intra-articular calcaneal fractures. Level of evidence: II.

24. Potenza V, Caterini R, Farsetti P, Bisicchia S, Ippolito E: Primary subtalar arthrodesis for the treatment of comminuted intra-articular calcaneal fractures. *Injury* 2010;41(7):702-706.

    The short-term and midterm results of seven patients with primary subtalar arthrodesis for a Sanders type IV fracture were reported. Level of evidence: IV.

25. Nosewicz T, Knupp M, Barg A, et al: Mini-open sinus tarsi approach with percutaneous screw fixation of displaced calcaneal fractures: A prospective computed tomography-based study. *Foot Ankle Int* 2012;33(11):925-933.

    Good to excellent functional and radiographic outcomes were found in 16 of 19 patients (19 fractures). Level of evidence: IV.

26. Magnan B, Bortolazzi R, Marangon A, Marino M, Dall'Oca C, Bartolozzi P: External fixation for displaced intra-articular fractures of the calcaneum. *J Bone Joint Surg Br* 2006;88(11):1474-1479.

27. Tomesen T, Biert J, Frölke JP: Treatment of displaced intra-articular calcaneal fractures with closed reduction and percutaneous screw fixation. *J Bone Joint Surg Am* 2011;93(10):920-928.

    A retrospective review of 37 patients found fairly good functional outcomes, although 46% of patients required removal of painful hardware. Level of evidence: IV.

28. DeWall M, Henderson CE, McKinley TO, Phelps T, Dolan L, Marsh JL: Percutaneous reduction and fixation of displaced intra-articular calcaneus fractures. *J Orthop Trauma* 2010;24(8):466-472.

    In a retrospective review, patients treated with percutaneous reduction had a lower incidence of deep infection than those treated with open reduction and internal fixation. Level of evidence: III.

29. Weber M, Lehmann O, Sägesser D, Krause F: Limited open reduction and internal fixation of displaced intra-articular fractures of the calcaneum. *J Bone Joint Surg Br* 2008;90(12):1608-1616.

In a retrospective review, 24 patients treated with limited open reduction and internal fixation of a displaced intra-articular fracture of the calcaneum were compared with 26 patients treated with the extensile lateral approach. Level of evidence: III.

30. Kline AJ, Anderson RB, Davis WH, Jones CP, Cohen BE: Minimally invasive technique versus an extensile lateral approach for intra-articular calcaneal fractures. *Foot Ankle Int* 2013;34(6):773-780.

A lower rate of wound complications (6% versus 29%) was found in patients treated using a minimally invasive technique rather than an extensile lateral approach. Level of evidence: III.

31. Femino JE, Vaseenon T, Levin DA, Yian EH: Modification of the sinus tarsi approach for open reduction and plate fixation of intra-articular calcaneus fractures: The limits of proximal extension based upon the vascular anatomy of the lateral calcaneal artery. *Iowa Orthop J* 2010;30:161-167.

Thirteen patients were treated using the sinus tarsi approach and followed for complications. A cadaver study defined the relevant vascular anatomy. Level of evidence: IV.

32. Schepers T, Ginai AZ, Van Lieshout EM, Patka P: Demographics of extra-articular calcaneal fractures: Including a review of the literature on treatment and outcome. *Arch Orthop Trauma Surg* 2008;128(10):1099-1106.

Demographic factors in intra-articular and extra-articular calcaneal fractures were compared. Level of evidence: III.

33. Hess M, Booth B, Laughlin RT: Calcaneal avulsion fractures: Complications from delayed treatment. *Am J Emerg Med* 2008;26(2):e1-e4.

Skin necrosis occurred after three calcaneal avulsion fractures because of a delay in treatment. Level of evidence: IV.

34. Lee SM, Huh SW, Chung JW, Kim DW, Kim YJ, Rhee SK: Avulsion fracture of the calcaneal tuberosity: Classification and its characteristics. *Clin Orthop Surg* 2012;4(2):134-138.

Calcaneal avulsion fractures in 20 patients were retrospectively reviewed, and a classification system was developed. Level of evidence: III.

35. Clare MP: Occult injuries about the subtalar joint, in Nunley J, Pfeffer GB, Sanders R, Trepman E, eds: *Advanced Reconstruction: Foot and Ankle.* Rosemont, IL, American Academy of Orthopaedic Surgeons, 2004, pp 385-391.

36. Della Rocca GJ, Nork SE, Barei DP, Taitsman LA, Benirschke SK: Fractures of the sustentaculum tali: Injury characteristics and surgical technique for reduction. *Foot Ankle Int* 2009;30(11):1037-1041.

A review of 19 surgically treated fractures of the sustentaculum tali found that open reduction and internal fixation through a medial approach was reliable and safe. Level of evidence: IV.

37. Lui TH: Endoscopic excision of symptomatic nonunion of anterior calcaneal process. *J Foot Ankle Surg* 2011;50(4):476-479.

This is a case report of symptomatic nonunion of an anterior process fracture treated with arthroscopic and endoscopic techniques.

38. Wiersema B, Brokaw D, Weber T, et al: Complications associated with open calcaneus fractures. *Foot Ankle Int* 2011;32(11):1052-1057.

A review of 127 open calcaneal fractures found an overall complication rate of 23.5%, which was lower than rates previously reported for open fractures. Level of evidence: III.

39. Firoozabadi R, Kramer PA, Benirschke SK: Plantar medial wounds associated with calcaneal fractures. *Foot Ankle Int* 2013;34(7):941-948.

Twelve open calcaneal fractures with a plantar medial wound were reviewed for complications and healing. Level of evidence: IV.

40. Borrelli J Jr, Silva MJ, Zaegel MA, Franz C, Sandell LJ: Single high-energy impact load causes posttraumatic OA in young rabbits via a decrease in cellular metabolism. *J Orthop Res* 2009;27(3):347-352.

A basic science study found that a single-impact load could lead to posttraumatic arthritis in rabbits by disrupting the extracellular matrix and causing a decrease in chondrocyte metabolism.

41. Borrelli J Jr, Tinsley K, Ricci WM, Burns M, Karl IE, Hotchkiss R: Induction of chondrocyte apoptosis following impact load. *J Orthop Trauma* 2003;17(9):635-641.

42. Borrelli J Jr, Torzilli PA, Grigiene R, Helfet DL: Effect of impact load on articular cartilage: Development of an intra-articular fracture model. *J Orthop Trauma* 1997;11(5):319-326.

43. Torzilli PA, Grigiene R, Borrelli J Jr, Helfet DL: Effect of impact load on articular cartilage: Cell metabolism and viability, and matrix water content. *J Biomech Eng* 1999;121(5):433-441.

44. Csizy M, Buckley R, Tough S, et al: Displaced intra-articular calcaneal fractures: Variables predicting late subtalar fusion. *J Orthop Trauma* 2003;17(2):106-112.

45. Flemister AS Jr, Infante AF, Sanders RW, Walling AK: Subtalar arthrodesis for complications of intra-articular calcaneal fractures. *Foot Ankle Int* 2000;21(5):392-399.

6: Foot and Ankle Trauma

46. Radnay CS, Clare MP, Sanders RW: Subtalar fusion after displaced intra-articular calcaneal fractures: Does initial operative treatment matter? *J Bone Joint Surg Am* 2009;91(3):541-546.

    A study of patients undergoing subtalar fusion found that patients initially treated with open reduction and internal fixation had better functional outcomes and fewer wound complications than those initially treated nonsurgically. Level of evidence: III.

47. Stephens HM, Sanders R: Calcaneal malunions: Results of a prognostic computed tomography classification system. *Foot Ankle Int* 1996;17(7):395-401.

48. Clare MP, Lee WE III, Sanders RW: Intermediate to long-term results of a treatment protocol for calcaneal fracture malunions. *J Bone Joint Surg Am* 2005;87(5):963-973.

49. Yu GR, Hu SJ, Yang YF, Zhao HM, Zhang SM: Reconstruction of calcaneal fracture malunion with osteotomy and subtalar joint salvage: Technique and outcomes. *Foot Ankle Int* 2013;34(5):726-733.

    A review of 26 calcaneal malunions treated with osteotomy and preservation of the subtalar joint found that functional and radiographic outcomes were satisfactory, with a relatively low complication rate. Level of evidence: IV.

6: Foot and Ankle Trauma

Chapter 26

Midfoot Injuries

David I. Pedowitz, MS, MD   Steven M. Raikin, MD

Introduction

The area of midfoot injury extends from the naviculocuneiform joints proximally to the tarsometatarsal (TMT) joints distally. Midfoot injury encompasses a wide spectrum of pathology from a subtle sprain incurred on an athletic field to a massive crush injury after a motor vehicle crash. Some patients are young but skeletally mature; others are of advanced age and often have poor bone quality. Keeping these distinctions in mind is paramount when making clinical decisions regarding these complex injuries.

Navicular Fractures

Although navicular fracture is not common, it is particularly important to understand. The navicular articulates with four bones in the foot, serves as the major attachment site for the posterior tibial tendon, and is responsible for significant midfoot motion. The navicular is named for its boatlike shape, which is concave from medial to lateral, concave from dorsal to plantar at the talonavicular joint, and convex at the naviculocuneiform joints. The navicular represents a transition zone from the mobile talonavicular joint, which allows the entire foot to pivot on the talus, to the stiff naviculocuneiform joints. Navicular fractures range from simple dorsal and medial avulsion to body and stress fractures. Any of these fractures, if missed, can lead to significant morbidity in the midfoot.

Avulsion Fractures

Dorsal capsular avulsion fracture, the most common type of navicular fracture, often is caused by acute plantar

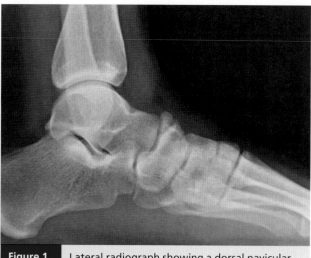

Figure 1   Lateral radiograph showing a dorsal navicular avulsion fracture.

flexion injury or ankle sprain. Typically, trauma to a portion of the strong dorsal talonavicular ligament causes avulsion of a small piece of the bone. This fracture is relatively benign and can be treated with immobilization in a walking boot for 6 to 8 weeks or until the patient is asymptomatic (**Figure 1**). Traditionally, treatment with a short period of immobilization has been recommended as leading to minimal disability, with fragment excision recommended if pain persists after immobilization.[1] A second recommendation is for a short period of immobilization with avoidance of weight bearing, in the presence of significant soft-tissue swelling and ecchymosis, to give the associated ligamentous injury ample time to heal.[2] If the avulsed fragment is a significant portion of the articular surface of the navicular, open reduction and internal fixation is indicated to minimize symptoms, the risk of posttraumatic arthritis, and the likelihood of subsequent midtarsal subluxation. Unfortunately, no clear criteria define the percentage of dorsal navicular involvement indicating that surgical intervention is necessary.

Avulsion fracture of the navicular tuberosity is the result of forceful eversion of the midfoot. Eversion tensions the posterior tibial tendon insertion, the tibionavicular ligament (the most anterior portion of the deltoid ligament), and the plantar calcaneonavicular

Dr. Pedowitz or an immediate family member is a member of a speakers' bureau or has made paid presentations on behalf of Integra Life Sciences; serves as a paid consultant to Tornier and Integra Life Sciences; and has received research or institutional support from Integra Life Sciences. Dr. Raikin or an immediate family member serves as a paid consultant to Biomet, and has received research or institutional support from Biomimetic.

6: Foot and Ankle Trauma

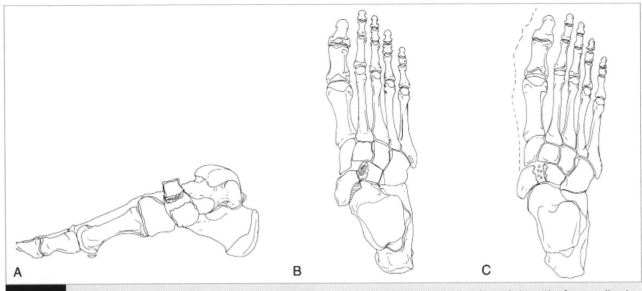

Figure 2 Schematic showing the three types of navicular fractures. **A,** Type I is best seen in a lateral view. The fracture line is in the coronal plane, there is no midfoot instability, and dorsal displacement is variable. **B,** Type II is best seen in an AP or oblique view. The fracture line is in the dorsolateral to plantarmedial plane, with medial displacement from the posterior tibial tendon. **C,** Type III is best seen in an AP view and is characterized by midbody comminution and valgus foot angulation as can be seen by comparing the medial column with its normal alignment demonstrated by the dashed line. (Reproduced from Ficke JR: Fractures and dislocation of the midfoot, in Pinzur MS, ed: *Orthopaedic Knowledge Update: Foot and Ankle* 4. Rosemont, IL, American Academy of Orthopaedic Surgeons, 2008, pp 107-114.)

spring ligament. Because of the broad insertion of the posterior tibial tendon throughout the plantar aspect of the midfoot, usually the tendon is not completely pulled off, and significant tuberosity displacement is rare. These fractures typically cause pain and ecchymosis medially and are easily seen on routine foot radiographs. Immobilization in a walking boot is used for 4 to 6 weeks. If a symptomatic nonunion develops, excision (a Kidner-type procedure) may be undertaken rather than internal fixation. Some experts recommend internal fixation for a fracture displaced more than 5 mm because of the risk of nonunion.[2]

An acute fracture should be distinguished from a type II accessory navicular. The accessory bone and the corresponding medial navicular body have more rounded edges than the fracture. These entities typically are treated in a similar fashion, however, based on the severity of the patient's symptoms.

Navicular Body Fractures

Fractures of the navicular body are uncommon because of the stability imparted by the position of the navicular between numerous bones. Such a fracture often is caused by a high-energy mechanism, as in a fall from a height or an axial load. The classification is based on fracture morphology: a type I fracture is in the coronal plane and has no misalignment of the midfoot; a type II fracture, the

most common type, has a dorsolateral to plantarmedial fracture line with the lateral fragment displaced dorsally; and a type III fracture is comminuted centrally or laterally within the navicular body (**Figure 2**). The foot collapses into abduction through the comminution. Many researchers suggest that displaced, comminuted fractures (all type II and III fractures) and larger fracture fragments benefit from internal fixation. As in all foot and ankle trauma, the integrity and suitability of the soft tissues for surgical intervention must be respected, and the surgery may need to be delayed 1 to 2 weeks. Temporary spanning external fixation may be necessary if there is gross instability. CT is particularly useful during surgical planning to fully appreciate the anatomy of the fracture fragments, especially in the presence of additional transverse tarsal and tarsometatarsal injuries.

Surgical treatment is done through a dorsal approach between the course of the anterior and posterior tibial tendons to facilitate visualization and evaluation. The saphenous vein and nerve must be avoided during the superficial dissection. Because the lateral aspect of the navicular is challenging to fully appreciate, usually it is beneficial to place the incision just medial to the anterior tibial tendon rather than more medially and closer to the posterior tibial tendon.

Simple fractures are fixed with lag screws. Screws may be placed medial to lateral or lateral to medial, depending on which placement will provide better fixation. If there is significant comminution, locked or minifragment plating of the navicular itself or temporary bridge plating of the medial column may be necessary.[3-5] Manipulation of fracture fragments may require the use of a small external fixator or Kirschner wire distractor, which eliminates the deforming forces on the navicular and improve visualization.

Late osteonecrosis may occur following these injuries and, in advanced stages, may lead to medial column collapse. Symptoms of posttraumatic arthrosis of the talonavicular joint can be treated with shoe wear modification, a stiff custom insert, or a rigid or rocker-bottom soled shoe. Some patients require delayed talonavicular, naviculocuneiform, or medial column arthrodesis.

Stress Fractures

The navicular bone historically was believed to be particularly susceptible to stress fracture because of the relative avascular zone in the central third of the bone. Recent arterial anatomic studies suggest that biomechanical and other clinical factors play a more significant role in the development of stress fractures than previously believed.[6] With explosive activity, this area undergoes considerable compression, which can cause stress responses including bone bruise, stress reaction, stress fracture, and complete fracture of the navicular. The diagnosis often is delayed because the symptoms are vague, insidious, and sometimes similar to those of a sprain. The fracture may be evaluated only after weeks or months of continued activity. Patients have poorly localized pain in the midfoot and usually are unable to perform the hop test, which requires jumping up and down on the involved forefoot. Radiographs of the foot should be carefully scrutinized for evidence of a fracture. Often the radiographs are normal, however, and a high index of suspicion as well as MRI confirmation are required. MRI is preferable to CT because CT can only document fractures with cortical disruption.

The treatment ranges from avoidance of weight bearing to early surgical intervention. The results of any treatment involving partial weight bearing appear to be inferior to those of complete avoidance of weight bearing or early surgical treatment, and therefore partial weight bearing should be discouraged. Although surgery may be the preferred initial treatment for a competitive athlete, avoidance of weight bearing and early surgical treatment appear to have similar results in the general population.[7,8]

Cuboid and Cuneiform Fractures

Cuboid Fractures

Through its articulation with the fourth and fifth metatarsal bases and the anterior process of the calcaneus, the cuboid forms an intercalary link from the lateral forefoot to the hindfoot. The medial column is relatively rigid. Conversely, the lateral column of the foot is quite mobile to accommodate ground reactive forces and the geometry of uneven surfaces. Fractures of the cuboid are believed to be rare because its bony surroundings offer some protection. Patients report lateral foot pain and difficulty in weight bearing. Lateral and plantar midfoot and hindfoot ecchymosis is common. Plain radiographs often are sufficient, but CT or MRI is recommended for surgical planning or evaluation to detect additional midfoot pathology.

Avulsion fractures and compression fractures are the two primary types of cuboid fractures. Avulsion fractures, which are more common, can occur even with mild to moderate foot and ankle sprains. These are capsular avulsions, and they can be treated nonsurgically with modified weight bearing in a fracture boot, as symptoms allow. Minimally displaced or nondisplaced cuboid fractures also can be treated nonsurgically and may benefit from a 4- to 6-week period of no weight bearing.

Although displaced fractures only rarely require surgical intervention, often they accompany more severe bony and soft-tissue midfoot Lisfranc injuries. Displaced fractures result from a direct crush or from an axial load in plantar flexion accompanied by eversion. In the second scenario, a so-called nutcracker fracture is produced when the cuboid is caught between the fourth and fifth metatarsal bases and the anterior process of the calcaneus, and it is cracked like a nut.[9] In these compression injuries, the lateral column is crushed and becomes shorter because it is no longer held out to length (**Figure 3**). These fractures carry a significant risk of collapse and painful malunion, and therefore surgery is believed to be beneficial.[10] However, no recommendations have been published as to the amount of lateral column shortening required to warrant urgent external fixation.[11]

The surgical options range from bone grafting with definitive internal fixation to temporary bridge plating or external fixation. Arthrodesis rarely is required but may be necessary if articular surfaces cannot be reconstructed. Although large studies of surgical treatment of compression injuries with lengthy follow-up are lacking, the importance of timely surgical intervention was underscored by midterm results suggesting that persistent symptoms often are caused by associated midfoot injuries.[12]

6: Foot and Ankle Trauma

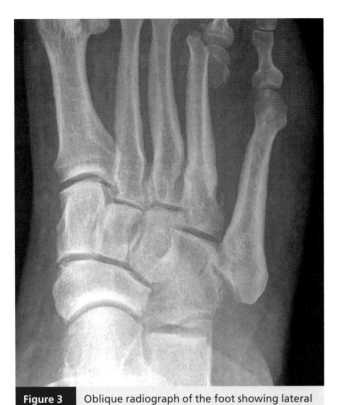

Figure 3 Oblique radiograph of the foot showing lateral dislocation of the fifth tarsometatarsal joint with a compression fracture of the cuboid.

Cuneiform Fractures

The cuneiforms are a relatively stable complex of bones between the navicular and the first three metatarsal bases. The strong intertarsal ligaments allow the cuneiforms only a small amount of motion. Accordingly, displaced fractures are rare and suggest the presence of a more sinister midfoot injury elsewhere. The mechanism usually is direct trauma, and patients have pain over the central to medial midfoot. Plain radiographs should be obtained, but MRI or CT often is needed to evaluate subtle fracture patterns because there is bony overlap on plain radiographs. A nondisplaced fracture is treated with a walking boot and modified weight bearing, as symptoms allow. A displaced fracture occasionally requires internal fixation and, when associated with a tarsometatarsal injury, is amenable to primary arthrodesis.

Tarsometatarsal Fractures

Tarsometatarsal injury can be ligamentous, bony, or both. Jacques Lisfranc de St. Martin in 1815 described a fracture-dislocation at the tarsometatarsal joints that occurred when a soldier caught his foot in a stirrup while dismounting his horse. Such injuries often were treated by amputation, and there is little similarity between classic descriptions and current understanding. Nonetheless, the tarsometatarsal joints often are called Lisfranc joints, and the terms tarsometatarsal injury and Lisfranc injury are used interchangeably.

Anatomy

The tarsometatarsal complex spans parts of the transverse and longitudinal arches of the foot and is stabilized by strong plantar ligaments and weaker dorsal ligaments. In the coronal plane, intrinsic stability is provided by the unique position of the second metatarsal base, which is recessed proximally between the medial and lateral cuneiforms. In the axial plane, the unique wedge shape of the bases of the metatarsals and their corresponding cuneiforms provide a bony congruity that maintains the transverse arch and confers tremendous stability.

The ligaments stabilizing the tarsometatarsal joints are dorsal, plantar, and interosseous. The interosseous ligaments are the strongest; they extend between each of the lateral four metatarsal bases but are conspicuously absent between the first two metatarsals. The first ray is connected to the second tarsometatarsal complex by the Lisfranc ligament, which extends from the medial base of the second and third metatarsals to the medial cuneiform, the plantar portion of which is the strongest and most important for midfoot stability.[13]

Little motion occurs at these articulations, but the tarsometatarsal joints provide sturdy bony attachment sites for the anterior and posterior tibial tendons. The dorsal neurovascular bundle, containing the dorsalis pedis artery and vein and the deep peroneal nerve, runs along the dorsum of the lateral second tarsometatarsal joint, just lateral to the extensor hallucis longus tendon.

Patient History and Physical Examination

Patients who have a nonneuropathic Lisfranc injury report swelling and midfoot pain and typically are incapable of weight bearing secondary to pain. The injury can result from low-energy or high-energy trauma that causes direct or indirect force onto the midfoot. Often the trauma occurs during a motor vehicle crash in which the midfoot sustains violent trauma or is crushed under great load. Lower energy sports injuries commonly have a twisting mechanism combined with an axial load and midfoot hyperdorsiflexion. To simplify the understanding of Lisfranc injuries, generally they are categorized as direct or indirect. Direct injury results from the application of load precisely over the tarsometatarsal complex, usually dorsally. Because the soft-tissue envelope overlying the tarsometatarsal complex is thin, it is important to be aware of concomitant soft-tissue injury, which can lead to compartment syndrome of the foot. Indirect injury is more common than direct injury and results from an

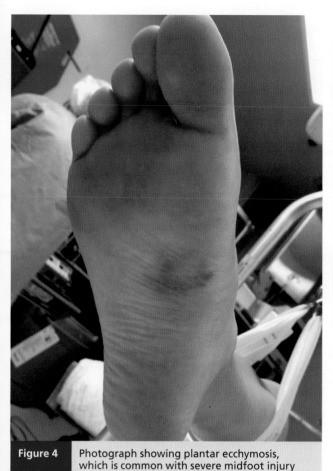

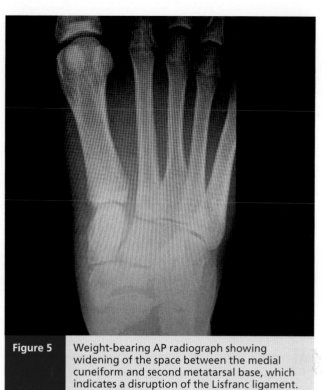

Figure 5   Weight-bearing AP radiograph showing widening of the space between the medial cuneiform and second metatarsal base, which indicates a disruption of the Lisfranc ligament.

Figure 4   Photograph showing plantar ecchymosis, which is common with severe midfoot injury or isolated lower energy injury to the midfoot complex.

axial load combined with twisting of the midfoot in plantar flexion. Indirect injury often occurs during soccer or American football, although occasionally it occurs when a stairstep is missed.

Because of the numerous mechanisms and tremendous variability in the forces causing the spectrum of tarsometatarsal injuries, it is necessary to maintain a high index of suspicion in patients with posttraumatic midfoot pain. More severe injury is easily diagnosed by the severity of swelling and gross displacement. Plantar ecchymosis, a cardinal feature of midfoot injury, always should suggest the need for further workup (Figure 4). On occasion, subtle injury causes only mild swelling and pain. A patient whose history and physical examination suggest a Lisfranc injury should receive prompt radiographic evaluation.

Diagnostic Studies
Plain weight-bearing radiographs of the injured and contralateral extremities should be obtained. Weight bearing often is difficult because of pain but is necessary because diastasis between the medial cuneiform

and base of the second metatarsal may not be evident on non–weight-bearing radiographs (Figure 5). If the radiographs are equivocal or nondiagnostic, CT is used to define bony injury and detect associated fractures. Three-dimensional CT reconstruction can be helpful for appreciating the geometry of the injury (Figure 6). MRI is useful for diagnosing a more subtle ligamentous injury, such as a Lisfranc tear or sprain, a bony contusion, or an occult fracture. MRI has high predictive value for midfoot instability[14] (Figure 7).

On weight-bearing AP radiographs, the medial border of the second metatarsal base should align with the corresponding medial border of the middle cuneiform. Failure to maintain this specific relationship indicates rupture of the strong plantar Lisfranc ligament. On an oblique foot radiograph, the medial border of the fourth metatarsal should align with the medial border of the cuboid. On a lateral radiograph, there should be no dorsal or plantar subluxation of the metatarsals relative to their corresponding cuneiforms or cuboid bone. Any dorsal displacement of the metatarsal bases is abnormal and must be distinguished from posttraumatic or degenerative bossing of the tarsometatarsal complex. A so-called fleck sign seen on radiographs or CT is indicative of a bony avulsion of the insertion of the Lisfranc ligament on the medial base of the second metatarsal (Figure 8). Because bone-to-bone healing is more reliable

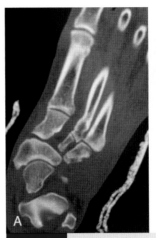
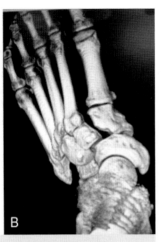

Figure 6   CT of a Lisfranc injury. **A,** Homolateral dislocation including a lateral shift of the cuneiforms. **B,** Three-dimensional reconstruction of the homolateral dislocation showing complete dislocation of the fourth and fifth metatarsals and a lateral shift of the medial cuneiform on the navicular.

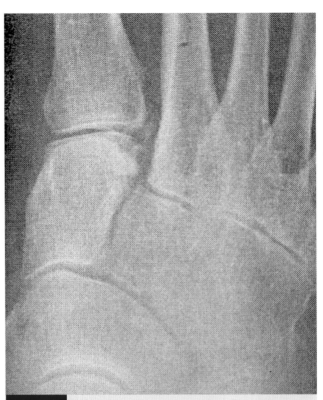

Figure 8   AP weight-bearing radiograph of the foot showing the fleck sign, which indicates avulsion of the origin of the Lisfranc ligament.

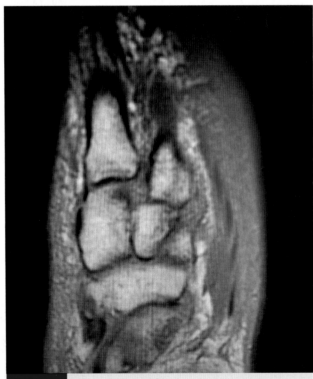

Figure 7   MRI of a Lisfranc injury showing a lateral deviation of the second metatarsal base.

Classification

Organizing Lisfranc injuries into specific groups with treatment algorithms is difficult because of tremendous variability in the severity of injury and the contribution of soft-tissue pathology. No single classification scheme appropriately balances ease of use and reproducibility with treatment recommendations and prognosis. A classification system originally devised by Quenu and Kuss[15] is predicated on the concept of the three columns of the foot (**Figure 9**). The medial column includes the first metatarsal, medial cuneiform, and navicular facet; the middle column, the second and third metatarsals, medial and lateral cuneiforms, and corresponding navicular facets; and the lateral column, the fourth and fifth metatarsals and cuboid. Type A injury has total incongruity with a homolateral dislocation. Type B injury has partial incongruity with an incomplete homolateral dislocation. Type C injury is divergent, with partial or total displacement. Although some clinicians find this classification system cumbersome to use, it provides a useful standard terminology for describing these injuries.

Treatment

The primary objective of the treatment of any Lisfranc injury is to achieve a pain-free, durable, and stable

than tendon-to-bone healing, the fleck sign is believed to suggest a good prognosis.

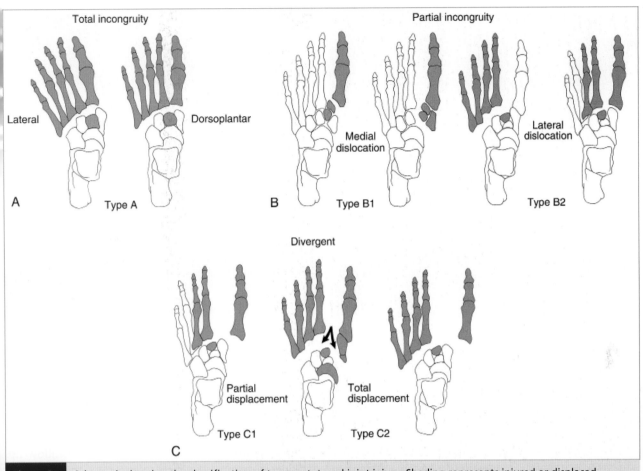

Figure 9 Schematic showing the classification of tarsometatarsal joint injury. Shading represents injured or displaced areas of the foot. **A,** In type A, total incongruity, all five metatarsals are displaced, with or without fracture at the base of the second metatarsal. The usual displacement is lateral or dorsolateral, and the metatarsals move as a unit. Type A injury is homolateral. **B,** In type B, one or more articulations remain intact. Type B1 represents partial incongruity with medial dislocation, and type B2 represents partial incongruity with lateral dislocation. The first metatarsal cuneiform joint may be involved. **C,** Type C is divergent, with partial (type C1) or total (type C2) displacement. The arrows in C2 represent the forces through the foot leading to a divergent pattern. (Reproduced from Watson TS, Shurnas PS, Denker J: Treatment of Lisfranc joint injury: Current concepts. *J Am Acad Orthop Surg* 2010;18[12]:718-728.)

plantigrade foot. This objective is achieved by anatomic reduction and adequate immobilization to ensure stability.

A patient with point tenderness over the area, normal plain weight-bearing radiographs, and MRI showing an abnormal Lisfranc ligament may have injured only the dorsal ligaments. With an intact plantar ligament, the appropriate treatment is rest and immobilization in a walking cast or boot, with weight bearing allowed as symptoms decrease, typically at 4 to 6 weeks. A course of physical therapy is useful for strengthening and gait training. After using a walking boot, many patients prefer to use a stiff insole or a carbon fiber insert, which somewhat restricts midfoot motion, before resuming their preinjury shoe wear.

Inability to obtain or maintain an anatomically reduced and stabilized Lisfranc complex leads to premature midfoot arch collapse and degenerative arthritis.[16] Surgical stabilization usually is required for an injury causing midfoot instability, such as a displaced fracture or disruption of the plantarmedial cuneiform to the second and third metatarsal base. Debate exists as to the optimal primary surgical treatment of Lisfranc injuries. The options include open reduction and internal fixation with transarticular screws and/or pins, open reduction and internal fixation with bridging plates and screws, and primary midfoot arthrodesis (**Figure 10**). Closed reduction with pinning or spanning external fixation is reserved for injury with severe soft-tissue compromise because of the difficulty of obtaining anatomic reduction without opening the dislocation site.[17]

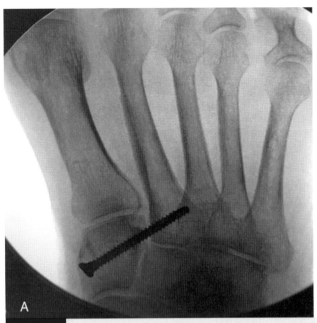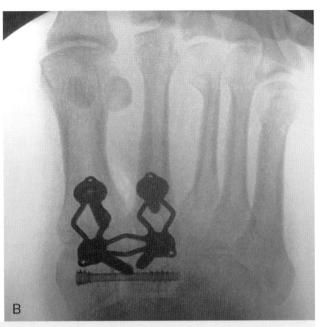

Figure 10   Intraoperative fluoroscopic images demonstrating open reduction and internal fixation of an isolated Lisfranc diastasis (**A**) and medial column primary arthrodesis (**B**).

Surgical Results and Prognosis

Proponents of open reduction and internal fixation believe that maintaining midfoot joint motion is essential for optimal long-term function and prevention of adjacent-segment degeneration. One study found that 28 of 30 patients with anatomic reduction of a Lisfranc injury had a good to excellent functional result.[18] However, none of 11 patients who underwent gait analysis had a normal gait pattern after anatomic reduction of a displaced Lisfranc injury.[19] As to the type and specific placement of hardware, no universal agreement exists. One of two general constructs may be followed: transarticular screw fixation or dorsal plate fixation. Advocates of transarticular screw fixation suggest that joint compression and alignment are easily achieved and, when necessary, screw removal is easily facilitated through percutaneous techniques. These surgeons argue that the removal of a dorsal plate is difficult and adds unnecessary morbidity to hardware removal. Those who favor dorsal plating mainly do so because transarticular screw fixation without arthrodesis causes significant articular chondral damage that may lead to premature posttraumatic midfoot arthritis. Of note, cadaver research has demonstrated that transarticular screw fixation and bridging-plate fixation have similar biomechanical strength for maintaining reduction.[20]

Proponents of primary midfoot fusion note that the medial column of the midfoot is inherently more stable and less mobile than the lateral column, and therefore little motion is lost through arthrodesis. A prospective, randomized study of 41 subacute, purely ligamentous Lisfranc injuries found that patients who underwent primary arthrodesis had significantly better scores on the American Orthopaedic Foot and Ankle Society midfoot scale than those who underwent open reduction and internal fixation.[21] At an average 46-month follow-up, patients who underwent arthrodesis rated their function at 92% of their preinjury level, compared with 65% of patients who underwent open reduction and internal fixation. Five patients who had open reduction and internal fixation later underwent arthrodesis secondary to persistent pain and deformity or osteoarthrosis. A similar randomized prospective study of 40 patients who underwent open reduction and internal fixation or fusion for treatment of Lisfranc fractures and/or ligamentous injuries reported no significant between-group differences on the Medical Outcomes Study Short Form–36 or Short Musculoskeletal Function Assessment at follow-up intervals extending 2 years after surgery.[22] A telephone survey of these patients at an average 53-month follow-up also found no between-group difference in satisfaction rates. However, 78.6% of patients who underwent open reduction and internal fixation required an additional surgical procedure (including planned removal of transarticular screws), compared with 16.7% of those who underwent fusion.[22]

Compartment Syndrome of the Foot

Although compartment syndrome of the foot is not common, severe trauma to the midfoot can lead to elevated intracompartmental pressures, which, if unrecognized, can cause soft-tissue injury beyond the injury from the initial trauma. Foot compartment syndrome recently was found to be most likely to occur when a crush mechanism was combined with a forefoot injury.[23] One study found Lisfranc injuries to be responsible for two thirds of the incidences of compartment syndrome of the foot.[24]

Compartment syndrome results from raised pressure within a closed fascial space that exceeds tissue capillary pressure and causes tissue hypoperfusion. The foot can be divided into nine compartments; on the plantar surface, medial, lateral, and central/superficial compartments exist. There are four interosseous compartments between the metatarsal shafts, and an adductor compartment in the proximal forefoot. A calcaneal compartment is found in the hindfoot. A septum divides the central compartment into superficial and deep compartments. The superficial compartment contains the flexor digitorum brevis muscle, and the deep calcaneal compartment contains the quadratus plantae muscle and lateral plantar nerve. The deep calcaneal compartment communicates directly with the deep posterior compartment of the leg.

Severe direct trauma or crush injury is responsible for many incidences of compartment syndrome. The classic signs and symptoms, consisting of pain out of proportion to the injury and pain with passive digital motion, are of little use in the setting of severe foot trauma because it is impossible to determine whether the pain is attributable to the injury or increased intracompartmental pressure. The diagnosis can be made by direct measurement of compartment pressures higher than 30 mm Hg or within 10 to 30 mm Hg of the patient's diastolic blood pressure. Decompression can be achieved through two dorsal incisions: a medial incision between the first and second metatarsals and a second incision between the fourth and fifth metatarsals. A medial incision may be needed to relieve pressure in the central and interosseous compartments. The use of a piecrust skin incision technique may be adequate if the compartment syndrome is the result of a massive subcutaneous hematoma. Repeat irrigation and débridement with secondary closure or skin grafting may be necessary if soft-tissue swelling precludes primary closure. Missed compartment syndrome can cause ischemic contracture, complex regional pain syndrome, and permanent loss of function. Therefore, a high index of suspicion for compartment syndrome is necessary in a patient with a severe crush and/or traumatic midfoot injury accompanied by profound swelling.

Summary

There are a myriad of injuries that can be seen in the midfoot. They range from subtle sprains and stress fractures,

to high-energy fracture dislocations and compartment syndrome. Because there is such a great range in presentation and severity, the evaluating surgeon must have a high index of suspicion for these injuries in order to minimize the morbidity of missed pathology. Only after the injury is recognized can the optimal treatment strategy be selected based on the best available data and clinical science.

Annotated References

1. Chapman M: Fractures and fracture dislocations of the ankle and foot, in Mann RA, ed: *DuVries' Surgery of the Foot,* ed 4. St Louis, MO, Mosby,1978.

2. Jackson JB, Ellington JK, Anderson RB: Fractures of the midfoot and forefoot, in Coughlin MJ, Saltzman CL, Anderson RB, eds: *Mann's Surgery of the Foot and Ankle,* ed 9. Philadelphia, PA, Mosby-Elsevier, 2014, pp 2154-2186.

3. Cronier P, Frin JM, Steiger V, Bigorre N, Talha A: Internal fixation of complex fractures of the tarsal navicular with locking plates: A report of 10 cases. *Orthop Traumatol Surg Res* 2013;99(4, suppl):S241-S249.

   A prospective case study found successful union of comminuted navicular fractures treated with locked plates.

4. Evans J, Beingessner DM, Agel J, Benirschke SK: Minifragment plate fixation of high-energy navicular body fractures. *Foot Ankle Int* 2011;32(5):S485-S492.

   Minifragment plate fixation of navicular body fractures in 24 patients led to union of all fractures, although 4 (17%) underwent hardware removal.

5. Schildhauer TA, Nork SE, Sangeorzan BJ: Temporary bridge plating of the medial column in severe midfoot injuries. *J Orthop Trauma* 2003;17(7):513-520.

6. McKeon KE, McCormick JJ, Johnson JE, Klein SE: Intraosseous and extraosseous arterial anatomy of the adult navicular. *Foot Ankle Int* 2012;33(10):857-861.

   A cadaver study of the intraosseous and extraosseous blood supply to the navicular using latex injection found dense posterior tibial and dorsalis pedis contributions to an extensive intraosseous vascular network.

7. Mann JA, Pedowitz DI: Evaluation and treatment of navicular stress fractures, including nonunions, revision surgery, and persistent pain after treatment. *Foot Ankle Clin* 2009;14(2):187-204.

   A systematic review of the literature regarding evaluation, management, and results of navicular stress fractures is presented. Although there is a frequent delay in diagnosis and difficulty in selecting the proper imaging techniques for these fractures, there are good results with surgical management.

6: Foot and Ankle Trauma

8. Torg JS, Moyer J, Gaughan JP, Boden BP: Management of tarsal navicular stress fractures: Conservative versus surgical treatment: A meta-analysis. *Am J Sports Med* 2010;38(5):1048-1053.

   A systematic review of the literature found that nonsurgical management without weight bearing should be considered the standard of care for navicular stress fractures. No advantage was found to surgical treatment over no weight bearing, and a statistical trend favored no weight bearing over surgery.

9. Hermel MB, Gershon-Cohen J: The nutcracker fracture of the cuboid by indirect violence. *Radiology* 1953;60(6):850-854.

10. Brunet JA, Wiley JJ: The late results of tarsometatarsal joint injuries. *J Bone Joint Surg Br* 1987;69(3):437-440.

11. Borrelli J Jr, De S, VanPelt M: Fracture of the cuboid. *J Am Acad Orthop Surg* 2012;20(7):472-477.

    The natural history, evaluation, and management of cuboid fractures were described, including surgical technique.

12. Weber M, Locher S: Reconstruction of the cuboid in compression fractures: Short to midterm results in 12 patients. *Foot Ankle Int* 2002;23(11):1008-1013.

13. Kaar S, Femino J, Morag Y: Lisfranc joint displacement following sequential ligament sectioning. *J Bone Joint Surg Am* 2007;89(10):2225-2232.

14. Raikin SM, Elias I, Dheer S, Besser MP, Morrison WB, Zoga AC: Prediction of midfoot instability in the subtle Lisfranc injury: Comparison of magnetic resonance imaging with intraoperative findings. *J Bone Joint Surg Am* 2009;91(4):892-899.

    MRI was found to be accurate for detecting traumatic Lisfranc ligament injuries and predicting Lisfranc joint complex instability when the plantar Lisfranc ligament bundle was used as a predictor. The usefulness of MRI for the diagnosis of an injury to the Lisfranc and adjacent ligaments was assessed.

15. Quenu E, Kuss G: Etude sur les luxations du metatarse (luxations metatarsotarsiennes) du diastasis entre le 1er et le 2e metatarsien. *Rev Chir* 1909;39:281-336, 720-791, 1093-1134.

16. Myerson MS, Fisher RT, Burgess AR, Kenzora JE: Fracture dislocations of the tarsometatarsal joints: End results correlated with pathology and treatment. *Foot Ankle* 1986;6(5):225-242.

17. Schepers T, Oprel PP, Van Lieshout EM: Influence of approach and implant on reduction accuracy and stability in lisfranc fracture-dislocation at the tarsometatarsal joint. *Foot Ankle Int* 2013;34(5):705-710.

    The authors looked at 28 patients with Lisfranc injuries treated either closed or open Kirschner wire fixation alone or open with Kirschner wires, screws, and/or plates. Open reduction and internal fixation with screws or plate resulted in better reduction and better maintenance of reduction in both low- and high-energy Lisfranc injuries. Level of evidence: III.

18. Arntz CT, Veith RG, Hansen ST Jr: Fractures and fracture-dislocations of the tarsometatarsal joint. *J Bone Joint Surg Am* 1988;70(2):173-181.

19. Wiss DA, Kull DM, Perry J: Lisfranc fracture-dislocations of the foot: A clinical-kinesiological study. *J Orthop Trauma* 1987;1(4):267-274.

20. Alberta FG, Aronow MS, Barrero M, Diaz-Doran V, Sullivan RJ, Adams DJ: Ligamentous Lisfranc joint injuries: A biomechanical comparison of dorsal plate and transarticular screw fixation. *Foot Ankle Int* 2005;26(6):462-473.

21. Ly TV, Coetzee JC: Treatment of primarily ligamentous Lisfranc joint injuries: Primary arthrodesis compared with open reduction and internal fixation. A prospective, randomized study. *J Bone Joint Surg Am* 2006;88(3):514-520.

22. Henning JA, Jones CB, Sietsema DL, Bohay DR, Anderson JG: Open reduction internal fixation versus primary arthrodesis for lisfranc injuries: A prospective randomized study. *Foot Ankle Int* 2009;30(10):913-922.

    A prospective randomized clinical study compared open reduction and internal fixation to arthrodesis at 24-month clinical and radiographic follow-up. Arthrodesis of tarsometatarsal joint injuries was found to result in a significant reduction in the rate of follow-up surgical procedures.

23. Thakur NA, McDonnell M, Got CJ, Arcand N, Spratt KF, DiGiovanni CW: Injury patterns causing isolated foot compartment syndrome. *J Bone Joint Surg Am* 2012;94(11):1030-1035.

    A review of 364 patients with an isolated foot compartment syndrome found the highest incidence after a crush injury combined with a forefoot injury, followed by an isolated crush injury.

24. Myerson MS: Management of compartment syndromes of the foot. *Clin Orthop Relat Res* 1991;271:239-248.

Chapter 27

Forefoot, Sesamoid, and Turf Toe Injuries

Kenneth J. Hunt, MD

Introduction

The foot is a complex and durable biomechanical structure composed of 28 bones and their articulations. The foot is of integral importance to gait, and fractures of the foot can have a substantial effect on normal function. Forefoot injury is particularly likely to cause long-term pain and disability after multiple trauma.[1] A study from a level I trauma center found that 15% of patients involved in a motor vehicle crash had trauma to the foot and ankle, and these injuries often were severe.[2] Recent advances may improve the success and efficiency of treatment techniques and implants designed to restore function to patients with traumatic foot injury.

Evaluation of Forefoot Injuries

Given the complexity of the foot and the diversity of injuries, making the correct diagnosis depends on understanding the mechanism and location of the patient's injury. The location, magnitude, and duration of the symptoms must be determined. The patient may be able to point to a particular location of pain. A thorough history of any previous injury, surgical intervention, or underlying disease that could affect the feet is useful, especially if the patient has a history of diabetes, venous insufficiency, congenital or acquired deformity, or uses assistive devices. It is important to have a good understanding of the patient's functional demands, work and recreational activities, and needs during and after injury treatment.

Comparing the injured foot with the uninjured foot allows detection of any deviation from the patient's normal state. Inspection and palpation aid in locating the injured foot structures and ruling out involvement of other, uninjured structures. The associated joints should be assessed for active and passive ranges of motion. Resistive testing of the associated muscles ensures that the tendons are intact and the muscles are functional. The entire foot and ankle should be assessed for stability and alignment, particularly in comparison with the contralateral extremity. Documentation of neurovascular status should include assessment of pulses, capillary refill to the toes, reflexes, motor function of all muscle groups in the foot and leg, and all five major sensory nerves using light touch (with a paper clip or monofilament). In an acute injury, any suspicion of excessive or worsening pain, swelling, numbness and tingling, or coolness in the foot requires immediate reassessment of neurovascular status and possibly measurement of foot compartment pressure. Foot compartment syndrome may require decompression to mitigate complications.

Radiographs are imperative to assess for fractures and foot alignment. Three views of the foot typically are needed, and they should be weight bearing if tolerated by the patient. Additional views, including sesamoid views, are obtained as indicated. If the patient is unable to bear weight, a simulated weight-bearing view can be obtained with the patient seated or supine. High-quality radiographs are important to the diagnosis and treatment decision making; any low-quality radiographs should be retaken. Proper training of technical personnel can help improve the quality of radiographs.

Treatment of Forefoot Fractures and Turf Toe Injuries

Most, but not all, fractures of the forefoot can be successfully treated without surgery. Standard trauma principles include anatomic reduction of the fracture and any involved joints, with sufficiently rigid internal or external fixation. It is important to evaluate the associated soft tissues to avoid incisions in areas at high risk for skin necrosis, dehiscence, or other complications. A surgical procedure can be delayed until resolution of the soft-tissue injury sufficient to minimize the risk of complications.

Dr. Hunt or an immediate family member serves as a board member, owner, officer, or committee member of the American Orthopaedic Foot and Ankle Society and the National Orthopaedic Foot & Ankle Outcomes Research Network.

6: Foot and Ankle Trauma

Metatarsal Fractures

Metatarsal fractures are relatively common. Each of the five metatarsals functions in a different manner, and optimal fracture healing requires a different approach to the treatment of each metatarsal. With the exception of the proximal fifth metatarsal, only limited published studies are available on the indications for treating metatarsal fractures and the long-term results. Most metatarsal fractures are effectively treated without surgery, but surgical treatment typically is indicated for severe displacement, multiple fractures, intra-articular injury, an open wound, compartment syndrome, displaced fracture fragments creating risk to the skin, significant sagittal displacement in any ray, or significant transverse displacement in the first or fifth metatarsal. It is considerably less problematic to initially reduce and stabilize a fracture than to do so after malunion, nonunion, or a skin complication has developed.

First Metatarsal Fractures

The first metatarsal is wider, shorter, and stronger than the lesser metatarsals. It is more mobile because the ligaments and articulation at its base allow more motion. Unlike the lesser metatarsals, the first metatarsal does not have a stout transverse intermetatarsal ligament distally between adjacent metatarsal necks. The first metatarsal bears approximately one third of the body's weight through the forefoot. Displacement of the first metatarsal head in any direction disturbs the tripodlike weight-bearing complex of the anterior portion of the foot and impairs forefoot function. Because even a small malalignment can affect the distribution of weight during ambulation, it is important to tolerate almost no displacement in the coronal or sagittal plane. The primary goal of treatment of a fracture of the first metatarsal is to maintain the normal distribution of weight under all of the metatarsal heads.

Nonsurgical Treatment

A minimally displaced or nondisplaced fracture of the first metatarsal can be successfully treated nonsurgically. A short leg cast or a controlled ankle movement (CAM) walker boot allows protected weight bearing. A boot has the advantages of allowing adjustment, skin assessment, and direct application of ice and anti-inflammatory medications. The disadvantages of the boot include possible difficulty with fit or compliance. For an unstable injury, it is preferable to use a cast and avoid weight bearing for 4 to 6 weeks, until there is evidence of healing. Displacement or nonunion is rare, however, and more aggressive mobilization may enhance healing and recovery.[3] Early displacement of such a fracture can be detected by close follow-up. The patient should begin to use a comfortable, well-cushioned regular shoe as soon as the symptoms and soft tissues permit, and active and passive motion exercises of the toes should be initiated.

Surgical Treatment

The first ray should be carefully evaluated for displacement, particularly in the transverse and sagittal planes, because malunion can lead to painful weight bearing, transfer metatarsalgia, and difficulty in shoe fitting.[3] Percutaneous or open reduction of the fracture should be followed by internal or external fixation. Internal fixation can be achieved using Kirschner wires, lag screws, or a low-profile, small-caliber plate (a one-quarter semitubular plate held with 2.7-mm screws). The location and position of the plate are determined by the fracture extent and pattern as well as the placement of the incision.

A proximal first metatarsal fracture can be fixed using a bridge plate across the tarsometatarsal joint. External fixation can allow proper healing if there is significant comminution, particularly near the tarsometatarsal joint. Primary arthrodesis of the first tarsometatarsal joint is an option for a severe injury and has little impact on foot function.

After surgery, a well-padded short leg splint should be used initially. The toes should be left uncovered so that swelling and perfusion can be assessed and toe range-of-motion exercises can be initiated to avoid stiffness. When the wounds have healed (generally at 2 to 3 weeks), a short leg walking cast or CAM walker boot gradually can be used, with progressive weight bearing. Generally, patients are allowed to increase the amount of weight put onto the foot over 3 to 4 weeks, until it is possible to bear weight without pain. Fusion of the first tarsometatarsal joint may require a longer period of limited weight bearing. When there is clinical and radiographic healing of the fracture, the transition to a comfortable accommodative shoe can begin, with increasingly aggressive range-of-motion and resistance exercises. Most injuries heal within 2 to 3 months and leave little functional impairment.

Middle Metatarsal Fractures

Fracture of a middle (second, third, or fourth) metatarsal is common. The injury can occur in isolation or with other injuries from vehicular or other high-energy trauma. Often a middle metatarsal fracture has a direct mechanism such as a crush injury, a puncture wound, or axial loading of a plantarflexed foot. Heightened suspicion is necessary to identify the fracture in a patient with multiple injuries and to evaluate for open fracture, which is most common with a crush injury. A metatarsal fracture is classified by its location as a neck, shaft, or base fracture.

Metatarsal Neck Fractures

A metatarsal neck fracture is inherently less stable than a shaft or base fracture. Often the fracture is multiple, further decreasing fracture stability and the ability to maintain adequate alignment by closed means. In particular, sagittal plane deformity can lead to painful plantar callosities and dorsal exostosis and corns.[4] A nondisplaced or minimally displaced fracture can be treated with a hard-soled shoe and weight bearing as tolerated. A more displaced fracture initially should be treated with closed reduction under sedation, using finger traps and direct manipulation with pressure over the metatarsal heads. An unstable fracture or a fracture with persistent sagittal plane deformity should be treated with closed reduction and retrograde pinning with Kirschner wires, open reduction and antegrade-retrograde pinning, or internal fixation with a small-caliber plate (if the head fragment is sufficiently large). A longitudinal skin incision that allows simultaneous access to adjacent metatarsals is used.[5] As an alternative, fixation after closed reduction can be done by driving Kirschner wires from the intact fifth metatarsal neck into the adjacent fractured middle metatarsal necks.[6]

Metatarsal Shaft Fractures

As with a metatarsal neck fracture, a minimally displaced or nondisplaced metatarsal shaft fracture can be treated with a hard-soled shoe and weight bearing as tolerated. Moderate frontal plane deformity does not typically lead to functional complications, but sagittal plane deformity is more problematic. A malunited fracture with significant sagittal plane deformity can lead to painful plantar callosities and dorsal exostoses and corns. The typical apex dorsal deformity in a shaft fracture results from plantar flexion of the distal fragment produced by the strong flexor tendons. In general the more distal the fracture, the greater the apex dorsal deformity is, and the higher probability is that open reduction will be required.[7] As for every foot injury, the radiographic evaluation should include AP, lateral, and oblique views. Oblique views are particularly useful because the metatarsals are seen as superimposed on the lateral view.

Most diaphyseal fractures can be treated nonsurgically. The surgical indications generally are limited to metatarsal shortening, significant displacement or angulation, and multiple displaced metatarsal fractures. The methods of fixation include intramedullary Kirschner wires, small plates and screws, and external fixation. Kirschner wires are suitable for most fracture patterns except comminuted length-unstable fractures, for which plates and screws may be more appropriate (**Figure 1**). Kirschner wires and external fixation are particularly useful for fractures with significant soft-tissue injury.

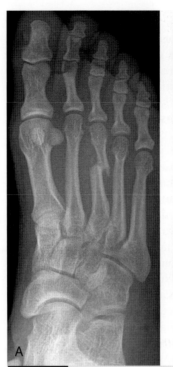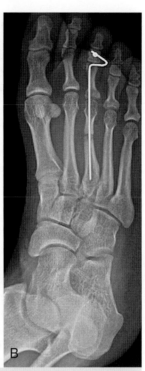

Figure 1 **A,** AP radiograph showing an open, displaced third metatarsal shaft fracture. **B,** Oblique radiograph showing the same third metatarsal shaft fracture treated using an intramedullary Kirschner wire.

After surgery a well-padded short leg splint should be applied, and the patient should not bear weight for 1 to 2 weeks, until acute swelling resolves. A walking short leg cast then can be applied if plantar pins are present. If no pins are present, the patient can gradually begin to use a CAM walker boot. After the initial 1 to 2 weeks, the patient is allowed to bear weight only through the heel. Pins are removed at the 4- to 6-week mark, based on evidence of fracture healing. In general, a relatively young patient will have radiographic healing earlier than an older patient.

Metatarsal Base Fractures

A metatarsal base fracture inherently is more stable than a shaft or neck fracture because of the shorter lever arm of the deforming flexor forces and the surrounding interosseous ligaments and capsular attachments.[4] Most base fractures are treated by closed means with a hard-soled shoe and weight bearing as tolerated. Care should be taken to rule out a Lisfranc variant injury before proceeding with closed treatment. Weight-bearing radiographs, if possible, or cross-sectional advanced imaging (MRI and/or CT) should be obtained to rule out such an injury (**Figure 2**). Open reduction and fixation should be considered if there is significant displacement, an open

6: Foot and Ankle Trauma

injury, or an unstable pattern (**Figure 3**). Fixation can be achieved with plates, screws, or percutaneous Kirschner wires. Plates spanning the metatarsophalangeal (MTP) joints can be considered. Primary fusion may be desirable for a comminuted intra-articular injury.

Fifth Metatarsal Fractures

Fifth metatarsal fractures account for approximately one quarter of all metatarsal injuries.[8] Fractures of the fifth metatarsal differ from those of the other lesser metatarsals in several respects. The fifth metatarsal is the only one with extrinsic tendon attachments; both the peroneus brevis and the peroneus tertius insert at the base of the fifth metatarsal. The fifth metatarsal has very little soft-tissue coverage on the lateral and plantar foot. There is a very strong ligamentous attachment to the plantar aponeurosis. The proximal fifth metatarsal has a vascular watershed area that creates a biomechanical and biologic environment in which fractures are common, often are difficult to treat, and can have problematic healing.[9]

A fifth metatarsal fracture can be classified as a proximal (base) fracture or a diaphyseal fracture. Each of these types has a unique etiology, treatment, and prognosis.[10] The management of a diaphyseal fracture is similar for all metatarsals. Most can be treated nonsurgically. The surgical indications generally are limited to shortening, malangulation, significant displacement, and multiple metatarsal fracture.

The proximal half (the base) of the fifth ray often is classified into three distinct fracture zones. Zone I includes the styloid process; zone II, the metadiaphyseal

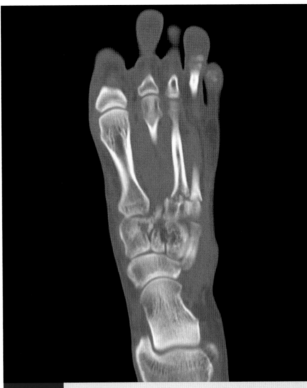

Figure 2 Axial CT showing fractures of the third and fourth metatarsal bases and the medial cuneiform.

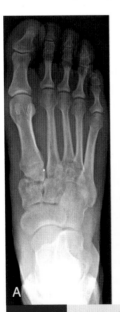
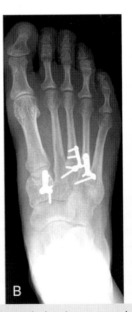
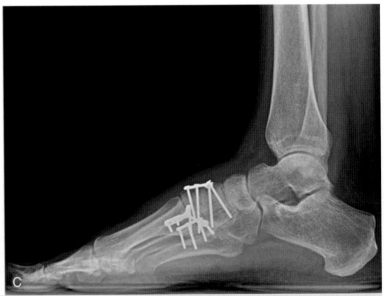

Figure 3 **A,** AP radiograph showing an unstable fracture pattern involving displaced fractures of the medial cuneiform and the third and fourth metatarsal bases. Postoperative (**B**) AP and (**C**) lateral radiographs showing reduction and plate fixation of all fractures.

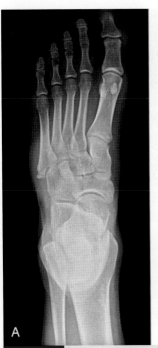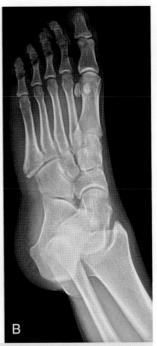

Figure 4	AP (**A**) and oblique (**B**) radiographs showing an avulsion fracture of the base of the fifth metatarsal.

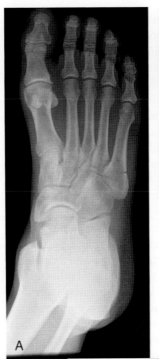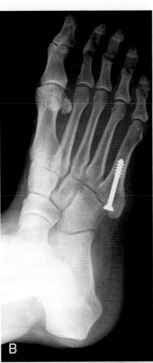

Figure 5	**A,** Oblique radiograph showing a Jones (metadiaphyseal) fracture of the fifth metatarsal. **B,** Oblique radiograph showing successful healing after percutaneous intramedullary screw fixation.

region; and zone III, the proximal diaphyseal region. Zones I, II, and III are subject to, respectively, an avulsion fracture (**Figure 4**), a Jones fracture (**Figure 5**), and (usually) a stress fracture.

Avulsion Fractures

Almost all fifth metatarsal fractures are avulsion fractures at the base.[11] This injury is believed to occur secondary to the forces exerted on the base by the strong attachment of the peroneus brevis and the lateral plantar aponeurosis. The plantar aponeurosis probably has a key role; these fractures are rarely displaced, and some fibers of the peroneus brevis remain intact.[12] The mechanism of injury usually is an acute inversion moment, as occurs when stepping off a curb. Many patients describe hearing a popping sound and have acute swelling, ecchymosis, and difficulty in ambulation. The location of tenderness and swelling determines whether a foot or ankle radiograph should be obtained to look for a fifth metatarsal avulsion fracture or another injury that can occur with the same mechanism, such as a fracture on the anterior process of the calcaneus or distal fibula.

Fifth metatarsal avulsion fractures typically are successfully treated without surgery by using a walking cast or walking boot. The transition to a stiff-soled but well-cushioned shoe is made when the swelling and pain have subsided, usually at 4 to 6 weeks. The progression of treatment often is based on clinical symptoms;

radiographs are not correlated with outcome, and radiographic healing can be prolonged or not occur. Most of these injuries clinically heal within 6 to 8 weeks. Painful nonunions are uncommon and are treated by excision of the fragment and repair of the peroneus brevis or, for larger fragments, by fixation and grafting. Primary internal fixation is reserved for fractures that include a large fragment entering the metatarsal-cuboid joint with more than 2 mm of displacement. Fixation usually is with a narrow tension band wire or a small-caliber lag screw.

Jones (Metadiaphyseal) Fractures

A fracture of the proximal metadiaphyseal junction of the fifth metatarsal, called a Jones fracture, occurs acutely with an adduction moment and axial loading causing an upward force on a plantar-flexed foot.[13] The mechanism is different from that of an avulsion fracture, in that a Jones fracture exits the intermetatarsal facet rather than the cuboid–fifth metatarsal articulation. Although a Jones fracture often can be successfully treated without surgery, nonunion and refracture are common and can be significant, especially for athletes.[14] It has been suggested that the location of the fracture and the high incidence of nonunion are secondary to the lack of blood supply to this region.[9]

6: Foot and Ankle Trauma

Successful nonsurgical treatment generally requires cast immobilization and avoidance of weight bearing over a prolonged (6-week) period. For this reason, Jones fractures often are treated surgically in young, active individuals. The treatment decision also is affected by whether the fracture represents acute or a stress injury, as can be accurately determined by the chronicity of symptoms, injury mechanism, radiographic evidence of sclerosis or nonunion at the fracture margins, and the presence of factors predisposing to stress fracture, such as cavovarus alignment.

Nonsurgical Treatment

Nonsurgical treatment is reserved for a nondisplaced fracture in a patient who is not an athlete and who chooses this treatment after discussing the risks and benefits of surgical treatment. A well-padded, non–weight-bearing cast or cast boot should be used. If healing is evident after 6 weeks, the patient begins to bear weight gradually during the next 2 to 3 weeks. Most fractures treated with this regimen progress to successful union. Surgical treatment should be considered if the symptoms persist and radiographic union is not seen at 10 weeks, or if there is a refracture.

Surgical Treatment

Percutaneous intramedullary screw fixation is the standard treatment for an acute displaced fracture or a fracture in a high-performance athlete.[15] Surgical treatment leads to a significantly shorter time to bone healing and return to sport than nonsurgical treatment.[16] Bone graft or other biologic supplementation can promote union in a chronic fracture, a nonunion, or a refracture.[14] Tension band techniques have been described but generally require a larger incision and more soft-tissue dissection than percutaneous screw fixation. The risks of surgical intervention include sural nerve injury, local wound problems including infection and delayed healing, iatrogenic fracture, and pain from the screw head. There is also risk of refracture, particularly in the presence of other mechanical or biologic risk factors.

Metatarsal Stress Fractures

Stress fracture is an overuse injury that occurs when activity repetition leads to a mismatch between bone microdamage and bone repair. Such injuries are common among active patients such as military recruits, athletes, and dancers, and often are related to a recent increase in activity level. The forefoot is especially vulnerable to stress fracture, and the metatarsals are commonly involved.[17,18] Both intrinsic and extrinsic factors can contribute to the development of stress fracture. The intrinsic factors include level of fitness, anatomic alignment, bone

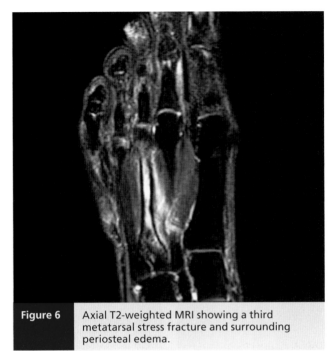

Figure 6   Axial T2-weighted MRI showing a third metatarsal stress fracture and surrounding periosteal edema.

morphology, menstrual pattern, and bone vascularity; the extrinsic factors include training regimen, shoe wear, and playing surface.[17,19] The fifth metatarsal is especially susceptible to stress fracture because of the poor blood supply to the metadiaphyseal junction, but all metatarsals are at risk.

Diagnosis of a metatarsal stress fracture is based on a characteristic history, the physical examination, and imaging findings. The key historical feature is pain of insidious onset, often correlated with a change in activity level or equipment. The patient's nutritional, endocrinologic, rheumatologic, and menstrual history should be obtained. Localized tenderness and soft-tissue swelling may be present on physical examination. Some authors recommend the use of a tuning fork as a diagnostic tool, but evidence of its efficacy is limited.[20] Imaging should begin with AP, lateral, and oblique foot radiographs. The characteristic radiographic findings include cortical radiolucent lines, periosteal reaction, callus formation, and focal sclerosis. The radiographic evidence of stress fracture may lag several weeks behind the clinical symptoms, and the diagnosis may need to be confirmed by repeating the plain radiographs weeks later. Advanced imaging studies also can confirm the diagnosis. CT, a technetium Tc 99m bone scan, and MRI are useful; MRI is the most sensitive test[21,22] (**Figure 6**).

Nonsurgical Treatment

The cornerstone of nonsurgical treatment is rest from the inciting activity. A CAM walker boot can be used for immobilization, but a short leg cast is preferred for a high-risk stress fracture such as a proximal fifth metatarsal stress fracture. Patients should avoid weight bearing for 6 to 8 weeks, depending on the severity of symptoms. A nutritional assessment should be done, and supplementation with calcium and vitamin D should be considered. If healing is delayed, extracorporeal shock wave therapy and teriparatide can be considered.[23,24] If appropriate, the patient can be referred to a metabolic bone disease specialist for a diagnostic workup and treatment of any identified disorder.

Surgical Treatment

Surgical treatment should be reserved for a high-level athlete, a patient with an established pseudarthrosis, or a patient with refracture. A preexisting foot deformity that creates a predisposition to metatarsal stress fracture, such as a cavovarus foot or metatarsus adductus, should be treated concomitantly, as necessary.[25,26] In general, rigid fixation with compression plating of the first through fourth metatarsals and intramedullary screw fixation of the fifth metatarsal are recommended. Autologous bone grafting can be used in the index operation, but there is no evidence to support the superiority of bone graft plus internal fixation over internal fixation alone for an acute stress fracture.

The initial postoperative immobilization is in a well-padded short leg splint with the toes uncovered. After 2 weeks, the splint can be removed, and the patient can begin partial weight bearing in a CAM walker boot. Low- and no-impact rehabilitation exercise to restore motion, strength, and fitness (such as cycling and swimming) can begin. At 6 weeks after surgery, the patient can return to full weight bearing and activity, provided there is clinical and radiographic evidence of fracture healing.

Toe Fractures

Fractures of the lesser toes are the most common fractures of the forefoot and account for 3.6% of all fractures in adults.[27,28] Almost all patients with such a fracture can be treated nonsurgically with no long-term pain or functional deficits.[28,29] Nonetheless, a thorough evaluation and radiographic workup should be done to evaluate for concomitant fractures, open fracture, nail bed injury, or other soft-tissue injury.

The most frequent mechanisms of lesser toe fractures are stubbing and crushing injuries, which account for 75% of the fractures, but penetrating trauma can also cause the injury.[28,30] The fifth toe accounts for half of all fractures of the lesser toes. A fracture of the fifth toe, sometimes called a night walker fracture, is produced by a direct abduction force and often is sustained while walking barefoot in the dark. Almost all phalangeal fractures are nondisplaced or minimally displaced. Extra-articular injuries are far more common than intra-articular injuries.

The treatment of lesser toe fracture is nonsurgical for almost all patients. A toe with mild or no fracture displacement or angulation can be treated with buddy taping, in which gauze sponges are placed between the affected toe and the adjacent toes, and the toes are strapped together with adhesive tape.[31] The patient should wear a stiff-soled shoe with an open toe box and is allowed to ambulate as tolerated. If there is deformity of the toe, closed reduction under local anesthesia is accomplished with longitudinal traction (manual or with finger traps) and angular correction, with a pencil in the web space serving as a fulcrum.

Surgical treatment is reserved for a patient with an open fracture, an unsuccessful closed reduction, or a grossly displaced, unstable fracture. The risks and benefits of surgery should be carefully weighed because a malunited phalangeal fracture is associated with minimal morbidity. As an alternative to surgical fixation, the patient can be offered exostectomy if the malunion becomes symptomatic.[32]

First MTP Joint Complex Injuries

The first (hallux) MTP joint is significantly larger than the lesser MTP joints. Several strong muscles (the abductor hallucis, the extensor hallucis brevis, the adductor hallucis, and the two flexor hallucis brevis tendons) attach to the base of the first proximal phalanx, and a robust plantar plate provides plantar stabilization of the joint. The plantar plate attaches to the base of the proximal phalanx and the metatarsal neck and is reinforced by a lateral transverse metatarsal ligament. The two slips of the flexor hallucis brevis tendon contain the sesamoid bones, which help support weight beneath the first metatarsal head during gait activity.[33]

Injury to the first MTP joint usually is the result of severe dorsiflexion with an axial-loading component and can range from a mild sprain to a turf toe injury (a severe sprain) or overt dislocation.[34] Normal motion in the hallux MTP joint is from 90° of dorsiflexion to 45° of plantar flexion. The first MTP joint is subject to compression injuries, fractures, sprains, and hyperextension injuries (turf toe injuries). Cartilage damage is common in the first MTP joint and can lead to hallux valgus or hallux rigidus and ultimately to osteoarthritis. Even seemingly minor injuries can lead to substantial disability.[34] Patients typically report significant pain, swelling, and stiffness in the toe. Routine standing AP, lateral, and oblique foot radiographs are necessary to detect injury to bones, joints, and sesamoid positioning (**Figure 7**).

Turf Toe Injuries

Turf toe injuries are relatively common in field athletes such as football, soccer, and lacrosse players. Although most patients recover with appropriate symptomatic care, some injuries are sufficiently debilitating to keep an athlete out of play for a season and may require surgical repair. It has not yet been proved whether an aggressive open repair has results superior to those of nonsurgical management, particularly because the postoperative rehabilitation can be quite prolonged.[34] A stretch of the capsuloligamentous complex with mild swelling and plantar medial tenderness is classified as a grade I injury; partial soft-tissue disruption with moderate swelling and diffuse tenderness is a grade II injury; and severe ligament injury with dorsal impaction of the first MTP articular surface, severe swelling, tenderness, and stiffness about the first MTP joint is a grade III injury.[35] Cartilage injury and bony impaction portend a relatively poor prognosis.

Contralateral comparison radiographs and stress dorsiflexion radiographs can be helpful for classifying the injury and, although most injuries remain stable, for detecting any retraction or injury of the sesamoids. MRI can be helpful for determining the extent of capsuloligamentous disruption.[36] Sprains and small capsular avulsions can be treated using hard-soled shoes or a carbon-fiber orthotic device to limit dorsiflexion until symptoms are resolved. The recovery period typically is 2 to 4 weeks. A grade I or II injury is treated in a short CAM walker boot or postoperative shoe, with 3 to 4 weeks of physical therapy to improve range of motion and reduce swelling, followed by a return to sports using a protective steel or carbon-fiber insole (a turf toe plate), as symptoms allow. Taping of the hallux in plantar flexion can be useful. A custom-made total-contact insole also can prevent further injury. A grade III injury may require significantly longer for recovery than a grade I or II injury. Surgical treatment is indicated if there is a large or incarcerated intra-articular fragment, joint incongruity, complete disruption of the plantar structures, gross instability, or retraction of the sesamoids. These injuries have been associated with late arthrosis and stiffness.[37]

Surgical treatment of a turf toe injury generally entails open repair of the plantar plate to restore congruity to the hallux MTP joint complex. A medial approach is used for the tibial sesamoid and a plantar approach is used for the fibular sesamoid. It is vital to identify and protect the sensory nerves. An injury through the sesamoid bones (a displaced fracture) should be repaired at the time of surgery. Flexor hallucis brevis tendon avulsion from the proximal phalanx can be repaired to the proximal

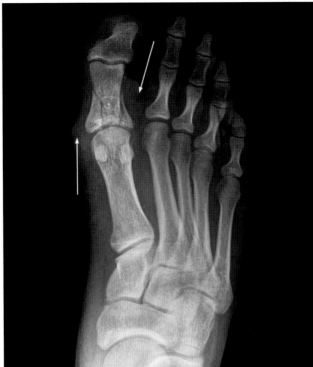

Figure 7 AP radiograph showing a comminuted intra-articular fracture of the hallux proximal phalanx after a gunshot wound. The entry and exit wounds are seen as soft-tissue shadows (arrows).

phalanx with suture anchors. The abductor hallucis tendon can be used to augment the plantar plate repair if there is significant loss of healthy collagen.

First MTP Joint Dislocations

First MTP joint dislocation is rare and most often occurs in a dorsal direction as a result of a high-energy hyperextension mechanism. Plain radiographs usually are sufficient for diagnosing a first MTP joint dislocation and associated injuries. The plantar plate typically is disrupted at its proximal attachment beneath the metatarsal; it becomes situated above the metatarsal head, along with the phalanx and sesamoids. Relocation can be blocked by the intact collateral ligaments and the abductor and adductor tendons. Although prompt closed reduction should be attempted, the injury often requires open reduction. Closed reduction can be attempted with digital block anesthesia. The interphalangeal joint is extended, longitudinal traction is applied, and plantar translation reduces the joint.

Open reduction usually is successful and stable and can be followed by restricted dorsiflexion in a stiff-soled shoe or a short CAM walker boot for 3 to 4 weeks, with early range-of-motion exercises. Open reduction is required if the joint is unstable or incongruent as a result of bony or soft-tissue interposition after attempted reduction. Kirschner wire fixation should be added. The wire can be removed at 3 to 4 weeks, and range-of-motion exercises can be initiated. Postreduction radiographs and a range-of-motion examination should be done to confirm stability, congruity, and clearance of soft-tissue interposition.

Sesamoid Injuries

The sesamoids are an important part of the great toe flexor mechanism and have a function similar to that of the patella in the quadriceps mechanism of the knee. The sesamoids support the first metatarsal head and the first MTP joint from pressure during weight bearing and provide a lever arm to the flexor hallucis brevis tendons to plantar flex the proximal phalanx. Each sesamoid is approximately 7 to 10 mm long and slightly oblong. The dorsal surfaces of the sesamoids articulate with the plantar aspect of the first metatarsal head. The strong intersesamoid ligament connects the two sesamoids and extends to the deep transverse intermetatarsal ligament. The flexor hallucis longus tendon runs between the two sesamoid bones, ultimately attaching to the distal phalanx. Typically, the medial (tibial) sesamoid is more centrally located beneath the first metatarsal head than the lateral (fibular) sesamoid and it probably bears more weight, making it more prone to injury such as sesamoiditis or stress fracture.

Sesamoid injury can cause tremendous pain and disability. Dancers and runners are particularly susceptible to traumatic stress fracture in the sesamoids from repeated impact and tension. Dancers and runners who train and perform in thin-soled shoes, the use of which is a recent trend among runners, are vulnerable to these injuries because they land on a hard surface with the toes dorsiflexed. Sesamoid injuries are evaluated with a routine set of AP, lateral, and axial sesamoid radiographs of the foot, which allow assessment of the congruity of each metatarsal-sesamoid articulation, the status of the cartilage surfaces, and any fracture displacement. The patient typically has mild swelling, stiffness of the MTP joint, and point tenderness over the involved sesamoid. Passive or active hyperextension exacerbates the pain by stretching the entire sesamoid apparatus. Resisted plantar flexion also can be painful.

Sesamoiditis

Sesamoiditis is characterized by pain, tenderness, inflammation, and possible cartilage injury at the metatarsal head–sesamoid articulation. This syndrome typically is caused by repetitive stress on the sesamoids and MTP joint apparatus, as occurs during dancing, running, and jumping. Sesamoiditis is aggravated by improper tracking of the sesamoids under the metatarsal head or by progressive metatarsus varus. Plantar flexion of the first metatarsal and overactivity of the long peroneal tendon, called peroneal overdrive, can overload the sesamoids and produce pain similar to that of sesamoiditis. Such underlying conditions must be identified and treated.

Sesamoid Fractures

Fracture of a sesamoid can result from tension force on the sesamoid apparatus or from a direct acute or repetitive impact force on the sesamoid itself. Most sesamoid fractures have a simple transverse pattern with minimal displacement and sharp fracture edges. An acute fracture must be differentiated from a symptomatic bipartite sesamoid. Many features of bipartite sesamoids can be distinguished on comparison plain radiographs: bilaterality and medial location (in 85% and 10%, respectively, of patients with bipartite sesamoids), smooth edges, large size, obliquity of the radiolucent line on radiographs (rather than transverse lines more typical of fracture), and lack of callus.

Treatment of Sesamoid Injuries

Acute fracture and suspected stress fracture of the sesamoids usually are treated by immobilizing the hallux in a spica cast for 3 to 6 weeks, ideally with the toe in plantar flexion. The patient should avoid weight bearing for at least the first 3 weeks. The cast should be followed by protection in a short CAM walker boot and initiation of range-of-motion exercises. If a sesamoid fracture does not heal with casting and/or if pain persists beyond 6 months, sesamoidectomy or bone grafting of the fracture is indicated. Sesamoiditis usually is successfully treated in a similar fashion. Subsequent use of an orthotic device that offloads the affected sesamoid with a metatarsal pad and a recess for the sesamoid can help prevent reinjury.

Little published information is available on open reduction and internal fixation and bone grafting of a sesamoid nonunion. Bone grafting and fixation of a sesamoid fracture is as likely to lead to union as splinting alone. A standard approach is used, a small hole is drilled into the center of the fracture site with a burr, and the fracture site is filled with cancellous autograft. Interfragmentary compression can be obtained with a 1.5-mm screw if the fragments are sufficiently large. This procedure is technically challenging, and the opportunity to gain experience in this technique is limited. Postoperatively, the great toe and the short flexor mechanism are splinted in a plantarflexed position. Protected weight bearing can begin after 6 weeks.

Every attempt should be made to salvage the sesamoids, particularly if the patient is an athlete. Sesamoidectomy is used only if the patient has severe and painful osteonecrosis or a nonhealing or comminuted fracture. Sesamoidectomy requires a precise surgical technique in which the sesamoid is carefully removed from its capsule without disrupting the tendon. If the fracture is small and at one of the poles, partial excision of the smaller sesamoid fragment can be done. For a lateral (fibular) sesamoid excision, a plantar approach between the first and second metatarsal heads is recommended to minimize painful scar formation. Care must be taken to avoid and protect the digital nerve, which traverses the MTP joint immediately adjacent to the sesamoid, because injury to this nerve can be quite debilitating. A direct medial approach is used for a medial (tibial) sesamoid excision, again avoiding the dorsal and plantar digital sensory nerve branches. After the bone is removed, the tendon is repaired or imbricated before wound closure. The toe is splinted in a protected position for 4 to 6 weeks before weight bearing and rehabilitation with dorsiflexion exercises are initiated.

Disability may result after sesamoidectomy, and pain-free function is not always restored. Excision of the lateral sesamoid can cause medial drift and a cock-up deformity (hallux varus). Removal of the medial sesamoid can create hallux valgus. Careful repair of the flexor hallucis brevis tendon can help prevent these complications. A transfer lesion may develop if the remaining sesamoid becomes painful from the extra weight it must support, despite an intact flexor mechanism.

Summary

Fractures and other injuries to the forefoot are common and can substantially affect normal function. A careful history and physical examination with appropriate radiographic studies can lead to an accurate and complete diagnosis. With an understanding of their mechanisms and natural history, these injuries can be successfully treated, and function usually can be restored. If surgical treatment is indicated to restore function, an in-depth knowledge of anatomy, surgical approaches, and postoperative rehabilitation can optimize the outcome. Careful attention should be paid to the mechanical and nutritional factors that can affect healing.

Acknowledgment

The author thanks Garet Comer, MD, for his assistance in the writing of this chapter.

Annotated References

1. Turchin DC, Schemitsch EH, McKee MD, Waddell JP: Do foot injuries significantly affect the functional outcome of multiply injured patients? *J Orthop Trauma* 1999;13(1):1-4.

2. Wilson LS Jr, Mizel MS, Michelson JD: Foot and ankle injuries in motor vehicle accidents. *Foot Ankle Int* 2001;22(8):649-652.

3. Digiovanni CW, Benirschke SK, Hansen ST: Foot injuries, in Browner BD, Jupiter JB, Levine AM, Trafton PG, eds: *Skeletal Trauma: Basic Science, Management, and Reconstruction, ed 3*. Philadelphia, PA, WB Saunders, 2003, pp 2375-2492.

4. Armagan OE, Shereff MJ: Injuries to the toes and metatarsals. *Orthop Clin North Am* 2001;32(1):1-10.

5. Schenck RC Jr, Heckman JD: Fractures and dislocations of the forefoot: Operative and nonoperative treatment. *J Am Acad Orthop Surg* 1995;3(2):70-78.

6. Donahue MP, Manoli A II: Technical tip: Transverse percutaneous pinning of metatarsal neck fractures. *Foot Ankle Int* 2004;25(6):438-439.

7. Sisk TD: Fractures, in Edmonson AS, Crenshaw AH, eds: *Campbell's Operative Orthopaedics, ed 6*. St Louis, MO, Mosby, 1980.

8. Heckman JD: Fractures and dislocations of the foot, in Rockwood CA, Green DP, Bucholtz RW, Heckman JD, eds: *Rockwood and Green's Fractures in Adults, 4th ed*. Philadelphia, PA, Lippincott-Raven, 1996, pp 2267-2405.

9. Smith JW, Arnoczky SP, Hersh A: *The intraosseous blood supply of the fifth metatarsal: Implications for proximal fracture healing. Foot Ankle* 1992;13(3):143-152.

10. Zwitser EW, Breederveld RS: Fractures of the fifth metatarsal: Diagnosis and treatment. *Injury* 2010;41(6):555-562.

    Fifth metatarsal fractures were reviewed, including diagnostic workup and current treatments.

11. Dameron TB Jr: Fractures and anatomical variations of the proximal portion of the fifth metatarsal. *J Bone Joint Surg Am* 1975;57(6):788-792.

12. Richli WR, Rosenthal DI: Avulsion fracture of the fifth metatarsal: Experimental study of pathomechanics. *AJR Am J Roentgenol* 1984;143(4):889-891.

13. Jones RI: I: Fracture of the base of the fifth metatarsal bone by indirect violence. *Ann Surg* 1902;35(6):697-700, 2.

14. Hunt KJ, Anderson RB: Treatment of Jones fracture non-unions and refractures in the elite athlete: Outcomes of intramedullary screw fixation with bone grafting. *Am J Sports Med* 2011;39(9):1948-1954.

   A retrospective study described outcomes of Jones fracture nonunions and refractures in elite athletes. Bone-grafting technique was described.

15. Porter DA, Duncan M, Meyer SJ: Fifth metatarsal Jones fracture fixation with a 4.5-mm cannulated stainless steel screw in the competitive and recreational athlete: A clinical and radiographic evaluation. *Am J Sports Med* 2005;33(5):726-733.

16. Polzer H, Polzer S, Mutschler W, Prall WC: Acute fractures to the proximal fifth metatarsal bone: Development of classification and treatment recommendations based on the current evidence. *Injury* 2012;43(10):1626-1632.

   A review of acute fractures of the base of the fifth metatarsal included the current evidence for treatment.

17. Cosman F, Ruffing J, Zion M, et al: Determinants of stress fracture risk in United States Military Academy cadets. *Bone* 2013;55(2):359-366.

   Data on risk factors for stress fractures among military cadets were discussed.

18. Jones BH, Thacker SB, Gilchrist J, Kimsey CD Jr, Sosin DM: Prevention of lower extremity stress fractures in athletes and soldiers: A systematic review. *Epidemiol Rev* 2002;24(2):228-247.

19. Shindle MK, Endo Y, Warren RF, et al: Stress fractures about the tibia, foot, and ankle. *J Am Acad Orthop Surg* 2012;20(3):167-176.

   The incidence, risk factors, and management of stress fractures in competitive athletes are reviewed. The management challenges associated with high-risk fractures, including those of the proximal fifth metatarsal, also are reviewed.

20. Lesho EP: Can tuning forks replace bone scans for identification of tibial stress fractures? *Mil Med* 1997;162(12):802-803.

21. Gaeta M, Minutoli F, Scribano E, et al: CT and MR imaging findings in athletes with early tibial stress injuries: Comparison with bone scintigraphy findings and emphasis on cortical abnormalities. *Radiology* 2005;235(2):553-561.

22. Boden BP, Osbahr DC: High-risk stress fractures: Evaluation and treatment. *J Am Acad Orthop Surg* 2000;8(6):344-353.

23. Alvarez RG, Cincere B, Channappa C, et al: Extracorporeal shock wave treatment of non- or delayed union of proximal metatarsal fractures. *Foot Ankle Int* 2011;32(8):746-754.

   A prospective study suggested that high-energy extracorporeal shock wave treatment is effective and safe for treating nonunion or delayed healing of a proximal metatarsal fractures.

24. Raghavan P, Christofides E: Role of teriparatide in accelerating metatarsal stress fracture healing: A case series and review of literature. *Clin Med Insights Endocrinol Diabetes* 2012;5:39-45.

   A retrospective study and literature review suggested that teriparatide may accelerate fracture healing, especially in patients who are at risk for impaired fracture healing.

25. Carreira DS, Sandilands SM: Radiographic factors and effect of fifth metatarsal Jones and diaphyseal stress fractures on participation in the NFL. *Foot Ankle Int* 2013;34(4):518-522.

   A web-based review suggested that Jones fracture is not associated with a patient's number of years playing in the National Football League. Players were more likely to have radiographic abnormalities in the coronal plane with varus alignment than in the sagittal plane.

26. Rongstad KM, Tueting J, Rongstad M, Garrels K, Meis R: Fourth metatarsal base stress fractures in athletes: A case series. *Foot Ankle Int* 2013;34(7):962-968.

   This is a case study of fourth metatarsal base fractures in 11 athletic patients.

27. Court-Brown CM, Caesar B: Epidemiology of adult fractures: A review. *Injury* 2006;37(8):691-697.

28. Van Vliet-Koppert ST, Cakir H, Van Lieshout EM, De Vries MR, Van Der Elst M, Schepers T: Demographics and functional outcome of toe fractures. *J Foot Ankle Surg* 2011;50(3):307-310.

   A study of 339 patients with toe fractures revealed no statistically significant associations between outcome and a particular toe, number of fractured toes, fracture type and location, articular involvement, or patient sex, age, body mass index, smoking habits, or diabetes. Satisfaction depended on age and sex.

29. Schnaue-Constantouris EM, Birrer RB, Grisafi PJ, Dellacorte MP: Digital foot trauma: Emergency diagnosis and treatment. *J Emerg Med* 2002;22(2):163-170.

30. Mittlmeier T, Haar P: Sesamoid and toe fractures. *Injury* 2004;35(2, Suppl 2):SB87-SB97.

31. Hatch RL, Hacking S: Evaluation and management of toe fractures. *Am Fam Physician* 2003;68(12):2413-2418.

32. Coughlin MJ: Common causes of pain in the forefoot in adults. *J Bone Joint Surg Br* 2000;82(6):781-790.

33. McCormick JJ, Anderson RB: Turf toe: Anatomy, diagnosis, and treatment. *Sports Health* 2010;2(6):487-494.

6: Foot and Ankle Trauma

The clinical diagnosis and treatment of turf toe injuries were reviewed.

34. Frimenko RE, Lievers W, Coughlin MJ, Anderson RB, Crandall JR, Kent RW: Etiology and biomechanics of first metatarsophalangeal joint sprains (turf toe) in athletes. *Crit Rev Biomed Eng* 2012;40(1):43-61.

The biomechanics of turf toe injury were reviewed.

35. McCormick JJ, Anderson RB: The great toe: Failed turf toe, chronic turf toe, and complicated sesamoid injuries. *Foot Ankle Clin* 2009;14(2):135-150.

This review article examines the current evidence pertinent to the incidence, epidemiology, and management of turf toe injuries and sesamoid injuries. Particular attention is paid to surgical indications and techniques.

36. Crain JM, Phancao JP, Stidham K: MR imaging of turf toe. *Magn Reson Imaging Clin N Am* 2008;16(1):93-103, vi.

Imaging modalities for turf toe injuries was reviewed.

37. Rodeo SA, O'Brien S, Warren RF, Barnes R, Wickiewicz TL, Dillingham MF: Turf-toe: An analysis of metatarsophalangeal joint sprains in professional football players. *Am J Sports Med* 1990;18(3):280-285.

Tendon Disorders and Sports-Related Foot and Ankle Injuries

SECTION EDITOR:

SUSAN N. ISHIKAWA, MD

Chapter 28

Disorders of the Anterior Tibial, Peroneal, and Achilles Tendons

Thomas Padanilam, MD

Anterior Tibial Tendon Disorders

The anterior tibial tendon originates along the anterolateral tibia and inserts onto the medial aspect of the first metatarsal and medial cuneiform. It functions concentrically during the swing phase of gait to dorsiflex the ankle and allow clearance of the foot. At heel strike, the tendon works in an eccentric fashion to control the progression to the foot's flat position. The anterior tibial tendon also assists with inversion of the foot.

Rupture of the anterior tibial tendon is relatively uncommon, and most studies involved only a small number of patients.[1,2] A normal anterior tibial tendon rarely ruptures except as a result of a laceration or sudden force. Spontaneous rupture occurs secondary to a degenerative process, usually in men age 50 to 70 years.[1] The causes of degeneration include impingement, inflammatory arthritis, diabetes mellitus, infection, chronic microtrauma, ischemia, hyperparathyroidism, systemic lupus erythematosus, gout, obesity, and oral or local steroid therapy.[3] The usual site of an anterior tibial tendon rupture is 0.5 cm to 3 cm proximal to its insertion, where the tendon passes under the inferior extensor retinaculum. Formerly this location was believed to be a vascular watershed area within the tendon, but microvascular studies have not found such an area.[4]

Anterior tibial tendon rupture appears in two forms. In relatively young patients an acute onset of symptoms occurs after penetrating injury or severe trauma; in patients older than 50 years, a moderately forceful plantar flexion stress can bring on the symptoms. The second form is seen in relatively sedentary patients older than 50 years with a several-month history of atraumatic foot drop. The rupture may have a prodrome of swelling, or it may follow a minor misstep or a twisting injury of the ankle. The signs and symptoms of the second form of anterior tibial tendon injury can be confusing.[1] The injury may be masked by a rapid resolution of any initial pain and compensation by the other extensor muscles. As a result, the diagnosis of rupture often is missed or delayed.[3] Pain may be minimal after the initial episode and is not a major factor for many patients who seek treatment. A patient is likely to report a foot slap or unsteady gait, limping, or increased fatigue with walking.

Physical examination findings include gait abnormalities such as a footslap or footdrop. It may be possible to palpate the proximal stump of the anterior tibial tendon as a mass along the anteromedial aspect of the ankle. Dorsiflexion of the ankle reveals a loss of tendon contour compared with the contralateral limb. Most patients are able to use the remaining, functioning tendons for dorsiflexion, but careful testing will reveal a strength deficit in comparison with the contralateral limb. Increased extension at the metatarsophalangeal joint of the toes may be observed as the extensor tendons attempt to compensate for loss of dorsiflexion power.

Both surgical and nonsurgical treatments have been recommended, but the optimal treatment remains controversial. One study found no difference in outcomes after surgical or nonsurgical treatment.[5] The patients treated nonsurgically had an average age of 74 years and had low physical demands; most of the patients treated surgically had an average age of 55 years and were more physically active. No relevant randomized prospective studies have been published. The available research is primarily composed of case reports and small studies, most of which recommended early direct repair to restore function.[5-7] This procedure may be particularly beneficial for a relatively young, active patient with a traumatic injury to the tendon. Direct tendon repair may be possible within the first few months after injury.[3] The retracted tendon end usually becomes entrapped at the distal extent of the superior extensor retinanculum.[2,6] Direct repair can be done end to end with a grasping stitch using a Krackow, Kessler, or Bunnell technique. If the tendon is avulsed off the insertion site, suture anchors or soft-tissue interference screws can be used for reattachment.

Dr. Padanilam or an immediate family member has stock or stock options held in Eli Lilly and Pfizer.

Late treatment after an atraumatic rupture should be individualized based on the patient's activity level. A patient with low physical demands or a significant medical comorbidity may benefit from nonsurgical treatment. The use of an ankle-foot orthosis can facilitate foot clearance during the swing phase of gait and decrease fatigue during prolonged ambulation. Some patients find brace treatment overly restrictive and opt not to use it.[3] In a delayed surgical procedure, end-to-end repair may not be feasible because of adhesions and lack of excursion of the tendon ends, and an interpositional graft is likely necessary. A variety of methods have been described for treating chronic ruptures, including Achilles tendon grafting or transfer of the extensor hallucis longus, extensor digitorum longus, plantaris, or peroneus tertius tendon.[2,3,6,7]

A 2009 retrospective review evaluated the results of surgical treatment of 19 anterior tibial tendon ruptures in 18 patients.[6] Eight tendons had an early repair, and 11 had a delayed repair; 7 were treated with a direct repair, and 12 required the use of an interpositional graft. The plantaris tertius tendon was most commonly used for grafting, followed by the extensor digitorum longus tendon. Patients in both the early repair group and the late repair group had significant improvement in scores on the American Orthopaedic Foot and Ankle Society (AOFAS) measure. Manual testing revealed normal dorsiflexion strength in 15 of the 19 ankles. Tendon repair was recommended for all patients with an unsteady gait, weakness, or fatigability because of lack of dorsiflexion strength. A 2010 retrospective review of 15 surgically treated anterior tibial tendon ruptures in 14 patients found significant improvement in postoperative AOFAS and Medical Outcomes Study 36-Item Short Form scores.[7] Five tendons were repaired primarily, and 10 had a tendon transfer; 9 of the transfers used the extensor hallucis longus tendon. There was no difference in the outcomes of patients with a primary repair and those who required a tendon transfer. Strength testing using a dynamometer and comparison with the uninjured contralateral limb found deficits in dorsiflexion strength in all patients.

No randomized prospective studies are available to guide the treatment of anterior tibial tendon ruptures; only case reports and relatively small retrospective case studies have been published. Patients with an atraumatic injury who have low physical demands and seek treatment after a delay can be treated nonsurgically, but most researchers favor surgical treatment of patients who have relatively high physical demands.[2,3,5-7] In patients undergoing late treatment, an interpositional graft usually is required.

Peroneal Tendon Disorders

The peroneal tendons originate as muscle bellies in the lateral compartment of the leg and become tendinous as they pass through a fibro-osseous tunnel posterior to the lateral malleolus. The peroneal tendons share a sheath that bifurcates at the level of the peroneal tubercle of the lateral calcaneus. The peroneus longus runs posterolateral to the peroneus brevis and turns sharply at the tip of the fibula, passing under the trochlear process of the calcaneus and along a groove in the plantar surface of the cuboid to insert on the plantar base of the first metatarsal. The peroneus brevis muscle belly is lower and lies between the posterior fibula and the peroneus longus tendon in the fibro-osseous tunnel before turning under the tip of the fibula to insert on the fifth metatarsal base. The peroneal tendons function as the major evertors and pronators of the ankle. In addition, the peroneus longus plantar flexes the first metatarsal.

A typical peroneal tendon disorder is classified as peroneal tendinitis without subluxation of the tendons, peroneal tendinitis with subluxation of the peroneal tendons at the level of the superior retinaculum, or stenosing tenosynovitis of the peroneus longus in the area of the peroneal tubercle, os peroneum, or cuboid tunnel. Peroneal tendon injuries can be missed because they often occur in conjunction with a lateral ankle sprain, with only vague symptoms along the lateral ankle.[8] A patient with an acute injury may report having twisted the ankle. Symptoms of subluxation often can be concealed by the pain and swelling associated with a lateral ankle sprain. Swelling posterior to the lateral malleolus occurs with peroneal instability, tearing, and synovitis. Symptoms of tenosynovitis can be brought on by a change in activity level. A patient with a dislocation often reports pain and a popping sensation along the lateral retromalleolar area.

A careful physical examination often is the most important step in making the appropriate diagnosis. Acute subluxation may present with ecchymosis posterior to the lateral malleolus, and it may be associated with tenderness over the insertion of the superior retinaculum. Pain and a sensation of instability in the lateral retromalleolar area can be reproduced with active eversion and dorsiflexion of the ankle.[9] Palpable snapping or crepitus may be evident during this maneuver. Synovitic thickening appears to be the most reliable sign of a peroneal tendon tear.[10] Pain with forced plantar flexion and inversion may be seen with synovitis. Pain is not always present with a peroneal tendon tear, but it may be possible to elicit pain with resisted eversion. A tear may cause tenderness along the course of the tendon. A longitudinal tear can cause early fatigability but not weakness.[11] A peroneus longus tear can cause pain with resisted plantar flexion

7: Tendon Disorders and Sports-Related Foot and Ankle Injuries

of the first metatarsal. A patient with suspected peroneal tendon pathology should undergo an assessment for concomitant ankle instability and varus malalignment of the hindfoot.

A plain radiograph may reveal an avulsion fracture of the lateral aspect of the distal fibula and suggest a peroneal tendon subluxation. Hypertrophy of the peroneal tubercle suggests peroneal tendon impingement. Fracture or migration of the os peroneum proximal to the calcaneocuboid joint may indicate a peroneus longus tear. The role of MRI in the evaluation of peroneal tendon pathology is unclear. A normal peroneus brevis tendon can appear to be partially torn because of an increase in signal intensity on T1-weighted images (the so-called magic angle effect). Tendon subluxation may be difficult to detect on MRI, especially if the subluxation is intermittent. A study of MRI in 133 patients found that radiologists detected only 56% of the peroneus brevis tears present at surgery.[12] In 82 patients who underwent surgery for lateral ankle instability, the positive predictive value of MRI for peroneal tendons was 66.7%.[13] Overreliance on MRI was found to lead to unnecessary surgical procedures.

Peroneal Tendon Subluxation

Acute peroneal tendon dislocation usually is associated with a traumatic event during a sports activity involving rapid changes in direction. The mechanism of injury is somewhat controversial; both inversion and extreme dorsiflexion have been suggested as the ankle position at the time of injury. An eccentric contraction of the peroneal tendons against resistance causes avulsion of the superior peroneal retinaculum off the fibula, often with periosteum or a cortical bone fragment off the lateral aspect of the fibula. The periosteum is elevated, creating a pouch in which the dislocated tendons sit.

The onset of chronic peroneal tendon subluxation usually is insidious and occurs after an untreated acute dislocation.[9] Recurrent subluxation from behind the lateral malleolus attenuates the superior retinaculum and often is associated with a split tear of the peroneus brevis tendon as it is caught between the fibrocartilaginous rim and the peroneus longus tendon. Often there is associated tenosynovitis.

Acute peroneal tendon dislocation that spontaneously reduces can be treated with immobilization. The reported success rate of nonsurgical treatment is approximately 50%.[14] Relatively young patients with high physical demands are treated surgically. Recurrent subluxation of the peroneal tendons can be associated with longitudinal tearing in the peroneus brevis, which should be treated during the instability surgery. Surgical treatment options for peroneal tendon subluxation include reconstruction of the superior peroneal retinaculum, rerouting of the tendons under the calcaneofibular ligament, reconstruction of the retinaculum with a portion of the Achilles tendon, and a groove-deepening procedure. An isolated repair or reconstruction of the retinaculum is ideal for an acute dislocation in which the tissue is unlikely to be compromised.[14] In chronic dislocation, compromised retinacular tissue may require augmentation of the retinaculum with additional tissue or routing of the tendon under the calcaneofibular ligament.

The retromalleolar groove, in which the tendons rest, usually is concave, but it is flat or convex in 10% to 20% of patients.[15] The flat or convex shape contributes to peroneal tendon instability, and a groove-deepening procedure is considered if the patient has a flat or convex configuration of the posterior fibula. The extent of impaction or deepening is adjusted until it is sufficient to prevent dislocation of the tendons with ankle manipulation. A variety of techniques have been described. A recent technique uses tendoscopy to deepen the groove.[9] Seven patients with peroneal dislocation had the retromalleolar groove deepened with a burr and tendoscopy. Four patients had detachment of the superior retinaculum at the site of the fibular insertion, but surgical repair was not attempted. At an average 15.4-month follow-up, none of the patients had recurrent subluxation, and five reported an excellent outcome. Although the procedure was claimed to lead to less morbidity and more rapid recovery than an open procedure, the study included no control group for comparison.

Recent research has questioned the association between groove morphology and peroneal subluxation.[15-17] A retrospective MRI study of 39 ankles after surgical treatment of peroneal tendon dislocation classified the shape of the retromalleolar groove as concave, convex, or flat.[17] No significant difference was found on MRI between the treated ankles and 39 ankles without peroneal tendon dislocation. The superior peroneal retinaculum inserts into a fibrocartilaginous rim on the posterolateral fibula, which helps to deepen the retromalleolar groove, and the study authors suggested that this rim has a significant role in stabilizing the tendons. A cadaver study found that the peroneal tunnel has two components; an osseous component is formed by the retromalleolar groove, and a medial soft-tissue component is formed by the posterior intermuscular septum of the leg[16] (**Figure 1**). The study concluded that the retromalleolar groove is shallow and unable to accommodate the peroneal tendons and suggested that splitting the soft-tissue component may be as effective as groove deepening.

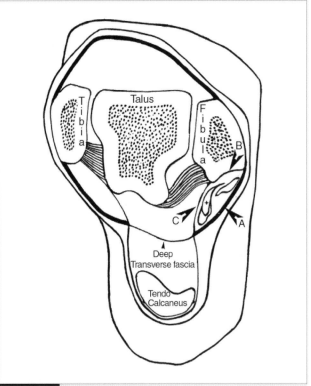

Figure 1 Schematic drawing showing a horizontal section through the superior peroneal tunnel. The boundaries of the tunnel are the superior peroneal retinaculum (**A**), the retromalleolar groove (**B**), and the posterior intermuscular septum (**C**). (Reproduced with permission from Athavale SA, Vangara SV: Anatomy of the superior peroneal tunnel. *J Bone Joint Surg Am* 2011;93:564-571.)

Peroneal Tenosynovitis

Peroneal tenosynovitis, also called peritendinitis, usually results from repetitive or prolonged activity or from trauma to the peroneal tendons. Peroneal tenosynovitis may be the result of stenosis of the synovial sheath, which can occur in the presence of a hypertrophied peroneal tubercle or other anatomic factors such a cavovarus foot, osseous calcaneal tunnel, presence of a peroneus quadratus muscle, and an incompetent superior peroneal retinaculum. Tenosynovitis usually occurs at a location where the tendon changes direction, such as behind the lateral malleolus, at the trochlear process, or under the cuboid. Tenosynovitis can be exacerbated by the presence of a space-occupying structure such as a low-lying peroneus brevis muscle belly or peroneus quartus tendon.

The initial treatment often is nonsurgical and may include activity modification, NSAIDs, physical therapy, a lateral-wedge orthotic device, or an ankle brace. If the condition does not improve, short-term immobilization with a boot or a short leg cast can be considered. Nonsurgical management is effective in most patients, but

surgical treatment may be indicated if nonsurgical treatment is unsuccessful. Surgical treatment involves débridement of inflamed tenosynovium, release of any areas of stenosis or compression around the tendon, removal of any space-occupying structures such as a low-lying peroneus brevis muscle belly or peroneus quartus tendon, and repair or débridement of pathologic tendon. In addition, any associated ankle or tendon instability or hindfoot malalignment should be corrected.

Peroneal Tendon Tears

Peroneal tendon tears may be associated with chronic ankle instability, peroneal tendon subluxation or dislocation, cavovarus hindfoot, a prominent peroneal tubercle, or an accessory tendon. These tears are believed to be caused by acute or repetitive mechanical trauma. Peroneus brevis tears are reported to be more common than peroneus longus tears.[8] Peroneus brevis tears most often occur at the distal portion of the lateral malleolus, where the peroneus longus tendon compresses the peroneus brevis tendon against the lateral malleolus.[14]

In the absence of an acute rupture, usually the treatment is nonsurgical and of 2 to 6 months' duration.[11] If surgical treatment is indicated, it is important to recognize that peroneal tendon injuries can be associated with other injuries. All 30 patients who had arthroscopic evaluation of the ankle at the same time as peroneal tendon repair were found to have intra-articular pathology.[8] Extensive scar tissue was the most common diagnosis, followed by synovitis and soft-tissue impingement. The absence of a comparison group in this study makes it difficult to determine the true benefit of arthroscopy.

Peroneal tendon tears typically are longitudinal rather than transverse, although transverse tears can occur.[10] The low-lying muscle belly of the peroneus brevis has been implicated as a contributor to peroneal tendon tears. A study of 115 cadaver specimens found that peroneus brevis tears were more common if the peroneus musculotendinous junction was relatively proximal.[18] The traditional recommendation is for débridement and tubularization of tears involving less than 50% of the tendon diameter and for débridement and tenodesis of larger tears.[10] Another algorithm recommends débridement and tubularization if both tendons are grossly intact, tenodesis if one tendon is not usable, and grafting rather than tendon transfer if both tendons are not usable and there is proximal peroneal muscle excursion[19] (**Figure 2**). Rupture of both tendons is uncommon (**Figure 3**). A staged procedure in which Hunter rod placement is followed by flexor hallucis longus (FHL) tendon transfer 3 months later has been used for chronic concomitant peroneal ruptures.[20] A recent study in which eight patients with concomitant tears of both tendons were treated with

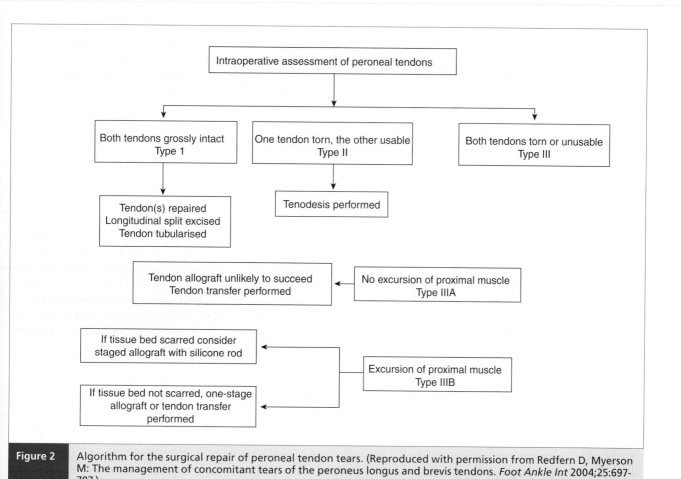

Figure 2   Algorithm for the surgical repair of peroneal tendon tears. (Reproduced with permission from Redfern D, Myerson M: The management of concomitant tears of the peroneus longus and brevis tendons. *Foot Ankle Int* 2004;25:697-707.)

a single-stage flexor digitorum longus (FDL) or FHL transfer found significant postoperative improvement in functional outcome and pain scores; seven patients rated their outcome as excellent.[21] The study authors concluded that, although both transfers were successful, the FHL transfer provided greater strength and a better outcome. This finding is consistent with that of a recent study to compare the relative strength of the calf muscles; the FHL transfer was found to be stronger than the peroneus longus or peroneus brevis transfer and much stronger than the FDL transfer.[22]

Achilles Tendon Disorders

The functional importance of the Achilles tendon is suggested by its status as the strongest and thickest tendon in the body. The Achilles tendon is formed by the two heads of the gastrocnemius and the soleus and inserts into the posterior aspect of the calcaneus. The slightly medial to midline insertion allows the tendon to provide some inversion in addition to its primary role of plantar flexion of the ankle. The tendon does not have a true synovial sheath; instead, it is surrounded by a paratenon, which

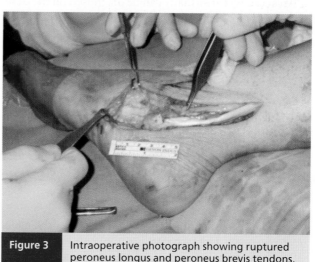

Figure 3   Intraoperative photograph showing ruptured peroneus longus and peroneus brevis tendons. The tendon ends are retracted, with gapping between the ends.

is a thin gliding membrane continuous proximally with the fascial envelope of the muscle. The paratenon is a highly vascular structure that, along with the surrounding muscle complex, provides blood flow to the tendon. An area of relative hypovascularity within the tendon 2 to 6 cm from the calcaneal insertion may be predisposed to degenerative changes and rupture. The Achilles tendon is subjected to forces as high as 6 to 10 times body weight during activities such as running. These factors, combined with the function of the gastrocnemius-soleus complex–soleus complex in crossing the knee, ankle, and subtalar joint, may help explain the high incidence of degenerative changes and injuries to the Achilles tendon.

Acute Achilles Tendon Ruptures

Achilles tendon rupture is most common in men age 30 to 50 years. A recent retrospective review of 331 patients with Achilles tendon rupture found that 83% were men, the average age was 46.4 years, and the mechanism of injury involved a sports activity in 68%.[23] Most Achilles tendon ruptures occur 2 to 6 cm from the insertion of the tendon; proximal ruptures account for only 10% to 15% of all Achilles tendon ruptures.[24] Ruptures at the insertion are rare and are associated with a factor such as Haglund deformity, a history of insertional Achilles tendinosis, or prior steroid therapy in the area. The common mechanism of rupture is a forced eccentric loading of the plantar-flexed foot. The exact cause of Achilles tendon rupture remains unclear, but it has been associated with inflammatory or autoimmune disorders, systemic or injectable steroid use, collagen abnormality, exposure to fluoroquinolones, repetitive microtrauma, metabolic disorders, and overpronation of the foot.

An acute rupture usually can be diagnosed on the basis of the patient's history and physical examination. Most patients have a history of a traumatic event and describe a feeling of being kicked in the heel. Walking and stair climbing or descending may be difficult. Examination reveals decreased plantar flexion strength, swelling around the tendon and loss of tendon contour, a palpable gap, lack of ankle movement when the calf is squeezed (the Thompson test), and an increased dorsiflexion position of the ankle when the patient is prone and the knee is bent to 90° (**Figure 4**).

The treatment of an acute Achilles rupture remains controversial. Nonsurgical treatment traditionally has consisted of prolonged immobilization in plantar flexion, with avoidance of weight bearing. Advocates of nonsurgical treatment emphasize the complications of surgical treatment, including wound-healing issues. Surgical treatment traditionally has been recommended for active patients because of the belief that rerupture rates are higher after nonsurgical treatment. Recent studies have attempted to answer the question of whether surgical or nonsurgical treatment is superior.

In a 2011 restrospective study of 945 patients with a nonsurgically treated Achilles tendon rupture, the

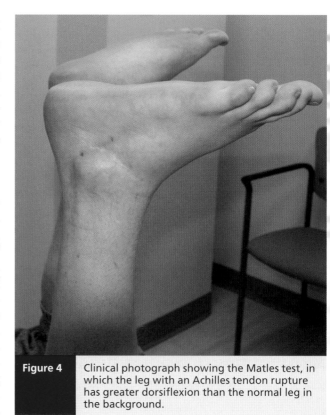

Figure 4 Clinical photograph showing the Matles test, in which the leg with an Achilles tendon rupture has greater dorsiflexion than the normal leg in the background.

decision for nonsurgical treatment was based on a palpation finding that the tendon ends were well approximated.[25] Patients were treated with an equinus cast for 4 weeks, a walker boot for the subsequent 4 weeks, and finally physical therapy. All patients were able to return to work and a preinjury level of sports activity. The rerupture rate was 2.8%. Almost all of the patients (99.4%) reported a good or excellent result. A historical control group of surgically treated patients was studied for comparison.

A 2011 retrospective study of 363 patients who underwent an identical functional rehabilitation program after surgical or nonsurgical treatment found a rerupture rate of 1.4% after surgical treatment and 8.6% after nonsurgical treatment.[24] The study was limited by the absence of standardized criteria for assignment to a treatment group. The patients who were surgically treated tended to be younger and have higher physical demands than those who were nonsurgically treated, or they had sought treatment more than 24 hours after injury. The study findings included no functional or outcome measures. Another study evaluated the functional outcomes of 80 patients who were randomly assigned to surgical or nonsurgical treatment.[26] No significant between-group difference was found in peak torque or total work at 1-year follow-up. Patients in both groups had decreased peak torque, however, in comparison with the uninjured leg.

Cast immobilization was used for 6 weeks after surgery and for 10 weeks in nonsurgical treatment. The rerupture rates (5.4% in the patients who were surgically treated and 10.3% in those who were nonsurgically treated) were not considered to be statistically significantly different.

Early mobilization has been emphasized in the treatment of Achilles tendon ruptures. A randomized study of 97 patients evaluated functional outcomes when early mobilization was used after surgical or nonsurgical treatment.[27] All treatment was initiated within 72 hours of injury, and patients in both groups used a removable boot after 2 weeks of immobilization in a short leg equinus cast. The rerupture rate was 4% in patients who were surgically treated and 12% in those who were nonsurgically treated. Functional testing at 6-month follow-up revealed much better results in the patients who were surgically treated, but at 12-month follow-up the only significant between-group difference was that patients in the surgical group performed better in the heel rise test. A randomized study of surgical and nonsurgical treatment in 144 patients evaluated functional outcomes after an accelerated functional rehabilitation program that began 2 weeks after injury.[28] No significant between-group difference was found in range of motion, strength, or rerupture rate. A meta-analysis of 10 randomized studies concluded that the risk of rerupture was equivalent after surgical or nonsurgical treatment of an Achilles tendon rupture if early motion was used during nonsurgical treatment.[29] If early motion was not used, the risk reduction with surgery was 8.8%. No significant difference was found in range of motion, strength, calf circumference, or functional outcome.

Recent research on the surgical treatment of Achilles tendon ruptures has focused on the use of minimally invasive repair techniques and early mobilization. Historically, minimally invasive and percutaneous techniques have been criticized as leading to relatively high rates of rerupture and sural nerve injury.[30-32] A retrospective study evaluated the use of immediate weight bearing in 52 patients.[30] After surgery using a modified percutaneous approach, the limb was placed in a cast, and immediate weight bearing was allowed. A boot with a heel lift was substituted after 2 weeks, and exercises were started. At an average 28-month final follow-up, 47 patients (90%) were able to return to their desired level of activity, and the average AOFAS score was 90. Four patients had sural neuritis, which resolved within 6 months. No reruptures were observed. A study of 15 elite athletes found that all were able to return to their sport after a minimally invasive repair.[32] Thirteen patients had no pain but did have a subjective perception of reduction in calf strength, two had wound-healing difficulty, and none had sural nerve injuries. The study

concluded that percutaneous repair is safe and effective for treating Achilles tendon rupture in elite athletes. In a randomized prospective study comparing open repair with the use of a commercially available percutaneous repair device, all 40 patients regained Achilles tendon function.[31] No between-group difference was found in maximal calf circumference, ankle dorsiflexion, or the ability to perform heel rises. The complication rate was 5% in the patients treated with a percutaneous repair and 35% in those treated with an open repair. No reruptures or sural nerve injuries were found in either group of patients. There were fewer incidences of local tenderness, skin adhesion, and tendon thickening in the patients who received a percutaneous repair.

Early motion was evaluated after open repair in a retrospective study of 107 patients, 96 (90%) of whom received no immobilization and started exercise 3 to 5 days after surgery.[33] Patients were able to resume heavy labor and sports activity an average 13 weeks after surgery. No rerupture, gap formation, or tendon elongation was noted. The study concluded that early motion may facilitate the proliferation, transportation, and alignment of tendon cells, thereby leading to an improvement in the overall reconstruction of the tendon.

Chronic Achilles Tendon Ruptures

An estimated 10% to 25% of Achilles tendon ruptures are neglected or not immediately identified.[34] The patient risk factors for delayed diagnosis include age older than 55 years, a high body mass index, and injury unrelated to sports activity.[23] Although there is no clear demarcation between acute and chronic rupture, a rupture estimated to have been present for 4 to 6 weeks is likely to have characteristics consistent with chronic rupture. Chronic rupture is more challenging to treat than acute rupture because of the presence of a gap between the tendon ends, retraction and scarring of the calf muscle, and loss of muscle contractility.

The patient may have vague symptoms that are not specific to the Achilles tendon region. There may be a sense of weakness or unsteadiness in gait, rather than pain. Difficulty in stair climbing and walking uphill is common. Loss of tendon contour is seen on examination. Some patients have sufficient reparative tissue to make palpation of a gap difficult. The Thompson test usually is positive but is less reliable than with acute rupture. The Matles test also usually is positive. Most patients are unable to perform a single-leg heel rise.

Retraction and scarring of tendon ends mean that nonsurgical restoration of the physiologic tension of the gastrocnemius-soleus complex is difficult. The use of an ankle-foot orthosis should be considered for a patient who is a poor surgical candidate because of significant comorbidities. A patient with minimal functional deficits also may benefit from nonsurgical treatment. The benefit of physical therapy is in recruiting other muscle groups to compensate for the loss of Achilles tendon function.

Surgical treatment of a chronic rupture involves the restoration of continuity to tendon ends that have retracted and created irreducible gaps. The available surgical techniques include tendon mobilization, turndown flaps, tendon advancement, tendon transfer, free-tissue transfer, and synthetic graft.[34] A 2- to 3-cm gap can be effectively treated using tendon mobilization and stretching of the proximal musculature, followed by end-to-end repair. The use of turndown flaps involves freeing a strip of tendon from the proximal tendon stump and weaving it through the distal and proximal tendon ends. In a recent study, significant histopathologic changes were found in three biopsy specimens taken from the site of Achilles tendon rupture and locations within the tendon proximal and distal to the rupture.[35] This finding may have implications for the use of turndown flaps. A V-Y tendon advancement can be used for gaps of less than 5 cm, and tendon transfers can be used for gaps of less than 6 cm. Two years after transfer of the peroneus brevis tendon through a limited approach, all 32 patients had returned to work and leisure activities.[36] Six were rated as having an excellent outcome, and 24 had a good outcome. Loss of eversion strength was found objectively on examination but was not subjectively reported by patients. The FHL tendon transfer has several reported advantages including limited donor morbidity, greater strength than a peroneus brevis transfer, an axis of pull similar to that of the Achilles tendon, and improved vascularity of reconstruction with presence of the low-lying muscle belly[22] (Figure 5). The use of a free-tissue transfer such a semitendinosus graft has had good results for the treatment of tendon gaps larger than 6 cm.[37] A recent study reported excellent results in 62 of 72 patients with a chronic rupture at the insertion of the Achilles tendon when the gastrocnemius aponeurosis was used to reconstruct the insertion.[38] Most studies of synthetic grafts have been small and comparative evaluation therefore is difficult. Although surgical treatment of chronic ruptures has led to improved outcomes, patients continue to have strength deficits in comparison with the contralateral limb. A variety of techniques have been studied, but the small numbers of patients, combined with variations in patient selection, gap measurements, postoperative regimens, and outcome measurements, create difficulty in comparing data and making firm recommendations.

Achilles Tendinopathy

Achilles tendinopathy is described as insertional or noninsertional. Noninsertional tendinopathy is further

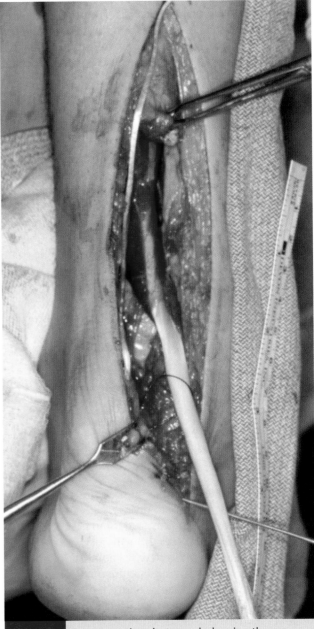

Figure 5 Intraoperative photograph showing the use of a harvested FHL tendon to treat a chronic Achilles tendon rupture.

classified as peritendinitis, peritendinitis with tendinosis, or tendinosis. Tendinosis is a chronic, noninflammatory, degenerative process of the tendon that is associated with decreased vascularity, repetitive microtrauma, and aging. The associated etiologic factors can include diabetes, hypertension, steroid use, obesity, and estrogen exposure. Patients range from relatively young and active patients with peritendinitis caused by overuse to patients older than 50 years with tendinosis combined with peritendinitis of varying severity. Patients with peritendinitis have diffuse swelling and tenderness along the course of the tendon. Patients with tendinosis typically have pain and swelling along a nodular area within the tendon. Tenderness to palpation often is present along the area of tendon thickening. The patient may have difficulty performing a single-leg heel rise. MRI and ultrasound can be useful for defining the location and extent of disease.

Nonsurgical management is effective in 70% to 75% of patients.[39,40] Modalities including rest, NSAIDs, activity modification, and eccentric strengthening frequently are used. Immobilization in a short leg cast or boot may be beneficial if the condition is recalcitrant. Injectable therapies are gaining popularity for treating Achilles tendinosis, using agents such as platelet-rich plasma, autologous blood, sclerosing agents, protease inhibitors, hemodialysate, corticosteroids, and prolotherapy. A recent systematic review of nine randomized controlled studies involving the use of injectable therapies found only one study meeting the quality criteria.[40] Most patients treated with an injectable therapy were found to have mild to moderate clinical benefit, but patients in placebo and control groups had similar improvements. The effectiveness of extracorporeal shock wave therapy (ESWT) was evaluated in a systematic meta-analysis of four randomized controlled studies and two pre-post studies.[41] The studies were inconsistent in participant characteristics as well as dosages and impulses per session. Four studies found statistically significant improvement in functional outcomes, and the meta-analysis concluded that the evidence was satisfactory to show the effectiveness of ESWT for treating chronic Achilles tendinopathy.

Surgical treatment may be indicated for refractory Achilles tendinosis after 6 months of unsuccessful nonsurgical treatment. The traditional surgical treatment consists of removing diseased portions of the tendon. Augmentation with FHL tendon transfer may be needed if more than 50% of the tendon is removed. A prospective study of 56 patients who had FHL transfer for insertional or noninsertional Achilles tendinopathy found significant improvement in functional outcome scores at 24-month follow-up, and 32 patients (57%) had no hallux weakness.[42] Most of the patients in this study were described as sedentary. The study authors expressed concern that relatively young, active patients might notice functional deficits associated with great toe weakness.

Minimally invasive paratenon release also has been suggested for treating Achilles tendinopathy. In a retrospective case study of 26 patients, percutaneous release of adhesions between the paratenon and tendon was followed by instillation of methylprednisolone and bupivacaine into the paratenon.[43] At an average 13-month follow-up, 73% of tendons were pain free or had significant improvement in pain. The study authors suggested that the release of adhesions in this procedure disrupts the neovascularization process and allows tendon healing. A retrospective review of the outcomes of 39 runners found that 30 runners (77%) reported a good or excellent outcome an average 17 years after ultrasound-guided multiple percutaneous tenotomies for Achilles tendinosis.[44] Two studies of the results of isolated gastrocnemius lengthening for Achilles tendinopathy found clinical improvement in all patients without loss of plantar flexion strength.[45,46] Comparison with other studies is difficult, however, because of the limited characterization of the extent of tendon involvement.

Insertional Achilles tendinopathy ranges from peritendinitis to tendinosis. Isolated peritendinitis tends to occur in relatively young and athletic individuals and can be caused by overuse, hill running, an interval training program, or a training error. Insertional tendinosis is more common in individuals older than 50 years with varying levels of activity. Patients often have concomitant symptoms from retrocalcaneal bursitis and Haglund deformity. Inflammatory arthropathies may contribute to the etiology and especially should be considered in a younger patient with bilateral symptoms. The initial symptoms usually are morning stiffness, posterior heel pain, and swelling with activity, progressing to constant pain. Often the patient has swelling along the posterior heel. Active and passive limitation of dorsiflexion may be present. The location of the tenderness can help distinguish among retrocalcaneal bursitis, Haglund deformity, and insertional tendinosis; all three sometimes are present. Radiographs may show calcification within the insertion of the tendon. Traditionally, a Haglund deformity was considered to be most common in patients with insertional tendinopathy, but a recent retrospective radiographic study challenged this belief.[47] No significant difference was found in the radiographic parameters of Haglund deformity between patients with or without insertional Achilles tendinosis. Calcification of the tendon insertion was present in 73% of patients.

The initial treatment, often including rest, NSAIDs, and activity modification, is effective in most patients.[39] Eccentric exercises are less effective for treating insertional tendinopathy than noninsertional tendinopathy.[41] A randomized controlled study found a 28% improvement in patients treated with eccentric exercise, compared with a 64% improvement in those treated with ESWT.[48] A prospective study of 103 patients treated using an ankle-foot orthosis and a home stretching program found improvement in 91 patients (88%). The average duration of treatment was 163 days.[49]

Surgical treatment may be indicated if symptoms are not relieved after 6 to 12 months of nonsurgical management. Surgical treatment is directed toward the

7: Tendon Disorders and Sports-Related Foot and Ankle Injuries

underlying pathologic changes. The techniques include débridement of the Achilles tendon insertion, débridement of the retrocalcaneal bursa, and posterosuperior calcaneal ostectomy. Several approaches have been described including medial, lateral, combined medial and lateral, endoscopic, J-shaped, transverse, and central tendon splitting; few data suggest the superiority of one approach over another. As much as 50% of the Achilles tendon insertion can be detached without significantly increasing the risk of rupture. With additional exposure, suture anchors may be needed to secure the tendon. Patients with significant degenerative changes of the tendon may require extensive débridement and augmentation with FHL tendon transfer (**Figure 6**). After extensive débridement, 6 to 12 months often is required for recovery. The lack of a standardized method for assessing the severity of the condition makes it difficult to compare studies and provide firm recommendations.

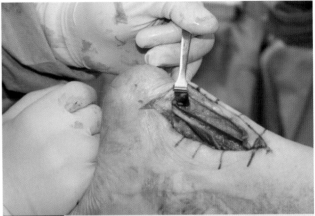

Figure 6 Intraoperative photograph showing the use of a harvested FHL tendon to augment the Achilles tendon after extensive débridement.

Summary

Acute and chronic injuries of the anterior tibial, peroneal, and Achilles tendons can cause significant pain and disability. Physical examination usually allows an accurate diagnosis, but MRI may be helpful if the diagnosis is questionable. Many of these tendon injuries can be successfully treated without surgery, especially in patients with low physical demands. If surgical treatment is required, an open, minimally invasive, or endoscopic procedure can be chosen, depending on the type and severity of the injury. A return to occupational and recreational activities is possible for most patients within 3 to 6 months of surgical treatment.

Annotated References

1. Khoury NJ, el-Khoury GY, Saltzman CL, Brandser EA: Rupture of the anterior tibial tendon: Diagnosis by MR imaging. *AJR Am J Roentgenol* 1996;167(2):351-354.

2. Tucker S, Sammarco GJ, Sammarco VJ: Surgical repair of tibialis anterior tendon rupture. *Tech Foot & Ankle* 2012;11:39-44.

   A technique for repairing anterior tibial tendon ruptures was described, in which end-to-end repair and repair with interpositional graft were used.

3. Ouzounian TJ, Anderson R: Anterior tibial tendon rupture. *Foot Ankle Int* 1995;16(7):406-410.

4. Geppert MJ, Sobel M, Hannafin JA: Microvasculature of the tibialis anterior tendon. *Foot Ankle* 1993;14(5):261-264.

5. Markarian GG, Kelikian AS, Brage M, Trainor T, Dias L: Anterior tibialis tendon ruptures: An outcome analysis of operative versus nonoperative treatment. *Foot Ankle Int* 1998;19(12):792-802.

6. Sammarco VJ, Sammarco GJ, Henning C, Chaim S: Surgical repair of acute and chronic tibialis anterior tendon ruptures. *J Bone Joint Surg Am* 2009;91(2):325-332.

   In a retrospective study of 18 patients treated surgically for rupture of the anterior tibial tendon, patients who underwent early or late repair both had significant improvement. Fifteen patients had normal dorsiflexion strength with manual testing. Level of evidence: IV.

7. Ellington JK, McCormick J, Marion C, et al: Surgical outcome following tibialis anterior tendon repair. *Foot Ankle Int* 2010;31(5):412-417.

   In a retrospective case study of 14 patients who were treated surgically, 5 tendons were repaired primarily and 10 received a tendon transfer. Using a dynamometer, dorsiflexion strength was found to be weaker than in the contralateral limb. Level of evidence: IV.

8. Bare A, Ferkel RD: Peroneal tendon tears: Associated arthroscopic findings and results after repair. *Arthroscopy* 2009;25(11):1288-1297.

   All 30 patients who underwent arthroscopic evaluation of the ankle at the time of peroneal tendon repair had at least one intra-articular lesion, and 80% had extensive scar tissue. Level of evidence: IV.

9. Vega J, Batista JP, Golanó P, Dalmau A, Viladot R: Tendoscopic groove deepening for chronic subluxation of the peroneal tendons. *Foot Ankle Int* 2013;34(6):832-840.

   Seven patients with recurrent subluxation of the peroneal tendon underwent a tendoscopic groove deepening. At an average 15.4-month follow-up, none of the patients had recurrent subluxation, and five reported an excellent outcome. Level of evidence: IV.

10. Krause JO, Brodsky JW: Peroneus brevis tendon tears: Pathophysiology, surgical reconstruction, and clinical results. *Foot Ankle Int* 1998;19(5):271-279.

11. Crates J, Barber FA: Treatment of longitudinal mid-substance tears of peroneal tendons. *Curr Orthop Pract* 2012;23(2):86-90.

    The diagnosis and treatment of longitudinal tears of the peroneal tendons were reviewed.

12. O'Neill PJ, Van Aman SE, Guyton GP: Is MRI adequate to detect lesions in patients with ankle instability? *Clin Orthop Relat Res* 2010;468(4):1115-1119.

    All 133 patients had MRI before 135 surgeries for ankle instability. The radiologist detected only 56% of peroneus brevis tears seen intraoperatively. Level of evidence: IV.

13. Park HJ, Cha SD, Kim HS, et al: Reliability of MRI findings of peroneal tendinopathy in patients with lateral chronic ankle instability. *Clin Orthop Surg* 2010;2(4):237-243.

    The positive predictive value of MRI for peroneal tendinopathy was 66.7%, and the negative predictive value was 88.4%. Overreliance on MRI should be avoided because it may lead to unnecessary surgery.

14. Philbin TM, Landis GS, Smith B: Peroneal tendon injuries. *J Am Acad Orthop Surg* 2009;17(5):306-317.

    A review article outlined the diagnosis and treatment of peroneal tendon injuries.

15. Grear B, Richardson D: Morphology of the malleolar fibular groove: Implications in peroneal tendon pathology. *Curr Orthop Pract* 2012;23(2):91-93.

    Lateral malleolar anatomy was reviewed in relation to peroneal tendon pathology. Only limited evidence supported the assumption that the morphology of the fibular groove plays a role in peroneal tendon pathology.

16. Athavale SA, Swathi, Vangara SV: Anatomy of the superior peroneal tunnel. *J Bone Joint Surg Am* 2011;93(6):564-571.

    A study of 58 cadaver specimens found the floor of the peroneal tunnel to have a lateral retromalleolar groove and a medial portion formed by distal part of the posterior intermuscular septum of the leg. Both components were believed to stabilize the peroneal tendons.

17. Adachi N, Fukuhara K, Kobayashi T, Nakasa T, Ochi M: Morphologic variations of the fibular malleolar groove with recurrent dislocation of the peroneal tendons. *Foot Ankle Int* 2009;30(6):540-544.

    An MRI review of 39 ankles was performed after surgical treatment of peroneal tendon dislocation. MRI of 39 ankles without peroneal tendon dislocation was used as a control group. No significant between-group difference in retromalleolar groove morphology was noted. Level of evidence: III.

18. Unlu MC, Bilgili M, Akgun I, Kaynak G, Ogut T, Uzun I: Abnormal proximal musculotendinous junction of the peroneus brevis muscle as a cause of peroneus brevis tendon tears: A cadaveric study. *J Foot Ankle Surg* 2010;49(6):537-540.

    A study of 115 cadaver ankles found that the peroneus brevis musculotendinous junction was more proximal than the tip of the lateral malleolus in specimens with peroneus brevis tears. The retromalleolar groove was shallower in this group.

19. Redfern D, Myerson M: The management of concomitant tears of the peroneus longus and brevis tendons. *Foot Ankle Int* 2004;25(10):695-707.

20. Wapner KL, Taras JS, Lin SS, Chao W: Staged reconstruction for chronic rupture of both peroneal tendons using Hunter rod and flexor hallucis longus tendon transfer: A long-term followup study. *Foot Ankle Int* 2006;27(8):591-597.

21. Jockel JR, Brodsky JW: Single-stage flexor tendon transfer for the treatment of severe concomitant peroneus longus and brevis tendon tears. *Foot Ankle Int* 2013;34(5):666-672.

    Seven of eight patients treated with a single-stage FHL or FDL tendon transfer for tears of both peroneal tendons had an excellent outcome. The FHL transfer provided greater strength and better outcomes. Level of evidence: IV.

22. Jeng CL, Thawait GK, Kwon JY, et al: Relative strengths of the calf muscles based on MRI volume measurements. *Foot Ankle Int* 2012;33(5):394-399.

    MRI was used to perform volume measurements of all calf muscles in 10 normal men. The peroneus longus and peroneus brevis were equal in strength, and the FHL was stronger than either.

23. Raikin SM, Garras DN, Krapchev PV: Achilles tendon injuries in a United States population. *Foot Ankle Int* 2013;34(4):475-480.

    A retrospective study of 331 patients treated for Achilles tendon rupture over a 10-year period found that a delayed diagnosis was most likely in patients older than 55 years, patients with a non–sports-related injury, and patients with a high body mass index. Sixty-eight percent of patients had a sports-related injury.

24. Gwynne-Jones DP, Sims M, Handcock D: Epidemiology and outcomes of acute Achilles tendon rupture with operative or nonoperative treatment using an identical functional bracing protocol. *Foot Ankle Int* 2011;32(4):337-343.

    In a study of 363 consecutive patients treated for acute Achilles rupture from 1999 to 2008, patients with high physical demands and those who sought treatment more than 24 hours after injury were treated surgically. The rerupture rate was 1.4% in patients who were surgically treated and 8.6% in those who were nonsurgically treated. Level of evidence: III.

7: Tendon Disorders and Sports-Related Foot and Ankle Injuries

25. Wallace RG, Heyes GJ, Michael AL: The non-operative functional management of patients with a rupture of the tendo Achillis leads to low rates of re-rupture. *J Bone Joint Surg Br* 2011;93(10):1362-1366.

   Of 945 patients treated with 4 weeks of equinus casting followed by 4 weeks in a walker boot, 2.8% had a rerupture, and 939 had a subjective good to excellent result. All patients returned to their preinjury level of sports activity.

26. Keating JF, Will EM: Operative versus non-operative treatment of acute rupture of tendo Achillis: A prospective randomised evaluation of functional outcome. *J Bone Joint Surg Br* 2011;93(8):1071-1078.

   A study of 80 patients found no significant difference in peak torque or total work after surgical or nonsurgical treatment. Cast immobilization was used for 6 weeks after surgery and for 10 weeks in nonsurgical treatment. The difference in rerupture rates (5.4% in patients who were surgically treated and 10.3% in those who were nonsurgically treated) was not statistically significant.

27. Nilsson-Helander K, Silbernagel KG, Thomeé R, et al: Acute Achilles tendon rupture: A randomized, controlled study comparing surgical and nonsurgical treatments using validated outcome measures. *Am J Sports Med* 2010;38(11):2186-2193.

   In 97 patients randomly assigned to surgical or nonsurgical treatment, treatment was initiated within 72 hours of injury. No functional difference was noted after treatment. Early mobilization of Achilles tendon rupture was found to be beneficial. The optimal treatment (surgical or nonsurgical) remains under debate. Level of evidence: I.

28. Willits K, Amendola A, Bryant D, et al: Operative versus nonoperative treatment of acute Achilles tendon ruptures: A multicenter randomized trial using accelerated functional rehabilitation. *J Bone Joint Surg Am* 2010;92(17):2767-2775.

   A randomized prospective study of 144 patients treated surgically or nonsurgically for acute Achilles rupture, with accelerated functional rehabilitation, found no significant between-group difference in range of motion, strength, or rerupture rate. Level of evidence: I.

29. Soroceanu A, Sidhwa F, Aarabi S, Kaufman A, Glazebrook M: Surgical versus nonsurgical treatment of acute Achilles tendon rupture: A meta-analysis of randomized trials. *J Bone Joint Surg Am* 2012;94(23):2136-2143.

   The risk of rerupture was equivalent after surgical or nonsurgical treatment of acute Achilles tendon rupture if early motion was used during nonsurgical treatment. If early motion was not used, the risk reduction with surgery was 8.8%. No significant difference in functional outcome was noted. Level of evidence: I.

30. Patel VC, Lozano-Calderon S, McWilliam J: Immediate weight bearing after modified percutaneous Achilles tendon repair. *Foot Ankle Int* 2012;33(12):1093-1097.

   In a study of 52 patients with an Achilles tendon rupture treated less than 14 days after injury, repair was followed by casting and weight bearing to tolerance. No reruptures occurred, and 90% were able to return to the desired level of activity. Level of evidence: IV.

31. Aktas S, Kocaoglu B: Open versus minimal invasive repair with Achillon device. *Foot Ankle Int* 2009;30(5):391-397.

   A prospective study of 40 patients randomly assigned to open repair or mini-open repair with the Achillon device (Integra Life Sciences) found no between-group functional difference. Those treated with the Achillon device had fewer complications (5%) than those treated with an open repair (35%). Level of evidence: I.

32. Maffulli N, Longo UG, Maffulli GD, Khanna A, Denaro V: Achilles tendon ruptures in elite athletes. *Foot Ankle Int* 2011;32(1):9-15.

   A retrospective review of percutaneous repair of acute Achilles tendon rupture in 17 elite athletes found that all patients were able to return to their preinjury sport, and that 13 of 15 patients had no pain around the Achilles tendon at final follow-up. Level of evidence: IV.

33. Jielile J, Sabirhazi G, Chen J, et al: Novel surgical technique and early kinesiotherapy for acute Achilles tendon rupture. *Foot Ankle Int* 2012;33(12):1119-1127.

   A retrospective study of Achilles tendon rupture in 107 patients treated with an open repair technique found no reruptures, gap formation, or tendon elongation at 60-day follow-up. Most patients did not have postoperative splinting. Level of evidence: IV.

34. Padanilam TG: Chronic Achilles tendon ruptures. *Foot Ankle Clin* 2009;14(4):711-728.

   A review article outlined the diagnosis and treatment of chronic Achilles tendon ruptures.

35. Maffulli N, Longo UG, Maffulli GD, Rabitti C, Khanna A, Denaro V: Marked pathological changes proximal and distal to the site of rupture in acute Achilles tendon ruptures. *Knee Surg Sports Traumatol Arthrosc* 2011;19(4):680-687.

   During repair of an acute Achilles tendon rupture, biopsy samples were taken from the rupture site as well as sites proximal and distal to the rupture in 29 consecutive patients. Significant histopathologic changes were found at all three sites.

36. Maffulli N, Spiezia F, Longo UG, Denaro V: Less-invasive reconstruction of chronic Achilles tendon ruptures using a peroneus brevis tendon transfer. *Am J Sports Med* 2010;38(11):2304-2312.

   After peroneus brevis transfer was used to treat chronic Achilles tendon rupture with a gap smaller than 6 cm, all 38 patients returned to preinjury work and leisure activities. There was objective loss of eversion strength but no subjective loss. Level of evidence: IV.

37. Sarzaeem MM, Lemraski MM, Safdari F: Chronic Achilles tendon rupture reconstruction using a free semitendinosus tendon graft transfer. *Knee Surg Sports Traumatol Arthrosc* 2012;20(7):1386-1391.

Free semitendinosus graft was used to treat chronic Achilles tendon rupture with a gap larger than 6 cm. The 11 patients had a good result. Level of evidence: IV.

38. Pavan Kumar A, Shashikiran R, Raghuram C: A novel modification of Bosworth's technique to repair zone I Achilles tendon ruptures. *J Orthop Traumatol* 2013;14(1):59-65.

After chronic Achilles tendon rupture was treated using the gastrocnemius aponeurosis to reconstruct the insertion, 62 of 78 patients had an excellent result. The rupture was at the insertion in 72 patients, and 44 patients had a steroid injection before rupture.

39. Paavola M, Kannus P, Paakkala T, Pasanen M, Järvinen M: Long-term prognosis of patients with Achilles tendinopathy: An observational 8-year follow-up study. *Am J Sports Med* 2000;28(5):634-642.

40. Gross CE, Hsu AR, Chahal J, Holmes GB Jr: Injectable treatments for noninsertional Achilles tendinosis: A systematic review. *Foot Ankle Int* 2013;34(5):619-628.

Most patients treated with injectable therapies for Achilles tendinosis had a mild to moderate clinical benefit, but similar improvements also occurred in patients in the placebo and control groups. Level of evidence: II.

41. Al-Abbad H, Simon JV: The effectiveness of extracorporeal shock therapy on chronic Achilles tendinopathy: A systematic review. *Foot Ankle Int* 2013;34(1):33-41.

A meta-analysis found overall satisfactory evidence for the effectiveness of ESWT for improving pain and function in chronic Achilles tendinopathies. Level of evidence: I.

42. Schon LC, Shores JL, Faro FD, Vora AM, Camire LM, Guyton GP: Flexor hallucis longus tendon transfer in treatment of Achilles tendinosis. *J Bone Joint Surg Am* 2013;95(1):54-60.

A prospective study of 56 patients with insertional or midsubstance Achilles tendinosis found significant improvement in functional scores after treatment with FHL tendon transfer. At 24-month follow-up, 57% did not have hallux weakness and 76% did not have lack of balance caused by hallux weakness.

43. Naidu V, Abbassian A, Nielsen D, Uppalapati R, Shetty A: Minimally invasive paratenon release for non-insertional Achilles tendinopathy. *Foot Ankle Int* 2009;30(7):680-685.

Twenty-six patients underwent treatment of noninsertional Achilles tendinopathy with surgical instillation of methylprednisolone and bupivacaine in the paratenon. At average 13-month follow-up, 73% of tendons were pain free or had significant improvement. Level of evidence: IV.

44. Maffulli N, Oliva F, Testa V, Capasso G, Del Buono A: Multiple percutaneous longitudinal tenotomies for chronic Achilles tendinopathy in runners: A long-term study. *Am J Sports Med* 2013;41(9):2151-2157.

Thirty-nine runners were reviewed at an average 17-year follow-up after percutaneous ultrasound-guided multiple tenotomies for Achilles tendinopathy, and 77% reported a good to excellent result. Twenty were active runners with an average level of sport and function at 60% of baseline status.

45. Kiewiet NJ, Holthusen SM, Bohay DR, Anderson JG: Gastrocnemius recession for chronic noninsertional Achilles tendinopathy. *Foot Ankle Int* 2013;34(4):481-485.

Twelve patients underwent isolated gastrocnemius recession for noninsertional Achilles tendinopathy. The seven patients seen at follow-up had no significant difference in calf strength or circumference compared with the nonsurgical side. All seven expressed satisfaction.

46. Duthon VB, Lübbeke A, Duc SR, Stern R, Assal M: Noninsertional Achilles tendinopathy treated with gastrocnemius lengthening. *Foot Ankle Int* 2011;32(4):375-379.

In a prospective case study, localized Achilles tendinopathy of at least 1 year's duration was treated with gastrocnemius lengthening in 14 patients. All clinical scores were improved after surgery. Plantar flexion strength was equal to that of the contralateral limb. Level of evidence: IV.

47. Kang S, Thordarson DB, Charlton TP: Insertional Achilles tendinitis and Haglund's deformity. *Foot Ankle Int* 2012;33(6):487-491.

A retrospective study of insertional Achilles tendinitis in 44 patients compared their radiographic measurements with those of patients in a control group. There was no between-group difference in measurement parameters for Haglund deformity. Level of evidence: III.

48. Rompe JD, Furia J, Maffulli N: Eccentric loading compared with shock wave treatment for chronic insertional Achilles tendinopathy: A randomized, controlled trial. *J Bone Joint Surg Am* 2008;90(1):52-61.

Fifty patients with Achilles tendinopathy were randomly allocated to receive either eccenteric loading exercises or repetitive low-energy shock wave therapy. All patients had received some treatment for 3 months prior to the study. Patients who underwent shock wave therapy showed significantly greater favorable results.

49. Johnson MD, Alvarez RG: Nonoperative management of retrocalcaneal pain with AFO and stretching regimen. *Foot Ankle Int* 2012;33(7):571-581.

The authors present a retrospective review of 103 patients treated for posterior heel pain with an AFO brace and a stretching program. Ninety-one patients (88%) had sufficient pain relief to avoid surgical treatment.

7: Tendon Disorders and Sports-Related Foot and Ankle Injuries

Chapter 29

Sports-Related Injuries of the Foot and Ankle

Mark J. Berkowitz, MD

Introduction

Acute traumatic injuries and cumulative stress injuries involving the foot and ankle can affect the sports participation and performance of both elite competitive athletes and people engaged in recreational or fitness activities. A thorough understanding of common injuries of the foot and ankle allows a logical and organized approach to treating these injuries and facilitates the patient's return to play.

Ankle Anatomy

The stability of the ankle is the result of a combination of anatomic factors having osseous, ligamentous, and musculotendinous components. The ankle generally is described as a mortise in which the talus is housed in the dome-shaped tibial plafond and the medial, lateral, and posterior malleoli. The talus is wider anteriorly than posteriorly, so that the ankle intrinsically is most stable in the dorsiflexed position when the wider portion of the talus is engaged in the mortise. Conversely, in the plantarflexed position, the narrower posterior talus is engaged in the mortise, and the ankle therefore is more unstable. It is in the plantarflexed position that the stability of the ankle most depends on the lateral ligament complex. Not surprisingly, most acute inversion sprains occur when the ankle is somewhat plantarflexed.

The lateral ankle ligament complex primarily is composed of the anterior talofibular ligament (ATFL) and the calcaneofibular ligament (CFL). The ATFL is the primary ligamentous stabilizer of the ankle; it prevents anterior translation of the plantarflexed ankle. The ATFL is the structure most commonly injured in an acute ankle sprain. The CFL is a collateral ligament that stabilizes both the ankle and the subtalar joint. In relatively severe inversion sprains, the CFL is injured with the ATFL.

The peroneal musculotendinous unit is an important contributor to ankle stability. The peroneal tendons rapidly contract to resist and prevent excessive inversion stress. The peroneal complex also provides important proprioceptive feedback that enables an athlete to instinctively sense and control the position of the foot and ankle in space.

Acute Lateral Ankle Ligament Injuries

Acute lateral ankle sprain is one of the most common injuries sustained during sports activity. An epidemiologic study of ankle sprains reported that more than three million sprains occurred during the 4-year study period and that more than half of these injuries occurred during athletic activity.[1] Acute ankle sprain was most common in individuals age 10 to 19 years. Boys and men age 15 to 24 years sustained more ankle sprains than girls and women in the same age range, but women older than 30 years sustained more sprains than their male counterparts.

An acute ankle sprain causes a variable amount of mechanical injury to the lateral ligament complex of the ankle. Such an injury can lead to lingering symptoms such as instability and pain, which can impede or preclude return to play. Proper initial management minimizes the risk of long-term morbidity and speeds the resumption of athletic participation.

Patient History and Physical Examination

Successful treatment of an acute ankle sprain begins with a careful history and meticulous physical examination. Important components of the history include the time since injury and whether the patient can tolerate weight bearing, believes the injury is improving, or had an earlier sprain of the same ankle. The physical examination should document the location and severity of swelling and ecchymosis. Probably the most important component of the physical examination is assessing the location of tenderness to palpation. After an acute lateral ankle ligament injury, swelling, ecchymosis, and tenderness usually are noted over the ATFL and CFL in the region just anterior and distal to the tip of the fibula. However, tenderness should be checked over several different structures to look for signs that could implicate an alternative or associated diagnosis. Laterally, the distal tibiofibular syndesmosis, lateral malleolus, peroneal tendons, fifth metatarsal, anterior process of the calcaneus, and lateral process of the talus should be palpated in addition to the lateral ligament complex. Medially, the medial malleolus, deltoid ligament, sustentaculum tali, and navicular should be examined and assessed for tenderness. Routine palpation of the Achilles tendon, tibialis anterior tendon, and midfoot articulations should be included; injury to these structures sometimes is neglected when a diagnosis of ankle sprain is presumed. These physical examination findings can be obscured by diffuse swelling and poorly localized tenderness during the first 10 to 14 days after an acute ankle inversion injury. Often it is important to repeat the examination 10 to 14 days later, when the findings will be more specific and revealing.

Instability tests such as the anterior drawer and talar tilt tests generally do not have a significant role in the evaluation of an acute ankle sprain. With an acute injury, the ankle often is too swollen and uncomfortable to allow an unguarded and accurate assessment of stability. The results of these tests generally do not affect the initial treatment of an acute sprain, and they should be reserved for evaluating chronic ankle instability.

Radiographic Evaluation

Appropriate radiographic studies are helpful for avoiding a misdiagnosis and facilitating a prompt diagnosis of associated injuries. In the emergency department, the Ottawa ankle rules provide guidance as to whether radiographs are necessary or can be deferred. Ankle radiographs are indicated if the presence of a fracture is suggested by tenderness along the distal 6 cm of the posterior edge of the fibula or the tip of the lateral malleolus, tenderness along the distal 6 cm of the posterior edge of the tibia or the tip of the medial malleolus, or inability to tolerate weight bearing for at least four steps. In the absence of these findings, the diagnosis usually is an acute sprain, and radiographs are unnecessary. Adherence to these guidelines reduces the patient's cost, time in the emergency department, and exposure to radiation.

The Ottawa ankle rules were designed for implementation and use in the emergency department. However, many patients who sustain an acute lateral ankle ligament injury are evaluated by an orthopaedic surgeon in an outpatient clinical office several days to a few weeks after injury. In this more specialized environment, the threshold for radiographic evaluation is lower because the definitive

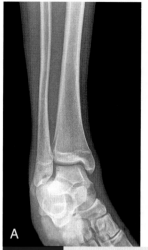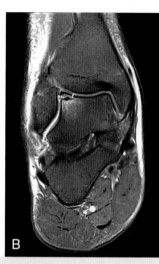

Figure 1   **A,** Mortise ankle radiograph in a patient with an acute ankle sprain. Lucency in the lateral talar dome suggests a fracture. **B,** MRI confirms that the patient has an acute unstable lateral talar osteochondral fracture.

diagnosis and treatment plan are based on the evaluation. An orthopaedic surgeon should obtain a weight-bearing series of foot and ankle radiographs for most patients with an acute lateral ankle sprain. Weight-bearing views provide substantially better imaging of relevant osseous structures than non–weight-bearing views and thereby minimize the possibility of missing an injury. Simulated weight-bearing views can be obtained at the initial evaluation if full weight bearing is too painful. Obtaining full weight-bearing views is deferred until symptoms improve. The AP and mortise ankle radiographs of the ankle should be evaluated for medial clear space and syndesmotic widening, malleolar fracture, lateral process of talus fracture, and talar osteochondral fracture (**Figure 1**). The lateral views of the ankle and foot reveal a dorsal talar avulsion fracture or the presence of an os trigonum. The AP foot view reveals a navicular fracture or Lisfranc injury, and the oblique foot view reveals an anterior process of the calcaneus fracture or a fifth metatarsal fracture. Radiographic and physical examination findings always must be correlated to provide an accurate and complete diagnosis.

CT and MRI have limited indications in the evaluation of an acute ankle sprain. CT is used to detect an associated fracture suspected on the basis of plain radiographs; these include fracture of the lateral process of the talus and the anterior process of calcaneus, posterior talar fracture, and osteochondral fracture. CT provides an accurate assessment of fracture size, displacement, and comminution that ultimately can guide treatment. MRI rarely is indicated to evaluate an acute ankle sprain and should be obtained only if suspicion is high for an osteochondral lesion of the talus or an associated soft-tissue injury such as an Achilles tendon rupture or peroneal tendon dislocation. MRI is useful for distinguishing a preexisting chronic osteochondral lesion from an acute osteochondral fracture. MRI was found to be superior to physical examination for the detection of syndesmotic injuries.[2]

Classification and Treatment

Acute lateral ankle sprains are graded based on the involved ligaments and the severity of the structural injury to the lateral ligament complex. A grade I acute sprain is a minor injury to the ATFL characterized by microscopic tears in the ligament fibers without gross structural damage. In a grade II sprain, partial macroscopic structural damage has occurred without complete loss of integrity; a grade II sprain primarily affects the ATFL, but the CFL may be involved to a lesser extent. A grade III sprain involves complete rupture of the lateral ligament complex, with loss of integrity of both the ATFL and the CFL.

The severity of a lateral ankle sprain affects both its treatment and prognosis. Patients with a grade I or II sprain typically do not require crutches and are able to perform activities of daily living with minimal discomfort. A grade I or II sprain appears to recover best when an early rehabilitation regimen is implemented. In fact, a recent randomized controlled study demonstrated that grade I and II sprains achieve earlier recovery when an immediate functional range of motion protocol is initiated compared with early immobilization.[3] The timing of the patient's return to sports activity primarily is based on the level of discomfort and ability to perform necessary sport-specific activities. Generally, the patient can return to sports 2 to 6 weeks after a grade I or II ankle sprain, with the use of a protective brace and initiation of peroneal strengthening and proprioceptive exercises aimed at preventing reinjury.

Patients with a grade III injury often initially experience discomfort during ambulation and while performing activities of daily living. A period of immobilization and protected weight bearing often is beneficial. A prospective randomized study compared the efficacy of four different modes of immobilization (tubular compression sleeve, walking boot, stirrup brace, cast) for the initial treatment of an acute grade III ankle sprain.[4] Somewhat surprisingly, the results favored initial cast immobilization for a severe ankle sprain. Patients who had initial casting experienced the most rapid overall recovery, with less pain and an earlier return to activity. The use of a walking boot was found to confer no significant benefit over that of a tubular compression sleeve. However, the physician must weigh the early benefits of casting against the reality that cast immobilization often is poorly tolerated by the patient.

After the initial pain, swelling, and discomfort have resolved over 2 to 4 weeks, a patient with a grade III sprain receives a functional brace, and formal physical therapy is initiated to decrease swelling, improve range of motion, and restore strength to the ankle. With symptom improvement, the therapeutic exercises gradually advance to proprioceptive exercises and sport-specific functional drills. Plyometric drills should be incorporated into the rehabilitation program because they are superior to standard peroneal strengthening exercises for restoration of subjective ankle stability and resumption of athletic participation.[5] The return to sport after a grade III sprain typically requires 6 to 12 weeks of rehabilitation.

Although nonsurgical functional rehabilitation for a grade III ankle sprain remains the standard of care in North America, a body of evidence from Europe suggests that superior results are possible when an acute grade III sprain is surgically treated.[6,7] A meta-analysis of 27 studies revealed less giving way and overall better functional results when the initial treatment of grade III sprains was surgical rather than nonsurgical.[6] A subsequent prospective, randomized comparison of surgical treatment and functional rehabilitation in grade III ankle sprains found comparable functional results and fewer recurrent sprains in the patients treated surgically.[7] Additional high-quality studies are necessary before surgical treatment can supplant functional rehabilitation as the treatment of choice for grade III ankle sprains.

Chronic Lateral Ankle Ligament Injuries

With proper treatment, most patients who sustain an acute lateral ankle sprain successfully recover and return to their desired sports and preinjury level of activity. However, the outcome of a lateral ankle sprain, particularly a grade III injury, is not always favorable. A multiple database study of acute ankle sprains found that as many as 33% of patients still had pain 1 year after injury, and as many as 34% of patients sustained a recurrent sprain within a 3-year period after the initial injury.[8] The evaluation of a patient with chronic symptoms after ankle ligament injury must help identify the source of the lingering symptoms and initiate appropriate nonsurgical treatment. When necessary, surgical intervention is required to facilitate a return to sports.

Patient History

In general, the history and physical examination must be more thorough and meticulous for a patient with a chronic lateral ankle ligament injury than for a patient with an acute sprain. The history should elicit details of the initial injury, subsequent reinjury, and current symptoms. It is important to assess whether the patient's symptoms primarily involve instability, pain, or both. A detailed characterization of the instability and pain components of the patient's symptoms should be sought. The duration, frequency, and severity of instability episodes should be recorded and should include the number of sprains per month or year. The examiner should assess whether the recurrent sprains occur only during sports activities or also during activities of daily living. Patients with severe chronic instability may report frequent sprains with seemingly innocuous mechanisms such as stepping on a pebble, a curb, or a crack in a sidewalk. The examiner should record the extent of earlier treatment, including physical therapy, and to what extent bracing controls the instability.

The timing, severity, and location of the pain component should be assessed. The patient should be asked whether pain is present constantly or only after a sprain. Patients sometimes report surprisingly little pain after recurrent ankle sprains because of the overall laxity of the ligaments. Other patients report pain as the primary symptom and describe episodes in which pain precipitates the ankle's giving way. This type of pain should alert the examiner to the possibility that functional instability symptoms are the result of concomitant pathology. It is particularly important for the patient to identify the location of the pain as specifically as possible. Determining whether the pain primarily is medial, anterolateral, or retrofibular will suggest the most likely causes and guide the choice of imaging.

Physical Examination

The physical examination of a patient with symptoms of chronic instability must be equally meticulous. The goals are to characterize the severity of ligament laxity, identify sources of pain, and assess for anatomic factors that predispose the patient to instability or affect the response to treatment. Ankle ligament laxity is assessed using the anterior drawer and talar tilt maneuvers. The anterior drawer test is used to assess the integrity of the ATFL and is performed with the ankle in a resting equinus position. This position of relative plantar flexion orients the fibers of the ATFL in line with the examiner's pull. The examiner stabilizes the tibia above the ankle with one hand, wraps the other hand around the heel, and translates the foot and ankle anteriorly on the stationary tibia. The examiner can feel the extent of anterior translation and can see a dimpling of the skin over the ATFL if significant laxity is present. The talar tilt maneuver assesses the laxity of the CFL. It is important to perform this maneuver with the ankle in a relatively neutral position to orient the CFL vertically and allow it to be tested as a

true collateral ligament of the ankle. Failure to adequately dorsiflex the ankle during the talar tilt test can make it difficult to distinguish normal subtalar motion from true talar tilt. Again, the examiner secures the tibia with one hand, positions the ankle in neutral with the other hand, and exerts an inversion stress on the ankle and hindfoot. Placing a thumb beneath the fibula allows the examiner to feel the talus tilt within the ankle mortise. With both of these tests, it is crucial to examine the contralateral side as well as the general laxity of other joints. Hyperextension of knees, elbows, and fingers can point to the presence of general ligamentous laxity, which can predispose a patient to recurrent instability. The Beighton criteria for joint hypermobility are used in identifying patients with signs of generalized laxity, which can significantly affect the outcome of treatment.

The foot and ankle should be examined for strength, range of motion, tenderness, swelling, and gait, in addition to ligament laxity. The presence of claw toes or weak ankle dorsiflexion and eversion may suggest the presence of a neurologic condition such as Charcot-Marie-Tooth disease. Isolated peroneal weakness with painful resisted eversion often accompanies a peroneal tendon tear. Tenderness, swelling, popping, or frank subluxation of the peroneal tendons provides further evidence of a peroneal tendon injury. Decreased passive ankle dorsiflexion may result from the presence of distal tibial osteophytes or a gastrocnemius-soleus complex contracture. Limited passive subtalar inversion can be a clue to the presence of a tarsal coalition.

It is critical to assess for cavovarus deformity while the patient is standing and walking. The importance of early diagnosis of cavovarus deformity cannot be overstated because these patients are at substantially increased risk for ankle inversion injury, are more likely than other patients to experience chronic symptoms, and are less likely to have a successful outcome after standard nonsurgical or surgical treatment. When a patient with cavovarus alignment is examined from the front, a so-called peek-a-boo heel sign can be seen, in which the medial portion of the heel pad is visible (Figure 2). When examined from the back, the heel is seen to be in frank varus, with weight bearing concentrated on the lateral border of the foot. If a plantarflexed first ray can be seen while the patient is seated, the examiner should perform the Coleman block test. The patient is observed from behind while standing on a 1-inch block with the first ray allowed to hang off the edge of the block. Improvement in hindfoot varus during this test suggests that first ray plantar flexion is driving the hindfoot deformity and that correcting the first ray will produce concomitant correction of the hindfoot. If the hindfoot varus is not corrected or only

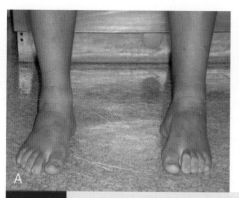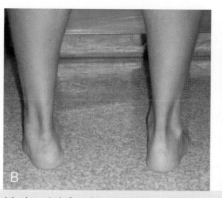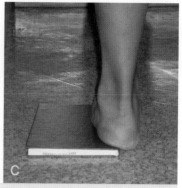

Figure 2 Clinical photographs of a patient with chronic left ankle instability and cavovarus. **A,** The so-called peek-a-boo heel sign. **B,** Hindfoot varus as seen from behind, with weight bearing on the outer border of the heel. **C,** Correction of hindfoot varus with the Coleman block test.

partially corrected during Coleman block testing, additional hindfoot correction will be required.

Radiographic Evaluation
Standard weight-bearing radiographs of the ankle and foot are used to evaluate a patient for chronic lateral ligament injury. AP and mortise views of the ankle should be scrutinized for lucent lesions in the talar dome that may signify osteochondral injury. The physician also should look for a large avulsion fracture off the distal tip of the fibula, which may accompany chronic ATFL injury. The lateral radiograph allows detection of anterior distal tibial osteophytes that can cause anterior ankle impingement. Radiographs can provide confirmation of subtle cavovarus malalignment. On a lateral radiograph of the foot, a cavus arch is suggested by a positive Meary angle formed by the axis of the talus and the axis of the first metatarsal. In cavovarus, a lateral radiograph fails to capture the talus in true profile, the fibula appears posterior, and the posterior facet is extremely well visualized, as in a Broden view. An AP foot radiograph may reveal so-called stacking of the metatarsals or metatarsus adductus. Each of these radiographic signs should raise the examiner's suspicion for concomitant malalignment.

Stress evaluation of the ankle involves the anterior drawer and talar tilt maneuvers done with fluoroscopy or plain radiography. Stress images are useful if it is desirable to quantify the severity of the instability, as for a research study. Stress fluoroscopy also is helpful for distinguishing true talar tilt from subtalar motion (**Figure 3**).

MRI has a more significant role in chronic lateral ankle ligament injuries than in acute injuries. MRI is recommended if the patient's history, physical examination, or plain radiographs suggest the possibility of osteochondral lesions of the talus or peroneal tendon injury. MRI also is indicated if the patient has poorly defined ankle pain because it can reveal conditions such

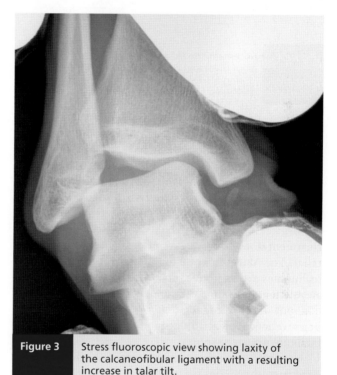

Figure 3 Stress fluoroscopic view showing laxity of the calcaneofibular ligament with a resulting increase in talar tilt.

as anterolateral soft-tissue impingement lesions.[9] If possible, 1.5- or 3.0-Tesla MRI should be obtained; the image resolution of open MRI is inadequate to provide meaningful information.

Treatment
The treatment of a patient with chronic lateral ankle ligament injury begins with nonsurgical interventions designed to improve ankle stability and decrease pain. Bracing should be implemented for a high-risk sports activity, such as basketball, volleyball, or tennis, or for any activity performed on uneven ground, such as hiking or lawn mowing. A course of neuromuscular physical therapy designed to optimize peroneal tendon strength,

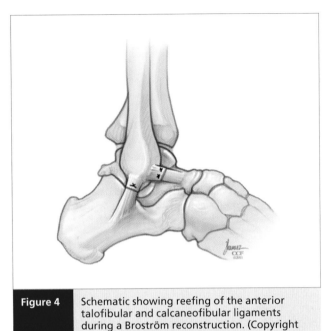

Figure 4   Schematic showing reefing of the anterior talofibular and calcaneofibular ligaments during a Broström reconstruction. (Copyright Cleveland Clinic, Cleveland, OH.)

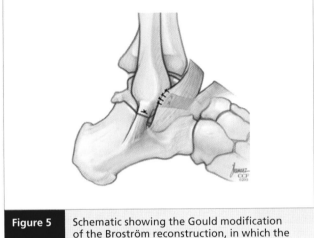

Figure 5   Schematic showing the Gould modification of the Broström reconstruction, in which the extensor retinaculum is incorporated into the ligament repair. (Copyright Cleveland Clinic, Cleveland, OH.)

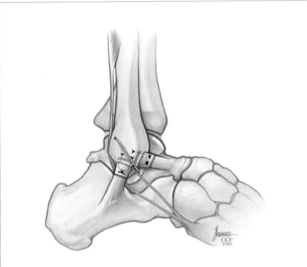

Figure 6   Schematic showing the modified Broström-Evans procedure, in which the anterior half of the peroneus brevis serves as a checkrein against excessive inversion. (Copyright Cleveland Clinic, Cleveland, OH.)

balance, and proprioception should be used unless previously completed. However, the long-term success of such a protocol for controlling instability symptoms is uncertain.[10] Unfortunately, nonsurgical treatments often do not adequately control symptoms, particularly in patients who desire to return to an active athletic lifestyle.

Surgical intervention may be indicated if nonsurgical treatment does not provide sufficient stability and pain relief. The four types of lateral ligament reconstruction techniques are anatomic, anatomic-augmented, nonanatomic tenodesis, and anatomic free tendon graft. The goals of all surgical strategies and techniques are to improve mechanical ankle stability, decrease pain, and facilitate return to sports.

The preferred technique for lateral ankle ligament reconstruction remains the anatomic Broström technique. This is the most commonly used technique, and it is successful in treating chronic instability in most patients.[11,12] This technique involves incising and reefing the ATFL alone or both the ATFL and CFL to eliminate the laxity and elongation produced by chronic inversion injuries[13] (Figure 4). The ligament can be reefed midsubstance in a vest-over-pants fashion or reefed directly to the fibula using drill holes or suture anchors.[14] The inferior extensor retinaculum can be advanced to the fibula (the Gould modification) to stabilize the CFL and the subtalar joint[15] (Figure 5).

The modified Broström-Evans anatomic-augmented procedure also has achieved excellent clinical results, particularly in high-level athletes.[16] Stability is added to a standard modified Broström procedure by transferring

half of the peroneus brevis tendon to the fibula. The orientation of this tendon transfer is approximately midway between the axes of the ATFL and the CFL. The tendon is placed through a bone tunnel in the fibula and is stabilized with an interference screw to serve as a checkrein against excessive ankle and hindfoot inversion (Figure 6). This procedure is particularly useful in a patient who is a high-demand athlete, is undergoing revision surgery, or has tenuous ligamentous tissue.

The modified Broström-Evans technique has been much more successful than older, nonanatomic tenodesis

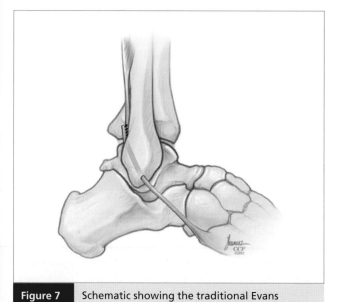

Figure 7 Schematic showing the traditional Evans procedure, in which the entire peroneus brevis is transferred. The result can be excessive stiffness. (Copyright Cleveland Clinic, Cleveland, OH.)

Figure 8 Schematic showing a free tendon graft reconstruction using hamstring autograft or allograft fixed in bone tunnels to recreate the orientation of the native anterior talofibular and calcaneofibular ligaments. (Copyright Cleveland Clinic, Cleveland, OH.)

procedures such as the traditional Evans tenodesis, in which the entire peroneus brevis tendon is transferred to the fibula at a right angle to the axis of the subtalar joint (**Figure 7**). This type of nonanatomic tenodesis procedure has largely been abandoned because it produces excessive peroneal weakness and stiffness of the subtalar joint. The current use of a nonanatomic tenodesis procedure is limited to patients with a neurologic condition and low functional demands.

Anatomic free tendon graft procedures generally use autograft or allograft hamstring tendon placed through bone tunnels in the talus, fibula, and calcaneus.[17-19] The tendon is routed in such a way as to re-create the anatomic orientation of the ATFL and CFL (**Figure 8**). This preservation of anatomic ligament orientation provides maximal ankle stability while avoiding excessive subtalar stiffness. As in the modified Broström-Evans procedure, the tendon generally is secured in the bone tunnels using interference screws. A free tendon augmentation procedure is indicated for a patient who is a high-level athlete, is undergoing revision surgery, or has generalized ligamentous laxity or severely attenuated ligamentous tissues.

If substantial cavovarus malalignment is identified before surgery, consideration should be given to including a realignment in the lateral ligament reconstruction procedure. The threshold for a cavovarus realignment is poorly defined and ultimately is based on clinical judgment, but patients with uncorrected cavovarus are at significant risk of gradually stretching out even the

stoutest lateral ligament reconstruction.[20] Thus, cavovarus malalignment should be included in the surgical plan if it is believed to be a contributor to the patient's instability or pain. Other commonly used procedures to correct cavovarus are plantar fascia release, dorsiflexion first metatarsal base closing-wedge osteotomy, lateralizing calcaneal tuberosity osteotomy, and peroneus longus to peroneus brevis transfer.

Chronic lateral ankle ligament injuries rarely occur in isolation, and a high incidence of concomitant intra-articular and extra-articular pathology has been observed.[21-24] These concomitant abnormalities often explain the pain that accompanies chronic ankle instability and must be considered during surgical reconstruction. Intra-articular pathology such as soft-tissue impingement lesions, distal tibial osteophytes, loose bodies, synovitis, and osteochondral lesions of the talus are best treated arthroscopically. Thus, many surgeons routinely perform ankle arthroscopy in conjunction with lateral ankle ligament reconstruction.[21,22]

Peroneal tendon abnormalities are common in patients with chronic ankle instability.[23] In 28% of patients undergoing lateral ligament reconstruction, abnormalities such as a peroneal tendon tear, tenosynovitis, or peroneal tendon subluxation or dislocation were found as well as symptomatic anatomic variants such as a low-lying peroneus brevis muscle belly or a peroneus quartus.[23] Untreated peroneal tendon abnormalities also were found to be associated with unsuccessful surgical treatment.

Therefore, a low threshold is recommended for exploring the peroneal tendons during ligament reconstruction.

Syndesmotic Sprains

Most ankle sprains are caused by inversion injury that primarily involves the lateral ankle ligaments. A mechanism of injury primarily involving eversion and external rotation changes the anatomy, character, and severity of the injury. Such a high ankle sprain must be distinguished from a lateral ankle sprain and treated in a different manner.

Patient History and Physical Examination
Obtaining an accurate history is critical to diagnosis of a high ankle sprain. The patient should be prompted to describe the mechanism of injury if possible, and it may be helpful to ask the patient to demonstrate the perceived mechanism of injury on the contralateral side. The clinician should suspect a high ankle sprain if the patient describes the ankle having turned or rotated outward rather inward. The location of maximal discomfort must be identified. Pain usually is localized to the lateral ankle after an inversion injury, but with a high ankle sprain the patient may describe more pain in the medial ankle and/or more proximally along the anterolateral leg.

During the physical examination the clinician should attempt to elicit pain by palpating along the deltoid ligament and the distal tibiofibular syndesmosis as well as, more proximally, the interosseous membrane and the proximal fibula. A syndesmotic sprain can be revealed by a positive squeeze test, in which the examiner compresses the tibiofibular joint in a mediolateral direction approximately 5 to 6 cm proximal to the ankle joint. Pain with this maneuver strongly suggests a syndesmotic injury. Similarly, external rotation stress applied to the ankle can be used to evaluate for injury to the deltoid ligament and syndesmosis, with reproduction of pain suggesting a high ankle sprain. These maneuvers have high specificity for syndesmotic injury when positive but have overall low sensitivity.[2] Thus, the examiner cannot rule out syndesmotic injury based on physical examination alone.

Radiographic Evaluation
The radiographic evaluation of a suspected high ankle sprain includes the standard three ankle views, preferably while the patient is bearing weight. Simulated weight bearing can be used if the pain is severe. The lateral radiograph should be closely scrutinized for evidence of a posterior malleolar avulsion fracture, which can accompany a high ankle sprain. Similarly, AP and mortise radiographic views must be assessed for signs of syndesmotic widening.

On the AP radiograph, the tibiofibular overlap should be at least 1 cm. On the mortise view, the tibiofibular clear space should be less than 1 mm. Abnormalities in these measurements suggest syndesmotic instability. A full-length tibiofibular radiograph should be included to evaluate for a proximal fibular fracture, as in a Maisonneuve-type injury.

Additional imaging is indicated if suspicion is high for syndesmotic instability but the radiographs are inconclusive. Axial CT of both ankles side by side can reveal even small amounts of widening or incongruity of the tibiofibular articulation. Alternatively, axial MRI can reveal structural injury to the anterior tibiofibular ligament as well as to the posterior syndesmotic ligaments and posterior malleolus.[2] Fluid-sensitive axial sequences reveal substantial edema within the interosseous membrane in the setting of a high ankle sprain.

CT and MRI provide more information than plain radiographs, but they are static studies that may miss dynamic instability of the syndesmosis. External rotation stress radiography or stress fluoroscopy is recommended if suspicion of instability remains high. To ensure an accurate test, a stress examination requires adequate relaxation and pain control, which can be challenging to achieve in the clinic. Thus, examination under anesthesia in the operating room should be considered if suspicion is high for an unstable syndesmosis (**Figure 9**).

Classification
High ankle sprains are classified based on the severity of injury to the deltoid ligament and the syndesmotic complex. A grade I sprain involves only microscopic structural damage. A grade II sprain involves macrostructural damage without loss of stability or subluxation. In a grade III sprain, complete ligamentous injury is accompanied by demonstrable widening of the syndesmosis and possibly by medial joint space widening.

Treatment
The treatment of a grade I or II syndesmotic sprain resembles that of an acute lateral ankle sprain, with several important differences. Because pain and swelling are often more severe and weight bearing takes longer to reestablish after a high ankle sprain than after an acute lateral sprain, a period of immobilization as long as 4 to 6 weeks should be considered. Initial cast immobilization may provide greater initial pain relief than the use of a prefabricated removable boot and can facilitate early recovery.[4] When the initial pain and swelling have subsided and weight bearing has been restored, standard functional rehabilitation protocols are initiated to restore range of motion, strength, balance, gait, and proprioception. Return to sports usually takes twice as long as after a lateral ankle

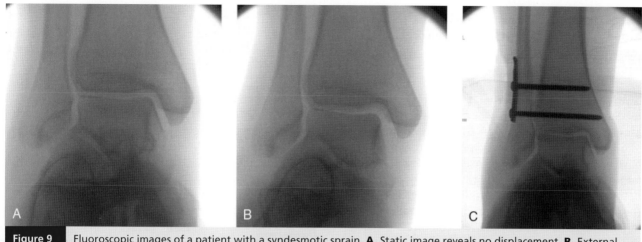

Figure 9   Fluoroscopic images of a patient with a syndesmotic sprain. **A,** Static image reveals no displacement. **B,** External rotation stress image, taken with the patient under anesthesia, reveals mortise and syndesmotic instability. **C,** Image after stabilization with syndesmotic screws.

sprain, and early in the treatment the patient should be counseled about the long recovery period.

A grade III syndesmotic sprain is unstable and requires surgical stabilization. Stabilization procedures traditionally use solid metal tibiofibular transfixion screws to immobilize the syndesmosis and mortise in an anatomic position so as to facilitate subsequent healing of the deltoid and syndesmotic ligaments. Despite extensive research, there is no consensus as to the size and number of screws to be used, the number of cortices to engage, and whether or when to remove the screws.[25]

A nonabsorbable suture button device has been used to stabilize the tibiofibular joint.[26] Suture stabilization theoretically avoids several difficulties associated with screw fixation. Proponents argue that suture devices provide more flexible fixation, thus facilitating restoration of normal tibiofibular biomechanics without implant removal or the potential for implant breakage.[27] A recent study also found that syndesmotic malreduction was less common when a suture button device was used, compared with traditional metal screws.[28] However, complications have been reported with the use of suture button devices, including stitch abscesses, loss of reduction, and osteolysis around the suture.[29] Until high-quality comparative research is completed, screw fixation remains the gold standard for syndesmotic stabilization.

A 6- to 12-week period of protected avoidance of weight bearing is required to facilitate ligament healing after surgical stabilization of a grade III high ankle sprain. Syndesmotic screws generally are left in place a minimum of 3 to 4 months. At that time, the surgeon must decide whether to remove or retain the screws. Removal requires a second surgical procedure and risks loss of reduction if ligament healing is incomplete. Retention may lead to restriction of ankle motion, screw breakage,

or osteolysis around the screws. One study found no negative effect with retention of syndesmotic screws, even if a screw later broke.[30] Although tibiofibular screws may be retained without consequence in nonathletes, consideration should be given to planned removal approximately 4 months after surgery in a patient who is an athlete.[30] This timing avoids the risk of broken hardware or ankle motion restriction while allowing adequate time for ligament healing. Functional rehabilitation is subsequently initiated, with a return to sports expected approximately 6 to 8 months after surgical treatment.

Stress Fractures of the Foot and Ankle

Athletes in training are susceptible to overuse injuries of the foot and ankle, including stress fracture. A stress fracture is distinguished from a traumatic fracture by its origin in repetitive, cumulative stress rather than in a single traumatic event. The most common sites of stress fracture in the foot and ankle are the distal tibia, malleoli, navicular, metatarsals, and sesamoids.[31]

Patient History and Physical Examination

The clinician should seek clues in the patient history that suggest a stress fracture. A change in the character, duration, or intensity of training is a major risk factor for stress fracture in athletes. Examples include the addition of hills or sprints for a jogger or a rapid increase in mileage for a distance runner. Similarly, an important change in shoe wear, such as an abrupt switch to a minimalist-type running shoe, should raise the examiner's suspicion for a stress fracture.[32] The physician should ask whether the patient has a history of osteoporosis or osteopenia and obtain a baseline 25-hydroxy vitamin D level if stress fracture is strongly suspected.[33]

The character of the pain caused by a stress fracture is variable. Some patients experience pain primarily during training and are relatively pain free during activities of daily living. The symptoms may have been present for several weeks to months. This type of pain suggests a slowly evolving stress fracture. Early in the process, focal tenderness to palpation may be minimal, and the patient must run or jump to reproduce the symptoms.

Some patients describe mild prodromal symptoms that have become acutely worse during training. Often these patients have pain with activities of daily living or may be unable to tolerate any weight bearing. Palpation of the affected bone reliably reproduces the pain. This level of pain suggests a complete stress fracture.

In addition to the location of tenderness, the examiner should look for evidence of malalignment, which can predispose an individual to stress fracture. For example, fibular stress fracture may be associated with hindfoot valgus. More commonly, cavovarus malalignment is associated with medial malleolar or fifth metatarsal stress fracture. A plantarflexed first ray, as often is present in cavovarus malalignment, can have a role in sesamoid stress fracture. Identifying these predisposing factors early in the treatment increases the likelihood of a successful outcome.

Radiographic Evaluation

It is critical to understand that radiographs may be negative during the early stages of a stress fracture. Follow-up radiographs 2 to 4 weeks after treatment is initiated generally are more revealing. If a stress fracture is present, the follow-up radiographs will show early callus formation and periosteal reaction consistent with initial bone healing (**Figure 10**). However, if the follow-up radiographs remain negative for fracture, another diagnosis should be considered, or more sophisticated imaging studies performed. MRI is particularly useful because it can show intraosseous edema consistent with stress reaction in a bone before progression to a radiographically detectable stress fracture.

Treatment

Most stress fractures about the foot and ankle can be successfully treated with a combination of relative rest, activity modification, immobilization, and restricted weight bearing. Immobilization in a prefabricated fracture boot and the use of crutches usually are successful for treating the initial pain while maintaining an acceptable level of function and fitness. If the patient's vitamin D level is found to be low, supplementation with 50,000 IU weekly is initiated.[33] In general, symptoms substantially improve 3 to 4 weeks after initiation of treatment. Use of the fracture boot can be gradually discontinued at this time, and

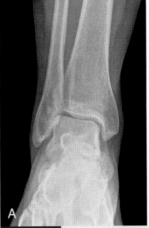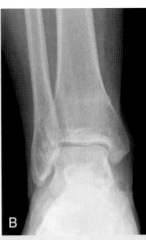

Figure 10 Radiographs of a patient with acute distal leg pain after running. **A,** Initial AP ankle radiograph showing no abnormality. The patient was found to have a vitamin D deficiency and was treated with restricted weight bearing and vitamin D supplementation. **B,** Follow-up AP ankle radiograph after 3 weeks of restricted weight bearing showing evidence of bone reaction consistent with a healing metaphyseal stress fracture.

a low-impact aerobic program can be initiated. For most fractures, clinical healing is achieved at 6 to 8 weeks, when a cautious return to a sports rehabilitation program can be started. As activity is resumed, it is critical to correct any training errors that may have precipitated the stress fracture. If malalignment is believed to have played a role in the development of the stress injury, appropriate shoe inserts should be prescribed. A patient with a sesamoid stress fracture benefits from wearing a shoe insert that incorporates relief beneath the first metatarsal head. A full return to sports generally requires 3 to 6 months of recovery, depending on the severity of the fracture and the specific physical demands of the sport.

Although nonsurgical treatment is indicated for most stress fractures of the foot and ankle, surgical intervention should be considered in specific situations. The most difficult-to-treat stress fractures in the foot and ankle are those of the medial malleolus, navicular, fifth metatarsal, and sesamoids.[31] These fractures have a relatively high risk of delayed healing or nonunion. In addition, the prolonged period of immobilization and restricted weight bearing necessary for successful nonsurgical treatment of these injuries often is poorly tolerated by athletic patients.

Stress fracture of the medial malleolus or navicular involves the ankle or talonavicular joint, respectively, and warrants aggressive surgical treatment. CT is used to accurately assess fracture completeness and displacement. A complete and/or displaced fracture should be treated surgically. Because most medial malleolar stress fractures are vertically oriented, they are best treated with compression screws and buttress plating. Débridement of the fracture and/or bone grafting may be necessary for a chronic injury, particularly if sclerosis or cystic change is noted on preoperative CT.

Navicular stress fractures are stabilized with compression lag screws. Because the fracture line typically is lateral, screws must be placed from lateral to medial to achieve adequate purchase and stability (**Figure 11**). A recent investigation into the intraosseous blood supply of the navicular challenged the traditional belief that the fracture line corresponds to a relatively avascular portion of the navicular.[34] If preoperative CT reveals substantial diastasis, displacement, cystic change, or sclerosis, open reduction and internal fixation through a dorsal approach is required, with liberal use of bone graft. A systematic literature review questioned the need for aggressive surgical treatment of navicular stress fractures.[35] No evidence was found to indicate that surgical treatment was preferred over nonsurgical treatment without weight bearing; both treatments were more successful than nonsurgical treatment with permitted weight bearing.

Indications for surgical treatment of a fifth metatarsal stress fracture include nonunion or delayed union as well as a desire to facilitate healing while minimizing the need for casting. A fifth metatarsal stress fracture is treated using the same intramedullary screw technique as for an acute Jones fracture. Intramedullary or extramedullary bone grafting can be considered for a chronic fracture with substantial sclerosis. However, bone grafting was found to be unnecessary in most fractures, even with a nonunion.[36] A sesamoid stress fracture can be treated with open reduction and internal fixation, partial excision, or complete excision, depending on the size of the fragments, the chronicity of the fracture, and the presence of avascular changes.

Midfoot Sprains

Injuries of the tarsometatarsal joint complex range in severity from a mild sprain to a severe crush injury. Although a midfoot sprain lies on the less severe end of the spectrum, this injury has the potential to render the midfoot unstable and cause lingering morbidity in an athlete.

Soccer and football players are particularly susceptible to a midfoot sprain because of the high-intensity sprinting, jumping, and cutting maneuvers involved in these sports. The mechanism of injury usually involves a dorsally directed abduction force applied to the plantarflexed foot and resulting in an awkward twisting motion. Particularly in football, another player may fall onto the back of the foot and ankle, again causing a dorsiflexion-abduction force to be applied to the foot. In

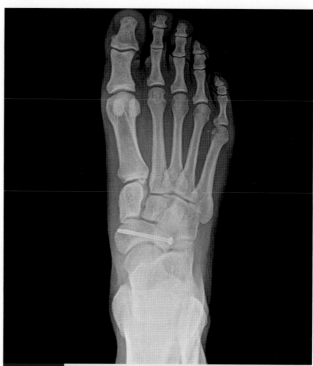

Figure 11 Postoperative AP foot radiograph of a navicular stress fracture treated using lateral-to-medial lag screw.

either scenario, the indirect force exerted on the foot produces injury of variable severity to the osseoligamentous structure of the midfoot. The ligamentous stability of the tarsometatarsal joint complex primarily is provided by the stout plantar ligaments, including the interosseous Lisfranc ligament that connects the medial cuneiform to the base of the second metatarsal. In a mild midfoot sprain, the relatively weak dorsal ligaments may be injured, producing pain but no subluxation or loss of stability. In a more severe sprain, injury to both the dorsal and plantar ligaments leads to tarsometatarsal joint subluxation and instability.

Patient History and Physical Examination

An athlete with a midfoot sprain has pain primarily on the dorsum of the midfoot. If the patient also reports significant pain in the lateral midfoot, the possibility of an associated cuboid fracture should be considered. Swelling, tenderness, and ecchymosis tend to occur dorsally over the midfoot. The presence of plantar midfoot ecchymosis particularly suggests a significant ligament injury to the tarsometatarsal joint complex. Dorsoplantar stressing of the metatarsals also may reproduce pain. Weight bearing may be difficult or impossible.

Radiographic Evaluation

No radiographic abnormalities are seen with a ligamentously stable midfoot sprain. On an AP radiograph of the foot, there is no widening between the medial cuneiform and the base of the second metatarsal, and the medial cortex of the second metatarsal base is collinear with the medial cortex of the middle cuneiform. On an oblique radiograph, the medial cortex of the fourth metatarsal is aligned with the medial border of the cuboid. The lateral radiograph also should show the dorsal cortices of the first and second metatarsals aligned with their respective cuneiforms. Widening of the Lisfranc joint, a fleck sign adjacent to the second metatarsal base, and/or lateral or dorsal subluxation of the tarsometatarsal joints, are each diagnostic of an unstable midfoot sprain.

Good-quality weight-bearing radiographs are essential. Obtaining weight-bearing radiographs can be particularly challenging after an acute injury, when weight bearing may be extremely painful, but non–weight-bearing radiographs are insufficiently sensitive for showing the subtle subluxations that can occur after a midfoot sprain. If plain radiographs are inconclusive, MRI should be considered. A high correlation was found between MRI and surgical findings after a suspected midfoot injury.[37] CT provides even greater osseous detail than MRI. Small avulsion fracture and subtle subluxation about the midfoot can be readily seen on CT. If static imaging studies are equivocal, stress fluoroscopy under local or general anesthesia can be used to assess the stability of the tarsometatarsal joint complex.

Treatment

The treatment of a midfoot sprain is dictated by the severity of the ligamentous injury. A dorsal sprain without instability or subluxation is treated nonsurgically with 4 to 6 weeks of immobilization in a cast or prefabricated boot and restricted weight bearing. As symptoms improve, weight bearing is begun with the use of a fracture boot for protection and support. For an athlete, a semirigid custom orthotic device subsequently can be used to facilitate the transition to regular shoes and resumption of activity. Return to sports typically is achieved 3 to 6 months after injury.

Unstable midfoot sprains, defined by the presence of any detectable subluxation, are treated surgically. The options for surgical treatment include open reduction and internal fixation as well as primary tarsometatarsal joint fusion. Prospective randomized studies found superior outcomes after primary fusion for primarily ligamentous midfoot injuries.[38,39] The benefits of primary fusion include reliable bony healing, decreased need for hardware removal, and decreased incidence of posttraumatic arthritis.

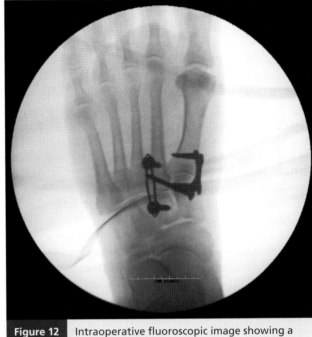

Figure 12 Intraoperative fluoroscopic image showing a midfoot sprain treated with a plate spanning the first tarsometatarsal joint and a staple spanning the second tarsometatarsal joint. The Lisfranc joint was stabilized with a lag screw.

Open reduction and internal fixation remains a viable alternative for athletes who want to return to competitive sports. Although flexibility of the tarsometatarsal joints is widely believed to be expendable, the putative benefits of open reduction and internal fixation include preservation of joint motion with improved balance, proprioception, and athletic performance. The traditional implants are transarticular metal screws. After anatomic reduction and screw fixation, immobilization without weight bearing is required for 6 to 8 weeks, with gradual resumption of protected weight bearing in a prefabricated boot. Hardware generally is removed 3 to 6 months after surgery and before initiation of a rehabilitation program. Return to sports after surgical treatment of an unstable midfoot sprain generally is achieved within 6 to 12 months.

To avoid iatrogenic joint damage associated with transarticular screws, surgeons have begun to use joint-spanning plates and staples to stabilize the tarsometatarsal joint complex (**Figure 12**). These devices are useful if the bone is osteoporotic or associated fractures compromise traditional screw fixation. Implant removal usually is required, however, and surgical dissection is more extensive when removing plates and staples than when removing screws only.

Nonabsorbable suture button devices have been used for fixation of unstable Lisfranc joint injuries.[40] The proposed benefits of suture stabilization include flexible fixation, which may allow an earlier return to weight bearing with a decreased risk of implant failure, as well as avoidance of routine hardware removal. Additional clinical studies are needed to evaluate the success of these implants in treating unstable midfoot injuries.

Summary

The foot and ankle are often injured during athletic activities, and acute or chronic ankle ligament injury can severely affect athletic performance and participation. These injuries can be challenging to treat, especially in high-level athletes for whom a rapid return to peak performance is of paramount importance. The initial treatment of an acute injury generally is nonsurgical. Immobilization in a cast or boot is followed by focused, sport-specific physical therapy, although some early evidence suggests that a severe (grade III) acute sprain may be best treated surgically. Treatment of a chronic sprain also begins with nonsurgical methods, but these may not be effective, and some type of lateral ligament reconstruction may be required. Syndesmotic (high) ankle sprain is a more severe injury and usually requires a longer treatment before return to sport. The initial treatment of a grade I or II syndesmotic sprain is similar to that of an acute lateral ligament sprain, but a grade III sprain is unstable and requires surgical stabilization. Midfoot sprains, which can cause significant disability in athletes, range from a mild sprain to a severe crush injury. Treatment of a midfoot sprain depends on its severity; a stable sprain is treated with immobilization and avoidance of weight bearing, and an unstable strain is treated surgically. Stress fractures are most common in the distal tibia, malleoli, navicular, metatarsals, and sesamoids. Most stress fractures of the foot and ankle can be successfully treated using a combination of relative rest, activity modification, immobilization, and restricted weight bearing. A stress fracture of the medial malleolus, navicular, fifth metatarsal, or sesamoids has a relatively high risk of nonunion and requires lengthy immobilization for healing. Surgery may be the preferred treatment in a high-performance athlete.

Annotated References

1. Waterman BR, Owens BD, Davey S, Zacchilli MA, Belmont PJ Jr: The epidemiology of ankle sprains in the United States. *J Bone Joint Surg Am* 2010;92(13):2279-2284.

   An extensive database review of ankle sprains found that sprains are most common in patients age 10 to 19 years. Sprains were more common in male than female patients age 15 to 24 years but were more common in women than men older than 30 years. More than 50% of ankle sprains occurred during athletic activity.

2. de César PC, Avila EM, de Abreu MR: Comparison of magnetic resonance imaging to physical examination for syndesmotic injury after lateral ankle sprain. *Foot Ankle Int* 2011;32(12):1110-1114.

   MRI revealed concomitant syndesmotic ligament injury in 17.8% of lateral ankle sprains. The squeeze test and external rotation stress test had low sensitivity but high specificity for syndesmotic injury in association with lateral ankle sprain.

3. Bleakley CM, O'Connor SR, Tully MA, et al: Effect of accelerated rehabilitation on function after ankle sprain: Randomised controlled trial. *BMJ* 2010;340:c1964.

   Immediate initiation of functional range-of-motion exercises after a grade I or II lateral ankle sprain was found to facilitate early resolution of symptoms and return to activity.

4. Lamb SE, Marsh JL, Hutton JL, Nakash R, Cooke MW; Collaborative Ankle Support Trial (CAST Group): Mechanical supports for acute, severe ankle sprain: A pragmatic, multicentre, randomised controlled trial. *Lancet* 2009;373(9663):575-581.

   Initial immobilization in a below-the-knee cast was found to have the greatest effect on early recovery after a grade III ankle sprain. Immobilization using a stirrup ankle brace also was beneficial. Use of a prefabricated walking boot had limited benefit over a simple compression sleeve.

5. Ismail MM, Ibrahim MM, Youssef EF, El Shorbagy KM: Plyometric training versus resistive exercises after acute lateral ankle sprain. *Foot Ankle Int* 2010;31(6):523-530.

   In comparison with traditional resistance exercises, incorporation of plyometric exercises into the rehabilitation protocol for lateral ankle sprains led to improved functional performance in athletes.

6. Pijnenburg AC, Van Dijk CN, Bossuyt PM, Marti RK: Treatment of ruptures of the lateral ankle ligaments: A meta-analysis. *J Bone Joint Surg Am* 2000;82(6):761-773.

7. Pihlajamäki H, Hietaniemi K, Paavola M, Visuri T, Mattila VM: Surgical versus functional treatment for acute ruptures of the lateral ligament complex of the ankle in young men: A randomized controlled trial. *J Bone Joint Surg Am* 2010;92(14):2367-2374.

   A prospective randomized comparison study of initial surgical repair and nonsurgical treatment of severe lateral ankle sprains revealed comparable long-term results. Surgical treatment appeared to decrease the likelihood of reinjury but was associated with an increased risk of arthritis.

8. van Rijn RM, van Os AG, Bernsen RM, Luijsterburg PA, Koes BW, Bierma-Zeinstra SM: What is the clinical course

of acute ankle sprains? A systematic literature review. *Am J Med* 2008;121(4):324-331, e6.

A meta-analysis of acute ankle sprains revealed that one-third of patients have residual symptoms at 1 year and one-third sustain additional sprains during the 3 years after a sprain.

9. Ferkel RD, Tyorkin M, Applegate GR, Heinen GT: MRI evaluation of anterolateral soft tissue impingement of the ankle. *Foot Ankle Int* 2010;31(8):655-661.

MRI was found to provide 78.9% accuracy in diagnosis, sensitivity of 83.3%, and specificity of 78.6% when used for the evaluation of anterolateral soft-tissue impingement of the ankle. A 33% incidence of associated diagnoses was noted.

10. de Vries JS, Krips R, Sierevelt IN, Blankevoort L, van Dijk CN: Interventions for treating chronic ankle instability. *Cochrane Database Syst Rev* 2011;8:CD004124.

Randomized controlled studies of nonsurgical and surgical treatments of chronic ankle instability were systematically reviewed.

11. Tourné Y, Mabit C, Moroney PJ, Chaussard C, Saragaglia D: Long-term follow-up of lateral reconstruction with extensor retinaculum flap for chronic ankle instability. *Foot Ankle Int* 2012;33(12):1079-1086.

A retrospective review of 150 patients an average 11 years after modified Broström-Gould lateral ligament reconstruction found that 93% were satisfied with the procedure. Only 4.8% had residual instability, and none had radiographic progression of arthritis.

12. Bell SJ, Mologne TS, Sitler DF, Cox JS: Twenty-six-year results after Broström procedure for chronic lateral ankle instability. *Am J Sports Med* 2006;34(6):975-978.

13. Lee KT, Park YU, Kim JS, Kim JB, Kim KC, Kang SK: Long-term results after modified Brostrom procedure without calcaneofibular ligament reconstruction. *Foot Ankle Int* 2011;32(2):153-157.

A retrospective review of 30 patients an average 10.6 years after modified Broström-Gould reconstruction without CFL reconstruction found that all patients achieved an excellent or good result.

14. Cho BK, Kim YM, Kim DS, Choi ES, Shon HC, Park KJ: Comparison between suture anchor and transosseous suture for the modified-Broström procedure. *Foot Ankle Int* 2012;33(6):462-468.

No significant clinical or functional differences were found when lateral ligament reconstruction was performed using suture anchors or transosseous sutures.

15. Behrens SB, Drakos M, Lee BJ, et al: Biomechanical analysis of Brostrom versus Brostrom-Gould lateral ankle instability repairs. *Foot Ankle Int* 2013;34(4):587-592.

A biomechanical study revealed no significant difference in initial stability between the traditional Broström repair and the modified Broström repair with incorporation of the extensor retinaculum.

16. Girard P, Anderson RB, Davis WH, Isear JA, Kiebzak GM: Clinical evaluation of the modified Brostrom-Evans procedure to restore ankle stability. *Foot Ankle Int* 1999;20(4):246-252.

17. Wang B, Xu XY: Minimally invasive reconstruction of lateral ligaments of the ankle using semitendinosus autograft. *Foot Ankle Int* 2013;34(5):711-715.

An excellent or good result was reported in 25 patients treated with hamstring autograft reconstruction of the lateral ankle ligaments using a minimally invasive technique. The average American Orthopaedic Foot and Ankle Society score had improved from 71.1 to 95.1 at an average 32.3-month follow-up.

18. Coughlin MJ, Schenck RC Jr, Grebing BR, Treme G: Comprehensive reconstruction of the lateral ankle for chronic instability using a free gracilis graft. *Foot Ankle Int* 2004;25(4):231-241.

19. Jeys LM, Harris NJ: Ankle stabilization with hamstring autograft: A new technique using interference screws. *Foot Ankle Int* 2003;24(9):677-679.

20. Fortin PT, Guettler J, Manoli A II: Idiopathic cavovarus and lateral ankle instability: Recognition and treatment implications relating to ankle arthritis. *Foot Ankle Int* 2002;23(11):1031-1037.

21. Sugimoto K, Takakura Y, Okahashi K, Samoto N, Kawate K, Iwai M: Chondral injuries of the ankle with recurrent lateral instability: An arthroscopic study. *J Bone Joint Surg Am* 2009;91(1):99-106.

Ankle arthroscopy in 93 patients with chronic instability was examined to determine risk factors for cartilage abnormalities. Patient age, talar tilt angle, and varus malalignment of the ankle were associated with an increased risk of severe chondral damage.

22. Ferkel RD, Chams RN: Chronic lateral instability: Arthroscopic findings and long-term results. *Foot Ankle Int* 2007;28(1):24-31.

23. Strauss JE, Forsberg JA, Lippert FG III: Chronic lateral ankle instability and associated conditions: A rationale for treatment. *Foot Ankle Int* 2007;28(10):1041-1044.

24. Crim JR, Beals TC, Nickisch F, Schannen A, Saltzman CL: Deltoid ligament abnormalities in chronic lateral ankle instability. *Foot Ankle Int* 2011;32(9):873-878.

Concomitant deltoid ligament injuries were found in 33 of 46 patients (72%) who underwent lateral ligament reconstruction. None of the patients had medial ankle pain.

25. Fractures and dislocations of the ankle, in Bucholz RW, Court-Brown CM, Heckman JD, Tornetta P III, eds: *Rockwood and Green's Fractures in Adults*, ed 7. Philadelphia, PA, Lippincott, Williams & Wilkins, 2009.

    This authoritative and comprehensive text presents thorough discussion of all aspects of ankle fracture evaluation and management.

26. DeGroot H, Al-Omari AA, El Ghazaly SA: Outcomes of suture button repair of the distal tibiofibular syndesmosis. *Foot Ankle Int* 2011;32(3):250-256.

    The use of suture button stabilization of the syndesmosis was reviewed in 24 patients a mean 20 months after injury. Successful stabilization and healing were achieved in all patients, but six (25%) required subsequent removal of the implant.

27. Klitzman R, Zhao H, Zhang LQ, Strohmeyer G, Vora A: Suture-button versus screw fixation of the syndesmosis: A biomechanical analysis. *Foot Ankle Int* 2010;31(1):69-75.

    A cadaver study found that the suture button device maintained reduction of the syndesmosis under cyclic loading. Suture button fixation also allowed more normal sagittal plane motion of the tibiofibular articulation than tricortical screw fixation.

28. Naqvi GA, Cunningham P, Lynch B, Galvin R, Awan N: Fixation of ankle syndesmotic injuries: Comparison of tightrope fixation and syndesmotic screw fixation for accuracy of syndesmotic reduction. *Am J Sports Med* 2012;40(12):2828-2835.

    Accuracy of syndesmotic reduction, as determined by postoperative CT, was compared in 46 patients treated with screw or suture button fixation. Five patients treated with screw fixation were found to have malreduction. No patient treated with suture button fixation had malreduction. Syndesmotic reduction was the major determinant of outcome.

29. Storey P, Gadd RJ, Blundell C, Davies MB: Complications of suture button ankle syndesmosis stabilization with modifications of surgical technique. *Foot Ankle Int* 2012;33(9):717-721.

    Eight of 102 patients treated with suture button stabilization of the syndesmosis required implant removal. Modifications of the technique were recommended to minimize complications.

30. Moore JA Jr, Shank JR, Morgan SJ, Smith WR: Syndesmosis fixation: A comparison of three and four cortices of screw fixation without hardware removal. *Foot Ankle Int* 2006;27(8):567-572.

31. Shindle MK, Endo Y, Warren RF, et al: Stress fractures about the tibia, foot, and ankle. *J Am Acad Orthop Surg* 2012;20(3):167-176.

    High-risk lower extremity stress fractures, including those of the tibial diaphysis, medial malleolus, navicular, and fifth metatarsal base, were thoroughly reviewed.

32. Salzler MJ, Bluman EM, Noonan S, Chiodo CP, de Asla RJ: Injuries observed in minimalist runners. *Foot Ankle Int* 2012;33(4):262-266.

    Ten patients sustained a stress-related foot injury (nine stress fractures, one plantar fascia rupture) after switching from traditional to minimalist running shoes.

33. McCabe MP, Smyth MP, Richardson DR: Vitamin D and stress fractures. *Foot Ankle Int* 2012;33(6):526-533.

    The role of vitamin D in normal bone metabolism and the association of vitamin D deficiency with stress fracture were reviewed. Supplementation guidelines were presented.

34. McKeon KE, McCormick JJ, Johnson JE, Klein SE: Intraosseous and extraosseous arterial anatomy of the adult navicular. *Foot Ankle Int* 2012;33(10):857-861.

    Vascular injection studies using 55 cadaver specimens determined avascular areas in the navicular. Only six specimens (11%) had a central-third avascular region. Other factors may play an important role in the development of navicular stress fractures.

35. Torg JS, Moyer J, Gaughan JP, Boden BP: Management of tarsal navicular stress fractures: Conservative versus surgical treatment. A meta-analysis. *Am J Sports Med* 2010;38(5):1048-1053.

    A meta-analysis of the available literature revealed no significant advantage to surgical treatment of navicular stress fractures compared with nonsurgical treatment without weight bearing. Weight-bearing nonsurgical treatment was inferior to both surgical treatment and non–weight-bearing nonsurgical treatment.

36. Habbu RA, Marsh RS, Anderson JG, Bohay DR: Closed intramedullary screw fixation for nonunion of fifth metatarsal Jones fracture. *Foot Ankle Int* 2011;32(6):603-608.

    Fourteen patients with a nonunion of a fifth metatarsal zone 2 fracture (a Jones fracture) had successful healing after intramedullary screw fixation without opening the nonunion site or using supplementary bone graft.

37. Raikin SM, Elias I, Dheer S, Besser MP, Morrison WB, Zoga AC: Prediction of midfoot instability in the subtle Lisfranc injury: Comparison of magnetic resonance imaging with intraoperative findings. *J Bone Joint Surg Am* 2009;91(4):892-899.

    MRI had high sensitivity, specificity, and positive predictive value for evaluation of the integrity of a Lisfranc ligament. A finding of a ruptured or grade II sprain of the Lisfranc ligament was strongly correlated with an intraoperative finding of instability.

38. Ly TV, Coetzee JC: Treatment of primarily ligamentous Lisfranc joint injuries: Primary arthrodesis compared with open reduction and internal fixation. A prospective, randomized study. *J Bone Joint Surg Am* 2006;88(3):514-520.

39. Henning JA, Jones CB, Sietsema DL, Bohay DR, Anderson JG: Open reduction internal fixation versus primary arthrodesis for Lisfranc injuries: A prospective randomized study. *Foot Ankle Int* 2009;30(10):913-922.

A study of primary arthrodesis with open reduction and internal fixation found comparable satisfaction and clinical outcomes in patients with Lisfranc injuries. Primary arthrodesis led to significantly fewer subsequent surgeries, mostly because hardware removal was avoided.

40. Panchbhavi VK, Vallurupalli S, Yang J, Andersen CR: Screw fixation compared with suture-button fixation of isolated Lisfranc ligament injuries. *J Bone Joint Surg Am* 2009;91(5):1143-1148.

A cadaver biomechanical study found that suture button stabilization of the Lisfranc joint was comparable to cannulated screw fixation.

Chapter 30

Osteochondral Lesions of the Talus

Wen Chao, MD   Erik Freeland, DO   Russell Dedini, MD

7: Tendon Disorders and Sports-Related Foot and Ankle Injuries

Introduction

Osteochondritis dissecans was originally described in 1888 as a process of loose body formation associated with articular cartilage and subchondral bone fracture in the hip and knee.[1] The first description of these lesions in the ankle was provided in 1922.[2] An original anatomic study in 1959 on cadaver limbs provided insight into the etiologic mechanism advancing the concept of trauma as a primary osteochondritis dissecans factor.[3] In addition, a staging system was developed based on radiographic and surgical parameters that are currently in use. Historically, a variety of terms including osteochondritis dissecans, transchondral talus fracture, and osteochondral talus fracture have been used to describe what are now universally referred to as osteochondral lesions of the talus (OLTs), a term that was introduced in 1994.[4]

Incidence

OLTs represent approximately 4% of all osteochondral lesions. In 1955, investigators reported a frequency of 6.5% in their series of 133 ankle sprains.[5] A 2011 epidemiologic study examining active-duty US military personnel found the overall occurrence of OLTs to be 27 per 100,000 patient years over a 10-year period.[6] This finding suggests that OLTs may be more common than previously considered. Several authors have reported that the incidence of bilateral lesions is approximately 10%.[3,7]

Medial osteochondral lesions are more common than lateral osteochondral lesions. Medial lesions have been described as deeper with extension into subchondral bone and they often develop into cystic lesions. Lateral lesions, which are more commonly associated with a traumatic injury, are described as shallow and have the tendency to become displaced.[3]

In 2007, MRIs of 428 ankles with talar osteochondral lesions were studied.[8] A grid system was used to identify the precise location of talar dome lesions. In contrast to the historically described anterolateral and posteromedial locations, the midtalar dome was involved in 80% of lesions. It was determined that the midmedial zone was the most common location (53%). The lesions in this location were the largest and deepest. The midlateral zone was the second most common zone (26%).[8]

In another study, the authors retrospectively reviewed the location, frequency, and size of OLTs on 77 MRI examinations based on a nine-zone grid. Their findings support the notion that the most common osteochondral lesions are not the traditionally described anterolateral and posteromedial lesions, but rather central medial and central lateral lesions. Additionally, it was determined that lesion location does not predict subject age, lesion chronicity or instability, or history of trauma. However, medial lesions were larger and lateral lesions were seen more commonly in association with ligamentous injury.[9] Using the same nine-zone grid described in 2007, investigators in 2012 performed a retrospective examination of all preoperative MRIs performed over a 4-year period in patients who underwent primary surgical management of symptomatic OLTs.[10] Their results supported findings published in 2007 and 2012; however, they noted that symptomatic surgically treated osteochondral defects of the talus were located in the lateral third of the talar dome almost twice as commonly as in the medial third (65% versus 35%).[10]

Clinical Presentation

An OLT diagnosis is rarely made immediately after an acute ankle injury. In most cases, the condition is associated with chronic ankle pain, especially after inversion injury to the lateral ligamentous complex. Patients presenting with an OLT often describe prolonged pain, recurrent ankle swelling, weakness, and continued subjective instability. Patients also may report mechanical symptoms including catching, clicking, and locking. The physical examination may reveal tenderness at the level of the ankle mortise anteriorly or posteriorly. The differential diagnosis is wide, but a high index of suspicion must be maintained for an OLT when evaluating patients with chronic ankle pain.[11,12]

Etiology/Pathoanatomy/Natural History

The etiology of an OLT may be nontraumatic or traumatic. Most authors believe that trauma has an integral role in the pathogenesis of most OLTs and that OLTs most likely represent the chronic phase of a compressed talar dome fracture. A single event of macrotrauma or repetitive microtrauma may elicit initiation of the lesion in a person who is already predisposed to talar dome ischemia. Endocrine or metabolic abnormalities, vasculopathy, and osteonecrosis are potential etiologic factors in nontraumatic OLTs.[13,14]

Subchondral cysts with overlying chondromalacia, osteochondral fragments, and loose bodies all represent various stages in the progression of OLTs. The development of a symptomatic OLT depends on various factors. The primary mechanism is damage and insufficient repair of the subchondral bone plate. Authors of a 2010 study theorized that water from compressed cartilage is forced into the microfractured subchondral bone during loading, which subsequently leads to localized increased fluid pressure within the subchondral bone. Local osteolysis can then predispose to the development of a subchondral cyst. The pain is believed to be a result of stimulation of the highly innervated subchondral bone under the cartilage defect.[11]

The precise natural history of OLTs is unclear. In a review of serial MRIs of 29 patients who had OLTs that were treated nonsurgically, 45% showed progression, 24% improved, and 31% remained unchanged.[15] The authors found that bone marrow edema and subchondral cysts are not reliable indicators of lesion progression.[15] Osteoarthritis of the ankle has been shown to be an uncommon final outcome.[16]

Imaging and Classification

In 1959, Berndt and Harty described the first staging system based on radiographic findings.[3] This classification system was later modified with the addition of stage V to describe lesions with a cystic component[17] (Figure 1). The overall correlation of radiographic assessment with arthroscopic findings has been found to be poor.[18]

Advanced imaging modalities have significantly increased the ability to accurately diagnose OLTs. CT scans are predominantly used as an adjunct for a more comprehensive evaluation of and preoperative planning

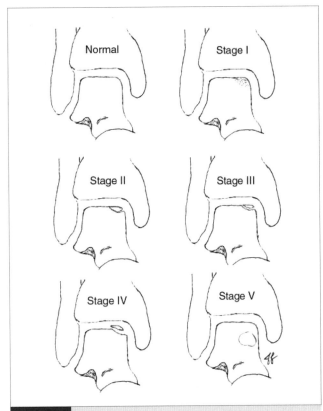

Figure 1 Loomer and associates' modification of the Berndt and Harty radiographic classification of osteochondral lesions of the talus. Stage I: Compression of subchondral bone. Stage II: Partially detached osteochondral fragment. Stage III: Completely detached osteochondral fragment remaining in fragment bed. Stage IV: Displaced osteochondral fragment. Stage V: Presence of cystic component. (Adapted from Loomer R, Fischer C, Lloyd-Schmidt R, et al: Osteochondral lesions of the talus. *Am J Sports Med* 1993;21:13-19.)

for known lesions[19] (Figure 2). In 1990, a four-stage system of classifying the lesions based on CT findings was described[20] (Figure 3). This classification system corresponds to stages described in the original classification by Berndt and Harty but also considers subchondral cyst formation, fragmentation, and the overall extent of osteonecrosis.

MRI is the preferred imaging study for detection of suspected OLTs that are not seen on initial plain radiographs[21] (Figure 4). It is also extremely useful for further evaluation of known OLTs. MRI provides improved three-dimensional localization and sizing of a lesion. It also aids in the assessment of stability and identification of a cystic component. MRI is also used to stage OLTs. In 1989, an MRI classification system based on the Berndt and Harty classification system was described.[22] This classification system was later revised primarily by

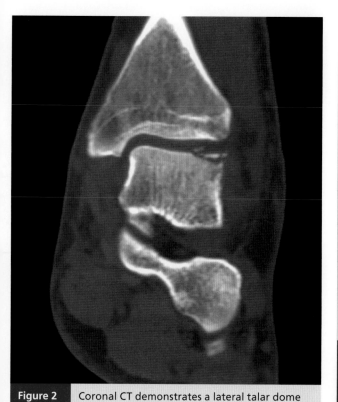

Figure 2 Coronal CT demonstrates a lateral talar dome osteochondral lesion.

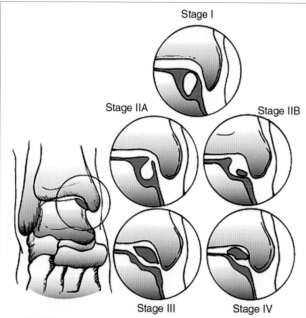

Figure 3 Ferkel and Sgaglione's CT classification of osteochondral lesions of the talus. Stage I: Cystic lesion within the dome of the talus, intact roof on all views. Stage IIA: Cystic lesion with communication to the talar dome surface. Stage IIB: Open articular surface lsion with overlying nondisplaced fragment. Stage III: Nondisplaced lesion with lucency. Stage IV: Displaced fragment. (Reproduced from Feinblatt J, Graves SC: Osteochondral lesions of the talus: Acute and chronic, in Pinzur MS, ed: *Orthopaedic Knowledge Update Foot and Ankle 4.* Rosemont, IL, American Academy of Orthopaedic Surgeons, 2008, pp 147-158.)

subdividing stage 2 based on the presence or absence of surrounding edema.[23] The same researchers reclassified lesions with subchondral cysts as stage 5.[23] In 2003, an MRI grading system based on an earlier arthroscopic grading system, the Mintz classification, was described[24] (Table 1). Fifty patients (52 OLTs) who had undergone both MRI and ankle arthroscopy were studied to examine the correlation between MRI and arthroscopic staging using the Mintz classification.[25] These authors concluded that MRI has accuracy of 81% in staging of OLTs, similar to the 83% accuracy depicted in Mintz's 2003 original article.[25] Pritsch and colleagues and the International Cartilage Repair Society[18,26] have described additional arthroscopic grading systems.

Nonsurgical Treatment

A trial of nonsurgical management for OLTs is typically appropriate for nondisplaced lesions. Several authors recommend a trial period minimum of 3 months;[27] however, there is no clear consensus on the ideal regimen. Nonsurgical treatment ranges from non–weight-bearing in a cast to protected weight bearing in a boot.[12] An updated systematic review in 2010 demonstrated that the use of immobilization over a period ranging from 3 weeks to 4 months demonstrated a 53% success rate.[28] Rest or activity modification alone was reported in three studies with a

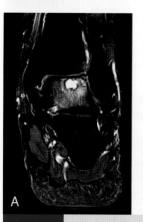
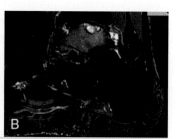

Figure 4 Coronal (**A**) and sagittal (**B**) T2-weighted images of the left ankle demonstrate a lateral talar dome osteochondral lesion.

45% success rate.[28] Published reports have demonstrated that a trial of nonsurgical management does not have a negative effect on later surgical treatment.[14,29]

Table 1

Mintz and Associates' MRI Classification Compared With Cheng's Arthroscopic Staging System for Osteochondral Lesions of the Talus

MRI	Arthroscopic
Grade 0: Normal	Stage A: Smooth, intact but soft
Grade I: Hyperintense but intact cartilage surface	Stage B: Rough surface
Grade II: Fibrillation of fissures not extending to bone	Stage C: Fibrillation or fissuring
Grade III: Flap present or exposed bone	Stage D: Flap present or exposed bone
Grade IV: Loose, nondisplaced fragment	Stage E: Loose, nondisplaced fragment
Grade V: Displaced fragment	Stage F: Displaced fragment

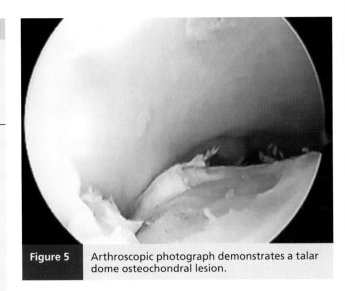

Figure 5 Arthroscopic photograph demonstrates a talar dome osteochondral lesion.

Surgical Treatment

Surgical intervention is indicated for acute displaced OLTs and for those refractory to nonsurgical care. The approach and objectives of surgery are variable and are determined by type of lesion. Goals may range from removal of a loose fragment to securing a larger fragment anatomically. Alternatively, the primary objective may be to create an environment amenable to fibrocartilaginous proliferation or resurfacing with hyaline cartilage.[12]

The primary traditional approach includes open ankle arthrotomy. Numerous exposure methods have been described, including several variations of medial malleolar osteotomies and distal tibial osteotomies along with combined anterior and posterior arthrotomies.[3,29-32] Open approaches produce significant tissue trauma and, as a result, may be associated with postoperative stiffness, prolonged rehabilitation time, and poor cosmetic appearance. Additionally, nonunion or malunion of the malleoli is a risk with approaches involving a malleolar osteotomy. Inadequate visualization of talar dome lesions, particularly posterior lesions, remains a primary limitation of any open approach.[3,29]

Ankle arthroscopy has been established as a useful tool in OLT diagnosis and treatment (**Figure 5**). When compared to an extensive open approach, arthroscopy provides superior visualization of the talar dome and improved access to the lesion. As a result of recent advances, arthroscopic management of OLTs is now the preferred technique.[12,33,34]

A wide variety of procedures that vary in complexity have been described for the treatment of OLTs. Treatment strategies generally are categorized as primary repair, reparative techniques, or restorative techniques. Marrow-inducing reparative treatments include abrasion arthroplasty, microfracture, and drilling techniques. Restorative techniques primarily include autologous chondrocyte implantation (ACI), osteochondral autologous transfer system (OATS) and mosaicplasty, and osteochondral allograft. Future directions in restorative techniques for OLTs include matrix/membrane ACI (MACI), collagen-covered ACI, arthroscopic allograft/autograft with platelet-rich plasma (PRP) implantation, stem cell–mediated cartilage implants, and scaffolds.[12,27,33]

A systematic review of 52 published reports describing the results of 65 treatment groups indicated that most recent publications on treatment of OLTs involve arthroscopic excision, curettage, and bone marrow stimulation (BMS), ACI, or OATS with success rates of 85%, 76%, and 87, respectively.[28] As a result, the authors recommended arthroscopic excision, curettage, and BMS as initial treatment because it is relatively inexpensive and is associated with low morbidity and a high success rate. However, because of diversity in the literature and highly variable treatment results, the authors could not draw definitive conclusions.[28]

When selecting the appropriate treatment option, several important variables should be considered. It is imperative to delineate, primarily from advanced imaging, the type, stability, and displacement of the lesion. Chronicity, size, location, and containment are other important factors to consider.

The prime variable to consider when choosing between a reparative versus a restorative technique is the size of the lesion. The prognostic significance of defect size on

MRI was examined in a large series of patients treated by arthroscopic marrow stimulation techniques.[35] The authors identified a cutoff point of 150 mm² for a defect size at which risk factors for poor outcomes became evident.[35] In a larger study, the subjective clinical outcomes of 130 patients after marrow stimulation for OLTs was retrospectively reviewed.[36] Numerous variables were examined, including patient age, body mass index, history of trauma, location, cystic nature, and containment of the lesion.[36] The authors found that lesion size larger than 1.5 cm² was the most important predictor of a poor outcome. Uncontained OLTs and age also contributed to overall outcome.[36] It was later demonstrated that patients with an uncontained shoulder-type osteochondral lesion, whether medial or lateral, have worse clinical outcomes with arthroscopic marrow stimulation techniques than those who have a contained nonshoulder-type lesion.[37] This was true even when the increased size of the shoulder-type lesion was taken into account. Using a novel three-dimensional geometric MRI profile of the osteochondral lesion, with emphasis on preoperative lesion depth and volume, it was determined that lesion depth of more than 7.8 mm and patient age older than 80 years were predictors of an unsatisfactory outcome following arthroscopic BMS.[38] It was suggested that lesion depth has a more significant association with clinical outcome than lesion area.[38]

Surgical Recommendations

Primary Repair
Primary repair of the OLT with internal fixation is indicated after acute osteochondral fracture of the talus and for larger lesions with intact articular cartilage. A 2003 systematic review of osteochondral defect treatment revealed a 73% success rate with this method.[27] More recent published studies regarding primary repair of OLTs are not available.

Arthroscopic BMS
For symptomatic OLTs that are smaller than 150 mm², the current recommendation is arthroscopic BMS with débridement, drilling, and microfracture or curettage of the lesion. The purpose of this procedure is to excise the loose or delaminated articular cartilage and to promote fibrocartilage formation over the defect. The fibrocartilaginous material is composed of mostly type 1 collagen rather than hyaline cartilage. The literature was reviewed to determine the prognostic factors affecting the clinical outcome after arthroscopic BMS and concluded that inferior clinical outcome is associated with lesions larger than 150 mm² and uncontained lesions.[39] The authors also found that advancing age and cystic formation may

not influence the outcome after surgery. A 2013 study[40] examined outcomes in 50 patients who had arthroscopic BMS for OLTs smaller than 150 mm². The study's authors concluded that medial lesions, especially uncovered medial lesions, were associated with worse outcomes than lateral lesions. Patients who were older than 40 years of age had inferior outcomes. No correlation was found between lesion size or body mass index and clinical outcome. In 2012, investigators examined the various techniques of arthroscopic BMS for the treatment of OLTs ranging in size from 0.9 cm² to 4.5 cm² in 198 patients.[41] All procedures involved excising the unstable cartilage and performing microfracture to depths of 2 to 4 mm and 3 to 4 mm apart. Excellent or good results were obtained in 81% of cases. Another study investigated the results of arthroscopic microfracture of OLTs in 22 patients, 18 of whom had no or mild occasional pain 2 years after surgery. MRI showed that most defects were completely (7) or partially (11) filled in.[42,43] Authors of a 2013 study described a four-step approach with synovectomy, débridement and microfracture, capsular shrinkage, and non–weight-bearing bracing for posttraumatic OLTs in 38 patients; 82% had good/excellent results and 71% experienced filling of the defect based on MRI obtained at 18 months after surgery.[43] A recent study examined the long-term result of arthroscopic treatment of osteochondral defect of the talus with a mean follow-up of 12 years.[44] The authors reported 74% good, 20% fair, and 6% poor results in this study group. In summary, the success rate of arthroscopic BMS for the treatment of OLTs is approximately 80%. Medial uncontained lesions have a worse prognosis compared to lateral lesions after arthroscopic BMS. Postoperative MRI can show evidence of filling of the defect.

Osteochondral Graft
For larger OLTs, osteochondral autograft or allograft can be used to fill the defect. Osteochondral autograft usually is obtained from the superior medial edge of the medial femoral condyle and bone plugs are transplanted into the prepared OLT defect. For lesions that are too large (>1.5 cm²), especially with a large cystic component involving the shoulder of the talus, osteochondral allograft can be used. When more than one plug is used, the technique is known as mosaicplasty. A new method with which to harvest periosteum-covered plugs from the iliac crest for transplantation into OLTs was described.[45] Thirteen patients experienced improvement of American Orthopaedic Foot and Ankle Society (AOFAS) score from a mean score of 47 preoperatively to 81 postoperatively. At the time of follow-up, plug consolidation was present in 9 of 11 ankles based on plain radiographic evaluation; however, arthroscopic evaluation revealed fibrocartilage

formation in only 4 ankles and periosteal hypertrophy in 5 ankles. The authors of a 2012 study[46] reported 95% good to excellent results in 52 patients with osteochondral autograft transplants. The osteochondral plugs were harvested from the lateral edge of the lateral trochlea of the femoral condyle. At the second-look arthroscopy a mean of 13 months after surgery, the incongruency at the medial malleolar osteotomy, presence of soft-tissue impingement, and uncovered areas around the graft were associated with poor results. The authors did not report any donor site morbidity at the ipsilateral knee.

Autologous Chondrocyte Implantation

ACI for the treatment of OLTs involves implantation of viable chondrocytes into the defect. In 1994, investigators[26] developed ACI for the treatment of osteochondral knee lesions. This is a two-stage procedure in which chondrocytes are harvested from the donor site and cells are implanted into the osteochondral defect. According to a 2012 study, lesions smaller than 137.6 mm^2 and age younger than 26 years were predictors of a better outcome at the time of second-look arthroscopy 1 year after ACI.[47] For the 38 patients in this study, sex, accompanying procedure, lesion depth and location, and preoperative AOFAS score did not influence healing of the cartilage. The 10-year follow-up results of ACI using MRI T2 mapping in 10 patients were reviewed, and it was determined that the regenerated cartilage had similar T2 mapping values as healthy hyaline cartilage.[48]

Matrix/Membrane Autologous Chondrocyte Implantation

The second generation of ACI, MACI, involves imbedding harvested and expanded autologous chondrocytes into a type I/III collagen bilayer or hyaluronic acid scaffold before implantation. As with ACI, MACI has been shown to result in formation of hyaline-like cartilage[49]; however, unlike ACI, MACI does not require a periosteal patch and the associated morbidity of periosteal harvest and possible hypertrophy. Moreover, there is no risk of chondrocyte cell leakage or uneven cell distribution within the talar defect because the chondrocytes are evenly embedded within the stable matrix and affixed to the defect with fibrin glue.[50] As a salvage procedure performed for ankles not affected by arthritis, "kissing lesions," instability, or axial defects that occur after failed débridement and curettage or microfracture, results to date are promising. A 2010 study[50]reported on 10 patients with full-thickness talar dome osteochondral lesions treated with MACI and observed improvement in physical function and pain as measured by the SF-36 and improved AOFAS hindfoot scores at 1 and 2 years in all patients. These authors noted that, unlike ACI, the MACI technique offers the advantage of no required malleolar osteotomy.[50] The authors of a 2012 study[51] treated 30 OLTs with an average size of 2.36 cm^2. Twenty-five MACI procedures were performed arthroscopically and only five necessitated a malleolar osteotomy because of the posterior location of the lesion. At an average of 45 months after surgery, 93.4% of patients had excellent or good results and 50% returned to sports 2 months postoperatively; investigators found good integration of the grafts as demonstrated by MRI. In another study,[52] 46 patients were treated arthroscopically; 80% experienced good or excellent results that were maintained over time and the return to sport rate was 86%. The authors of a 2011 study[53] described the use of a porcine-origin collagen matrix implanted in a single stage in one patient with a large (3 cm^2) OLT prepared with débridement and antegrade drilling. The patient had no pain and an AOFAS score of 100 at 1 year, full osseous consolidation of the graft, and a near-anatomic contour of the medial talar edge. Because this technique, termed autologous matrix-induced chondrogenesis, is a single-stage procedure involving mesenchymal cell invasion into a matrix as opposed to a two-stage procedure to harvest, expand, and embed chondrocytes into a matrix, the authors advocate this technique as a less morbid alternative to MACI for large lesions. A 2013 study[54] reported on the use of fibrin matrix-mixed gel-type ACI in the treatment of 38 OLTs, 34 of which had excellent, good, or fair subjective results. Analysis of chondrocyte regeneration by second-look arthroscopy at 12 months and MRI at 24 months after surgery revealed that 75% of OLTs were graded as normal or nearly normal.

Allograft Transplantation

Allograft transplantation, like ACI, can be used to treat larger lesions in patients who are too young or active for arthroplasty or arthrodesis; unlike ACI, however, this intervention obviates the need for a two-stage procedure and potential for donor site morbidity and it can be used to treat lesions involving large volumes of subchondral bone.[55] The use of both frozen and fresh talar allograft has been described.[56,57,] Despite good integration of frozen allograft into host bone, the process of cryopreservation may be associated with a decreased number of viable chondrocytes and may prove suboptimal compared to fresh allografts.[57] One long-term study with an average follow-up of 11 years reported that 6 of 9 patients treated with allograft transplants retained functional grafts, with the remaining 3 requiring conversion to arthrodesis.[58] A subsequent study reported 4-year midterm results in 13 patients with an average age of 30 years who underwent fresh allograft transplantation.[59] Although five of these patients required additional surgeries because of prominent hardware and soft-tissue impingement, all eventually had good results with 100% graft incorporation, improved pain and function, return to at least low-demand activities of daily living, and, in 11 patients, return to high-impact activities by 1 year.[59] Although showing promising results, these two studies may be limited by their small sample size. In contrast, the authors of a 2011 study were able to report their experience with 38 of 42 patients who underwent fresh allograft transplantation with an average follow-up of just over 3 years.[60] Although four grafts failed, the average pain and functional scores significantly improved, and 74% of the patients reported satisfaction with the procedure as good to excellent.[60] Tempering these positive clinical results, posttransplant MRI performed on a subset of 15 of these patients revealed that although there was little graft subsidence, instability, or loss of articular congruence, 80% of the grafts appeared to be unincorporated into surrounding native bone.[60] Other disadvantages of allograft transplantation include the cost and inconvenience of obtaining grafts from a tissue bank and the potential for transmission of disease and immunologic rejection, although preparation of grafts with pulsatile lavage to remove donor immunogenic cells may decrease this risk.[57,59]

Particulated Juvenile Cartilage

For OLTs typically larger than 100 mm^2, ACI/MACI and allograft transplant are particularly useful because they involve restoration of a hyaline or hyaline-like articular surface. However, these techniques are technically challenging and, for ACI, necessitate a two-stage procedure. A recently devised alternative is particulated juvenile cartilage implantation, in which prepackaged cartilage allograft from juvenile donors is placed directly into the talar lesion in a single-stage procedure. The authors of a 2013 study reported the use of this technique for 24 OLTs judged unlikely to respond well to BMS alone.[61] The average lesion size and depth were 125 mm^2 and 7 mm, respectively, and 16 of the 24 lesions were uncontained. Lesions were approached according to surgeon preference, either arthroscopically or by limited arthrotomy. The technique involved applying a thin layer of fibrin glue to the prepared lesion surface, followed by the particulated juvenile cartilage, and finally covering the cartilage with a second thin layer of fibrin glue after which the ankle was ranged to mold the construct. Although the retrospective nature of the study precluded comparison to preoperative functional outcome scores, postoperative results at an average of 16.2 months are encouraging, with 92% good or excellent results in lesions 10 to 15 mm in the largest dimension. In contrast, these investigators found only 56% good or excellent results in lesions at least 15 mm in size in the largest dimension, suggesting that particulated

juvenile cartilage may offer a good gap strategy for lesions larger than 100 mm^2 but smaller than 150 mm^2.

Future Directions

Stem Cell Therapy

Stem cell therapy holds great promise for OLT treatment but currently has limited applicability; it may be used as an adjunct to marrow stimulation treatment, however. Microfracture relies on penetration through the subchondral plate to underlying bone marrow with subsequent release of mesenchymal stem cells (MSCs) into the cartilage defect where they may differentiate into chondrocytes. Because density of MSCs within a patient's marrow appears to decline with age, the addition of MSCs previously harvested from other sites into the microfractured lesion may benefit older patients.[62] A recent study compared the outcomes of OLTs in older patients treated with either microfracture alone or with microfracture plus the addition of MSCs harvested from the gluteal fat pad.[63] These investigators found that patients older than 50 years experienced better improvement in pain, level of activity, and satisfaction when MSCs were used as an adjunct to microfracture compared to microfracture alone.[63]

Bone Marrow–Derived Cells

The transformation of human MSCs toward the chondrocyte lineage requires the complex interaction of MSCs with their physiologic environment, including the extracellular matrix, local adhesion molecules, cytokines, growth factors, and chemokines.[64] Because both MSCs and many of these essential factors exist in autologous bone marrow, concentrated bone marrow aspirate may provide a new strategy for articular cartilage restoration. A prospective study of 48 patients with lesions larger than 150 mm^2 and less than 5 mm deep showed that a single-step arthroscopic procedure in which iliac crest harvested bone marrow aspirate was imbedded within a collagen or hyaluronic acid scaffold and implanted into prepared talar defects using a platelet-rich fibrin gel resulted in improved AOFAS scores within a range comparable to that achieved with other widely used treatment techniques.[64] Moreover, second-look arthroscopy in three asymptomatic patients demonstrated complete integration of the graft and macroscopic appearance of new cartilage that was similar to surrounding native cartilage. Two more patients underwent arthroscopic chondroplasty to treat MRI-demonstrated cartilage hypertrophy; histologic analysis of these two patients showed varying degrees of tissue remodeling toward a hyaline cartilage lineage. MRI T2 mapping corroborates the success of this technique in regenerating articular cartilage; as much as

78% of regenerated tissue demonstrated relaxation times comparable to that achieved with hyaline as opposed to fibrocartilage.[65]

Platelet-Rich Plasma

In vitro studies demonstrate that PRP may increase chondrocyte proliferation and production of collagen, and stimulate MSC migration, proliferation, and chondrogenic differentiation.[66] In addition, PRP has been shown to suppress many of the catabolic mediators present in inflammatory intra-articular environments that would otherwise add to further cartilage injury and inhibit cartilage regeneration. Despite the theoretical rationale for its use, it remains to be seen what role, if any, PRP will play in treatment of OLTs.

Summary

Nonsurgical and surgical OLT treatments continue to pose challenges. The success rate of surgical treatment is dependent on many variables such as lesion size, location, and containment and patient age. As research on articular cartilage restoration continues, future OLT treatments will improve.

Annotated References

1. Konig F: Über freie Korper in den Gelenken. *Dtsch Z Chir* 1888;27:90.

2. Kappis M: Weitere Beitrange zur traumatisch-mechanischen Entstehung der "spontanen" Knorpelablosungen (sogen. Osteochondritis dissecans). *Dtsch Z Chir* 1922;171:c13.

3. Berndt AL, Harty M: Transchondral fracture fractures (osteochondritis dissecans) of the talus. *J Bone Joint Surg Am* 1959;41:988-1020.

4. Ferkel RD, Fasulo GJ: Arthroscopic treatment of ankle injuries. *Orthop Clin North Am* 1994;25(1):17-32.

5. Bosien WR, Staples OS, Russell SW: Residual disability following acute ankle sprains. *J Bone Joint Surg Am* 1955;37-A(6):1237-1243.

6. Orr JD, Dawson LK, Garcia EJ, Kirk KL: Incidence of osteochondral lesions of the talus in the US military. *Foot Ankle Int* 2011;32(10):948-954.

   An epidemiologic study examining the active-duty United States military population found an overall incidence of OLT of 27 per 100,000 patient years over a 10-year period. This suggests that OLTs may be more common than previously considered. Level of evidence: IV.

7. Hermanson E, Ferkel RD: Bilateral osteochondral lesions of the talus. *Foot Ankle Int* 2009;30(8):723-727.

   A database search of 526 patients treated between 1984 and 2007 found that the overall incidence of bilateral involvement was 10%. Most patients with bilateral involvement had the OLT located on the medial side. Level of evidence: IV.

8. Raikin SM, Elias I, Zoga AC, Morrison WB, Besser MP, Schweitzer ME: Osteochondral lesions of the talus: Localization and morphologic data from 424 patients using a novel anatomical grid scheme. *Foot Ankle Int* 2007;28(2):154-161.

9. Hembree WC, Wittstein JR, Vinson EN, et al: Magnetic resonance imaging features of osteochondral lesions of the talus. *Foot Ankle Int* 2012;33(7):591-597.

   These authors retrospectively reviewed the location, frequency, and size of OLTs of the talus on 77 MRI examinations based on a nine-zone grid. These findings support the notion that the most common osteochondral lesions are not the traditionally described anterolateral and posteromedial lesions, but rather central medial and central lateral lesions. Investigators also found that lesion location does not appear to predict subject age, lesion chronicity, history of trauma, or lesion instability. However, medial lesions were larger and the lateral lesions were seen more commonly in association with ligamentous injury.

10. Orr JD, Dutton JR, Fowler JT: Anatomic location and morphology of symptomatic, operatively treated osteochondral lesions of the talus. *Foot Ankle Int* 2012;33(12):1051-1057.

    Using the same nine-zone grid described by Elias et al, these investigators performed a retrospective examination of all preoperative MRIs performed over a 4-year period in patients who underwent primary surgical management of symptomatic OLTs. Their results supported those of Elias and Hembree; however, they noted that symptomatic surgically treated osteochondral defects of the talus were located in the lateral third of the talar dome almost twice as commonly as in the medial third (65% versus 35%). Level of evidence: IV.

11. van Dijk CN, Reilingh ML, Zengerink M, van Bergen CJ: Osteochondral defects in the ankle: Why painful? *Knee Surg Sports Traumatol Arthrosc* 2010;18(5):570-580.

    The development of symptomatic osteochondral defects is dependent on various factors. The primary mechanism is damage and insufficient repair of the subchondral bone plate. These authors theorize that water from compressed cartilage is forced into the microfractured subchondral bone during loading, which subsequently leads to localized increased fluid pressure within the subchondral bone. Local osteolysis can then predispose to the development of a subchondral cyst. The pain is believed to be a result of stimulation of the highly innervated subchondral bone under the cartilage defect.

12. Ferkel RD, Dierckman BD, Phisitkul P: Arthroscopy of the foot and ankle, in Coughlin MJ, Saltzman CL, Anderson RB, eds: *Surgery of the Foot and Ankle,* ed 9. Philadelphia, PA, Elsevier, 2014, pp 1748-1758.

13. Saxena A, Eakin C: Articular talar injuries in athletes: Results of microfracture and autogenous bone graft. *Am J Sports Med* 2007;35(10):1680-1687.

14. Flick AB, Gould N: Osteochondritis dissecans of the talus (transchondral fractures of the talus): Review of the literature and new surgical approach for medial dome lesions. *Foot Ankle* 1985;5(4):165-185.

15. Elias I, Jung JW, Raikin SM, Schweitzer MW, Carrino JA, Morrison WB: Osteochondral lesions of the talus: Change in MRI findings over time in talar lesions without operative intervention and implications for staging systems. *Foot Ankle Int* 2006;27(3):157-166.

16. Bauer M, Jonsson K, Lindén B: Osteochondritis dissecans of the ankle. A 20-year follow-up study. *J Bone Joint Surg Br* 1987;69(1):93-96.

17. Loomer R, Fisher C, Lloyd-Smith R, Sisler J, Cooney T: Osteochondral lesions of the talus. *Am J Sports Med* 1993;21(1):13-19.

18. Pritsch M, Horoshovski H, Farine I: Arthroscopic treatment of osteochondral lesions of the talus. *J Bone Joint Surg Am* 1986;68(6):862-865.

19. Zinman C, Wolfson N, Reis ND: Osteochondritis dissecans of the dome of the talus. Computed tomography scanning in diagnosis and follow-up. *J Bone Joint Surg Am* 1988;70(7):1017-1019.

20. Ferkel RD, Sgaglione NA, DelPizzo W, et al: Arthroscopic treatment of osteochondral lesions of the talus: Long-term results. *Orthop Trans* 1990;14:172-173.

21. Loredo R, Sanders TG: Imaging of osteochondral injuries. *Clin Sports Med* 2001;20(2):249-278.

22. Anderson IF, Crichton KJ, Grattan-Smith T, Cooper RA, Brazier D: Osteochondral fractures of the dome of the talus. *J Bone Joint Surg Am* 1989;71(8):1143-1152.

23. Hepple S, Winson IG, Glew D: Osteochondral lesions of the talus: A revised classification. *Foot Ankle Int* 1999;20(12):789-793.

24. Mintz DN, Tashjian GS, Connell DA, Deland JT, O'Malley M, Potter HG: Osteochondral lesions of the talus: A new magnetic resonance grading system with arthroscopic correlation. *Arthroscopy* 2003;19(4):353-359.

25. Lee KB, Bai LB, Park JG, Yoon TR: A comparison of arthroscopic and MRI findings in staging of osteochondral lesions of the talus. *Knee Surg Sports Traumatol Arthrosc* 2008;16(11):1047-1051.

These authors prospectively investigated 50 patients (52 cases) who had undergone both MRI and ankle arthroscopy for OLTs to investigate the correlations between MRI and arthroscopic staging using the Mintz classification. They concluded that MRI has accuracy of 81% in staging of OLTs, similar to the 83% accuracy depicted in Mintz's 2003 original article.

26. Brittberg M, Winalski CS: Evaluation of cartilage injuries and repair. *J Bone Joint Surg Am* 2003;85-A(suppl 2):58-69.

27. Verhagen RA, Struijs PA, Bossuyt PM, van Dijk CN: Systematic review of treatment strategies for osteochondral defects of the talar dome. *Foot Ankle Clin* 2003;8(2):233-242, viii-ix.

28. Zengerink M, Struijs PA, Tol JL, van Dijk CN: Treatment of osteochondral lesions of the talus: A systematic review. *Knee Surg Sports Traumatol Arthrosc* 2010;18(2):238-246.

In a systematic review, the authors concluded that BMS is the treatment of choice for primary OLTs. However, in light of the diversity in the literature and high variability in treatment results, they state that no definitive conclusions can be drawn. A recent systematic review of 52 published reports describing the results of 65 treatment groups was published in 2010. These authors indicate that most of the recent publications on treatment of OLTs involve arthroscopic excision, curettage and BMS, ACI, and OATS. They scored success percentages of 85, 76, and 87, respectively. As a result, they recommend arthroscopic excision, curettage, and BMS as the first treatment of choice because it is relatively inexpensive and is associated with low morbidity and a high success rate.

29. Alexander AH, Lichtman DM: Surgical treatment of transchondral talar-dome fractures (osteochondritis dissecans). Long-term follow-up. *J Bone Joint Surg Am* 1980;62(4):646-652.

30. Alexander AH, Lichtman DM: Surgical treatment of transchondral talar-dome fractures (osteochondritis dissecans). Long-term follow-up. *J Bone Joint Surg Am* 1980;62(4):646-652.

31. Lee KB, Yang HK, Moon ES, Song EK: Modified step-cut medial malleolar osteotomy for osteochondral grafting of the talus. *Foot Ankle Int* 2008;29(11):1107-1110.

The modified step-cut medial malleolar osteotomy provided better results than traditional osteotomy in 10 patients studied.

32. Young KW, Deland JT, Lee KT, Lee YK: Medial approaches to osteochondral lesion of the talus without medial malleolar osteotomy. *Knee Surg Sports Traumatol Arthrosc* 2010;18(5):634-637.

The authors determined the area of the talus that can be accessed via anterior and posterior arthrotomy without medial malleolar osteotomy.

7: Tendon Disorders and Sports-Related Foot and Ankle Injuries

33. Giannini S, Vannini F: Operative treatment of osteochondral lesions of the talar dome: Current concepts review. *Foot Ankle Int* 2004;25(3):168-175.

34. Kim HN, Kim GL, Park JY, Woo KJ, Park YW: Fixation of a posteromedial osteochondral lesion of the talus using a three-portal posterior arthroscopic technique. *J Foot Ankle Surg* 2013;52(3):402-405.

   The authors discuss a three-portal posterior arthroscopic technique to access a posteromedial osteochondral talar lesion and osteochondral fragment fixation in the absence of transmalleolar drilling or malleolar osteotomy.

35. Choi WJ, Park KK, Kim BS, Lee JW: Osteochondral lesion of the talus: Is there a critical defect size for poor outcome? *Am J Sports Med* 2009;37(10):1974-1980.

   The authors examined the prognostic significance of defect size using MRI in a large series of patients treated by arthroscopic marrow stimulation techniques. They identified a cutoff point of 150 mm^2 for a defect size at which risk factors for poor outcomes became evident. Level of evidence: III.

36. Cuttica DJ, Smith WB, Hyer CF, Philbin TM, Berlet GC: Osteochondral lesions of the talus: Predictors of clinical outcome. *Foot Ankle Int* 2011;32(11):1045-1051.

   In this large study, the authors retrospectively reviewed the subjective clinical outcomes of 130 patients after marrow stimulation for OLTs. Numerous variables were examined, including patient age, body mass index, history of trauma, location, cystic nature, and containment of the lesion. They found that lesion size larger than 1.5 cm^2 was the most important predictor of a poor outcome. Uncontained OLTs and age were also shown to contribute to overall outcome. Level of evidence: IV.

37. Choi WJ, Choi GW, Kim JS, Lee JW: Prognostic significance of the containment and location of osteochondral lesions of the talus: Independent adverse outcomes associated with uncontained lesions of the talar shoulder. *Am J Sports Med* 2013;41(1):126-133.

   The authors demonstrated that patients with an uncontained shoulder-type osteochondral lesion, whether medial or lateral, have worse clinical outcomes following arthroscopic marrow stimulation techniques than those with a contained, nonshoulder-type lesion. This was true even when the increased size of the shoulder-type lesion was taken into account. Level of evidence: III.

38. Angthong C, Yoshimura I, Kanazawa K, et al: Critical three-dimensional factors affecting outcome in osteochondral lesion of the talus. *Knee Surg Sports Traumatol Arthrosc* 2013;21(6):1418-1426.

   Using a novel 3D-geometric MRI profile of the osteochondral lesion, with specific emphasis on preoperative lesion depth and volume, investigators found that lesion depth exceeding 7.8 mm and patient age older than 80 years predicted an unsatisfactory outcome following arthroscopic BMS. They argued that lesion depth has a more significant association with clinical outcome than lesion area. Level of evidence: III.

39. Choi WJ, Jo J, Lee JW: Osteochondral lesion of the talus: Prognostic factors affecting the clinical outcome after arthroscopic marrow stimulation technique. *Foot Ankle Clin* 2013;18(1):67-78.

   The authors report the prognostic factors affecting the clinical outcome after arthroscopic BMS after reviewing the literature. They conclude that an inferior clinical outcome is associated with lesions larger than 150 mm^2 and uncontained lesions. They also found that increasing age and cystic formation may not influence the outcome after surgery.

40. Yoshimura I, Kanazawa K, Takeyama A, et al: Arthroscopic bone marrow stimulation techniques for osteochondral lesions of the talus: Prognostic factors for small lesions. *Am J Sports Med* 2013;41(3):528-534.

   Fifty patients underwent arthroscopic BMS for OLTs smaller than 150 mm^2. The authors concluded that medial lesions, especially uncovered medial lesions, had worse outcomes than lateral lesions. Patients who were older than 40 years had inferior outcomes. No correlation was found between lesion size or body mass index and clinical outcomes. Level of evidence: IV.

41. Kok AC, Dunnen Sd, Tuijthof GJ, van Dijk CN, Kerkhoffs GM: Is technique performance a prognostic factor in bone marrow stimulation of the talus? *J Foot Ankle Surg* 2012;51(6):777-782.

   The authors evaluated various techniques of arthroscopic BMS for the treatment of OLTs sized between 0.9 cm^2 and 4.5 cm^2 in 198 patients. All procedures involved excision of unstable cartilage. With each procedure, microfracture to a depth of 2 to 4 mm and 3 to 4 mm apart was performed. The excellent/good result was 81%. Level of evidence: II.

42. Kuni B, Schmitt H, Chloridis D, Ludwig K: Clinical and MRI results after microfracture of osteochondral lesions of the talus. *Arch Orthop Trauma Surg* 2012;132(12):1765-1771.

   Twenty-two patients underwent arthroscopic microfracture. This study showed that 18 of 22 patients had no or mild occasional pain 2 years after surgery. MRI showed that the majority of the defect was completely (7) or partially (11) filled in. Level of evidence: IV.

43. Ventura A, Terzaghi C, Legnani C, Borgo E: Treatment of post-traumatic osteochondral lesions of the talus: A four-step approach. *Knee Surg Sports Traumatol Arthrosc* 2013;21(6):1245-1250.

   The authors reported a four-step approach with synovectomy, débridement and microfracture, capsular shrinkage, and non-weight–bearing bracing for posttraumatic OLTs in 38 patients. Eighty-two percent of the patients had good/excellent result. Seventy-one percent of the cases had filling of the defect based on MRI performed 18 months after surgeryLevel of evidence: IV.

44. van Bergen CJ, Kox LS, Maas M, Sierevelt IN, Kerkhoffs GM, van Dijk CN: Arthroscopic treatment of osteochondral defects of the talus: Outcomes at eight to twenty years of follow-up. *J Bone Joint Surg Am* 2013;95(6):519-525.

This study suggested that initial success of arthroscopic débridement and bone marrow stimulation for osteochondral defects of the talus are maintained over time. At a mean follow-up of 12 years, 74% of patients rated results as good, 20% as fair, and 6% as poor. Compared with the preoperative osteoarthritis classification, 67% of radiographs showed no progression and 33% showed progression by one grade. Level of evidence: IV.

45. Leumann A, Valderrabano V, Wiewiorski M, Barg A, Hintermann B, Pagenstert G: Bony periosteum-covered iliac crest plug transplantation for severe osteochondral lesions of the talus: A modified mosaicplasty procedure. *Knee Surg Sports Traumatol Arthrosc* 2014;22(6):1304-1310.

A new method of harvesting periosteum-covered plugs from the iliac crest and transplantation into the OLT was described. AOFAS scores of 13 patients improved from a mean score of 47 preoperatively to 81 postoperatively. At the time of follow-up, consolidation of the plug was present in 9 of 11 ankles based on plain radiographic evaluation. However, arthroscopic evaluation revealed fibrocartilage formation only in four ankles and periosteal hypertrophy in five ankles. Level of evidence: IV.

46. Kim YS, Park EH, Kim YC, Koh YG, Lee JW: Factors associated with the clinical outcomes of the osteochondral autograft transfer system in osteochondral lesions of the talus: Second-look arthroscopic evaluation. *Am J Sports Med* 2012;40(12):2709-2719.

The authors reported a 95% good to excellent result in 52 patients who underwent osteochondral autograft transplantation. The osteochondral plugs were harvested from the lateral edge of the lateral trochlea of the femoral condyle. At the second-look arthroscopy at a mean of 13 months after surgery, the incongruency at the medial malleolar osteotomy, presence of soft-tissue impingement, and uncovered areas around the graft were associated with poor result. The authors did not report any donor site morbidity at the ipsilateral knee. Level of evidence: IV.

47. Lee KT, Lee YK, Young KW, Park SY, Kim JS: Factors influencing result of autologous chondrocyte implantation in osteochondral lesion of the talus using second look arthroscopy. *Scand J Med Sci Sports* 2012;22(4):510-515.

A lesion smaller than 137.6 mm² and age younger than 26 years were associated with better outcomes at the time of second-look arthroscopy at 1 year after ACI. Authors of this 38-patient study found that sex, accompanied procedure, depth and location of the lesion, and preoperative AOFAS score did not influence healing of the cartilage.

48. Giannini S, Battaglia M, Buda R, Cavallo M, Ruffilli A, Vannini F: Surgical treatment of osteochondral lesions of the talus by open-field autologous chondrocyte implantation: A 10-year follow-up clinical and magnetic resonance imaging T2-mapping evaluation. *Am J Sports Med* 2009;37(suppl 1):112S-118S.

The authors reviewed 10-year follow-up results of ACI using MRI T2 mapping evaluation on 10 patients. This study showed that the regenerated cartilage had a similar T2 mapping value as healthy hyaline cartilage. Level of evidence: IV.

49. Ronga M, Grassi FA, Montoli C, et al: Treatment of deep cartilage defects of the ankle with matrix-induced autologous chondrocyte implantation (MACI). *Foot Ankle Surg* 2005;11:29-33.

50. Giza E, Sullivan M, Ocel D, et al: Matrix-induced autologous chondrocyte implantation of talus articular defects. *Foot Ankle Int* 2010;31(9):747-753.

As a salvage procedure following failed débridement and curettage or microfracture, the authors reported on 10 patients with full-thickness talar dome osteochondral lesions treated with MACI and observed improvement in both physical function and pain out to 2 years. Level of evidence: IV.

51. Magnan B, Samaila E, Bondi M, Vecchini E, Micheloni GM, Bartolozzi P: Three-dimensional matrix-induced autologous chondrocytes implantation for osteochondral lesions of the talus: Midterm results. *Adv Orthop* 2012;2012:942174.

The authors treated 30 talar osteochondral lesions with an average size of 2.36 cm². Twenty-five cases were performed arthroscopically and only five required a malleolar osteotomy because of the posterior location of the lesion. At an average of 45 months excellent or good results were obtained in 93.4% of patients, return to sport in 50% of patients at 2 months after surgery, and good integration of grafts as demonstrated by MRI was noted.

52. Giannini S, Buda R, Vannini F, Di Caprio F, Grigolo B: Arthroscopic autologous chondrocyte implantation in osteochondral lesions of the talus: Surgical technique and results. *Am J Sports Med* 2008;36(5):873-880.

The authors treated 46 patients arthroscopically and realized 80% good or excellent results that sustained over time and an 86% rate of return to sport. Level of evidence: IV.

53. Wiewiorski M, Leumann A, Buettner O, Pagenstert G, Horisberger M, Valderrabano V: Autologous matrix-induced chondrogenesis aided reconstruction of a large focal osteochondral lesion of the talus. *Arch Orthop Trauma Surg* 2011;131(3):293-296.

The authors present a case report on the use of a porcine-origin collagen matrix implanted in a single stage in one patient with a large (3 cm²) OLT. The technique, autologous matrix-induced chondrogenesis, may offer numerous advantages over MACI with similarly good results. Level of evidence: V.

54. Lee KT, Kim JS, Young KW, et al: The use of fibrin matrix-mixed gel-type autologous chondrocyte implantation in the treatment for osteochondral lesions of the talus. *Knee Surg Sports Traumatol Arthrosc* 2013;21(6):1251-1260.

   The authors reported on the use of fibrin matrix-mixed gel-type ACI the treatment of OLT. Thirty-eight patients were involved in the study. Thirty-four patients reported excellent, good, or fair outcomes. The authors analyzed chondrocyte regeneration by second-look arthroscopy at 12 months and MRI at 24 months after surgery. Level of evidence: V.

55. Winters BS, Raikin SM: The use of allograft in joint-preserving surgery for ankle osteochondral lesions and osteoarthritis. *Foot Ankle Clin* 2013;18(3):529-542.

   This is an overview of the use of allograft transplantation for patients with large OLTs who are too young to undergo arthrodesis.

56. Raikin SM: Stage VI: Massive osteochondral defects of the talus. *Foot Ankle Clin* 2004;9:737-744.

57. Tasto JP, Ostrander R, Bugbee W, Brage M: The diagnosis and management of osteochondral lesions of the talus: Osteochondral allograft update. *Arthroscopy* 2003;19(suppl 1):138-141.

58. Gross AE, Agnidis Z, Hutchison CR: Osteochondral defects of the talus treated with fresh osteochondral allograft transplantation. *Foot Ankle Int* 2001;22(5):385-391.

59. Hahn DB, Aanstoos ME, Wilkins RM: Osteochondral lesions of the talus treated with fresh talar allografts. *Foot Ankle Int* 2010;31(4):277-282.

   The authors provide midterm results in 13 younger patients who underwent fresh talar allograft transplantation. Although 5 of 13 required additional surgery to address prominent hardware and soft-tissue impingement, all patients eventually had good results with 100% graft incorporation and improved pain and function. They returned to at least low-demand activities of daily living, and, in 11 cases, returned to high-impact activities by 1 year. Level of evidence: IV.

60. El-Rashidy H, Villacis D, Omar I, Kelikian AS: Fresh osteochondral allograft for the treatment of cartilage defects of the talus: A retrospective review. *J Bone Joint Surg Am* 2011;93(17):1634-1640.

   This study evaluated 38 patients with a mean follow-up duration of 37.7 months. The mean AOFAS score increased significantly from 52 points preoperatively to 79 points postoperatively. Graft failure occurred in four patients. A postoperative MRI was completed on 15 patients showing graft subsidence in one patient, who also had graft failure. Graft incorporation was rated as fair or poor in 12 patients (80%). One-third of the grafts were also graded as unstable according to the De Smet criteria.

61. Coetzee JC, Giza E, Schon LC, et al: Treatment of osteochondral lesions of the talus with particulated juvenile cartilage. *Foot Ankle Int* 2013;34(9):1205-1211.

   The authors provide a retrospective report on a series of 24 ankles judged unlikely to respond well to BMS alone treated with particulated juvenile cartilage secured with fibrin glue. Their postoperative results at an average of 16.2 months were encouraging, with 92% good or excellent results in lesions greater than 10 mm but less than 15 mm in the largest dimension. In contrast, they found only 56% good or excellent results in lesions at least 15 mm in size in the largest dimension, suggesting that particulated juvenile cartilage may offer a good gap strategy for lesions larger than 1 cm^2 but smaller than 1.5 cm^2. Level of evidence: IV.

62. Nishida S, Endo N, Yamagiwa H, Tanizawa T, Takahashi HE: Number of osteoprogenitor cells in human bone marrow markedly decreases after skeletal maturation. *J Bone Miner Metab* 1999;17(3):171-177.

63. Kim YS, Park EH, Kim YC, Koh YG: Clinical outcomes of mesenchymal stem cell injection with arthroscopic treatment in older patients with osteochondral lesions of the talus. *Am J Sports Med* 2013;41(5):1090-1099.

   This study compared the outcomes of older patients with OLTs treated with either microfracture alone or with microfracture plus the addition of MSCs harvested from the gluteal fat pad. They found that among patients older than 50 years, there was greater improvement in pain, level of activity, and satisfaction when MSCs were used as an adjunct to microfracture versus microfracture alone. Level of evidence: III.

64. Giannini S, Buda R, Vannini F, Cavallo M, Grigolo B: One-step bone marrow-derived cell transplantation in talar osteochondral lesions. *Clin Orthop Relat Res* 2009;467(12):3307-3320.

   A prospective study of 48 patients with lesions larger than 1.5 cm^2 and less than 5 mm deep showed that a single-step arthroscopic procedure in which iliac crest harvested bone marrow aspirate was imbedded within a collagen or hyaluronic acid scaffold and implanted into prepared talar defects using a platelet-rich fibrin gel resulted in improved AOFAS scores comparable to those achieved using other widely used treatment techniques, complete integration of the graft, and a macroscopic appearance of new cartilage that was similar to surrounding native cartilage. Level of evidence: IV.

65. Battaglia M, Rimondi E, Monti C, et al: Validity of T2 mapping in characterization of the regeneration tissue by bone marrow derived cell transplantation in osteochondral lesions of the ankle. *Eur J Radiol* 2011;80(2):e132-e139.

   MRI T2 mapping corroborated the success of the implanted bone marrow aspirate technique described by authors of a 2009 study on regenerating articular cartilage. Level of evidence: IV.

66. Smyth NA, Murawski CD, Haleem AM, Hannon CP, Savage-Elliott I, Kennedy JG: Establishing proof of concept: Platelet-rich plasma and bone marrow aspirate concentrate may improve cartilage repair following surgical treatment for OLTs. *World J Orthop* 2012;3(7):101-108.

This is a discussion of the theoretic rationale for the use of PRP in treating OLTs.

Chapter 31

Arthroscopy of the Foot and Ankle

David Hakbum Kim, MD

Introduction

Ankle arthroscopy has become an essential part of orthopaedic foot and ankle practice during the past 25 years. Ankle arthroscopy originally was primarily a diagnostic tool, but it is now widely used as a definitive treatment modality. Although anterior arthroscopy continues to be the most common type of procedure, posterior ankle arthroscopy also is poised to become a routine orthopaedic foot and ankle procedure.

Anterior Ankle Arthroscopy

Low complication rates can be expected when modern methods of anterior ankle arthroscopy are used. In general, patients with a workers' compensation claim have a higher-than-average complication rate, and patients who do not have a specific preoperative diagnosis are likely to have a relatively poor outcome.[1,2]

Indications

The conditions most commonly treated with anterior ankle arthroscopy are anterolateral impingement, anteromedial impingement, osteochondral lesions of the talus and tibia, and symptomatic loose bodies (**Figure 1**). Anterior ankle arthroscopy also is used for arthroscopically assisted arthrodesis, ankle stabilization, and fracture reduction. Evacuation, irrigation, and débridement of a septic ankle joint can be accomplished arthroscopically. Arthroscopic treatment of impingement lesions after total ankle arthroplasty recently was described and is likely to become more common with the increasing popularity of total ankle arthroplasty procedures.[3,4]

Technique

Most ankle arthroscopies can be done as outpatient ambulatory surgery. The typical modern setup for ankle arthroscopy includes a noninvasive distraction device

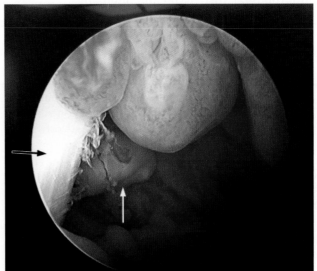

Figure 1 Arthroscopic photograph from the anterior ankle portal, showing a loose body (vertical arrow) in the posterior ankle. Synovitis also can be seen. Horizontal arrow points to the flexor hallucis longus tendon.

and a small joint arthroscope, usually 2.4 or 2.7 mm in diameter. A sterile backup arthroscope should be immediately available as a precaution against equipment malfunction. Gravity or an arthroscopic pump at a low setting can used for inflow. A thigh tourniquet typically is used. A padded thigh holder is useful for providing countertraction. Most complications are neurologic in origin, and prolonged use of traction should be avoided to prevent neurapraxia. Dorsiflexion of the ankle without traction helps the surgeon evaluate the anterior joint pouch by increasing its volume and may offer advantages over fixed distraction.[2,5]

An anteromedial portal is made at the joint level medial to the tibialis anterior tendon. The skin first is scratched or nicked, and a small hemostat is used to vertically spread the underlying soft tissue for entering the joint capsule. The saphenous nerve and vein can be put at risk with establishment of the anteromedial portal. The superficial peroneal nerve, which frequently can be seen through the skin, is at risk during establishment of the anterolateral portal. The superficial peroneal nerve moves 4 mm laterally when the ankle is brought from plantar flexion to neutral, and the anterolateral incision should be made medial to the visualized nerve to avoid iatrogenic damage.[6] Although the skin closure can be done according to surgeon preference, an improperly placed suture can irritate the intermediate branch of the superficial peroneal nerve.[1]

Anterolateral Soft-Tissue Impingement

Anterolateral soft-tissue impingement by the anteroinferior tibiofibular (Bassett) ligament has been well described.[7] These lesions are believed to be caused by the formation and resorption of hematoma after an ankle sprain. The patient commonly reports a history of ankle sprains and swelling. MRI can be useful for ruling out other entities, but often the MRI findings do not contribute to making a correct diagnosis of anterolateral soft-tissue impingement.[8]

Anteromedial Impingement

Anteromedial impingement lesions can occur after repeated capsular traction injuries. The typical patient is a soccer player or a martial artist. Anteromedial osseous abnormality, if present, often can be seen on oblique radiographs of the foot. Arthroscopic resection of anteromedial impingement lesions was found to have a satisfactory outcome in 93% of patients.[9]

Ankle Arthrodesis

Fusion rates of more than 90% can be expected with arthroscopic ankle arthrodesis.[10] Although arthroscopic arthrodesis usually is reserved for patients without significant ankle deformity, a comparison study of ankles with or without major deformity found no difference in fusion rates.[10]

Ankle Stabilization

Arthroscopically assisted ankle stabilization procedures are increasingly being reported. A 95% rate of good to excellent outcomes was reported in 38 patients after a three-portal technique was used for reconstruction of the anterior talofibular ligament with extensor retinaculum reinforcement; the calcaneofibular ligament was not surgically treated.[11] A review of single-surgeon arthroscopic repair of lateral ankle instability in 28 patients found an average postoperative American Orthopaedic Foot and Ankle Society (AOFAS) score of 85 and a 29% complication rate. Preoperative AOFAS scores were not reported.[12]

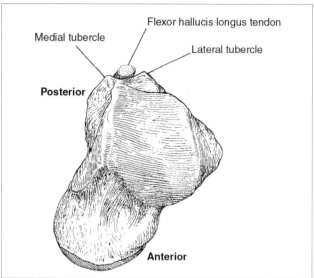

Figure 2   Drawing showing the medial tubercle (Cedell process) and lateral tubercle (Stieda process) of the posterior process of the talus. The flexor hallucis longus tendon is between the tubercles at the ankle joint level.

Posterior Ankle Arthroscopy

Posterior ankle arthroscopy is not as commonly used as anterior ankle arthroscopy, and most orthopaedic surgeons are relatively unfamiliar with this procedure.[13] The increasing number of reports on posterior ankle arthroscopy reflects an evolving interest among foot and ankle orthopaedic surgeons.[2,13-19]

Anatomy

The os trigonum, which is the unossified lateral tubercle of the posterior process of the talus, initially appears as a secondary ossification center at age 8 to 11 years. If the os trigonum fuses with the talus, the elongated projection is called the Stieda process. If fusion does not occur, synchondrosis connects the os trigonum to the posterolateral portion of the talus. The posterior process of the talus is composed of the medial tubercle (also called the Cedell process), which is the attachment for the posterior tibiotalar ligament, and the lateral tubercle (the Stieda process), which is the attachment for the posterior talofibular ligament. The flexor hallucis longus (FHL) tendon courses between the medial and lateral tubercles of the posterior process of the talus at the ankle joint level, and thus it serves as a major landmark during ankle arthroscopic procedures (**Figure 2**). The neurovascular structures should be safe from harm, provided that the surgery is lateral to the FHL. However, the occasional presence of an accessory muscle called the peroneocalcaneus internus muscle, or false FHL, can disorient an inexperienced arthroscopic surgeon and jeopardize the neurovascular structures.[14]

Indications

Several indications for posterior ankle arthroscopy have been described: débridement of posterior soft-tissue impingement of the ankle, microfracture of osteochondral lesions, excision of a symptomatic os trigonum–Stieda process, removal of loose bodies, visualization of structures not well seen in anterior ankle arthroscopy, and visualization during fracture reduction or arthrodesis.[2] Contraindications include an inadequate period of appropriate nonsurgical treatment, an infection, and an earlier open procedure that may have caused scarring around the vital structures. Relative contraindications include the presence of a vascular disease and severe edema.[15]

Technique

Isolated posterior ankle arthroscopy usually is done with the patient prone. After induction of general or spinal anesthesia and proper padding to prevent iatrogenic injury, the patient is positioned with the ankle distal to the edge of the operating table. A bump-type positioning device can be used under the distal tibia. A thigh tourniquet is applied and inflated (**Figure 3**). A large-bore (4.0-mm) arthroscope and shaver can be used outside the joint capsule to clear the soft-tissue envelope and create working space. A small joint arthroscope then can be used if needed. An arthroscopic pump, if used, should be set at 30 to 40 mm Hg. Although a minimally invasive distraction technique has been described, most routine setups do not include distraction.[16,17]

The posterolateral portal is made at the level of the tip of the fibula, along the lateral border of the Achilles tendon. The medial portal is made at the same level at the medial border of the Achilles tendon. The initial skin incision should be superficial and should be followed by vertical spreading of the underlying soft tissues to prevent iatrogenic injury to nearby structures. Fluoroscopy should be available to assist in portal placement, if needed. The arthroscope initially is introduced through the lateral portal. A blunt probe is introduced through the medial portal and directed toward the arthroscope until the instruments are in contact. The probe then follows the arthroscope to the posterior ankle joint.[17] An alternative technique has been described for introducing the instruments toward the fibula to avoid inadvertently damaging the medial neurovascular structures.[20] An anatomic study suggested keeping the ankle in neutral position and making the portals at the level of the tip of the fibula to avoid iatrogenic neurovascular injury.[21]

Combined anterior and posterior ankle arthroscopy may be indicated for some patients. The patient can be

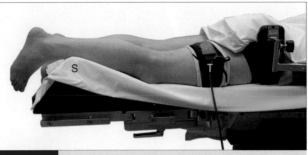

Figure 3 Photograph showing the setup for posterior ankle arthroscopy with the patient in the prone position. S = small support placed under the leg to allow the surgeon to control ankle movement. T = thigh tourniquet. (Reproduced from Niek van Dijk C, van Bergen C: Advancements in ankle arthroscopy. *J Am Acad Orthop Surg* 2008;16[11]:635-646.)

repositioned supine for anterior arthroscopy after the prone posterior arthroscopy, but this repositioning disrupts the procedure and requires an intraoperative delay. To avoid repositioning the patient, an experienced arthroscopic surgeon can consider other positioning options including the lateral decubitus, supine, and prone positions. In the lateral decubitus position, the leg is externally rotated over a leg holder for anterior ankle arthroscopy; the leg holder then is removed and the hip is internally rotated to facilitate posterior ankle arthroscopy.[22] After anterior ankle arthroscopy using the supine position, the leg holder is removed, and the leg is then externally rotated at the hip to allow access to the medial ankle. Two medial portals are made to accomplish posterior ankle arthroscopy.[23] When the prone position is used, the ankle is suspended on a shoulder-holding traction frame to allow combined anterior and posterior arthroscopy without repositioning the patient.[24]

Posterior Ankle Impingement

Posterior talar compression can occur in extreme plantar flexion when the posterior lip of the tibia closes against the superior border of the calcaneus. This condition most commonly occurs as a result of repetitive injury to these structures in dancers and soccer players. The patient often reports having posterior ankle pain while running downhill, wearing high heels, or dancing in the en pointe or demi pointe ballet position. In dancers, posterior impingement can be caused by pseudomeniscal transformation of the posterior transverse ligament.[25]

The location of the pain can be confused with that of a peroneal tendon condition. The os trigonum–Stieda process can be seen on imaging, but its presence is not sufficient to diagnose the condition. MRI typically shows edema of the Stieda process and increased effusion (**Figure 4**). After unsuccessful nonsurgical treatment,

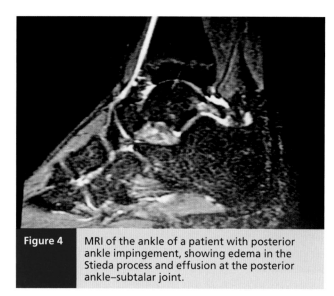

Figure 4 MRI of the ankle of a patient with posterior ankle impingement, showing edema in the Stieda process and effusion at the posterior ankle–subtalar joint.

injection to the area should be done to confirm the diagnosis before proceeding to surgery. The injection can be performed under fluoroscopic guidance. The anatomic goal of surgery for posterior ankle impingement is to remove the offending soft-tissue or osseous structures. An os trigonum causing posterior impingement can be débrided serially with a large burr or removed in its entirety through a separate working portal.

A bone tumor can occur at the posterior aspect of the talus, and an appropriate workup is necessary to avoid the incorrect use of posterior ankle arthroscopy in these patients.[26]

It is important to rule out the presence of concomitant FHL-related pathology. The FHL courses along the medial calcaneal wall after it passes posterior to the ankle joint and may not be readily accessible arthroscopically beyond the ankle joint unless the surgeon is highly experienced.

Arthroscopic treatment of posterior ankle impingement may lead to an earlier return to activities than an open procedure. A review of 12 procedures in athletes found a return to sports at 5.9 weeks and a return to full activity at 13 weeks.[18] After 16 posterior ankle arthroscopies, all patients had a good to excellent result at a mean 32-month follow-up, and 93% had returned to their earlier athletic activities at 5.8-month follow-up.[27] At 36-month follow-up after posterior ankle arthroscopy for osseous or soft-tissue impingement in 55 patients, the average AOFAS score had improved from 75 to 90, and the average time to return to sports was 8 weeks. The patients with a posttraumatic etiology fared worse than those with a repetitive etiology.[19] A recent review of 189 prone posterior ankle arthroscopic procedures with an average 17-month follow-up found an 8.5% rate of complications including dysesthesia, numbness, Achilles

tendon contracture, regional pain syndrome, infection, and cyst formation.[28]

Posteromedial Impingement
Hypertrophy of the posterior tibiotalar ligament after an injury that caused intra-articular impingement can be treated with posterior ankle arthroscopy. Other causes of posteromedial ankle pain include FHL tendon pathology and missed fracture of the Cedell process.[29] Because of the proximity of neurovascular structures, open treatment of these extra-articular conditions is recommended.[30] No conclusive data exist to support all-arthroscopic treatment of these conditions, and it should be avoided until the safety profile of the arthroscopic approach is firmly established.

Subtalar Arthroscopy

Indications
The conditions that may warrant subtalar arthroscopy include synovitis, sinus tarsi syndrome, loose bodies, and arthrofibrosis. If pain, swelling, catching, and locking continue despite a course of nonsurgical treatment, subtalar arthroscopy can be considered.[31] Confirmation of the diagnosis with an injection to the subtalar joint is an integral part of the preoperative workup. Subtalar arthroscopy also has been described for excision of coalitions, subtalar arthrodesis, and fracture reduction.[31-35]

Technique
The equipment and setup for subtalar arthroscopy are similar to those for anterior tibiotalar joint arthroscopy. A 70° arthroscope should be available to improve visualization in the confined space. A relatively small (such as 1.9-mm) arthroscope should be available for a tight joint. The anterior subtalar arthroscopy portal is made 2 cm anterior and 1 cm distal to the fibular tip, and the posterior portal is made 2 cm posterior and 1 cm proximal to the fibular tip. An accessory portal may be necessary. Alternatively, two-portal subtalar arthroscopy can be done using a posterior portal technique with the patient prone, as in a posterior ankle arthroscopy setup.

Subtalar Arthrodesis
Subtalar arthrodesis may be used to treat subtalar arthritis. Traditional open arthrodesis has a fusion rate of 84% to 95%, and a similar success rate can be expected after arthroscopic subtalar arthrodesis by an experienced arthroscopic surgeon.[32-34] The arthroscopic approach may offer advantages important for surgical success, especially in patients at high risk, including preservation of the talar blood supply and protection of the soft tissues from intraoperative damage. Patients with a severe deformity

should not be treated with the arthroscopic approach. The limits of deformity have not yet been defined, however.

Arthrofibrosis

Arthroscopic débridement of the joint can be considered as an alternative to subtalar arthrodesis for treating arthrofibrosis after calcaneal fracture.[35] In a retrospective study, 17 patients with painful stiffness after a Sanders type II or III calcaneal fracture were treated with arthroscopic débridement of the subtalar joint. The mean AOFAS score had increased from 50 to 80 points at 17-month follow-up. Although no immediate complications were noted, two patients subsequently underwent arthrodesis.[36]

First Metatarsophalangeal Joint Arthroscopy

Arthroscopy of the great toe metatarsophalangeal (MTP) joint is uncommon. The theoretic advantages of the procedure include less bleeding, lower infection, less scarring, better cosmesis, and more rapid recovery than in an open procedure. No studies have compared open and arthroscopic treatment of pathology of the first MTP joint.[37]

Indications

The reported indications for first MTP joint arthroscopy include unsuccessful nonsurgical treatment of hallux rigidus, focal chondral lesions, loose bodies, arthrofibrosis, and synovitis. The contraindications include local infection, severe joint disease, severe edema, and severe joint narrowing. The indications and contraindications continue to evolve.[31]

Technique

Traction can be provided using the sterile finger trap device or suspension holder commonly used in wrist arthroscopic procedures. Because of the small joint size, a short 1.9-mm to 2.4-mm arthroscope is used. Relatively small-diameter shavers (2.0 mm to 2.3 mm) are recommended. Dorsomedial and dorsolateral portals are made at the joint, avoiding the extensor hallucis longus tendon and the dorsomedial cutaneous branch of the superficial peroneal nerve. As in arthroscopy of other joints, a nick-and-spread technique is used to enter the MTP joint capsule from portals at the joint. A straight medial portal can be used to improve the ability to see the sesamoid–metatarsal head articulation.

Hallux Rigidus

Arthroscopic cheilectomy of the first MTP joint can be considered for removal of small osteophytes. The arthroscopic shaver can be used from the dorsomedial portal to improve visualization. The arthroscopic burr is used to remove the dorsal spur.[31] There are several reports reviewing the results of the great toe arthroscopy. Published reports on small cohorts reflect overall good to excellent results of 66% to 74%.[38,39]

First MTP Joint Arthrodesis

To preserve the soft-tissue envelope in patients who have a high risk of poor wound healing, arthroscopic arthrodesis of the first MTP joint can be considered. Only anecdotal reports and small studies have been published. Crossed cannulated screws are used in this procedure.

Intraoperative fluoroscopy and a high-angled small joint arthroscope should be readily available. A cadaver study found that the use of a third accessory medial portal led to more complete cartilage débridement than the two-portal technique.[40]

Tendoscopy

Although the intra-articular portion of the FHL is routinely seen during anterior and posterior ankle arthroscopic procedures, true diagnostic tendoscopic procedures of the ankle and hindfoot are uncommon. Most of the existing studies are from a limited number of institutions. As the technique and indications continue to evolve, tendoscopy may become more common. Visualization of the tendons and limited synovectomy can be facilitated by using tendoscopy, but more involved procedures are likely to be done using an open or a limited open technique.

Posterior Tibialis Tendon

Patients with medial ankle pain who have tenderness directly over the tendon sheath may have pathology involving the posterior tibialis tendon. Clinical suspicion is further elevated if the patient has difficulty or pain with single-toe heel raises. Posterior tibialis tendoscopy and synovectomy may be indicated in patients with early posterior tibialis tendon dysfunction but no hindfoot deformity after an unsuccessful course of nonsurgical treatment. The portals can be made approximately 2 cm proximal and 2 cm distal to the tip of the medial malleolus, directly superficial to the posterior tibialis tendon. With the use of a small joint arthroscope and shaver, tenosynovitis, vincula thickening, and partial tears can be débrided.[41]

Peroneal Tendons

The peroneal tendons are the primary dynamic lateral stabilizers of the ankle. Patients with ankle instability symptoms and pain located directly over the peroneal tendons are suspected to have pathology of the peroneal tendons. Pain and swelling over the tendons are typical.

True weakness of the peroneal tendons is uncommon. The peroneal tendons usually are explored with a lateral incision when the traditional open method is used. Intra-articular ankle joint pathology was found in all 30 patients with peroneal tendon pathology, and ankle arthroscopy was recommended.[42]

The indications for tendoscopy may include peroneal synovitis and small partial tears. The setup for peroneal tendoscopy is similar to that for anterior ankle arthroscopy, with the patient's leg positioned over a thigh holder. The distal portal is made 2 cm distal to the tip of the fibula, and the proximal portal is made 3 cm proximal to the tip of the fibula. Small shavers and low inflow are used.

Intrasheath subluxation of the peroneal tendon can be difficult to diagnose clinically, and MRI findings often are negative. Dynamic ultrasonography can be important for making the correct diagnosis. The common causes of intrasheath subluxation include the presence of a peroneus quartus or another accessory muscle, a low-lying muscle belly of peroneus brevis, and a nonconcave configuration of the posterior fibula surface. Endoscopic evaluation and groove deepening have been recommended, and a favorable outcome was reported in a study of six patients.[43]

Flexor Hallucis Longus Tendon

The intra-articular portion of the FHL is routinely seen during anterior and posterior ankle arthroscopic procedures. Although FHL sheath release to the sustentaculum tali level has been described, the entire fibro-osseous tunnel of the FHL is relatively difficult to visualize with endoscopic procedures.[28] Nearby neurovascular structures may be at risk during FHL tendoscopic procedures.[30,44] As the technique becomes more refined, routine endoscopic release of the fibro-osseous tunnel may be possible for treating stenosing tenosynovitis.

Achilles Tendon

Endoscopic bursectomy and calcaneoplasty are feasible with the patient in the prone position. A relatively large (4.0-mm) arthroscope can provide good inflow for visualization. Intraoperative minifluoroscopy is used to confirm the adequacy of bone removal, if needed.[45] High rates of wound dehiscence have been reported with the open technique, and therefore an endoscopic technique maybe preferred for treating some patients at high risk for wound dehiscence.[46]

Summary

The applications of foot and ankle arthroscopy continue to expand. Foot and ankle orthopaedic surgeons can anticipate further refinement of posterior ankle arthroscopic procedures and their use to treat tendons and relatively small joints.

Annotated References

1. Young BH, Flanigan RM, DiGiovanni BF: Complications of ankle arthroscopy utilizing a contemporary noninvasive distraction technique. *J Bone Joint Surg Am* 2011;93(10):963-968.

   A single surgeon's experience of ankle arthroscopy with noninvasive distraction in 294 patients was retrospectively reviewed. The overall complication rate was 6.8%, although the complication rate in patients with a workers' compensation claim was 21%. Level of evidence: IV.

2. van Dijk CN, van Bergen CJ: Advancements in ankle arthroscopy. *J Am Acad Orthop Surg* 2008;16(11):635-646.

   Arthroscopic approach to addressing talar OCD, and anterior and posterior impingement syndrome are reviewed. The authors also review published reports on arthroscopic treatment of various ankle conditions.

3. Kim BS, Choi WJ, Kim J, Lee JW: Residual pain due to soft-tissue impingement after uncomplicated total ankle replacement. *Bone Joint J* 2013;95(3):378-383.

   Seven patients underwent ankle joint arthroscopy after uncomplicated total ankle arthroplasty was required because of persistent pain. Soft-tissue impingement and fibrosis were confirmed. Arthroscopic débridement led to a satisfactory outcome in six patients.

4. Shirzad K, Viens NA, DeOrio JK: Arthroscopic treatment of impingement after total ankle arthroplasty: Technique tip. *Foot Ankle Int* 2011;32(7):727-729.

   Soft-tissue impingement after total ankle arthroplasty was treated with anterior ankle arthroscopy. Technical aspects of the surgery were described. Level of evidence: V.

5. Lozano-Calderón SA, Samocha Y, McWilliam J: Comparative performance of ankle arthroscopy with and without traction. *Foot Ankle Int* 2012;33(9):740-745.

   In 103 patients who underwent anterior ankle arthroscopy with or without traction, dorsiflexion of the ankle improved visualization of the anterior compartment. The complication rate was 4%. Level of evidence: II.

6. de Leeuw PA, Golanó P, Sierevelt IN, van Dijk CN: The course of the superficial peroneal nerve in relation to the ankle position: Anatomical study with ankle arthroscopic implications. *Knee Surg Sports Traumatol Arthrosc* 2010;18(5):612-617.

   A cadaver study revealed that the superficial peroneal nerve moves laterally as the ankle is brought from plantar flexion-inversion to neutral dorsiflexion. Making the anterolateral portal medial to the nerve was recommended.

7. Bassett FH III, Gates HS III, Billys JB, Morris HB, Nikolaou PK: Talar impingement by the anteroinferior tibiofibular ligament: A cause of chronic pain in the ankle after inversion sprain. *J Bone Joint Surg Am* 1990;72(1):55-59.

8. Brennan SA, Rahim F, Dowling J, Kearns SR: Arthroscopic debridement for soft tissue ankle impingement. *Ir J Med Sci* 2012;181(2):253-256.

 A single surgeon's experience of 41 anterior ankle arthroscopic procedures for soft-tissue impingement was reported. Thirty-four patients had a favorable result. Soft-tissue impingement was underreported on preoperative MRI.

9. Murawski CD, Kennedy JG: Anteromedial impingement in the ankle joint: Outcomes following arthroscopy. *Am J Sports Med* 2010;38(10):2017-2024.

 In 43 patients including 16 soccer players who underwent arthroscopic treatment of anteromedial impingement, the average AOFAS score improved from 63 to 91. The complication rate was 7%. Level of evidence: IV.

10. Gougoulias NE, Agathangelidis FG, Parsons SW: Arthroscopic ankle arthrodesis. *Foot Ankle Int* 2007;28(6):695-706.

11. Nery C, Raduan F, Del Buono A, Asaumi ID, Cohen M, Maffulli N: Arthroscopic-assisted Broström-Gould for chronic ankle instability: A long-term follow-up. *Am J Sports Med* 2011;39(11):2381-2388.

 Arthroscopic ankle reconstruction was performed by a single surgeon in 40 patients. At an average 9.8-year follow-up of 38 patients, 36 (95%) had a good to excellent result. Concomitant procedures such as microfracture of the talus did not influence the results. Level of evidence: IV.

12. Corte-Real NM, Moreira RM: Arthroscopic repair of chronic lateral ankle instability. *Foot Ankle Int* 2009;30(3):213-217.

 At 24.5-month follow-up, 28 patients who underwent arthroscopic ankle reconstruction had a 29% rate of complications, most of which were believed to be minor. Patients with a workers' compensation claim had lower AOFAS scores. Level of evidence: IV.

13. Ferkel RD: In which position do we perform arthroscopy of the hindfoot: Supine or prone? [Commentary]. *J Bone Joint Surg Am* 2012;94(5):e33.

 A perspective on the development of and current trends in posterior ankle arthroscopy was provided, with a recommendation for careful, deliberate, and gradual inclusion of the technique by experienced ankle arthroscopic surgeons.

14. Phisitkul P, Amendola A: False FHL: A normal variant posing risks in posterior hindfoot endoscopy. *Arthroscopy* 2010;26(5):714-718.

 The peroneocalcaneus internus muscle can be mistaken for the FHL during posterior ankle arthroscopy, thus endangering the medial neurovascular structures.

15. Gasparetto F, Collo G, Pisanu G, et al: Posterior ankle and subtalar arthroscopy: Indications, technique, and results. *Curr Rev Musculoskelet Med* 2012;5(2):164-170.

 A review of posterior ankle arthroscopy emphasizes the steep learning curve associated with the procedure.

16. Beals TC, Junko JT, Amendola A, Nickisch F, Saltzman CL: Minimally invasive distraction technique for prone posterior ankle and subtalar arthroscopy. *Foot Ankle Int* 2010;31(4):316-319.

 A 1.8-mm calcaneal traction pin with a frame was used to facilitate posterior ankle arthroscopy in 14 patients, with no complications. Level of evidence: IV.

17. van Dijk CN, de Leeuw PA, Scholten PE: Hindfoot endoscopy for posterior ankle impingement: Surgical technique. *J Bone Joint Surg Am* 2009;91(Suppl 2):287-298.

 The authors describe the setup and technique to avoid iatrogenic complications during posterior ankle arthroscopy. Schematic diagrams are used to illustrate the important technical concepts.

18. Noguchi H, Ishii Y, Takeda M, Hasegawa A, Monden S, Takagishi K: Arthroscopic excision of posterior ankle bony impingement for early return to the field: Short-term results. *Foot Ankle Int* 2010;31(5):398-403.

 Twelve patients with posterior ankle impingement were treated with posterior ankle arthroscopy using posterolateral and accessory posterior lateral portals. Lateral decubitus positioning was used. Distraction or posteromedial portals were not used. The average AOFAS score improved from 68 to 98 points. One complication (transient neuritis) was noted. The average return to sports was 5.9 weeks, and full activity was reached within 13 weeks. Level of evidence: IV.

19. Scholten PE, Sierevelt IN, van Dijk CN: Hindfoot endoscopy for posterior ankle impingement. *J Bone Joint Surg Am* 2008;90(12):2665-2672.

 Fifty-five patients with posterior ankle impingement were treated with two-portal ankle arthroscopic débridement. At 36-month follow-up, the AOFAS score had improved from 75 to 90. The average time to return to sports was 8 weeks. Patients whose symptoms were the result of overuse had a better response than those whose symptoms were posttraumatic. There was only one complication (transient neuritis). Level of evidence: IV.

20. Yoshimura I, Naito M, Kanazawa K, Ida T, Muraoka K, Hagio T: Assessing the safe direction of instruments during posterior ankle arthroscopy using an MRI model. *Foot Ankle Int* 2013;34(3):434-438.

MRI findings were reviewed to determine the safety of posterior portals for the major neurovascular structures of the hindfoot. Although the average distance to the neurovascular structures was 15 to 18 mm, the instruments should be directed toward the fibula to avoid iatrogenic damage to the medial neurovascular structures.

21. Urgüden M, Cevikol C, Dabak TK, Karaali K, Aydin AT, Apaydin A: Effect of joint motion on safety of portals in posterior ankle arthroscopy. *Arthroscopy* 2009;25(12):1442-1446.

    MRI was used at different ankle positions in 20 individuals. Portals made at the level of the tip of the fibula with the ankle in neutral position provided the greatest margin of safety for the posterior medial and lateral neural structures.

22. Hampton CB, Shawen SB, Keeling JJ: Positioning technique for combined anterior, lateral, and posterior ankle and hindfoot procedures: Technique tip. *Foot Ankle Int* 2010;31(4):348-350.

    Anterior ankle arthroscopy was completed by positioning the patient in the lateral decubitus position with the hip externally rotated. The leg holder was removed to facilitate lateral and posterior ankle procedures without totally repositioning the patient. Level of evidence: V.

23. Allegra F, Maffulli N: Double posteromedial portals for posterior ankle arthroscopy in supine position. *Clin Orthop Relat Res* 2010;468(4):996-1001.

    Anterior and posterior ankle arthroscopies were completed during the same procedure in 32 patients who were in the supine position. With the leg in a figure-of-4 position and with the use of two posteromedial portals, the posterior ankle arthroscopy was successfully completed without repositioning the patient. Level of evidence: IV.

24. Kim HN, Park YJ, Lee SY, Park YW: Three-portal ankle arthroscopy in prone position with ankle suspended: Technique tip. *Foot Ankle Int* 2012;33(11):1027-1030.

    The use of a shoulder-holding traction device was recommended for combined anterior and posterior ankle arthroscopy with the patient in the prone position.

25. Hamilton WG: Posterior ankle pain in dancers. *Clin Sports Med* 2008;27(2):263-277.

    Differential diagnosis, anatomy, as well as surgical and nonsurgical treatments of posterior ankle pain in elite dancers are extensively detailed.

26. Winters KN, Jowett AJ, Taylor H: Osteoid osteoma of the talus presenting as posterior ankle impingement: Case reports. *Foot Ankle Int* 2011;32(11):1095-1097.

    Osteoid osteoma mimicking posterior impingement was described in two patients. Level of evidence: V.

27. Willits K, Sonneveld H, Amendola A, Giffin JR, Griffin S, Fowler PJ: Outcome of posterior ankle arthroscopy for hindfoot impingement. *Arthroscopy* 2008;24(2):196-202.

    In a 23-patient study of posterior ankle arthroscopy, 16 procedure results were evaluated at 32-month follow-up. Patients had returned to work at 1 month and to sports at 5.8 months. There were no major complications. Level of evidence: IV.

28. Nickisch F, Barg A, Saltzman CL, et al: Postoperative complications of posterior ankle and hindfoot arthroscopy. *J Bone Joint Surg Am* 2012;94(5):439-446.

    A review of 189 prone posterior ankle arthroscopic procedures revealed an 8.5% complication rate at an average 17-month follow-up. Level of evidence: IV.

29. Kim DH, Berkowitz MJ, Pressman DN: Avulsion fractures of the medial tubercle of the posterior process of the talus. *Foot Ankle Int* 2003;24(2):172-175.

30. Keeling JJ, Guyton GP: Endoscopic flexor hallucis longus decompression: A cadaver study. *Foot Ankle Int* 2007;28(7):810-814.

31. Ferkel RD, Hammen JP: Arthroscopy of the ankle and foot, in Coughlin MJ, Mann RA, Saltzman CL, eds: *Surgery of the Foot and Ankle,* ed 8. Philadelphia, PA, Mosby Elsevier, 2007, pp 1641-1726.

32. Muraro GM, Carvajal PF: Arthroscopic arthrodesis of subtalar joint. *Foot Ankle Clin* 2011;16(1):83-90.

    Arthroscopic subtalar arthrodesis should be considered in patients with minimal to no deformities. Surgical technique and previously published results are reviewed.

33. El Shazly O, Nassar W, El Badrawy A: Arthroscopic subtalar fusion for post-traumatic subtalar arthritis. *Arthroscopy* 2009;25(7):783-787.

    A retrospective review of nine patients who were treated with arthroscopic subtalar fusion for posttraumatic arthritis found that all subtalar joints had achieved fusion at an average 28.4-month follow-up. The mean time to fusion was 11.4 weeks. There was only one complication (a neuroma). Level of evidence: IV.

34. Lee KB, Park CH, Seon JK, Kim MS: Arthroscopic subtalar arthrodesis using a posterior 2-portal approach in the prone position. *Arthroscopy* 2010;26(2):230-238.

    The results of arthroscopic arthrodesis using the prone position in 16 patients were reviewed at a mean 30-month follow-up. The union rate was 94% at 11 weeks. There was one nonunion. The average AOFAS score improved from 35 to 84. Level of evidence: IV.

35. Elgafy H, Ebraheim NA: Subtalar arthroscopy for persistent subfibular pain after calcaneal fractures. *Foot Ankle Int* 1999;20(7):422-427.

36. Lee KB, Chung JY, Song EK, Seon JK, Bai LB: Arthroscopic release for painful subtalar stiffness after intra-articular fractures of the calcaneum. *J Bone Joint Surg Br* 2008;90(11):1457-1461.

Seventeen patients with posttraumatic arthrofibrosis of the subtalar joint after intra-articular calcaneus fracture were treated with subtalar arthroscopy and débridement of fibrosis. The mean AOFAS score had improved from 49.4 to 79.6 at 16.8-month follow-up.

37. Carreira DS: Arthroscopy of the hallux. *Foot Ankle Clin* 2009;14(1):105-114.

Anatomy, indication, set up, and technique of hallux arthroscopy is described in this review paper. Results from previously published studies are reported.

38. Ferkel RD: Great toe arthroscopy, in Whipple TL, ed: *Arthroscopy: The Foot and Ankle.* Philadelphia, PA, Lippincott-Raven, 1996, pp 255-272.

39. van Dijk CN, Veenstra KM, Nuesch BC: Arthroscopic surgery of the metatarsophalangeal first joint. *Arthroscopy* 1998;14(8):851-855.

40. Vaseenon T, Phisitkul P: Arthroscopic debridement for first metatarsophalangeal joint arthrodesis with a 2- versus 3-portal technique: A cadaveric study. *Arthroscopy* 2010;26(10):1363-1367.

A cadaver study found that the use of three portals was superior to the use of two portals for arthroscopic cartilage débridement in first MTP joint preparation.

41. Khazen G, Khazen C: Tendoscopy in stage I posterior tibial tendon dysfunction. *Foot Ankle Clin* 2012;17(3):399-406.

Tendoscopy can be considered in patients with stage I posterior tibialis tendon dysfunction. The authors report good results in eight of nine patients. If tears are seen during the tendoscopy, limited open repair is recommended.

42. Bare A, Ferkel RD: Peroneal tendon tears: Associated arthroscopic findings and results after repair. *Arthroscopy* 2009;25(11):1288-1297.

All 30 patients with peroneal tendon pathology had intra-articular ankle joint pathology, and 80% had extensive intra-articular scarring on arthroscopy. Anterior ankle arthroscopy was recommended. Level of evidence: IV.

43. Vega J, Golanó P, Dalmau A, Viladot R: Tendoscopic treatment of intrasheath subluxation of the peroneal tendons. *Foot Ankle Int* 2011;32(12):1147-1151.

At 18.3-month follow-up, six patients who were treated with tendoscopy for intrasheath peroneal subluxation had mean AOFAS score improvement from 79 to 99. Level of evidence: IV.

44. Lui TH: Lateral plantar nerve neurapraxia after FHL tendoscopy: Case report and anatomic evaluation. *Foot Ankle Int* 2010;31(9):828-831.

Dorsiflexion of the ankle should be avoided in FHL tendoscopy, as dorsiflexion of the ankle brings the posterior tibial nerve closer to the arthroscope in this cadaver study.

45. van Dijk CN: Hindfoot endoscopy for posterior ankle pain. *Instr Course Lect* 2006;55:545-554.

46. Steenstra F, van Dijk CN: Achilles tendoscopy. *Foot Ankle Clin* 2006;11(2):429-438, viii.

Index

Index

deformity and, 160–162
etiology, 160
incidence, 160
nonsurgical treatment, 160–161
pain and, 160
pathophysiology, 159–160
primary arthrodesis for trauma, 163–164
malunion, 164
nonunion, 164
surgical treatment, 161–163
lateral column, 162–163, 163*f*
medial midfoot joints, 161–162, 162*f*
other osteotomies, 163
wound-healing complications, 163
Mintz classification, 389, 390*t*
Moberg osteotomy, 196, 197*f*
Modified Broström-Evans procedure, 376–377, 376*f*
Modified Jones procedure, cavovarus deformity, 58
Morton extensions, metatarsalgia, 218
Morton interdigital neuroma, 253–254, 254*f*
Morton neuroma, 213–214
surgical treatment, 220–221, 221*f*
Motor neuropathy, 68
MPPDN syndrome. *See* Medial plantar proper digital nerve syndrome
MRI. *See* Magnetic resonance imaging
MSCN. *See* Medial sural cutaneous nerve
MSCs. *See* Mesenchymal stem cells
MTP joint. *See* Metatarsophalangeal joint
Multiple myeloma, 259

N

Nail disorders, 228–229, 265*f*
anatomy of, 265
foot, 265–267
glomus tumor, 267
infectious conditions, 266
inflammatory conditions, 266–267
ingrown toenail, 267
lichen planus, 267
melanoma, 267
onychomycosis, 266
paronychia, 266
psoriasis, 266–267
subungual exostosis, 267
traumatic subungual hematoma, 265–266
tumors, 267
Navicular
accessory, 37–39
body fractures, 334–335, 334*f*
fractures, 333–335
stress, 335, 380–381, 381*f*
Necrotizing fasciitis, 229
Nerve conduction velocity (NCV), 90
Nerve syndromes
MPPDN, 97
plantar heel, 239–244

Neurilemoma, 254
Neurofibroma, 254
Neuromas
Morton, 213–214
surgical treatment of, 220–221, 221*f*
Morton interdigital, 253–254, 254*f*
recurrent, 89
Neuropathy
autonomic, 68
CMT disease, 53
diabetic, 67
motor, 68
peripheral, 230
sensory, 67–68
New Jersey Low-Contact Stress prosthesis, 129
Newton prosthesis, 129
Nodular fasciitis, foot and ankle, 253
Nondiabetic foot infections, 227–233
of ankle, 231–233, 232*f*
deep infections, 229–233
diagnosis, 227
of hindfoot, 231–233
history, 227
imaging studies, 227–228, 228*f*
laboratory studies, 228
of midfoot, 231–233
multidisciplinary management, 233
nail disorders, 228–229
physical examination, 227
soft-tissue infections, 229
Nononcologic excised malignant tumors, 260–261
Nonossifying fibromas, 257
Nonsteroidal anti-inflammatory drugs (NSAIDs)
for ankle arthritis, 111
hallux rigidus, 194–195
midfoot arthritis, 161
Nonunion
midfoot arthritis, 163, 164
talar neck fracture, 315
NSAIDs. *See* Nonsteroidal anti-inflammatory drugs
Nuclear medicine, 29

O

OA. *See* Osteoarthritis
OATS. *See* Osteochondral autologous transfer system
Ofloxacin, diabetic foot disease, 71
OLT. *See* Osteochondral lesion of the talus
Onychomycosis, 229–230
toenail, 266, 266*f*
treating, 266, 266*t*
Open reduction and internal fixation (ORIF), 164
intra-articular calcaneal fractures, 320–321
talar neck fracture, 312–313, 313*f*, 314*f*
Orthotic devices, 16–20
metatarsalgia, 218, 219*f*

Osseous grafting, 259
Osseous injury, 31–32, 31*f*
Osteoarthritis (OA), 107
ankle, 108
Osteoblastoma, 258
Osteochondral autologous transfer system (OATS), 390
Osteochondral graft, 391–392
Osteochondral lesion of the talus (OLT)
ACI for, 392
allograft transplantation, 392–393
arthroscopic BMS, 391
bone marrow-derived cells, 393–394
classification, 388–389, 388*f*, 389*f*, 390*t*
clinical presentation, 387–388
etiology, 388
future directions, 393–394
imaging, 388–389, 389*f*
incidence, 387
MACI, 392
natural history, 388
nonsurgical treatment, 389
osteochondral graft, 391–392
particulated juvenile cartilage, 393
pathoanatomy, 388
primary repair, 391
PRP, 394
stem cell therapy, 393
surgical recommendations, 391–393
surgical treatment, 390–391, 390*f*
Osteochondroma, 255–256
Osteochondrosis
Freiberg infraction, 44
Köhler disease, 43–44, 44*f*
Osteoid osteoma, 257–258
Osteomyelitis
calcaneus, 244
hallux, 230–231
lesser toe, 230–231
Osteonecrosis
talar neck fractures and, 313–315
treatment, 314–315
Osteonecrosis of the talus, 283–290
arthrodesis, 288–289
bone grafting, 287–288, 287*f*, 288*f*
core decompression, 286–287
diagnosis, 285
etiology, 283–285
Ficat and Arlet classification system for, 285, 286*t*
incidence, 283–285
nonsurgical treatment, 285–286, 286*f*
surgical treatment, 286–290
symptoms, 285
TAA, 289–290, 290*t*
talar body prostheses, 289–290, 289*f*
treatment algorithm, 290, 291*f*
Osteopenia, 74
Osteosarcoma, 258
Osteotomy
calcaneal, 59–60, 62*f*, 63*f*, 64*f*
Z-cut, 173, 175*f*
Cotton, 173, 174*f*
dorsiflexion, 59

Index

Dwyer closing-wedge, 59, 60*f*
hallux rigidus, 196–197, 197*f*
midfoot arthritis, 163
Moberg, 196, 197*f*
Z-calcaneal osteotomy, 173, 175*f*
Z-shaped, 59–60, 61*f*, 62*f*

P

PAB. *See* Pronation-abduction
Pain. *See also* Complex regional pain
    syndrome
    after amputation, 278
    forefoot, 213
    midfoot arthritis and, 160
    plantar heel, 237–244
Paronychia, 229–230, 266
Particulated juvenile cartilage, OLT, 393
Pediatric conditions
    accessory navicular, 37–39
    apophysitis, 43
    flexible flatfoot, 42–43
    of foot and ankle, 37–47
    osteochondrosis, 43–44
    tarsal coalition, 39–41
Peek-a-boo heel sign, 374
Percutaneous reduction and fixation, intra-
    articular calcaneal fracture, 323–324
Periarticular osteotomies
    ankle arthritis, 115–117
    background, 115–116
    results, 116–117
    technique, 116, 116*f*
Periosteal chondroma, 256
Peripheral nerve disease, 85–102
    CRPS, 97–100
    deep peroneal nerve entrapment, 93–94
    interdigital plantar neuralgia, 85–89
    LPN entrapment, 92–93
    MPN entrapment, 92
    MPPDN syndrome, 97
    SPN, 94–96
    sural nerve, 96–97
    TTS, 89–92
Peripheral neuropathy, 230
Peroneal communicating branch (PCB), 96
Peroneal tendon
    disorders, 358–361
    subluxation, 359, 360*f*
    tears, 360–361, 361*f*
    tendoscopy, 405–406
Peroneal tenosynovitis, 360
Peroneus brevis to peroneus longus
    tenodesis and lateral ligament
    reconstruction, cavovarus deformity,
    58–59
Pes cavus, 53
Pexiganan, diabetic foot disease, 71
Pigmented villonodular synovitis, 251–252
Pilon fractures
    classification, 302–303, 303*f*
    clinical evaluation, 302
    initial management, 303
    radiographic evaluation, 302

surgical treatment
    approaches to, 303–305, 304*f*
    external fixation, 305–306
    internal fixation, 305
Pirogoff amputation, 276
Plantar fascia, ruptured, 239
Plantar fascia release, cavovarus deformity,
    58
Plantar fasciitis, 238–239, 238*f*
    chronic, TTS with, 240–242, 242*f*
    treatment, 238–239
Plantar fibroma/fibromatosis, 253
Plantar heel
    disorders and treatment, 238–244
    nerve syndromes, 239–244
Plantar heel pain, 237–244
    calcaneal branches of tibial nerve and,
        243
    diagnosis, 237–238, 237*t*
    etiologies, 237, 237*t*
    foreign body in heel pad and, 244
    heel pad tumors and, 244
    LPN involvement in, 242
        first branch of, 242–243, 243*f*
    medial plantar nerve involvement and,
        243
    nerve syndromes, 239–244
    osteomyelitis of calcaneus and, 244
    physical examination, 237–238
    stress fractures of calcaneus and, 244
    sural nerve involvement in, 243–244
    TTS and, 239–240
        chronic plantar fasciitis with, 240–
            242, 242*f*
Plantar nerve branches
    lateral, 85
        plantar heel pain and, 242–243, 243*f*
    medial, 85
        plantar heel pain and, 243
    surgery and identifying/resecting, 88
Plantar space abscess, 230
Plantar warts, 267–268
Platelet-rich plasma (PRP), 153
    for ankle arthritis, 111
    OLT, 394
Posterior ankle arthroscopy
    anatomy, 402, 402*f*
    indications, 403
    posterior ankle impingement, 403–404,
        404*f*
    posteromedial impingement, 404
    technique, 403, 403*f*
Posterior ankle impingement, 403–404,
    404*f*
Posterior inferior tibiofibular ligament, 5
Posterior malleolus, 300, 301*f*
Posterior process fractures, 316
Posterior talofibular ligament (PTFL), 5
Posterior tibialis tendon, tendoscopy, 405
Posterior tibial tendon (PTT), 167
    stage II flexible dysfunction of, 18, 19*f*
Posterior tibial tendon dysfunction
    (PTTD), 167–176
    anatomy, 167
    ankle joint deformity and, 168, 170*f*

classification, 168, 168*f*, 169*f*
clinical presentation, 168
complications, 176
etiology, 167
examination, 168–170
imaging, 170–172
nonsurgical treatment, 172
pathophysiology, 167
stage I, 170, 171*f*
    surgical treatment for, 172
stage II
    Cotton osteotomy for, 173, 174*f*
    MDCO for, 173, 174*f*
    periarticular osteotomy options for,
        173–174
    surgical treatment for, 172–174,
        175*f*
    Z-calcaneal osteotomy for, 173, 175*f*
stage III, surgical treatment for, 174–
    175, 176*f*
stage IV, 170, 171*f*
    surgical treatment for, 175–176
surgical treatment, 172–176
talonavicular uncoverage, 173, 175*f*
TMT joint and, 168, 170*f*
Posterior tibial tendon transfer, cavovarus
    deformity, 59
Posteromedial impingement, 404
Posts, 15
Posttraumatic arthritis
    calcaneal fractures, 328–329
    talar neck fracture, 315
Pregabalin, CRPS, 99
Primary arthrodesis for type IV fractures,
    322
Pronation-abduction (PAB), 298
Pronation-external rotation (PER), 298
Prosthesis
    after amputation, 278
    New Jersey Low-Contact Stress, 129
    Smith, 129
    TAA, 129, 131
    talar body, 289–290, 289*f*
Prosthetic replacement
    foot and ankle, 259
    hallux rigidus, 199–200, 200*f*
    MTP joint, 199–200, 200*f*
PRP. *See* Platelet-rich plasma
Psoriasis
    skin, 268, 268*f*
    toenail, 266–267
PTFL. *See* Posterior talofibular ligament
PTT. *See* Posterior tibial tendon
PTTD. *See* Posterior tibial tendon
    dysfunction

R

Radiographs
    digital, 25
    plain, 25, 26
Radiolucencies, TAA, 135–136
Ray resections, 275–276
Recombinant human (rh) BMPs, 153

W

Z